Color Atlas of
Dermoscopy

Color Atlas of Dermoscopy

Horacio Antonio Cabo MD PhD
Head Professor of Dermatology
Universidad de Buenos Aires (UBA)
Buenos Aires, Argentina
Specialist in Dermatology
Universidad de Buenos Aires (UBA)
Head of Dermatology
Institute of Medical Research
Universidad de Buenos Aires (UBA)
Ex-President
The Argentine Society of Dermatology
Member
Executive Committee of Ibero-Latin Americano College
of Dermatology (CILAD) and
The Board of the International Dermoscopy Society (IDS)
Graz, Austria

Foreword

Fernando Stengel

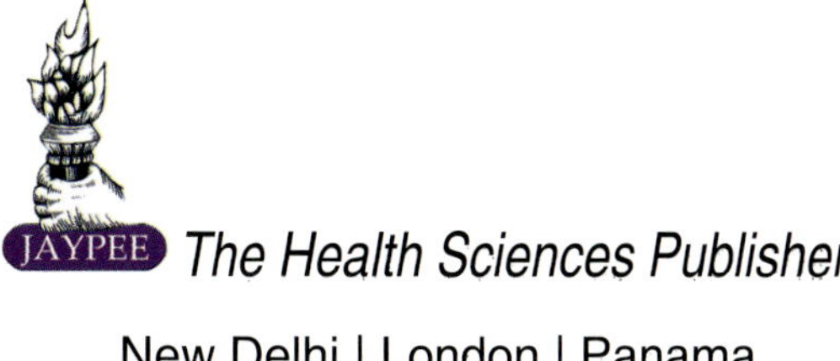

New Delhi | London | Panama

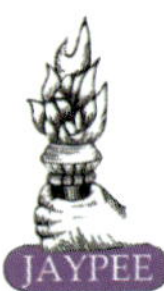

Jaypee Brothers Medical Publishers (P) Ltd

Headquarters
Jaypee Brothers Medical Publishers (P) Ltd.
4838/24, Ansari Road, Daryaganj
New Delhi 110 002, India
Phone: +91-11-43574357
Fax: +91-11-43574314
E-mail: jaypee@jaypeebrothers.com

Overseas Offices
J.P. Medical Ltd.
83, Victoria Street, London
SW1H 0HW (UK)
Phone: +44-20 3170 8910
Fax: +44(0)20 3008 6180
E-mail: info@jpmedpub.com

Jaypee-Highlights Medical Publishers Inc.
City of Knowledge, Bld. 235, 2nd Floor, Clayton
Panama City, Panama
Phone: +1 507-301-0496
Fax: +1 507-301-0499
E-mail: cservice@jphmedical.com

Jaypee Brothers Medical Publishers (P) Ltd.
17/1-B, Babar Road, Block-B, Shaymali
Mohammadpur, Dhaka-1207
Bangladesh
Mobile: +08801912003485
E-mail: jaypeedhaka@gmail.com

Jaypee Brothers Medical Publishers (P) Ltd.
Bhotahity, Kathmandu, Nepal
Phone: +977-9741283608
E-mail: kathmandu@jaypeebrothers.com

Website: www.jaypeebrothers.com
Website: www.jaypeedigital.com

Inquiries for bulk sales may be solicited at: jaypee@jaypeebrothers.com

Color Atlas of Dermoscopy

First Edition: **2017**

ISBN: 978-93-86056-30-6

Printed at Sanat Printers

Dedicated to

My wife, sons and daughters, grandchildren and my patients

Contributors

Giuseppe Albertini MD
Dermatologist
Italy

Zoe Apalla MD
Dermatologist
Greece

Giuseppe Argenziano MD PhD
Professor and Head
Dermatology Unit
University of Campania
Naples, Italy

Renato Marchiori Bakos MD PhD
Professor of Dermatology
Universidade Federal do Rio
Grande do Sul
Porto Alegre, Brazil

Elisa Benatti MD
Dermatologist
Italy

Stefania Borsari MD
Dermatologist
Italy

Gabriella Brancaccio MD
Dermatologist
Italy

Horacio A Cabo MD PhD
Head Professor of Dermatology
Universidad de Buenos Aires (UBA)
Buenos Aires, Argentina
Specialist in Dermatology
Universidad de Buenos Aires (UBA)
Head of Dermatology
Institute of Medical Research
Universidad de Buenos Aires (UBA)
Ex-President
The Argentine Society of Dermatology
Member
Executive Committee of
Ibero-Latin Americano College
of Dermatology (CILAD) and
The Board of the International
Dermoscopy Society (IDS)
Graz, Austria

Stefano Caccavale MD
Dermatologist
Italy

Nathalie De Carvalho MD
Dermatologist
Brazil

Teresa Deinlein MD
Dermatologist
University of Graz
Graz, Austria

Paula Friedman MD
Dermatologist
Department of Dermatology
Instituto de Investigaciones Médicas
'A Lanari'
University of Buenos Aires
Buenos Aires, Argentina

Alessio Gambardella MD
Dermatologist
Italy

Stefano Gardini MD
Dermatologist
Italy

Harald Kittler MD
AO Professor
Department of Dermatology
Medical University of Vienna
Vienna, Austria

Aimilios Lallas MD MSc PhD
Dermatologist-Venereologist
First Department
of Dermatology
Aristotle University
Thessaloniki, Greece

Caterina Longo MD
Professor of Dermatology
Dermatology Unit
University of Modena and Reggio
Emilia, Italy

Amalia Lupoli MD
Dermatologist
Italy

Marco Manfredini MD
Dermatologist
Italy

Carolina Marcucci MD
Dermatologist
Hospital Alvarez
Buenos Aires, Argentina

Elvira Moscarella MD
Dermatologist
Dermatology and Skin
Cancer Unit
Arcispedale S Maria Nuova
IRCCS Reggio
Emilia, Modena, Italy

Giovanni Pellacani MD
Full Professor and Chairman
Department of Dermatology
University of Modena and Reggio
Emilia, Modena, Italy

María Rosario Peralta MD
Dermatologist
University of Buenos Aires
Honorary Assistant
Medical Research Institute
University of
Buenos Aires
Buenos Aires, Argentina

Simonetta Piana MD
Dermatologist
Italy

Cliff Rosendahl MBBS PhD
Associate Professor
University of Queensland
Australia
Distinguished Visiting Professor
Tehran University of Medical
Sciences
Tehran, Iran

Lidia Rudnicka MD PhD
Professor
Department of Dermatology
President
Polish Dermatological Society
Chairman
Department of Dermatology
Medical University of Warsaw
Warsaw, Poland

Emilia Noemi Cohen Sabban MD
Dermatologist
Deputy Chief of the Instituto de
Investigaciones
Médicas A Lanari
University of Buenos Aires
Buenos Aires, Argentina
Assistant Professor
Department of Dermatology
University of Buenos Aires
Buenos Aires, Argentina

Gabriel Salerni MD PhD
Dermatologist, Doctor in Medicine
Universidad Nacional de Rosario
and Hospital Provincial del
Centenario de Rosario
Santa Fe, Argentina

Philipp Tschandl MD PhD
Dermatologist
Department of Dermatology
Medical University of Vienna
Vienna, Austria

Iris Zalaudek MD PhD
Dermatologist
Associate Professor
Division of Dermatology
Medical University of Graz
Graz, Austria
President
International Dermoscopy Society
Graz, Austria

Foreword

If you believe that augmenting your diagnostic skills with available, office-based and cheap hand-held intruments is your duty as a dermatologist, this book will prove helpful to you.

Drawn from personal experience and in association with a group of world-recognized experts, Professor Cabo covers the growing field of Dermoscopy, including melanocytic and nonmelanocytic lesions, benign and malignant total body follow-up photography, entomodermatoscopy, inflammatoscopy, tricoscopy, capillaroscopy and *in vivo* reflectance confocal microscopy.

The information in this state-of-the-art volume is presented in a simple manner, with the aid of clear diagrams, that emphasize the things one should look out for. Data are highlighted with the use of tables that single out the characteristic signs of each individual entity.

The authors present a user-friendly book, a practically rapid consultation reference in the office.

As the use of the dermatoscope expands, so have its applications widened, well beyond the original differential diagnosis of melanocytic lesions. The recognition of vascular patterns associated with nonpigmented (amelanotic) melanomas, the importance of diagnostic algorithms, the chapters on Revised Pattern Analysis and Chaos and Clues, all emphasize the fact that dermoscopy is a rapidly evolving diagnostic technique. Thus, to achieve high specificity and sensitivity, the method requires knowledge and hands-on expertise.

It is no surprise that colleagues with this wonderful hand-held device—a dermatoscope—would begin to visualize the normal and disease-related fauna on/in the skin superficial layers; that they would look at hairs, nailfolds and nailbed and 'dig into' inflammatory skin conditions. The results of their efforts are well represented in the corresponding chapters!

The main author of this book hopes that his readers may improve their dermoscopic skills for the benefit of their patients. *Color Atlas of Dermoscopy* is a step in the right direction.

Fernando Stengel MD
Ex-Assistant Professor
Skin & Cancer Unit
New York University
New York City, New York, USA
Ex-Chief
Department of Dermatology
Clinical Hospital
University of Buenos Aires
Buenos Aires, Argentina
Ex-Chief
Centro de Educación Médica e Investigaciones
Clínicas (CEMIC)
Buenos Aires, Argentina

Preface

Many years have passed since I began to use the dermatoscope with nonpolarized light.

For over twenty years, I have attended courses, I have read many journals and books, I have published articles, my own books, CD-ROMs, I have taught numerous courses, and presented hundreds of cases.

Today, I finish a much-cherished project, my first book in English.

Here I share all the experiences amassed in these years. I hope, dear reader, that you will find it useful to improve your dermoscopic learning for the benefit of your patients.

Horacio Antonio Cabo

Acknowledgments

To Estela Riviere for helping me in this project.

To all the contributors.

I thank **Mr Jitendar P Vij (Group Chairman)**, **Mr Ankit Vij (Group President)**, **Ms Chetna Malhotra Vohra (Associate Director–Content Strategy)**, **Ms Angima Shree (Senior Development Editor)** and the production team of **Jaypee Brothers Medical Publishers, New Delhi, India** for giving us a go-ahead at the very beginning and helping us in every way possible to bring out this book.

Contents

WHY USE THE DERMATOSCOPE

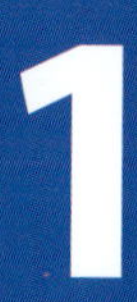

Horacio A Cabo

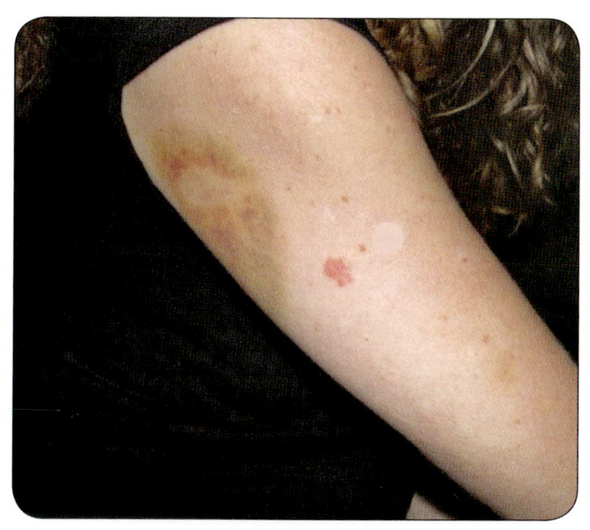

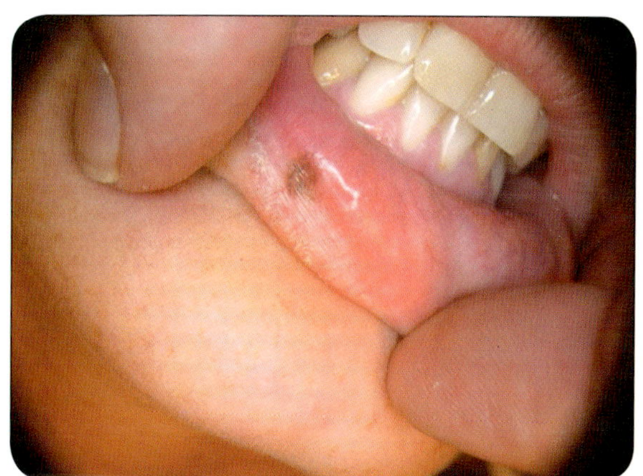

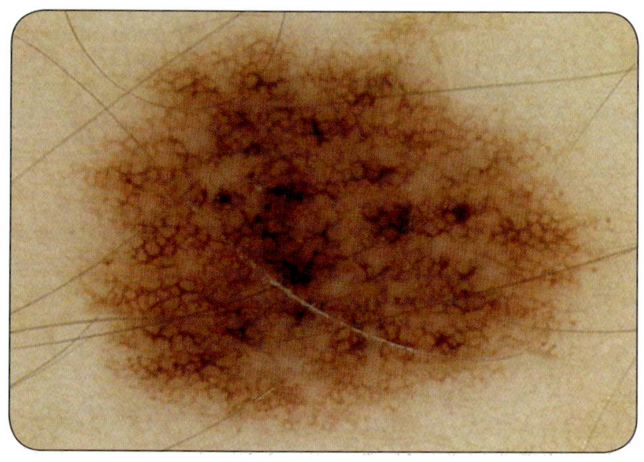

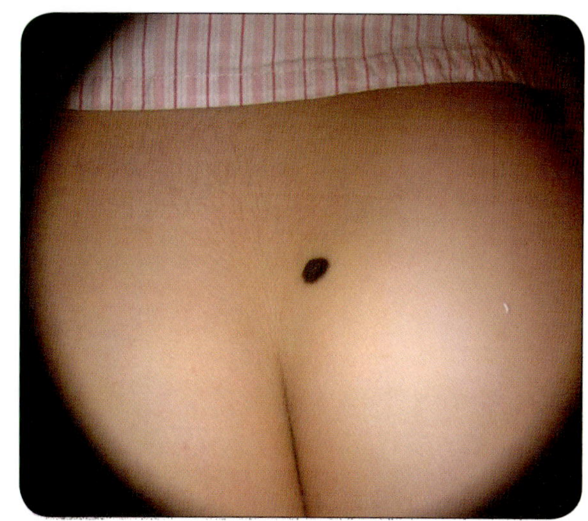

"Dermoscopy is a noninvasive technique that improves the clinical diagnosis of pigmented and nonpigmented lesions. This technique allows us to differentiate melanoma from other melanocytic and nonmelanocytic lesions according to new morphological criteria. Under clinical examination, many nevi and melanomas have clinical characteristics which sometimes make them look very similar. This happens with some melanocytic lesions. With the dermatoscope, benign or malignant patterns may be identified and in this manner, the diagnostic accuracy can be improved as compared with the clinical examination."

Dermoscopy is a noninvasive technique that improves the clinical diagnosis of pigmented and nonpigmented lesions.

It has been used for over 20 years and in this first chapter we will see briefly why we should incorporate it to our patients' routinely examination.

- This technique allows us to differentiate melanoma from other melanocytic and nonmelanocytic lesions according to new morphological criteria (Figs. 1.1 to 1.8).
- It is the merges of clinical dermatology (macroscopy) and dermatopathology (microscopy) (Figs. 1.9 to 1.14).
- Dermoscopy improves clinical diagnosis of pigmented skin lesions by 10–30% (Figs. 1.15 to 1.20 and Table 1.1).
- Dermoscopy improves the diagnosis of nail lesions (Figs. 1.21 to 1.25).
- Dermoscopy improves the diagnosis of palm and sole lesions (Figs. 1.27 and 1.28).
- Dermoscopy reduces the number of unnecessary cutaneous biopsies (40%).

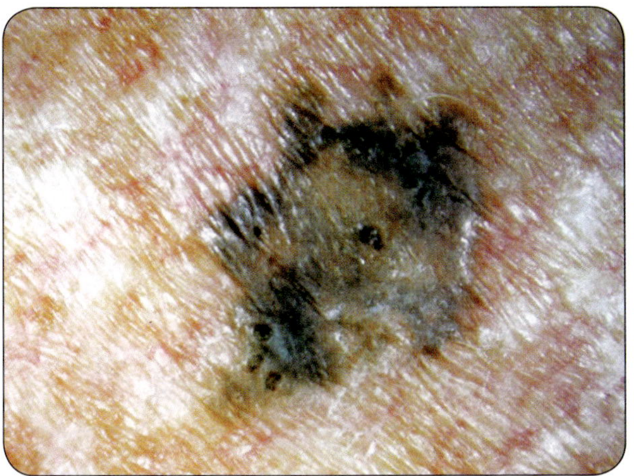

Fig. 1.1: Clinical image of a pigmented lesion where it is difficult to distinguish whether it is a melanocytic or a nonmelanocytic lesion.

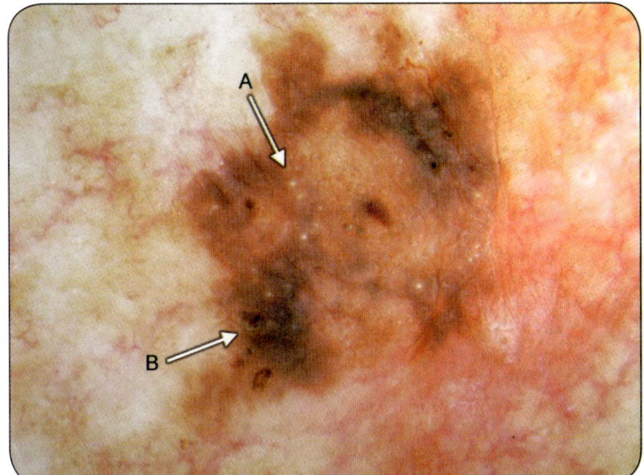

Fig. 1.2: Dermoscopic image of the lesion in Figure 1.1, where the criteria for seborrheic keratosis are clearly observable. (A) Multiple pseudocysts. (B) Pseudo follicular openings.

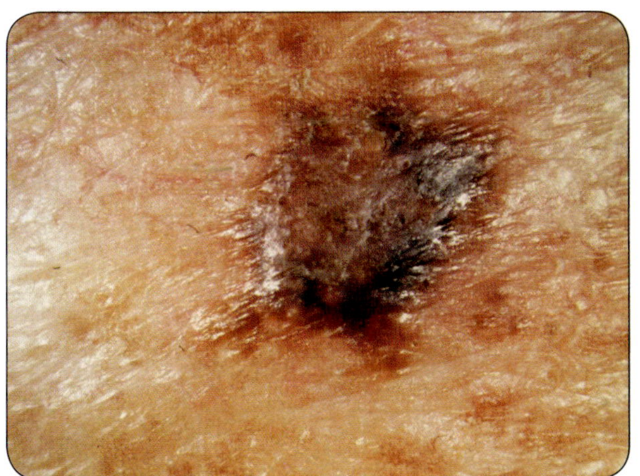

Fig. 1.3: Clinical image of a pigmented lesion where it is difficult to distinguish whether it is a melanocytic or a nonmelanocytic lesion.

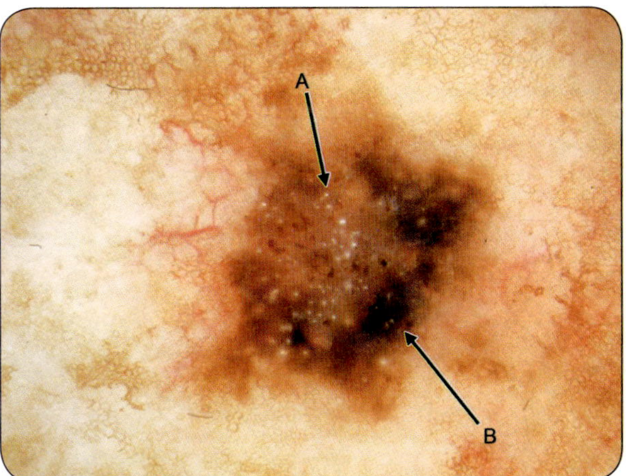

Fig. 1.4: Dermoscopic image of the lesion in Figure 1.3, where the criteria for seborrheic keratosis are clearly observable. (A) Multiple pseudocysts. (B) Pseudo follicular openings.

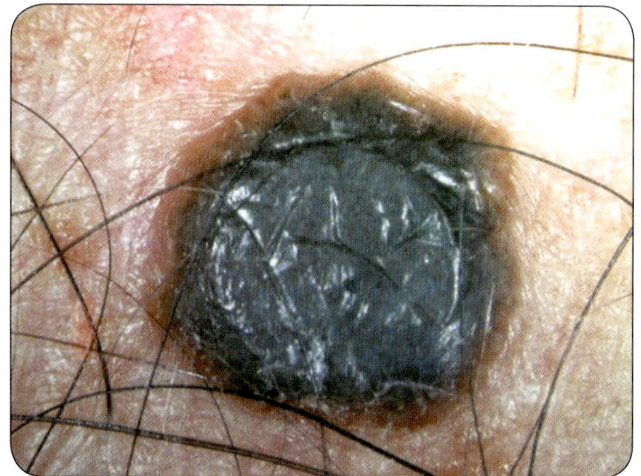

Fig. 1.5: Clinical image of a pigmented lesion where it is difficult to distinguish whether it is a melanocytic or a nonmelanocytic lesion.

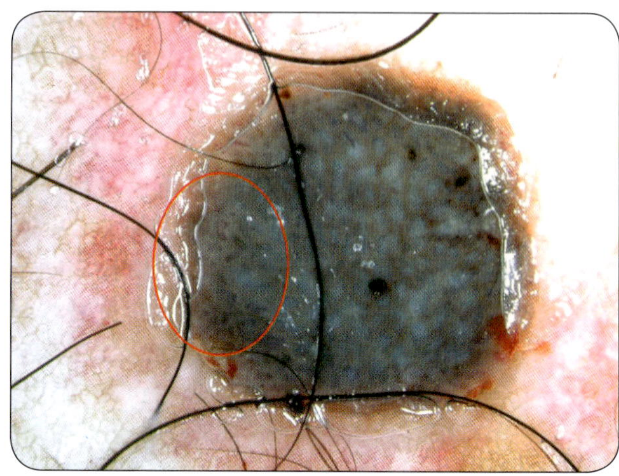

Fig. 1.6: Multiple hairpin vessels in the periphery (red circle).

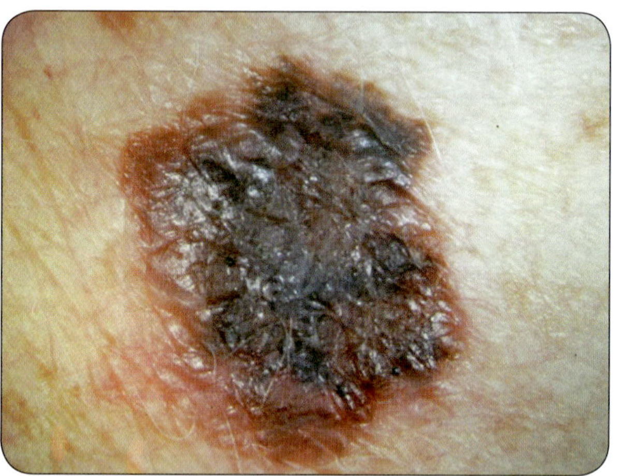

Fig. 1.7: Clinical image of a pigmented lesion where it is difficult to distinguish whether it is a melanocytic or a nonmelanocytic lesion.

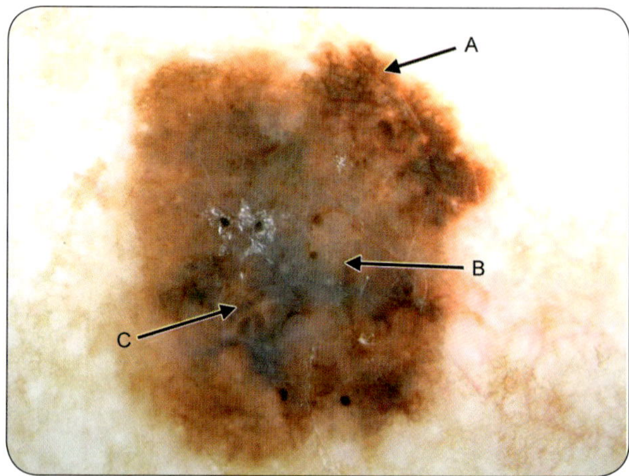

Fig. 1.8: Dermoscopic image of a melanoma. (A) Atypical pigment network. (B) Blue-white veil. (C) Negative pigment network.

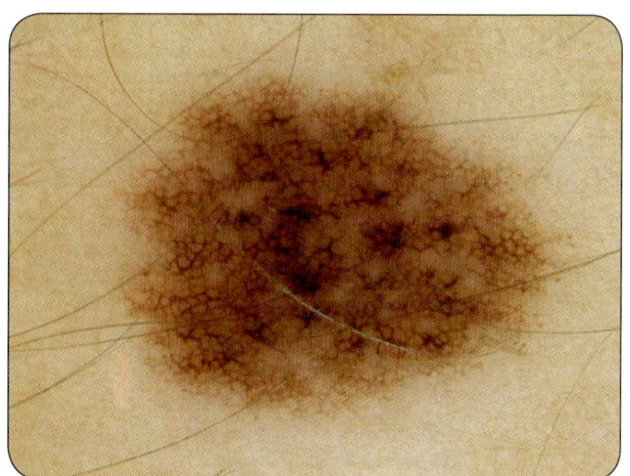

Fig. 1.9: Pigment network in a nevus with reticular pattern.

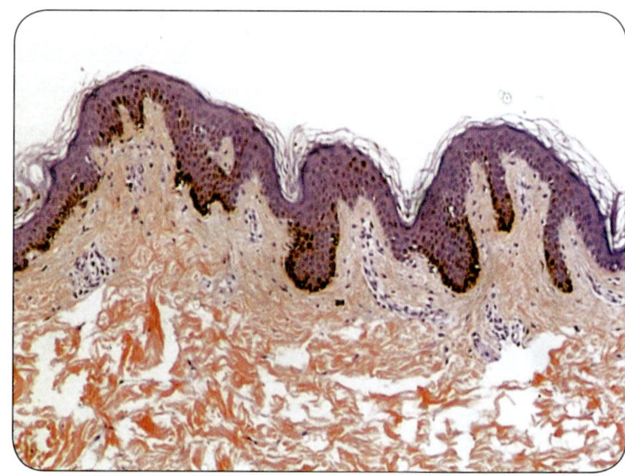

Fig. 1.10: Histological correlation of the pigment network.

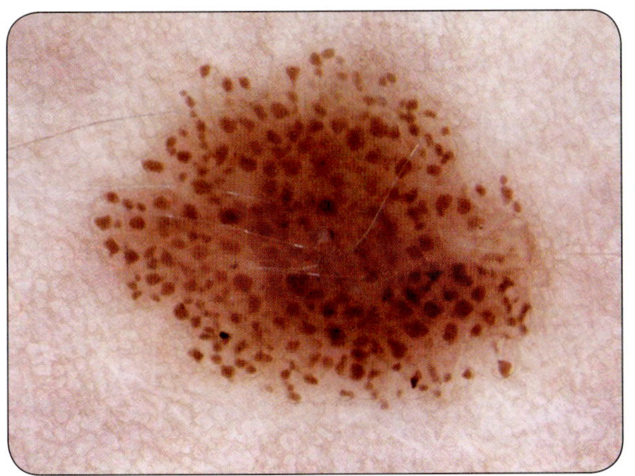

Fig. 1.11: Brown globules in a nevus with globular pattern.

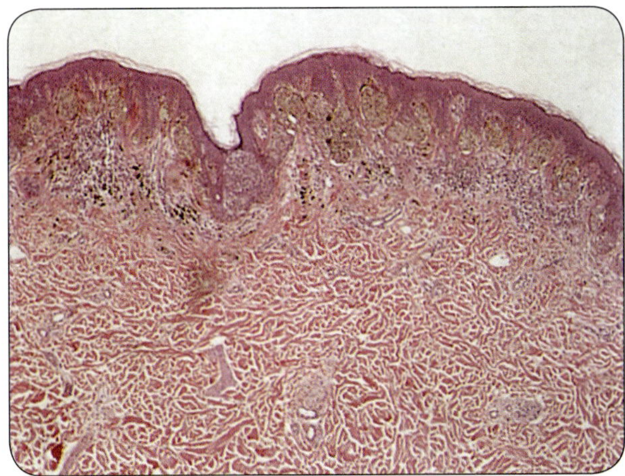

Fig. 1.12: Histological correlation of the globules.

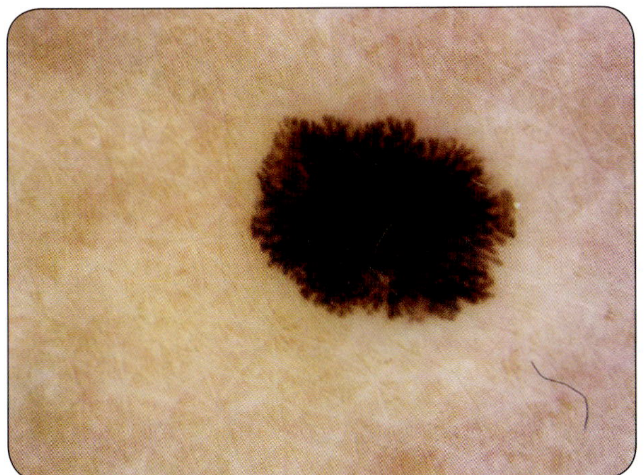

Fig. 1.13: Streaks or projections.

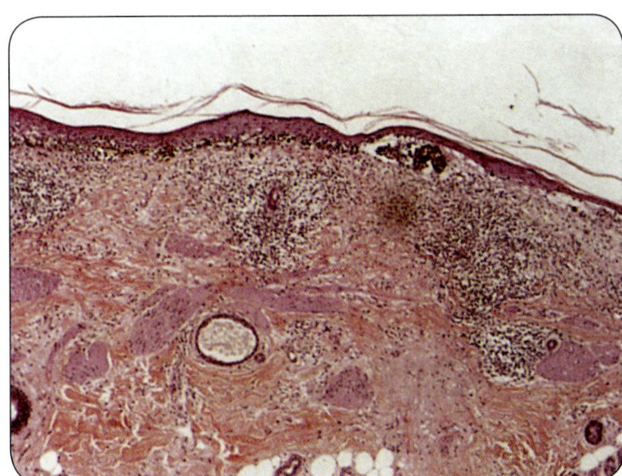

Fig. 1.14: Histological correlation of the streaks or projections.

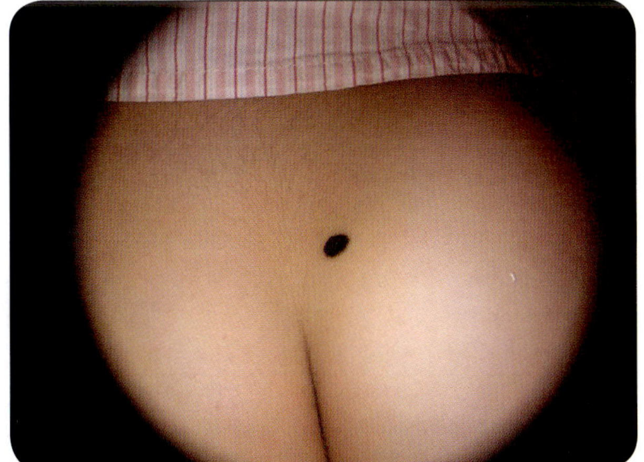

Fig. 1.15: Clinical image of a 12-year-old patient with a symmetrical black lesion, where it is difficult to perform a clinical diagnosis.

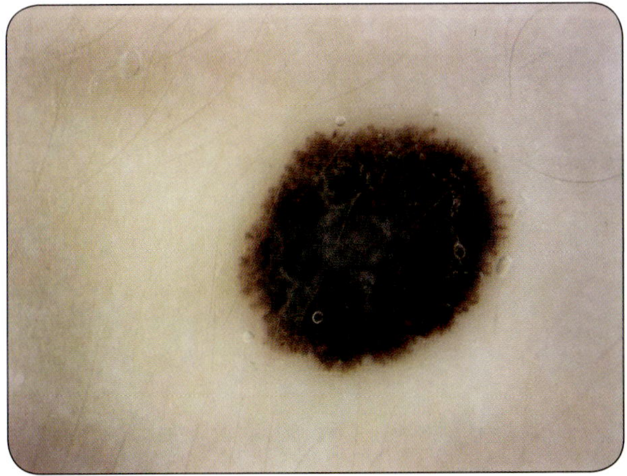

Fig. 1.16: Dermoscopic image where it is possible to observe the starburst pattern (peripheral projections over the whole lesion) typical of the Spitz nevus.

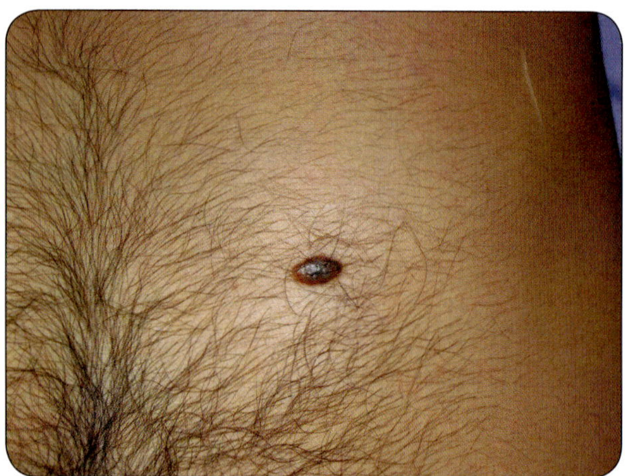

Fig. 1.17: Clinical image of a symmetrical raised lesion with multiple colors and difficult clinical diagnosis.

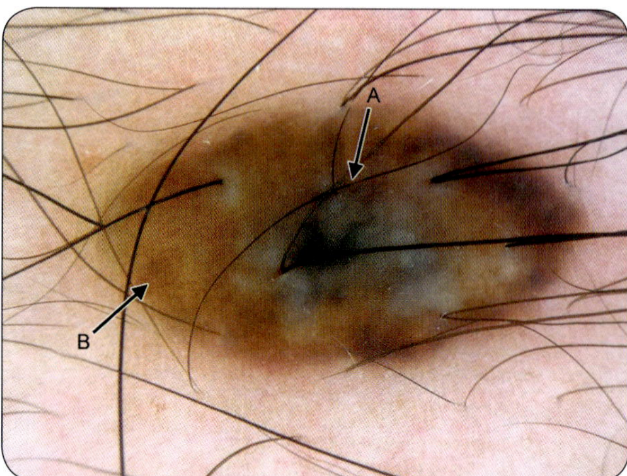

Fig. 1.18: Dermoscopic image of combined lesion with a diagnosis of combined nevus. The central area presents a homogeneous blue coloration (deep component) corresponding to a blue nevus, (A) and the periphery (superficial component) presents a pigment network corresponding to a compound nevus (B).

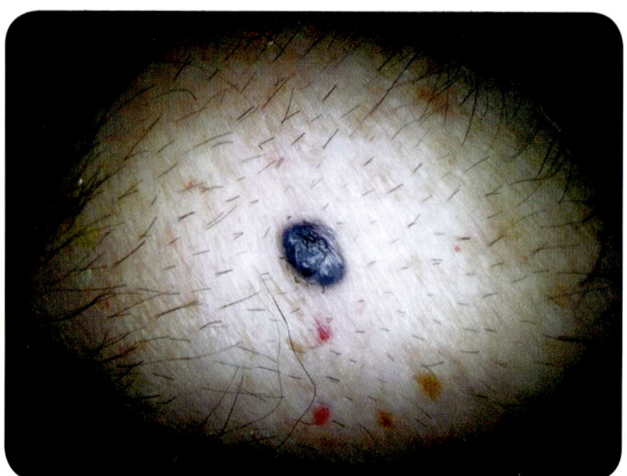

Fig. 1.19: Clinical image of a blue-black pigmented lesion with fast onset and difficult clinical diagnosis.

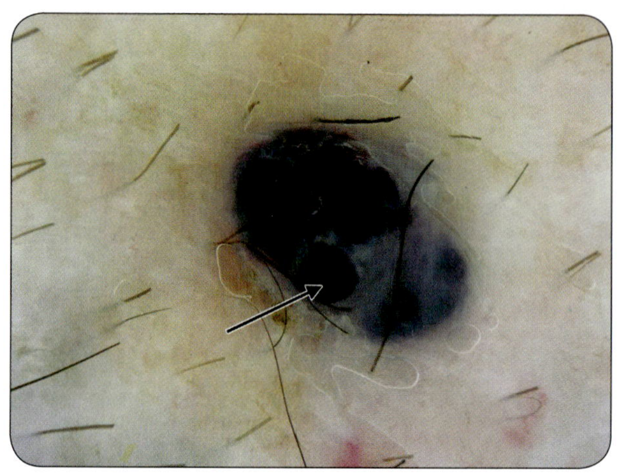

Fig. 1.20: Dermoscopic image of a hemangioma, with multiple red blue areas (lacunae).

Table 1.1: Diagnostic accuracy in pigmented lesions.	
Without dermatoscope (%)	65–85
With dermatoscope (%)	85–95
Dermoscopy improves clinical diagnosis (%)	10–30

- Dermoscopy decreases the benign/malignant ratio of excised lesions:
  - Predermoscopy 18:1 (we need to remove 18 benign lesions to find a melanoma)
  - Dermoscopy 4:1

- The diagnosis of melanoma with few dermoscopic characteristics has improved with the short-term and the long-term follow-up (Figs. 1.29 to 1.32).
- Dermoscopy with polarized light with or without contact has improved the diagnosis of nonpigmented lesions (Figs. 1.33 to 1.38).
- Dermoscopy improves the diagnosis of pigmented lesions of the mucosae (Figs. 1.39 to 1. 42).
- Dermoscopy has been shown to improve the treatment of pigmented lesions in children and adolescents and reduce the number of unnecessary excisions (Fig. 1.43).

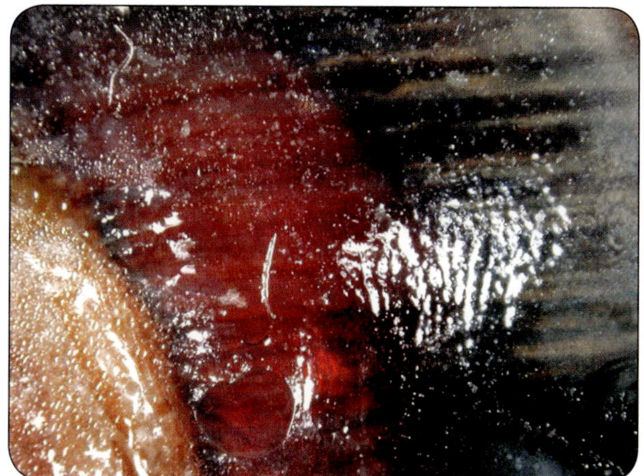

Fig. 1.21: Subungual hematoma.

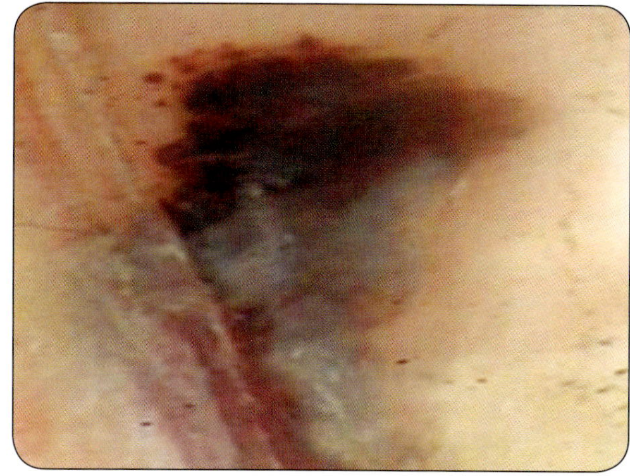

Fig. 1.22: Subungual hematoma.

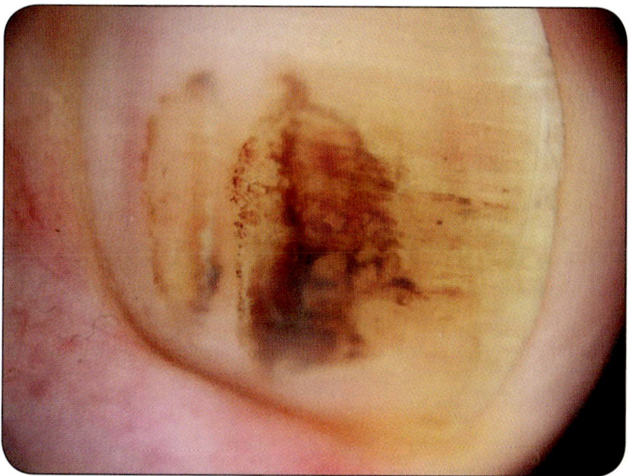

Fig. 1.23: Subungual hematoma.

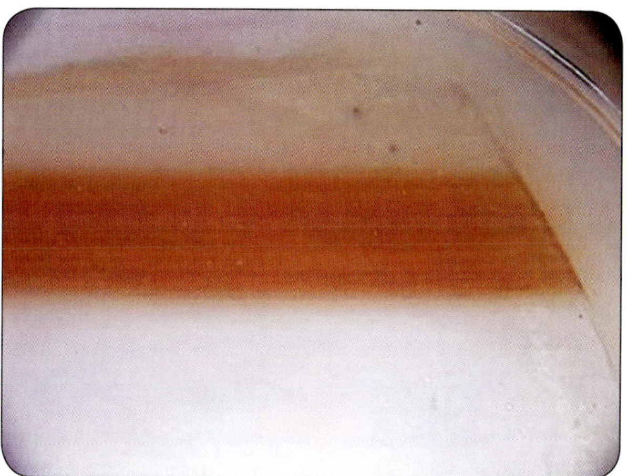

Fig. 1.24: Nevus: Brown background pigmentation with regular longitudinal bands.

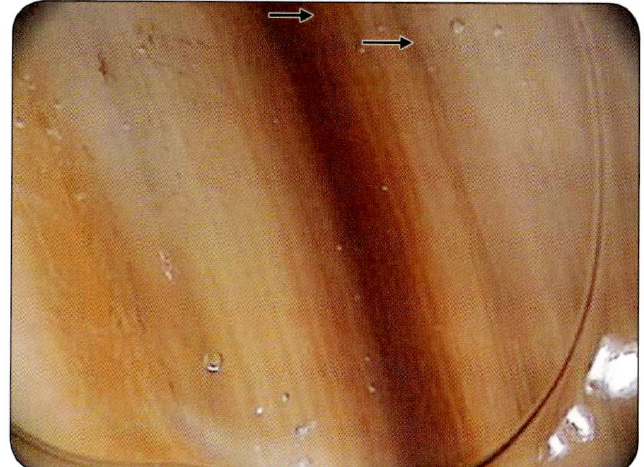

Fig. 1.25: Melanoma: Brown background pigmentation with irregular longitudinal bands (arrows).

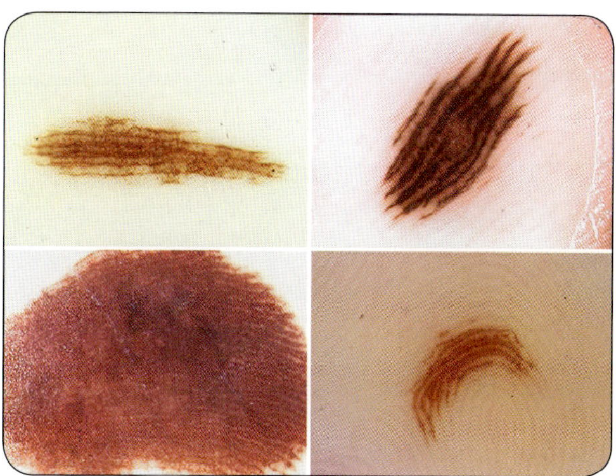

Fig. 1.26: Acral nevi with parallel furrow pattern.

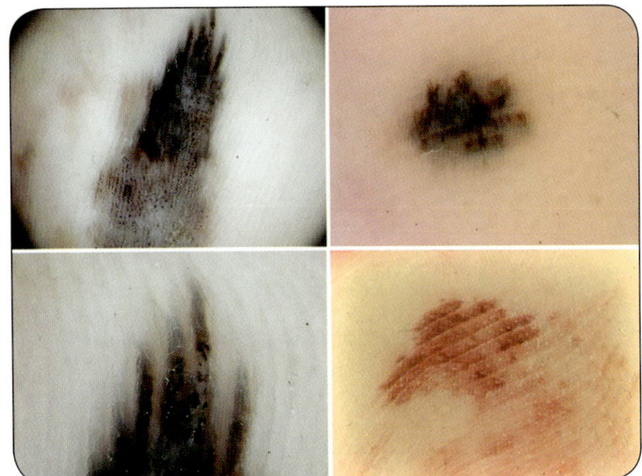

Fig. 1.27: Melanoma with parallel ridge pattern.

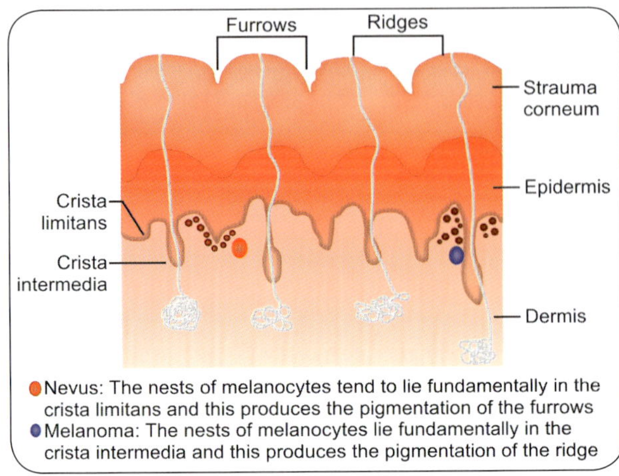

Fig. 1.28: Diagram of skin histology in acral areas.

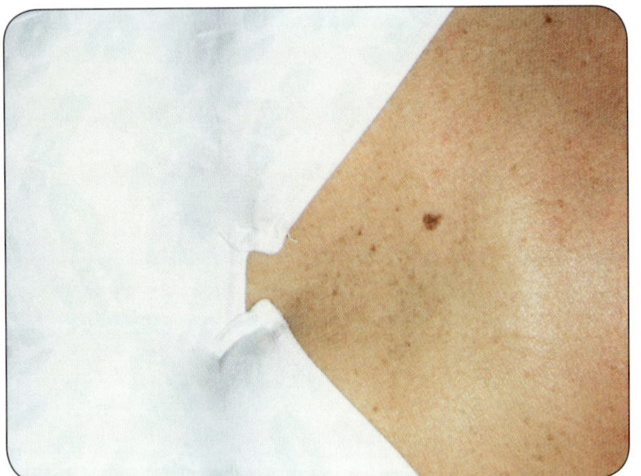

Fig. 1.29: Pigmented lesion in the neckline.

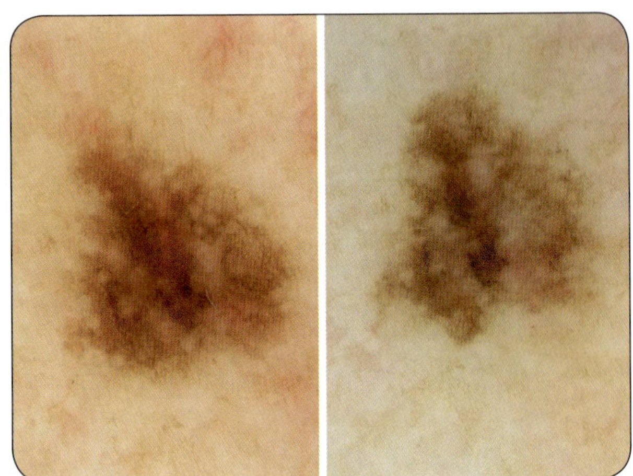

Fig. 1.30: Melanoma in situ in thorax. Dermoscopy of lesion in Figure 1.29 with patent changes in the digital follow-up.

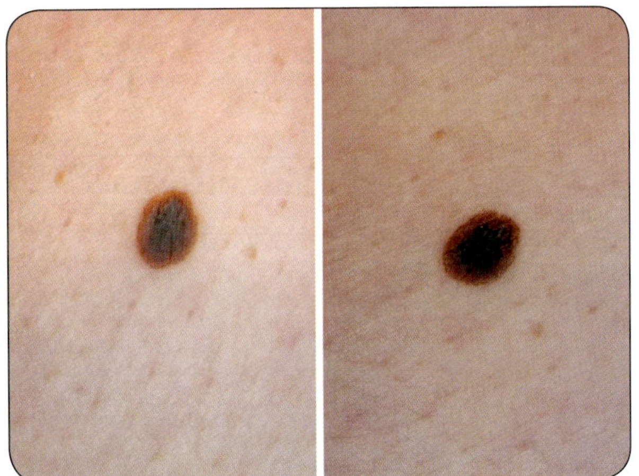

Fig. 1.31: Pigmented lesion in neckline showing clinical changes in 4 months.

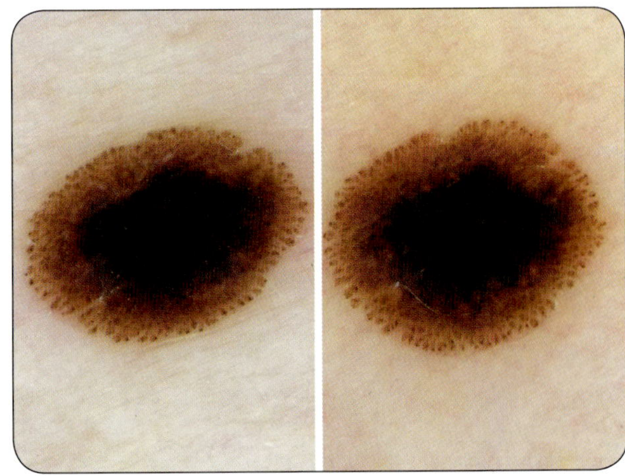

Fig. 1.32: Spreading superficial melanoma B 0.37. Dermoscopy of the lesion in Figure 1.31, showing obvious changes in the digital follow-up.

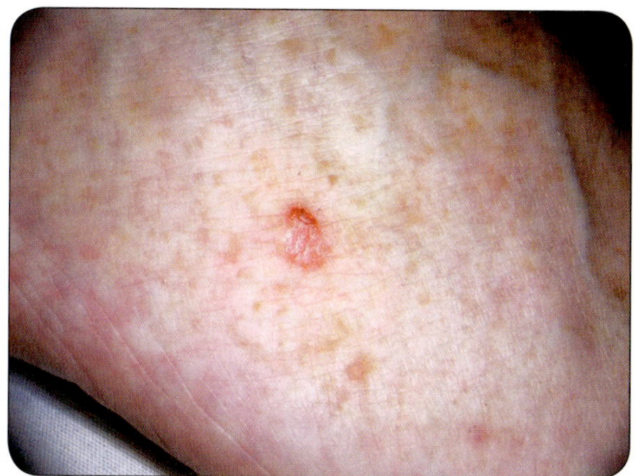

Fig. 1.33: Pink lesion in anterior foot of difficult clinical diagnosis.

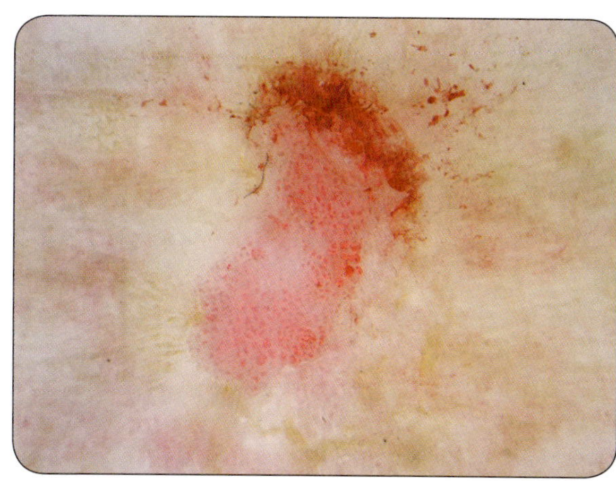

Fig. 1.34: Dermoscopy of the lesion in Figure 1.33, where it is possible to observe glomerular vessels with focal distribution. Diagnosis: squamous cell carcinoma.

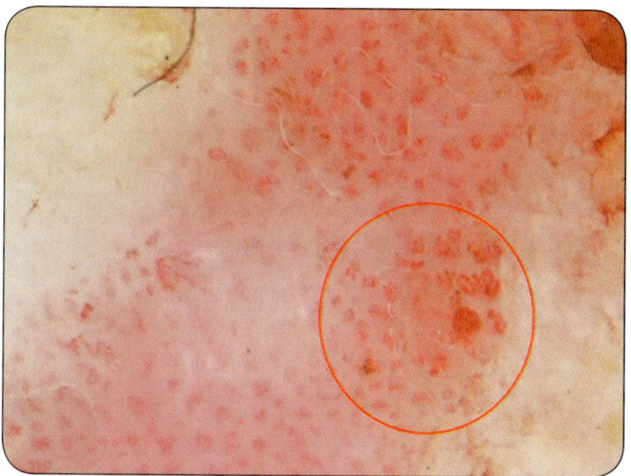

Fig. 1.35: Close-up view of Figure 1.34 (red circle shows glomerular vessels with focal distribution).

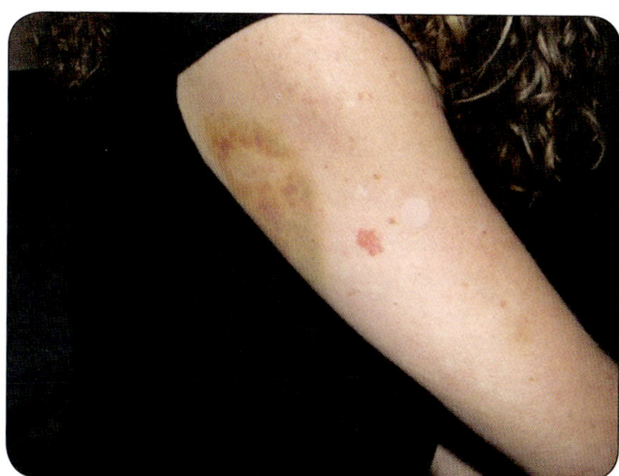

Fig. 1.36: Pink lesion in the right arm, difficult to diagnose clinically.

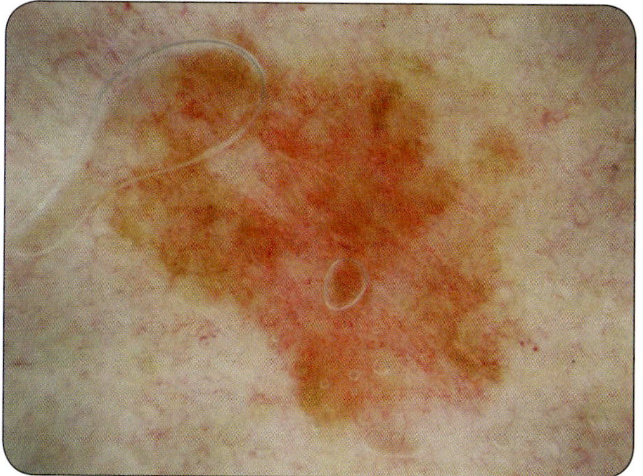

Fig. 1.37: Dermoscopy of lesion in Figure 1.36, where it is possible to observe irregular lineal and dot-like vessels. Diagnosis: Hypomelanotic melanoma.

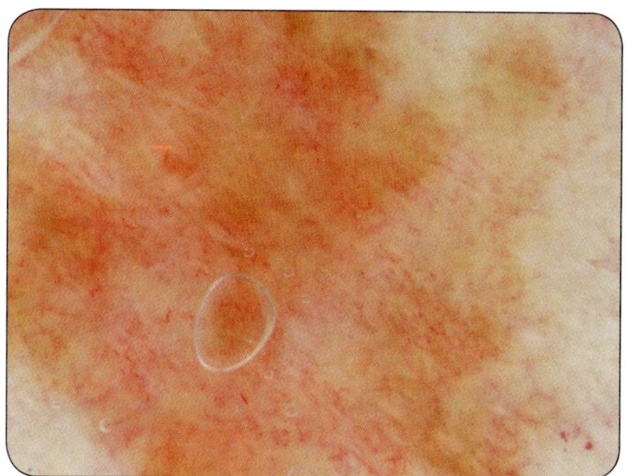

Fig. 1.38: Close-up view of Figure 1.37.

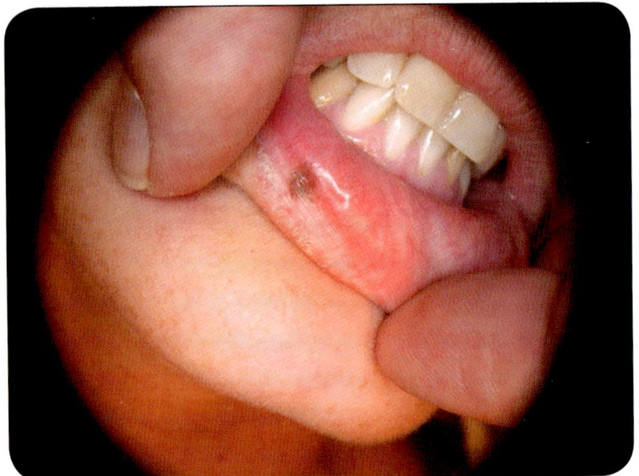

Fig. 1.39: Pigmented lesion on the lower lip, difficult to diagnose.

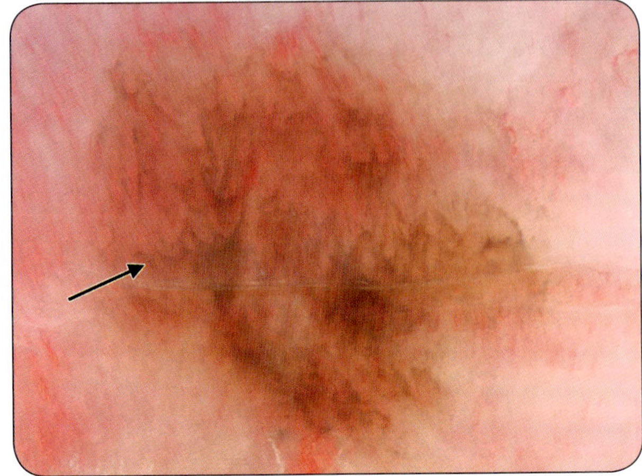

Fig. 1.40: Dermoscopy of lesion in Figure 1.39. Labial melanotic macula. Fish-scale pattern (arrow).

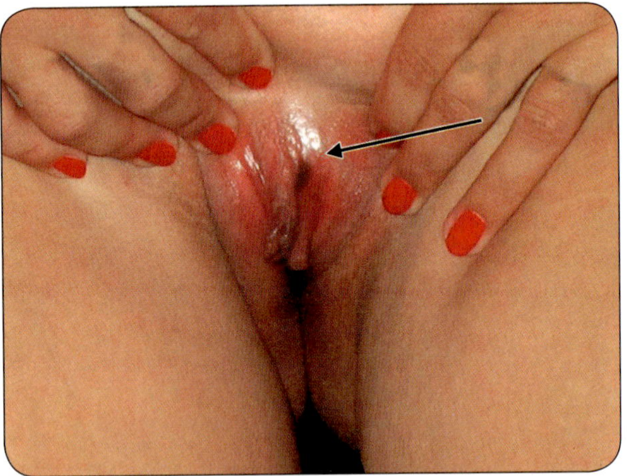

Fig. 1.41: Pigmented lesion on genitalia, difficult to diagnose (arrow).

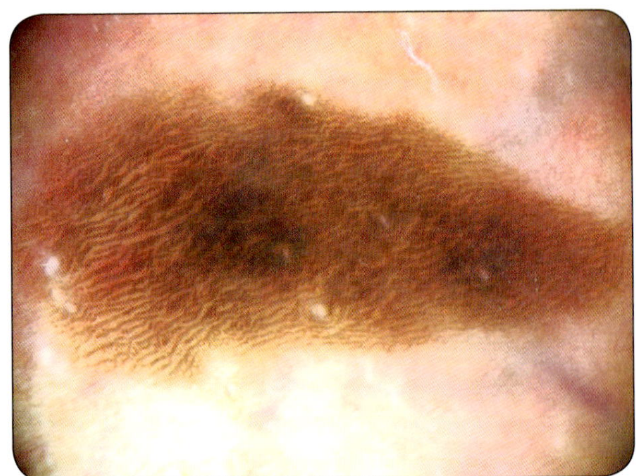

Fig. 1.42: Dermoscopy of the lesion in Figure 1.40. Genital melanotic macula. Fingerprint pattern.

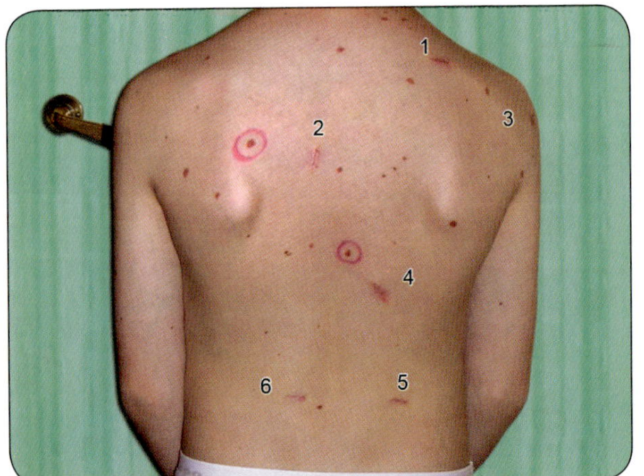

Fig. 1.43: A 12-year-old boy with multiple excisions of typical nevi (1–6). Example of what not to do.

Table 1.2: Comparative dermoscopic approach.
Predominant nevus pattern (signature nevus)
The different lesion
Clinically and dermoscopically (ugly duckling sign)
Dermoscopically (Little Red Riding Hood sign)

- Dermoscopy has been shown to improve the diagnosis of patients with multiple nevi using the comparative dermoscopic approach (Table 1.2).
  - Dermoscopy improves the diagnostic accuracy (specificity and sensitivity) of pigmented lesions (Figs. 1.44 and 1.45). Sensitivity is the capacity to detect melanomas.

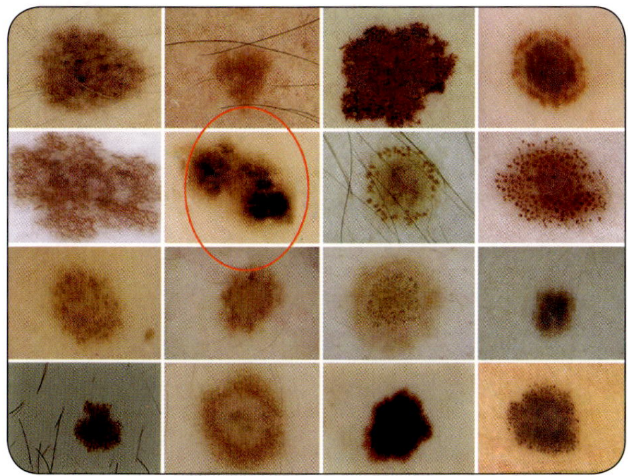

Fig. 1.44: Sensitivity: Capacity to detect melanoma. The lesion in the red circle is quickly identified as atypical and different from the other nevi.

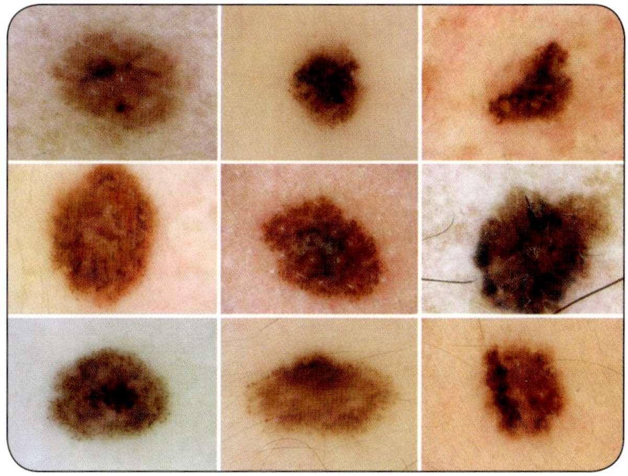

Fig. 1.45: Specificity: Capacity to detect nonmelanoma. In these examples, it is very difficult to distinguish atypical nevi from melanoma.

- Specificity is the capacity to detect nonmelanomas.
  - Sensitivity = TP/(TP + FN)
  - Specificity = TN/(TN + FP)
  - TP: true-positive results
  - TN: true-negative results
  - FN: false-negative results
  - FP: false-positive results—Lesions which were clinically diagnosed as melanoma and whose histopathological study proved them to be nevi.

Under clinical examination many nevi and melanomas have clinical characteristics which sometimes make them look very similar. This happens with some melanocytic lesions.

With the dermatoscope, benign or malignant patterns may be identified and in this manner the diagnostic accuracy can be improved as compared with the clinical examination.

SUGGESTED READING

Altamura D, Altobelli E, Micantonio T, et al. Dermoscopic patterns of acral melanocytic nevi and melanomas in a white population in central Italy. Arch Dermatol. 2006;142:1123.

Bauer J, Metzler G, Rassner G, et al. Dermoscopy turns histopathologist's attention to the suspicious area in melanocytic lesions. Arch Dermatol. 2001;137:1338-40.

Braun RP, Kaya G, Masouye I, et al. Histopathologic correlation in dermoscopy: a micropunch technique. Arch Dermatol. 2003;139:349-51.

Carli P, de Giorgi V, Chiarugi A, et al. Addition of dermoscopy to conventional naked-eye examination in melanoma screening: a randomized study. J Am Acad Dermatol. 2004;50:683-9.

Carli P, de Giorgi V, Crocetti E, et al. Improvement of malignant/benign ratio in excised melanocytic lesions in the "dermoscopy era": a retrospective study 1997-2001. Br J Dermatol. 2004;150(4):687-92.

Carli P, de Giorgi V, Soyer HP, et al. Dermoscopy in the diagnosis of pigmented skin lesions: a new semiology for the dermatologist. J Eur Acad Dermatol Venereol. 2000;14(5):353-69.

Haenssle HA, Krueger U, Vente C, et al. Results from an observational trial: digital epiluminescence microscopy follow-up of atypical nevi increases the sensitivity and the chance of success of conventional dermoscopy in detecting melanoma. J Invest Dermatol. 2006;126:980-5.

Johr RH, Izakovic J. Dermoscopy/ELM for the evaluation of nail-apparatus pigmentation. Dermatol Surg. 2001;27:315-22.

Kittler H, PehambeKittler H, Pehamberger H, et al. Diagnostic accuracy of dermoscopy. Lancet Oncol. 2002;3:159-65.

Menzies S, Zalaudek I. Why perform dermoscopy? The evidence for its role in the routine management of pigmented skin lesions. Arch Dermatol. 2006;142:1211-2.

Menzies SW. Cutaneous melanoma: making a clinical diagnosis, present and future. Dermatol Ther. 2006;19:32-9.

Menzies SW, Gutenev A, Avramidis M, et al. Short-term digital surface microscopic monitoring of atypical or changing melanocytic lesions. Arch Dermatol. 2001;137:1583-9.

Pehamberger H, Binder M, Steiner A, et al. In vivo epiluminescence microscopy: improvement early diagnosis of melanoma. J Invest Dermatol. 1993;100(3):356-62.

Skvara H, Teban L, Fiebiger M, et al. Limitations of dermoscopy in the recognition of melanoma. Arch Dermatol. 2005;141:155-60.

Tosti A, Argenziano G. Dermoscopy allows better management of nail pigmentation. Arch Dermatol. 2002;138:1369-70.

STRUCTURES, PATTERNS, CRITERIA AND COLORS

2

Horacio A Cabo

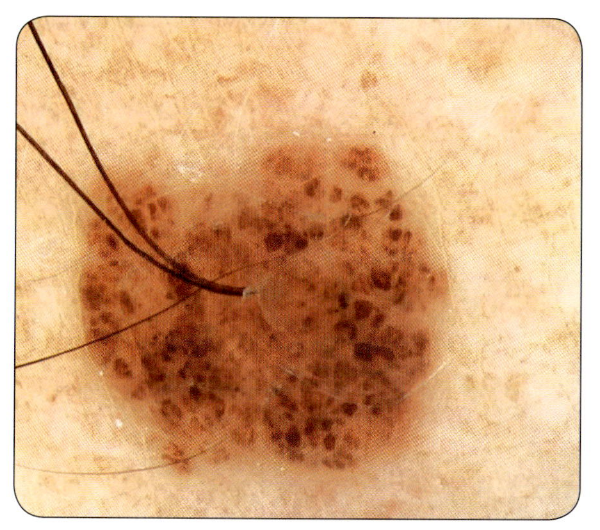

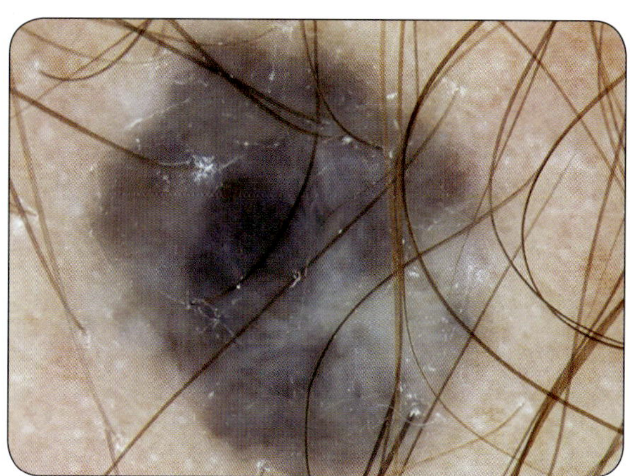

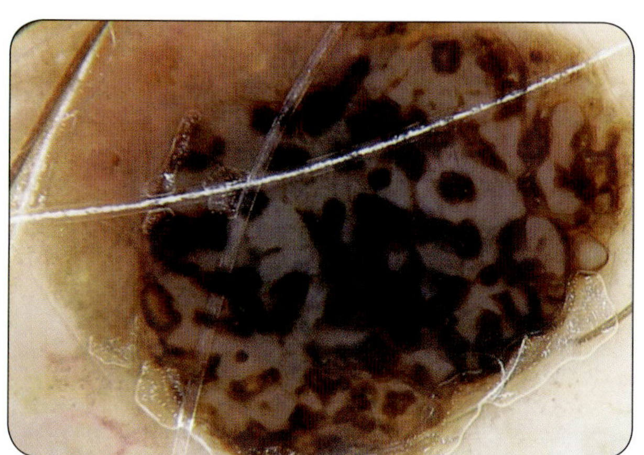

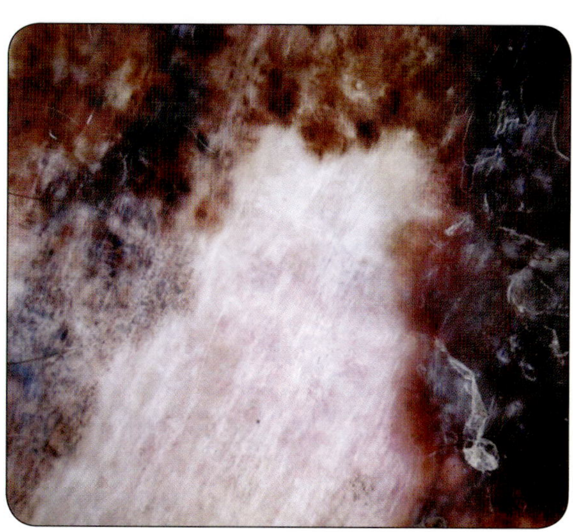

"" The multiple repetitions of a structure form a pattern.
When the structures are associated with certain pigmented lesions and their observation implies defining a given lesion, they are called criteria.
In this manner, there are criteria for melanocytic and nonmelanocytic lesions and such criteria will be explored in different chapters of this book.
Besides the structures, different colors can be observed which help, elaborate the dermoscopic diagnosis.
It is necessary to consider type, number, and color distribution.""

By modifying the optic characteristics of the skin, the dermatoscope makes it possible to see different shapes or structures that cannot be discerned with the naked eye (Fig. 2.1).

These shapes or structures are given a name to identify them. At the beginning, a metaphoric language was used; for example, "spoke-wheel areas" or "starburst"; but this made learning difficult for beginners. For some years now, this metaphoric language has been combined with or even replaced by a new morphologic one in which, as we will see hereunder, new terms are applied; so, for example, what used to be called brown globules and blue-gray ovoid nests are now given the morphologic names of Brown Areas and Blue-Gray Areas (Figs. 2.2 and 2.3).

In Chapter 12, we will see that there are five basic elements (lines, dots, areas, pseudopods, and circles) with which all dermoscopic structures can be described without using the metaphoric method (Fig. 2.4).

Just as under clinical examination we can recognize a papule or blister, under dermoscopic examination it is possible to recognize, for instance, pigment network or brown globules (Figs. 2.5 and 2.6).

Identifying all these dermoscopic structures is as necessary as recognizing basic dermatologic lesions. These structures are like the letters of the alphabets, and recognizing them makes it possible "to read" the different pigmented lesions with the dermoscope.

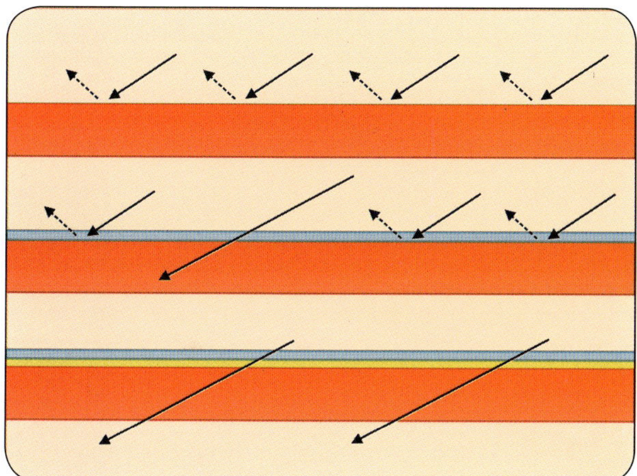

Fig. 2.1: Light reflection scheme.

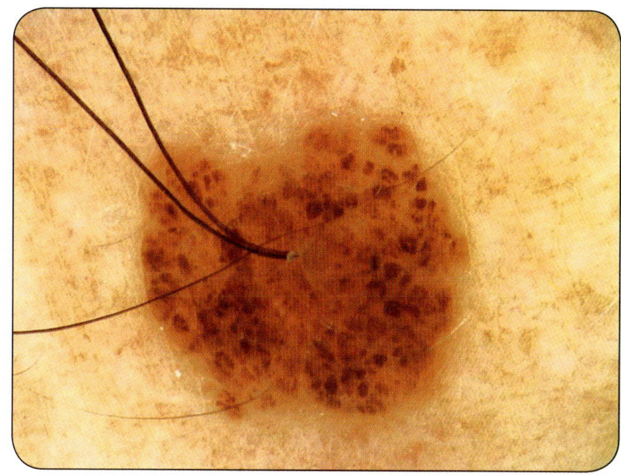

Fig. 2.2: Brown globules or brown areas (compound nevi).

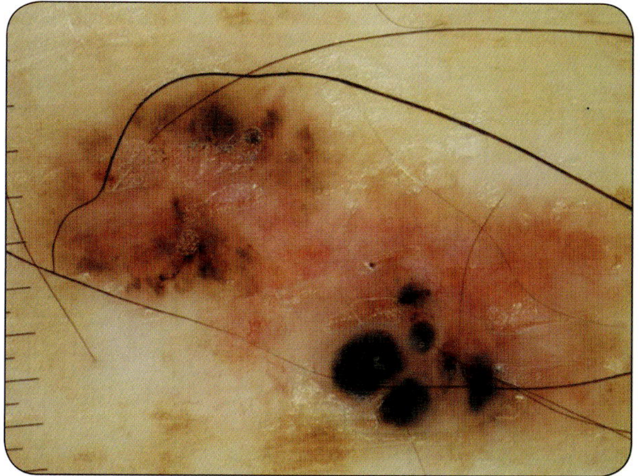

Fig. 2.3: Gray-blue ovoid nests or gray-blue areas (basal cell carcinoma).

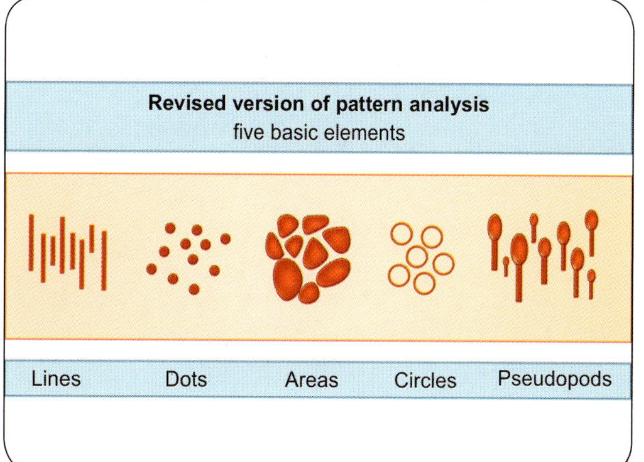

Fig. 2.4: Basic elements.

The multiple repetitions of a *structure* form a *pattern*. When the structures are associated with certain pigmented lesions and their observation implies defining a given lesion, they are called *criteria* (Fig. 2.7).

In this manner, there are criteria for melanocytic and nonmelanocytic lesions, as can be observed in Tables 2.1 to 2.4, and such criteria will be explored in different chapters of this book (Figs. 2.8 to 2.16).

Besides the structures, different colors can be observed which help elaborate the dermoscopic diagnosis.

Color is extremely important; just imagine having to differentiate brown globules from blue or red areas if we saw everything in black and white (Figs. 2.17 and 2.18).

It is necessary to consider type, number, and color distribution. Skin color is determined mainly by hemoglobin and melanin.

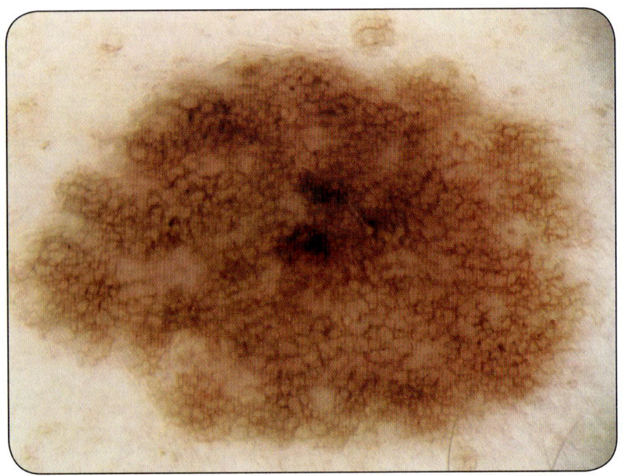

Fig. 2.5: Pigment network.

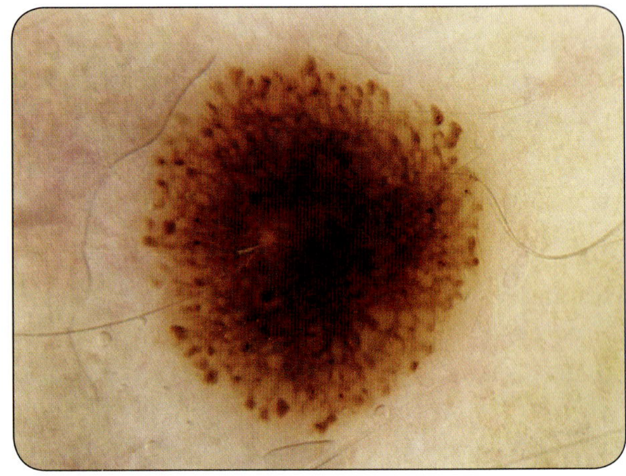

Fig. 2.6: Brown globules.

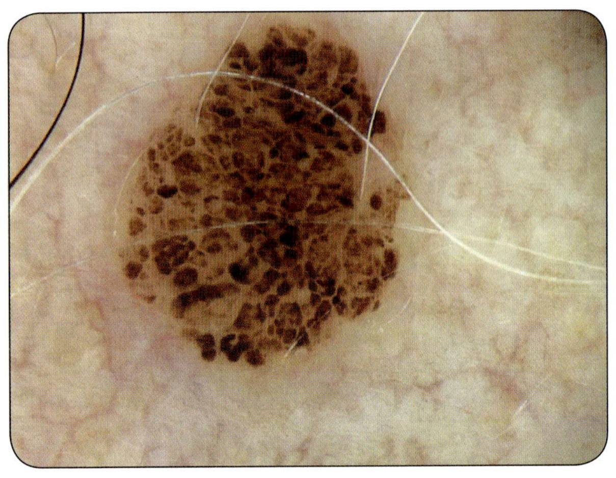

Fig. 2.7: Structure: globules; pattern: globular; "brown globules are a criterion for melanocytic lesions.

Table 2.1: Dermoscopic criteria for melanocytic lesions (Figs. 2.8 to 2.11).

Pigment network	Aggregated globules	Streaks or projections	Homogeneous blue pigmentation	Parallel pattern

Table 2.2: Dermoscopic criteria for seborrheic keratosis (Figs. 2.12 to 2.14).

Classic seborrheic keratosis	*Flat seborrheic keratosis (Lentigo solaris)*
Milia-like cysts	Fingerprint-like structures
Comedo-like openings (irregular ridges)	Moth-eaten border Jelly sign
Fissures and ridges (similar to brain surface)	
Vascular pattern	

Table 2.3: Dermoscopic criteria for basal cell carcinoma (Fig. 2.15).

Vascular pattern	*Blue-gray pigmentation*	*Ulceration*
Thick vessels with multiple branching or arborizing vessels	Leaf-like or digit-like structures	
	Big ovoid nests or structures	
	Multiple globules	
	Radiated areas	

Table 2.4: Dermoscopic criteria for angioma (Fig. 2.16).

Blue-red lacunes: round areas of blue or red color

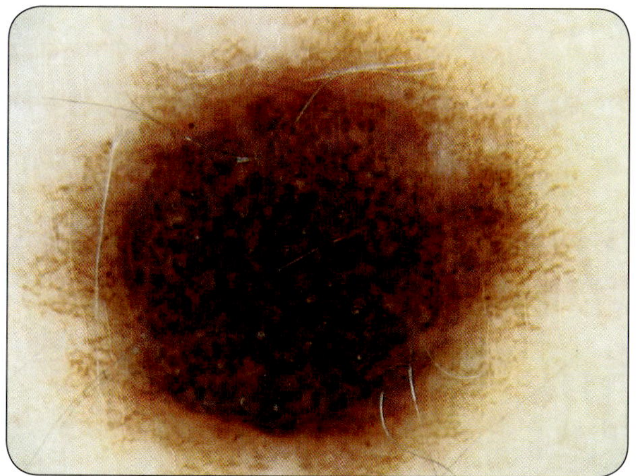

Fig. 2.8: Compound nevi. Pigment network and aggregated brown globules.

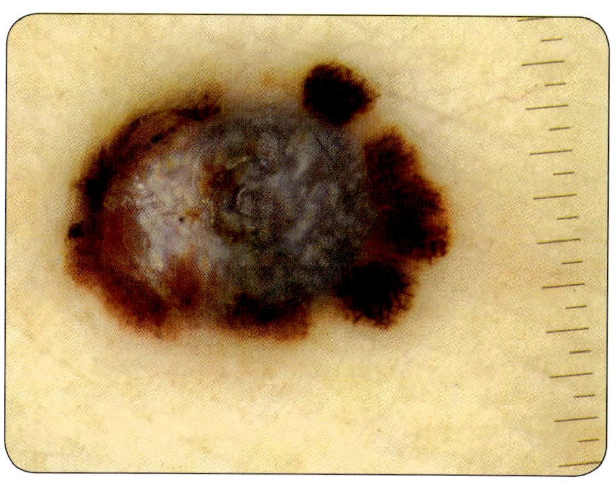

Fig. 2.9: Melanoma. Projections or streaks.

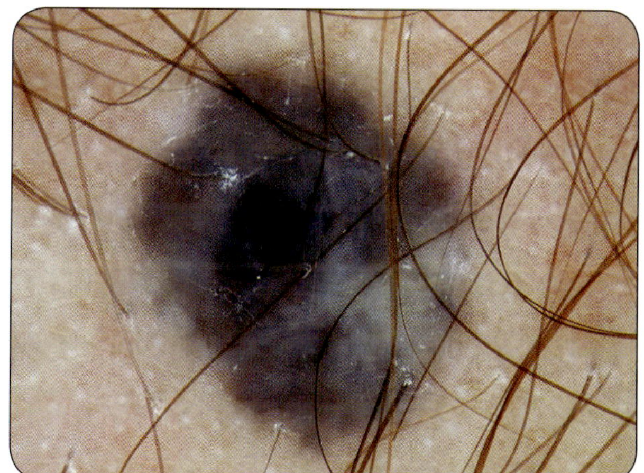

Fig. 2.10: Blue nevus. Homogeneous blue pigmentation.

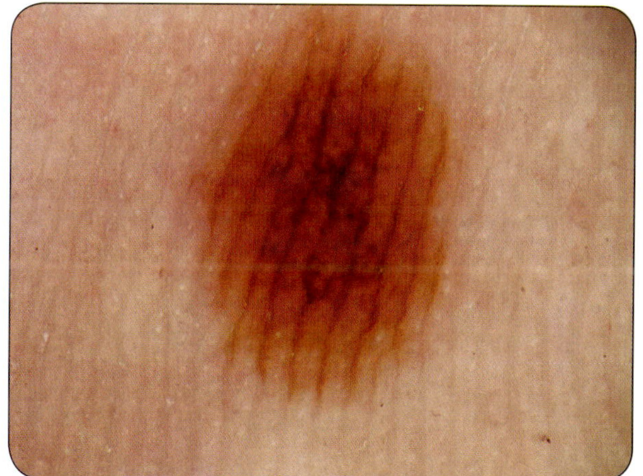

Fig. 2.11: Acral nevus. Furrow parallel pattern.

The different colors that can be observed are white, red, black, blue, gray, yellow, light brown, and dark brown and their combinations or variants. Colors red, pink, or blue-red, and occasionally light brown, are related to the vessels, with the presence of hemoglobin and the degree of oxidation (Fig. 2.19).

White color represents lack of pigment, atrophy, or fibrosis (Fig. 2.20), while yellow corresponds to keratin (Fig. 2.21).

Brown color is generally related to melanin. Depending on where it is located, melanic pigment will be visualized in different colors, due to the Tyndall effect (Fig. 2.22).

When it is located in the stratum corneum or epidermis, it looks black; if it lies in the dermoepidermal junction and in the papillary dermis, it looks dark brown or light brown; and if it is located in the dermis, it looks blue (Fig. 2.23).

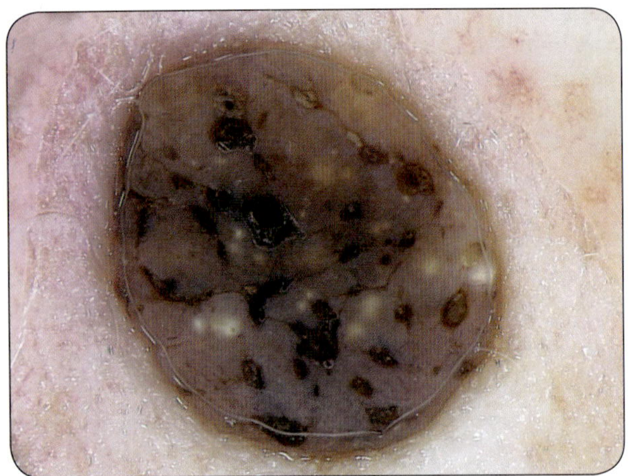

Fig. 2.12: Seborrheic keratosis. Multiple pseudocysts and pseudo-openings.

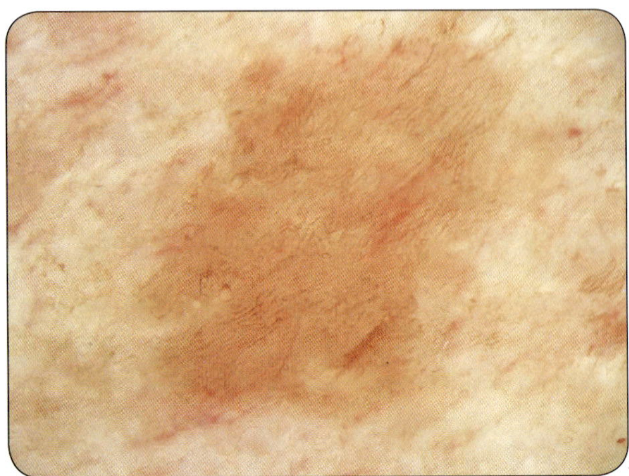

Fig. 2.13: Solar lentigo. Fingerprint-like structures and concave border.

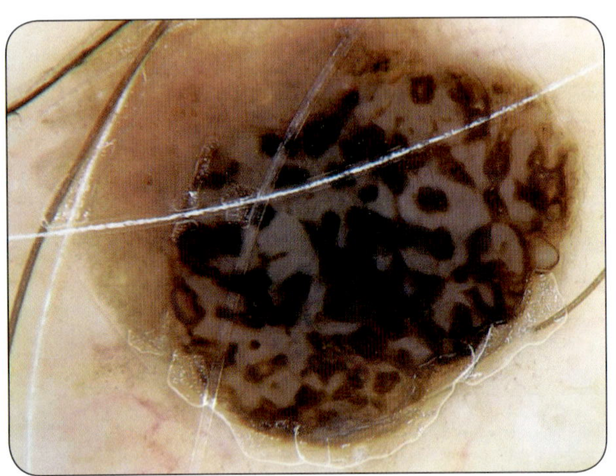

Fig. 2.14: Seborrheic keratosis. Brain-like pattern.

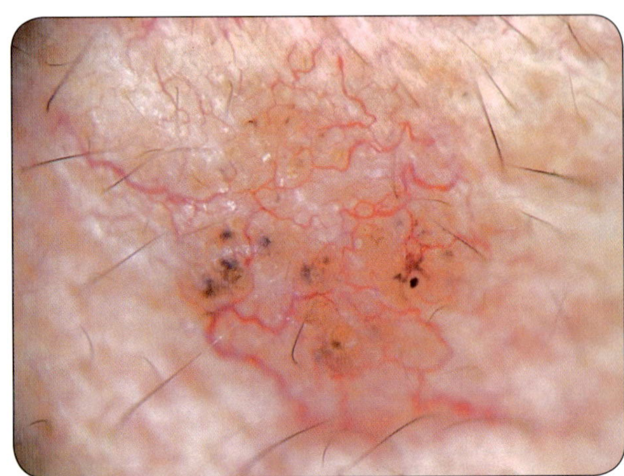

Fig. 2.15: Basal cell carcinoma. Arborizing vessels and blue-gray pigmentation.

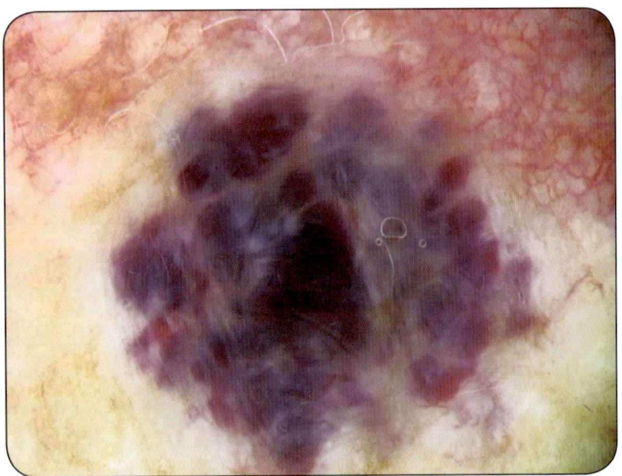

Fig. 2.16: Hemangioma. Red-blue areas.

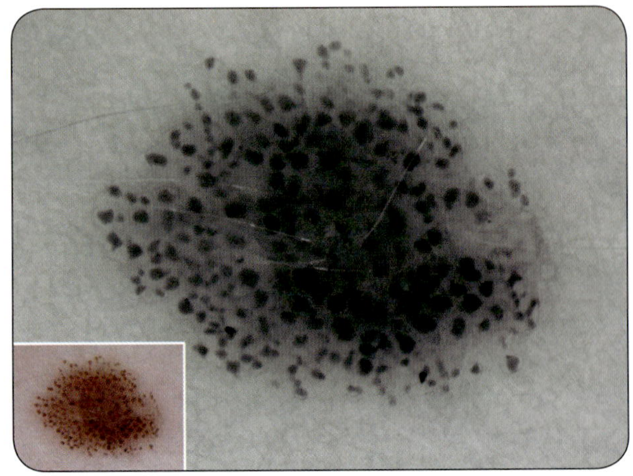

Fig. 2.17: Lesion in black and white. Diagnosis: Nevus.

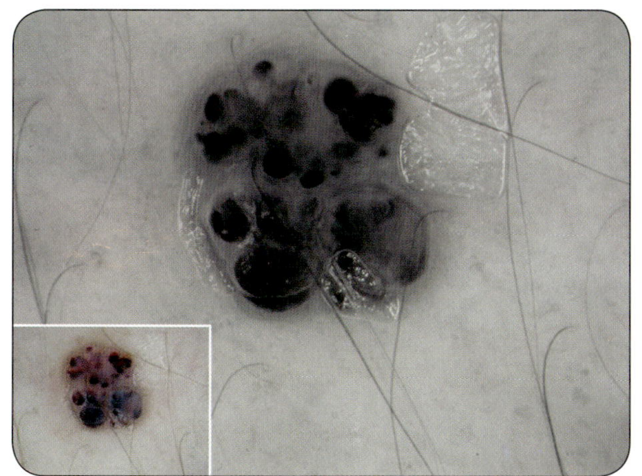

Fig. 2.18: Lesion in black and white. Diagnosis: angioma.

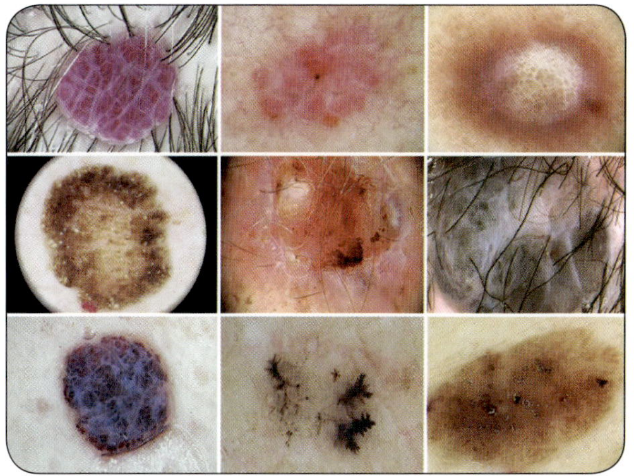

Fig. 2.19: Examples of different colors.

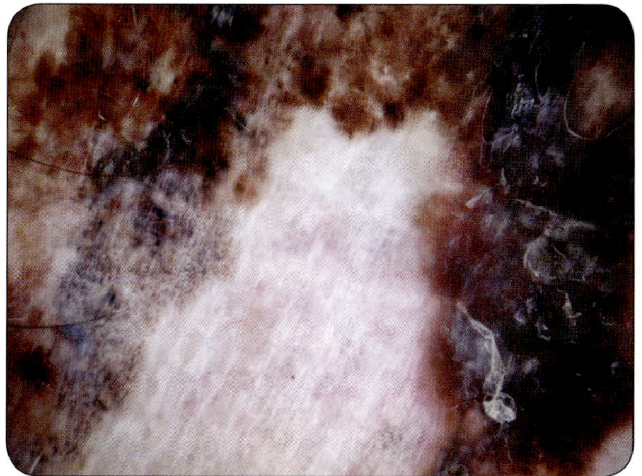

Fig. 2.20: Melanoma. White color.

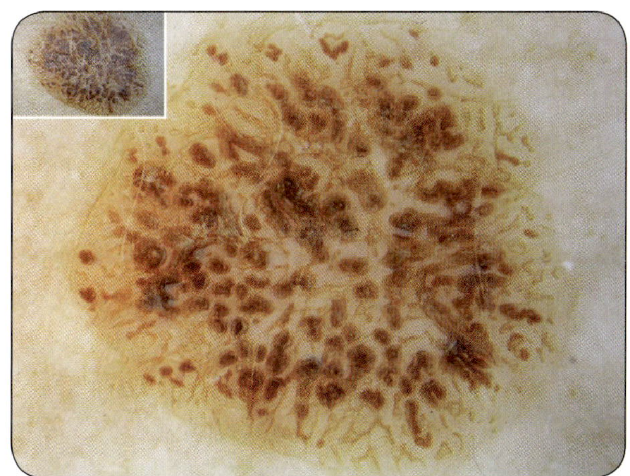

Fig. 2.21: Seborrheic keratosis. Yellow color.

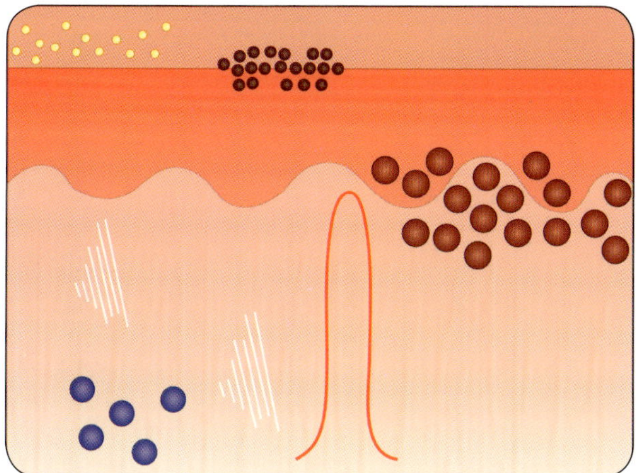

Fig. 2.22: Different colors seen with dermoscopy depending on localization (Tyndall effect).

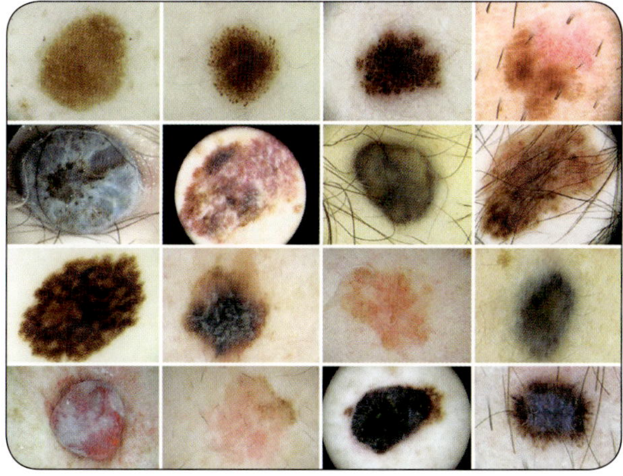

Fig. 2.23: Example of different colors due to melanic pigment.

SUGGESTED READING

Argenziano G, Soyer P, De Giorgio V, et al. Interactive Atlas of Dermoscopy. Milán: EDRA Medical Publishing & New Media; 2000.

Cabo H. Dermatoscopia. Buenos Aires: Weber Ferro; 2000.

Cabo H. Dermatoscopia, 2nd edition. Buenos Aires, Argentina: Ediciones Journal; 2012.

Johr R, Stolz W. Dermoscopy: An Illustrated Self-Assessment Guide, 2nd edition. New York: McGraw-Hill Education; 2015.

Jorh R, Soyer P, Argenziano G, et al. Dermoscopy. The Essentials (MOABT). New York: Elsevier Ltd; 2004.

Kittler H. Dermatoscopy. An Algorithmic Method Based on Pattern Analysis. 2011 Facultas Verlags- und Buchhandels AG facultas wuv Universitätsverlag, Austria www.facultas.wuv.at

Malvhey J, Puig S. Principles of Dermoscopy. Barcelona: Creaciones Gráficas; 2009.

Marghoob A, Braun R, Kopf A. Atlas of Dermoscopy. London: Taylor & Francis; 2005.

Menzies S, Crotty K, Ingvar C, et al. An Atlas of Surface Microscopy of Pigmented Skin Lesions. Sydney: McGraw-Hill Book Company; 1996.

Rabinovitz H, Kopf A. Dermoscopy: A Practical Guide. Miami: American Academy of Dermatology; 1999.

Soyer P, Argenziano G, Chimenti S, et al. Dermoscopy of Pigmented Skin Lesions. An Atlas Based on the Consensus Net Meeting on Dermoscopy. Milán: EDRA Medical Publishing & New Media; 2001.

Stolz W, Braun-Falco O, Bilek P, et al. Color Atlas of Dermatoscopy. USA: Blackwell Science; 1994.

Zalaudek I, Argenziano G, Giacomel J. Dermoscopy of nonpigmented skin tumors. Boca Raton, FL: CRC Press; 2016.

VASCULAR PATTERNS

3

Emilia Noemi Cohen Sabban, Horacio A Cabo

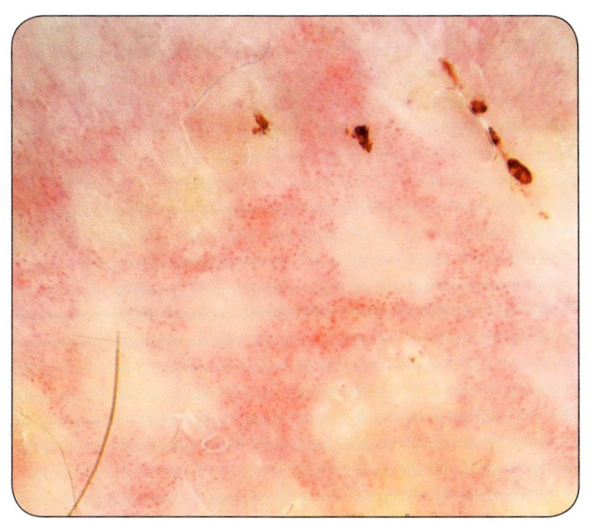

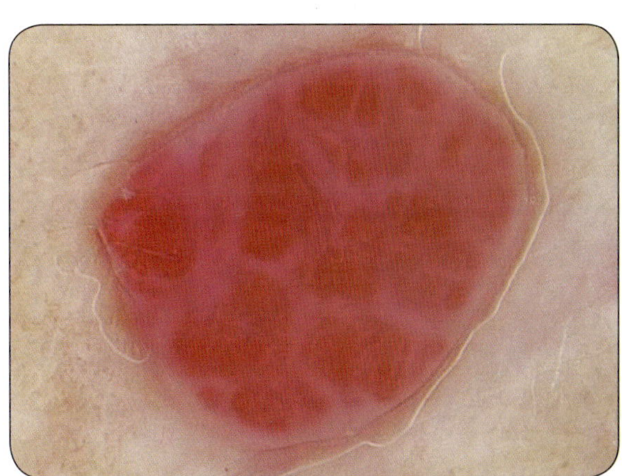

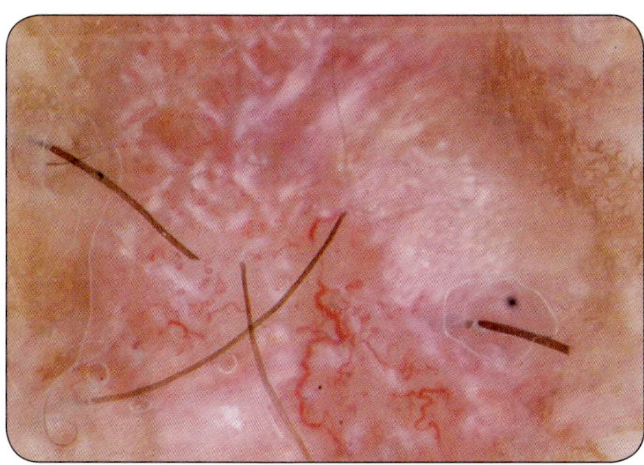

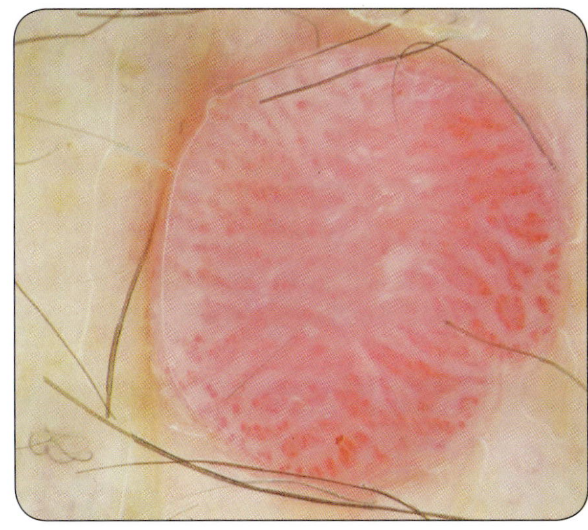

"In order to follow a diagnostic algorithm for dermoscopic lesions with blood vessels, it is recommended to perform the following steps:

- Observe the morphology of the blood vessels.
- Observe the arrangement of the blood vessels in the lesion.
- Differentiate a monomorphic pattern from a polymorphic one"

Initially, dermoscopy was performed using dermatoscopes with nonpolarized light, inserting an interphase liquid (oil or alcohol) between the skin and the glass plate of the dermatoscope and exerting pressure to visualize lesions (Fig. 3.1). This obviously produced a whitening effect and prevented the observation of vessels (Fig. 3.2). With the use of ultrasound or high-thickness ecograph gels and without applying so much pressure, vessels can be clearly observed, although they are difficult to register. With the coming of dermatoscopes with polarized light with or without contact, the different types of vessels and pink areas are easily observed (Figs. 3.3 and 3.4).

Dermoscopy of the vascular pattern of a lesion may be the only tool for the diagnosis of nonpigmented cutaneous tumors. The prevailing vascular pattern will also depend on tumor volume and progression. Therefore, a thin, more recent tumor will generally have a vascular pattern different from that of a thicker, more advanced one (Table 3.1).

Nevertheless, there are many benign and malignant lesions that can present similar vascular patterns. The color of the different vascular structures is pink, red, or sometimes bluish. The distribution and morphology of the vessels are very helpful for the clinical dermoscopic diagnosis.

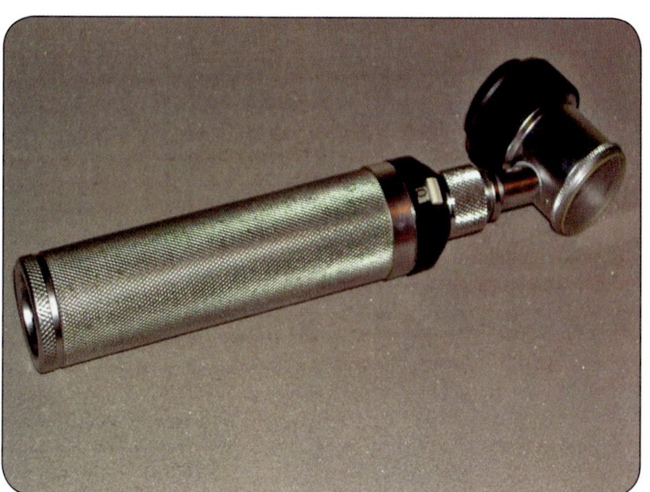

Fig. 3.1: Nonpolarized light dermatoscope.

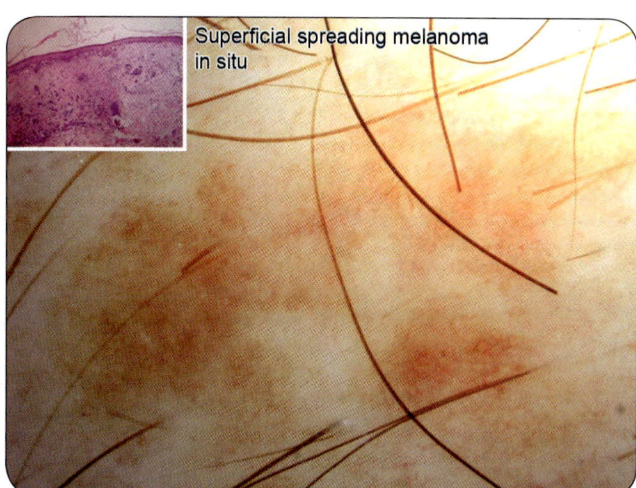

Fig. 3.2: Image of a hypomelanotic melanoma captured with a nonpolarized light dermatoscope.

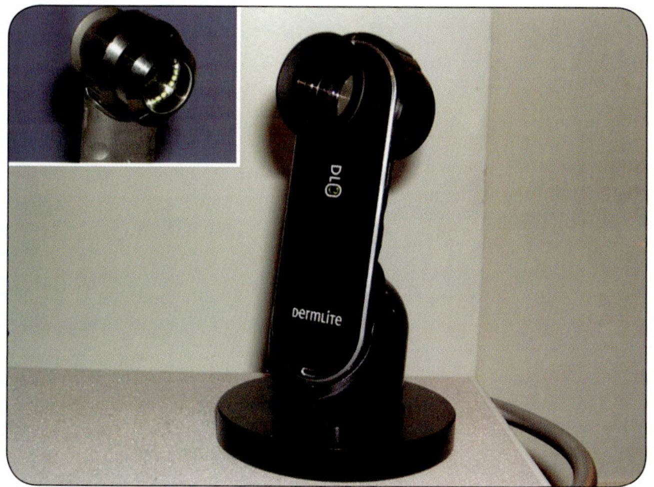

Fig. 3.3: Polarized light dermatoscope.

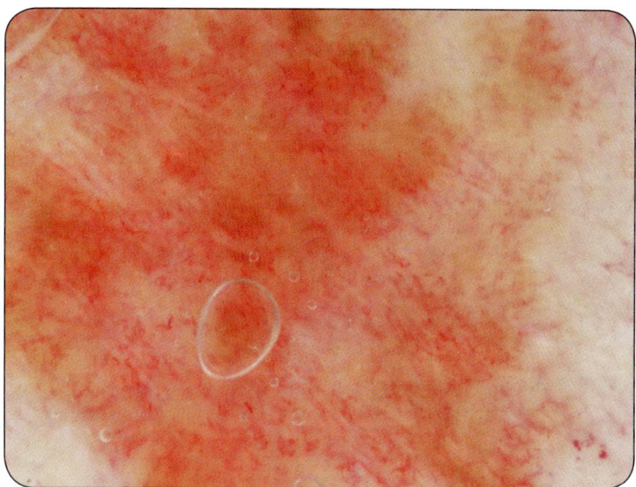

Fig. 3.4: Hypomelanotic melanoma image captured with a polarized light dermatoscope.

In order to follow a diagnostic algorithm for dermoscopic lesions with blood vessels, it is recommended to perform the following steps:

- Observe the morphology of the blood vessels.
- Observe the arrangement of the blood vessels in the lesion.

Table 3.1: Dermoscopy.
• Dermoscopy with nonpolarized light
• Dermoscopy with polarized light
– With contact
– Without contact

- Differentiate a monomorphic pattern from a polymorphic one (Figs. 3.5 to 3.7).

MORPHOLOGY

Depending on their position in the skin, vessels can be seen as round or linear.

Round or Dotted Vessels

- They can be small like *dots,* or larger, in which case they are called *clods* (*areas* or *globules*) (Figs. 3.8 and 3.9).
- *Lagoons or lacunae*: Large red *areas*, usually clustered, resembling lakes (Fig. 3.10).

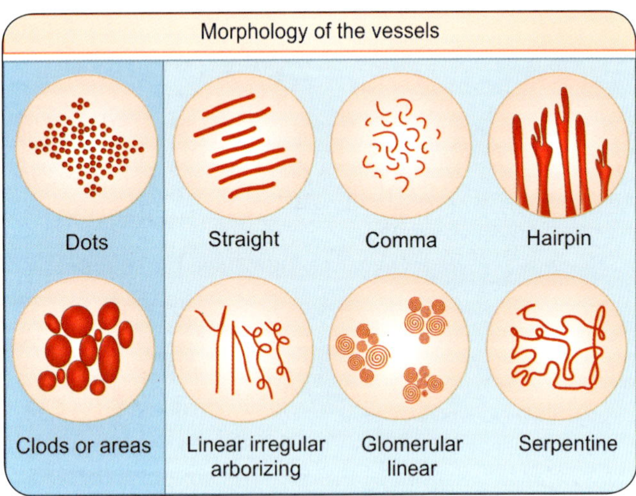

Fig. 3.5: Diverse vessel morphology.

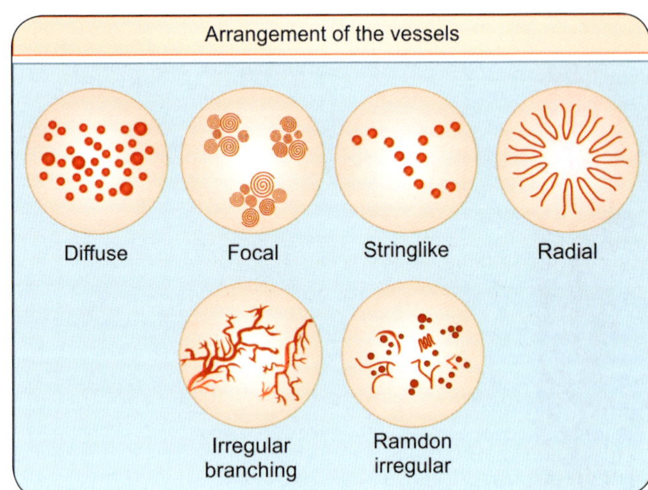

Fig. 3.6: Diverse vessel distribution.

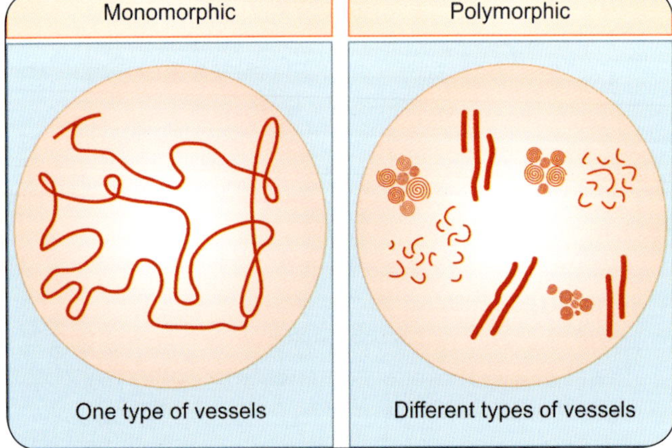

Fig. 3.7: Monomorphic and polymorphic patterns.

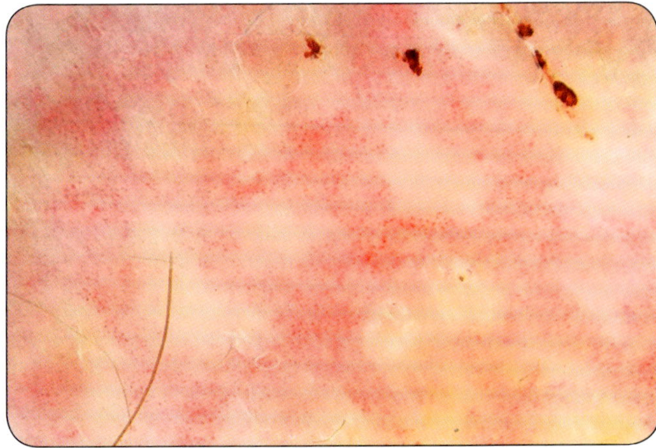

Fig. 3.8: Dotted vessels—psoriasis.

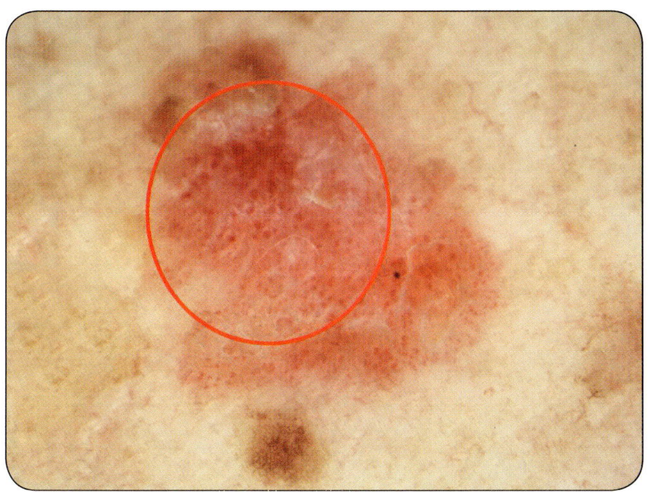

Fig. 3.9: Clod vessels (areas or globules) squamous cell carcinoma (red circle).

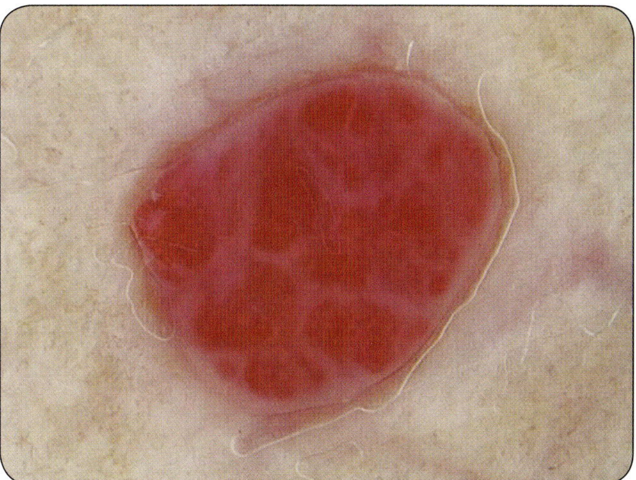

Fig. 3.10: Red lagoons—angioma.

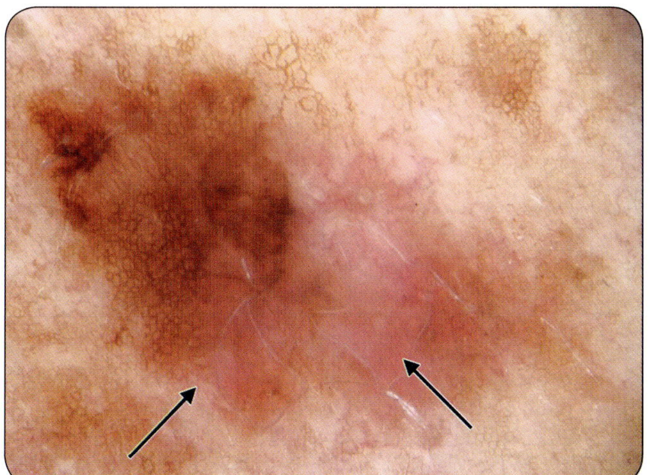

Fig. 3.11: Milky red areas—melanoma (arrows).

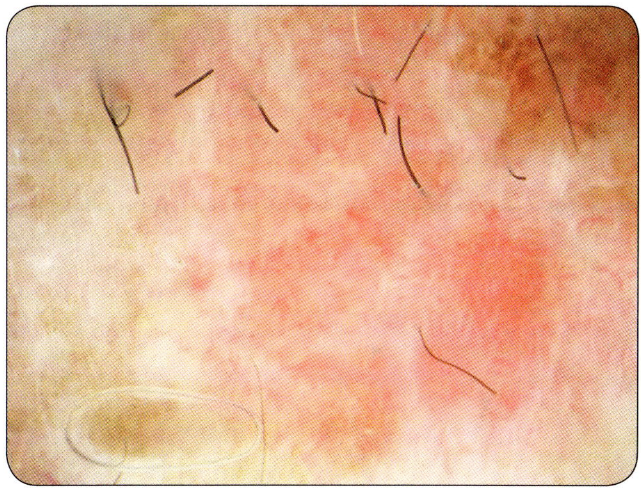

Fig. 3.12: Straight vessels—squamous cell carcinoma.

- *Milky red areas*: (Vascular reddening) Large blurred areas of milky red color. Within, we can observe other dermoscopic structures (Fig. 3.11).

Linear Vessels

They can be as follows:

- *Straight*: Linear, small and thin, regular or irregular (Fig. 3.12)
- *Arborizing*: Thick vessels that become thinner and arborized into narrow vessels like the branches of a tree (Figs. 3.13 and 3.14)
- *Comma-like*: Bending or curving vessels (Fig. 3.15)
- *Hairpin*: Vessels with a vascular knot, shaped like a handle, either fine or thick (Fig. 3.16)
- *Spiral or glomerular*: Vessels in a tight spiral, which can resemble areas or globules (Fig. 3.17)
- *Twisted or serpent-like*: With curves and lines, and generally very irregular (Fig. 3.18)

ARRANGEMENT

This can be as follows:

- *Diffuse*: Spreading over almost all of the lesion (Fig. 3.19)
- *Focal*: Appearing in different areas (Fig. 3.20)
- *Crown*: Lying in the periphery (comma-like) (Fig. 3.21)
- *Spoke wheel or radial*: Lying in the periphery (straight linear or hairpin) (Fig. 3.22)
- *Irregular randomly distributed*: Mostly irregular linear vessels (Fig. 3.23)

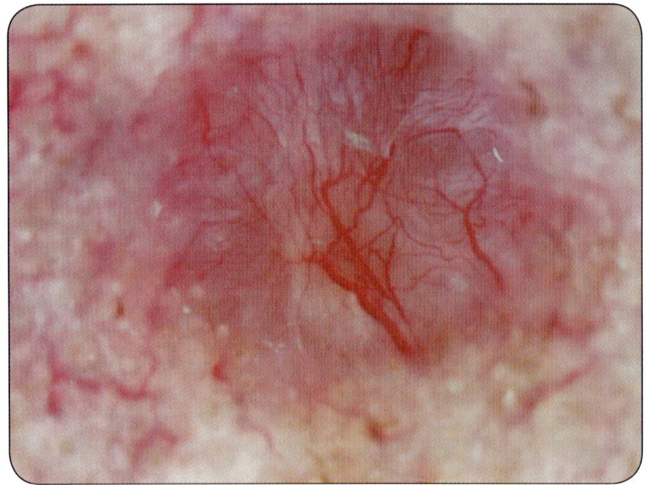

Fig. 3.13: Arborizing vessels—basal cell carcinoma.

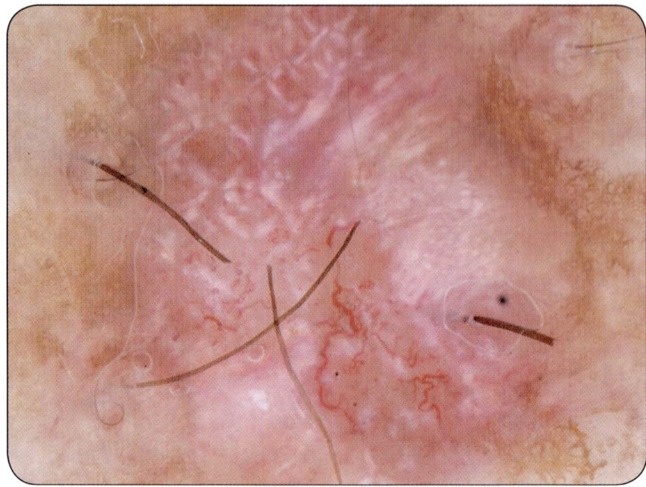

Fig. 3.14: Arborizing vessels—basal cell carcinoma.

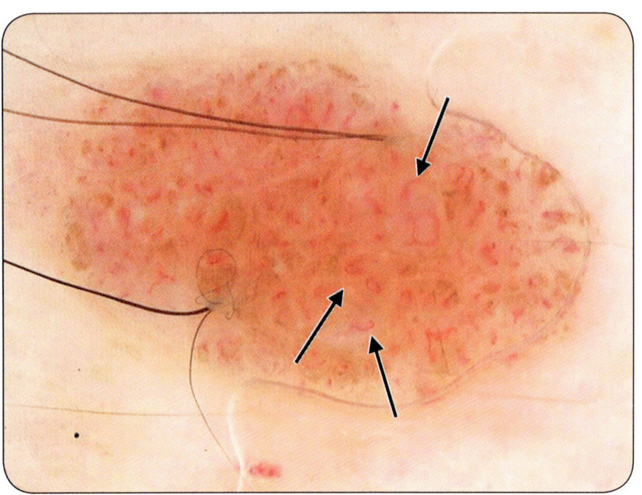

Fig. 3.15: Comma-like vessels—intradermal nevus (arrows).

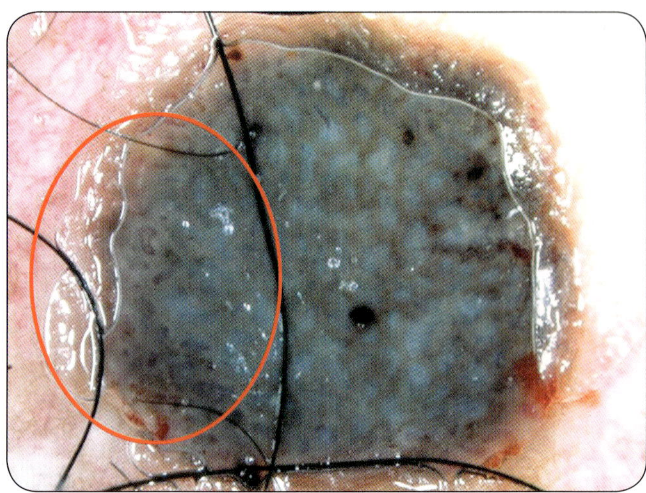

Fig. 3.16: Hairpin vessels—seborrheic keratosis (red circle).

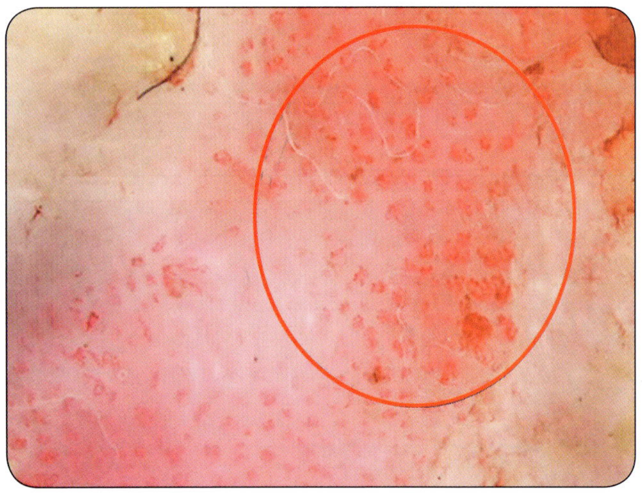

Fig. 3.17: Glomerular vessels—squamous cell carcinoma (red circle).

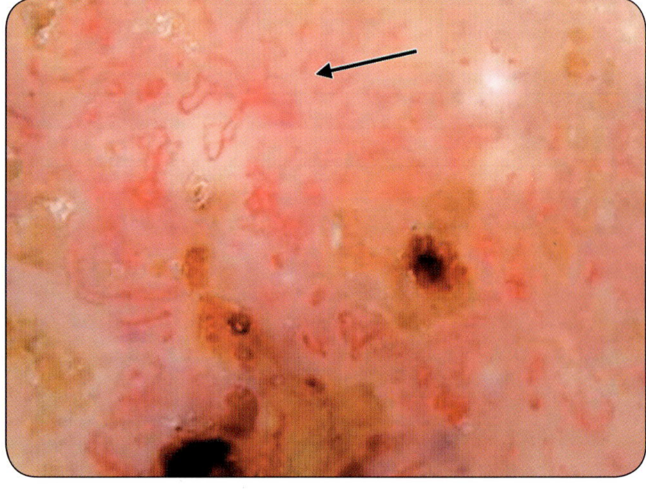

Fig. 3.18: Twisted vessels—melanoma (arrow).

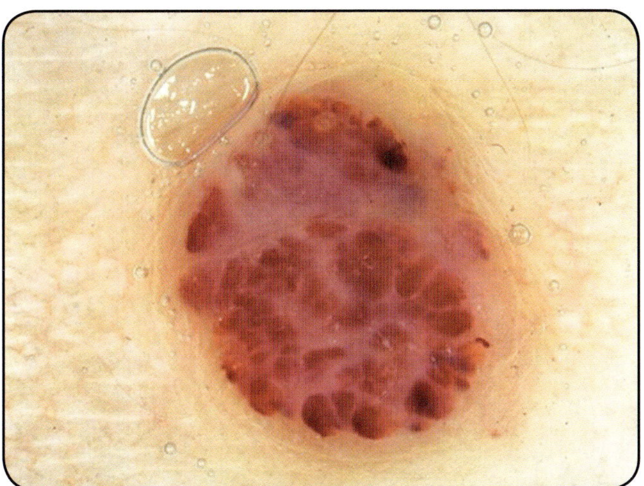

Fig. 3.19: Diffuse arrangement—hemangioma.

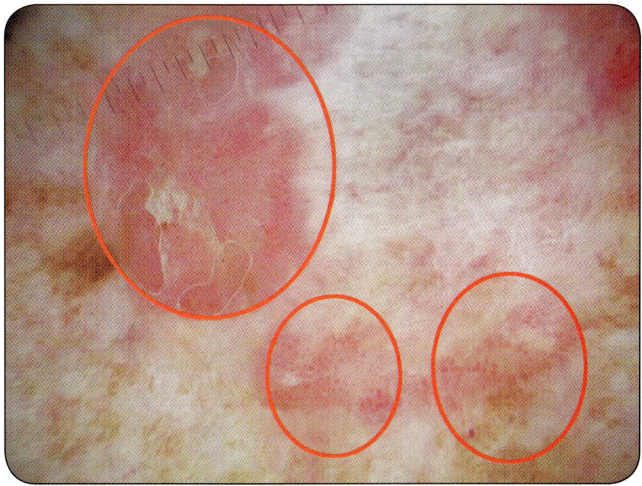

Fig. 3.20: Focal arrangement—squamous cell carcinoma (red circles).

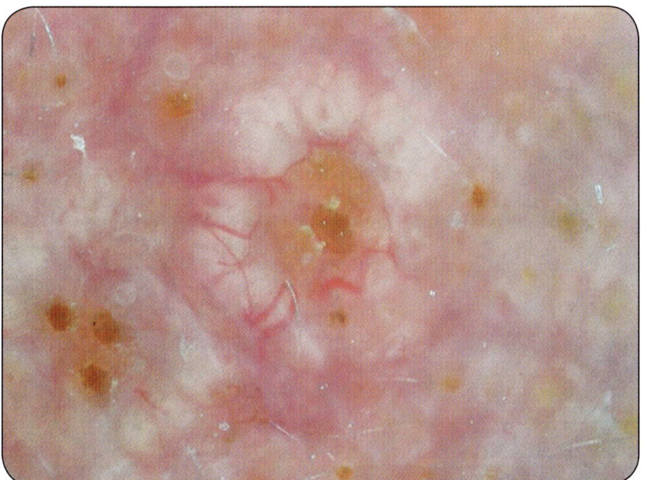

Fig. 3.21: Crown vessels—sebaceous hyperplasia.

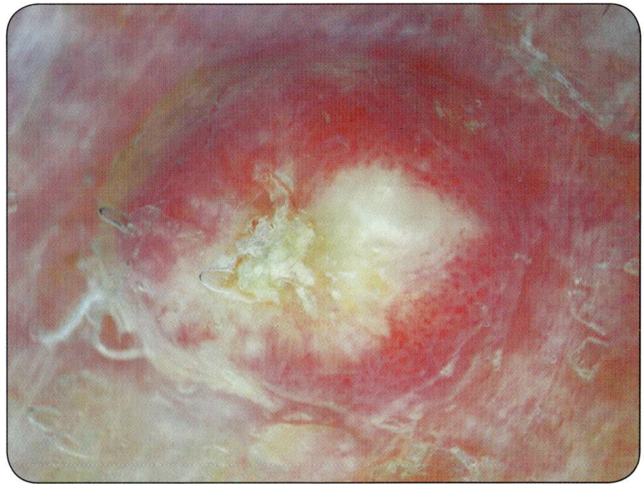

Fig. 3.22: Radial vessels—keratoacanthoma.

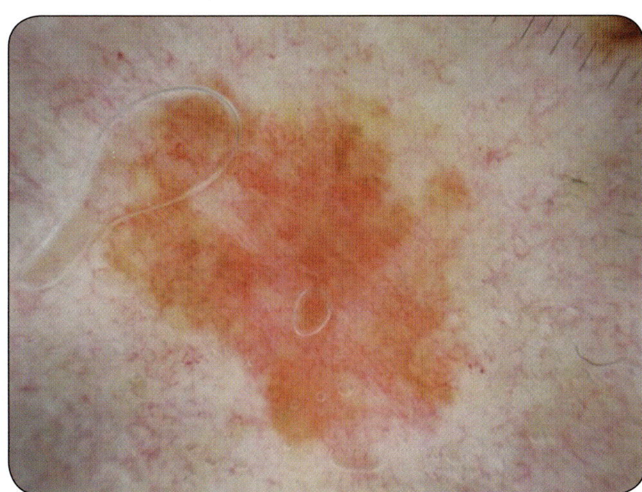

Fig. 3.23: Irregular randomly distributed vessels—hypomelanotic melanoma.

Since the morphology of the vessels can be the same for two or more types of tumors, their distribution in the lesion is sometimes the key to the diagnosis.

- *Crown curved linear vessels*: Sebaceous hyperplasia (Fig. 3.21).
- *Dot-like vessels in a string-of-pearls or rosary distribution*: Clear cell acanthoma (Fig. 3.24)
- *Focal or in-nest glomerular vessels:* Squamous carcinoma in situ or Bowen disease (Figs. 3.17 to 3.20)
- *Diffuse comma-like or curvilinear vessels*: Intradermal cellular nevus (Fig. 3.25)
- *Diffuse hairpin vessels*: Seborrheic keratosis (Fig. 3.26)
- *Hairpin vessels with radial peripheral distribution:* Keratoacanthoma, in which case we can also observe a structureless area, formed by a yellow-whitish keratotic central mass and thrombosed vessels (Fig. 3.27)

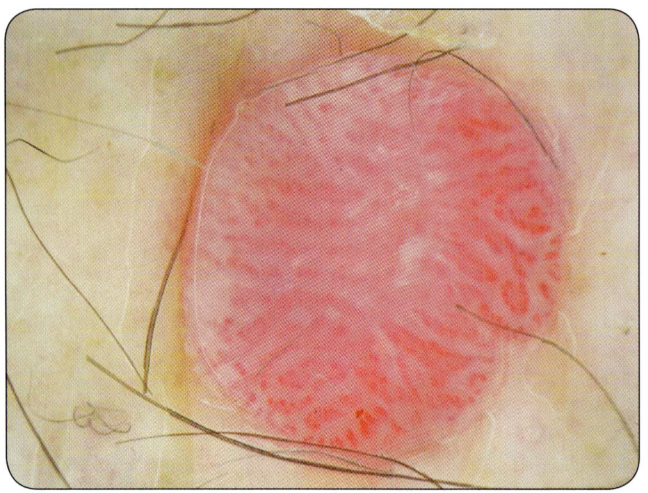

Fig. 3.24: Dot-like vessels in a string-of-pearls or rosary distribution—clear cell acanthoma.

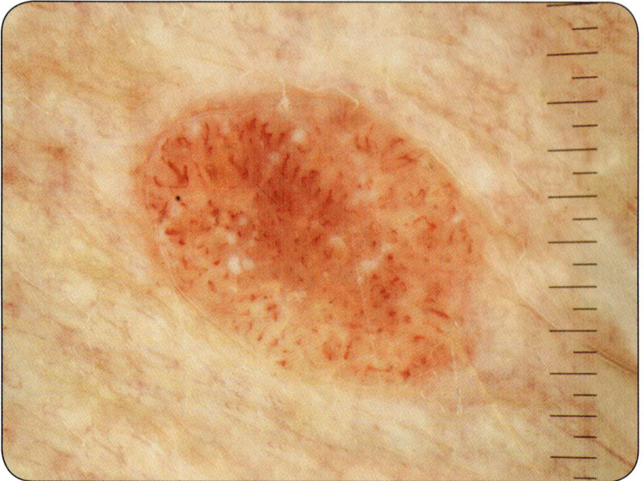

Fig. 3.25: Diffuse comma-like or curvilinear vessels—intradermal nevus.

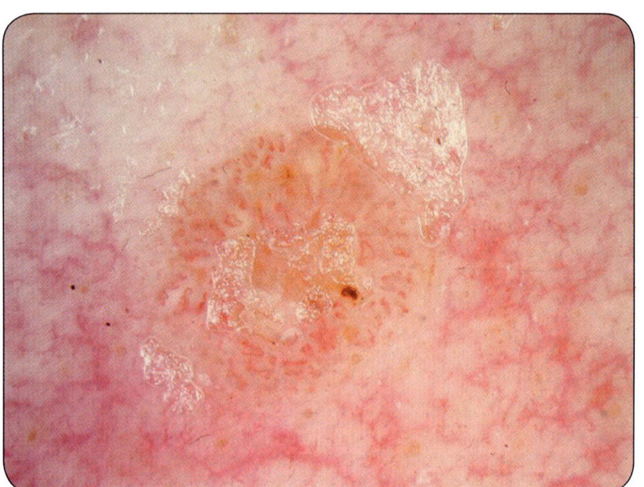

Fig. 3.26: Diffuse hairpin vessels—seborrheic keratosis.

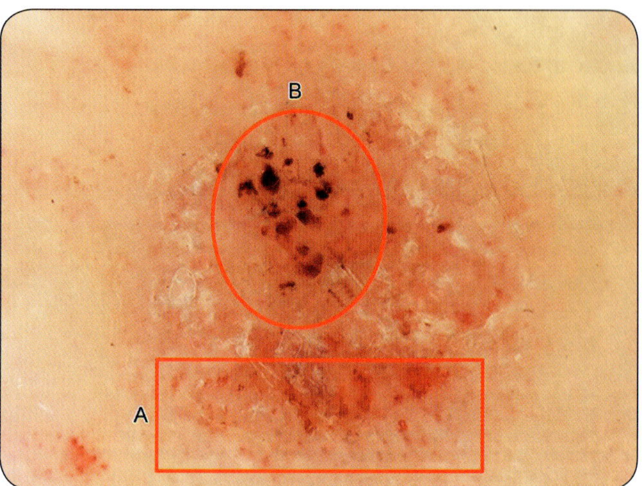

Fig. 3.27: Hairpin vessels with radial peripheral distribution (A) and structureless area, formed by a yellow-whitish keratotic central mass and thrombosed vessels (B) keratoacanthoma.

- *Arborizing vessels*: Basal cell carcinoma (Figs. 3.13 and 3.14)
- *Irregular distribution:* Hypomelanotic/amelanotic melanoma (HAM) (Fig. 3.28)

PATTERN

Monomorphic: Only one vessel type (Figs. 3.10 to 3.14).

Angioma, with its red areas (lacunae), is an example of monomorphic pattern in benign lesions. Basal cell carcinoma with its arborizing vessels is an example of monomorphic pattern in malignant lesions.

Polymorphic: This means the presence of two or more vessel morphologic types.

The most frequent combination is dot-like vessels and linear ones in different shapes, widths, and arrangements, which appear on milky red areas of HAM, generally of medium thickness. In thicker HAM, on the other hand, although the pattern is polymorphic, it is frequent to observe glomerular vessels, hairpin-shaped, twisted or linear, irregular and randomly distributed over milky red areas (Fig. 3.28).

Diagnosis of nonpigmented cutaneous lesions is a real challenge. Every pink lesion must arise suspicion of being

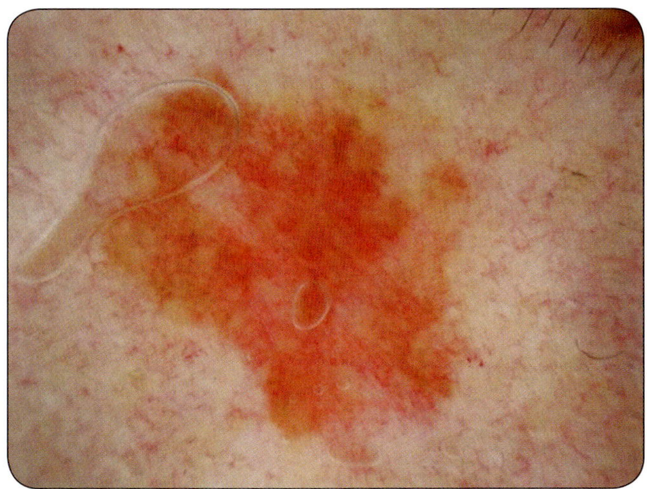

Fig. 3.28: Dot-like and linear vessels in different shapes, widths, and arrangements—hypomelanotic melanoma.

HAM, and therefore, following the vascular pattern diagnostic algorithm together with other dermoscopic characteristics of the lesion can be an invaluable tool (Table 3.2).

Table 3.2: Correlations between vessels morphology and diseases.

Main vessels morphology	*Disease*
Arborizing vessels	Basal cell carcinoma
Comma-like vessels	Intradermal nevi Congenital melanocytic nevi Dysplastic nevi
Crown vessels	Sebaceous hyperplasia Molluscum contagiosum
Dotted and globular vessels	Melanoma Spitz nevus Dysplastic nevus Light-cell acanthoma ("string-of-pearls" distribution) Psoriasis Squamous cell carcinoma Stasis dermatitis Warp (frequently with thrombosis)
Hairpin vessels: Narrow Thick Irregular	Seborrheic keratosis (Peripheral) Keratoacanthoma Melanoma Irritated seborrheic keratosis Spinal cell carcinoma Spitz nevus
Lacunae	Hemangiomas
Irregular lineal vessels	Melanoma Spitz nevus
Milky red areas/globules	Melanoma
Polymorphic vessels	Melanoma

SUGGESTED READING

Argenziano G, Zalaudek I, Corona R, et al. Vascular structures in skin tumors: a dermoscopy study. Arch Dermatol. 2004;140:1485-9.

Cabo H. Dermatoscopia, 2nd edition. Buenos Aires, Argentina: Ediciones Journal; 2012.

Kreusch JF. Vascular patterns in skin tumors. Clin Dermatol. 2002;20:248-54.

Malvehy J, Puig S. Principios de dermatoscopia. España: Dermoscop; 2009.

Pizzichetta MA, Talamini R, Stranganelli I, et al. Amelanotic/hypomelanotic melanoma: clinical and dermoscopic features. Br J Dermatol. 2004;150:1117-24.

Zaballos P, Ara M, Puig S, et al. Dermoscopy of sebaceous hyperplasia. Arch Dermatol. 2005;141:808.

Zalaudek I, Argenziano G, Giacomel J. Dermoscopy of non-pigmented skin tumors. Boca Raton, FL: CRC Press; 2016.

Zalaudek I, Kreusch J, Giacomel G, et al. How to diagnose non-pigmented skin tumors: a review of vascular structures seen with dermoscopy. Part I. Melanocytic skin tumors. JAAD. 2010;63:361-74.

Zalaudek I, Kreusch J, Giacomel G, et al. How to diagnose non-pigmented skin tumors: a review of vascular structures seen with dermoscopy. Part II. Nonmelanocytic skin tumors. JAAD. 2010;63:377-86.

DERMOSCOPY: A TWO-STEP PROCEDURE

4

Horacio A Cabo

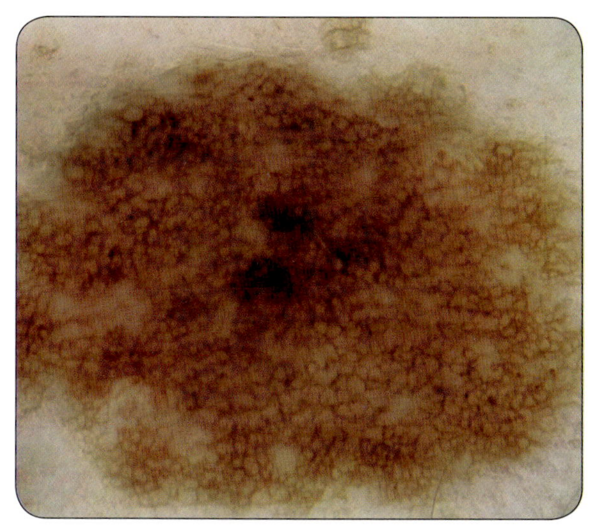

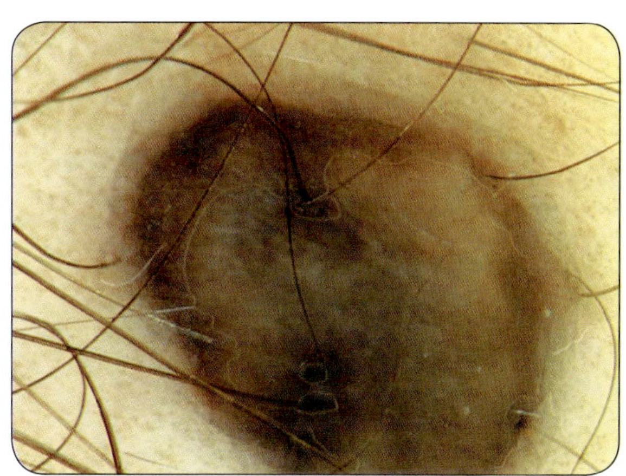

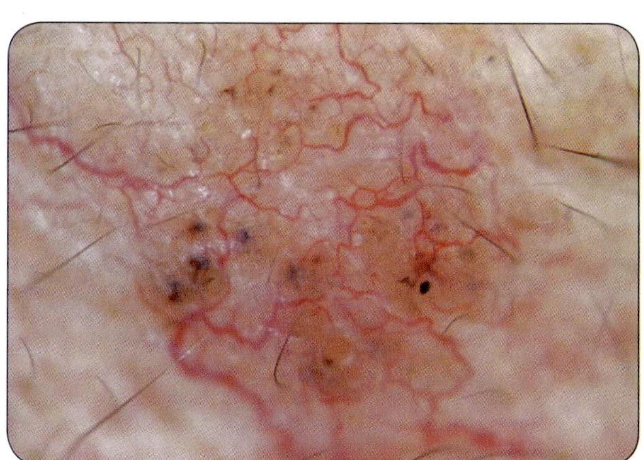

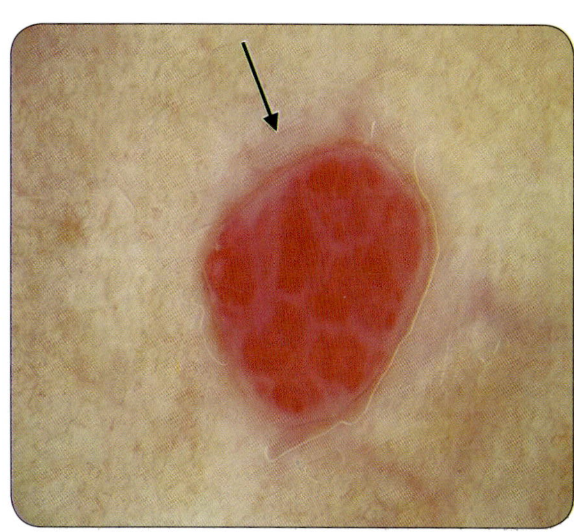

"Dermoscopic examination can be performed in two steps.
The first step aims at determining whether we are in the presence of a melanocytic lesion or a nonmelanocytic one. If it is a melanocytic lesion, we move on to the second step, which means determining if it is a melanoma, a benign melanocytic lesion or a suspicious or atypical melanocytic lesion."

Dermoscopic examination can be performed in two steps. The first step aims at determining whether we are in the presence of a melanocytic lesion or a nonmelanocytic one. If it is a melanocytic lesion, we move on to the second step, which means determining if it is a melanoma, a benign melanocytic lesion or a suspicious or atypical melanocytic lesion.

FIRST STEP

In the first step, it is very useful to apply the diagnosis algorithm as discussed in Table 4.1 and Figures 4.1 to 4.21.

It may happen that we are in the presence of a pigmented lesion, without the criteria for melanocytic lesions nor for nonmelanocytic ones. This is an unspecified lesion without definite criteria. The majority of these cases are atypical melanocytic nevi or melanoma.

Recently, a modification has been proposed to the diagnosis algorithm for the first step, by adding the vascular patterns (Figs. 4.5 and 4.6) which were described in Chapter 3.

SECOND STEP

In this step, we must examine the different criteria and structures, in order to determine if it is a benign lesion or a melanoma.

There are different diagnosis methods, which are described in detail in Chapter 10.

These algorithms are very similar as regards sensitivity and specificity, which make them all extremely useful. The only requirements to use them are sound knowledge and good mastery in the chosen method. Table 4.2 lists the best-known diagnosis methods.

Table 4.1: Diagnosis algorithm.

1. Criteria for melanocytic lesions:
    - Pigment network
    - Brown globules
    - Streaks or projections
    - Homogeneous blue pigmentation
    - Parallel pattern
2. Criteria for seborrheic keratosis:
    - Multiple pseudocysts
    - Multiple pseudo follicular openings
    - Fissures and ridges (brain-like appearance)
    - Vascular pattern with peripheral hairpin vessels
3. Criteria for basal cell carcinoma:
    - Vascular pattern:
        - Large arborizing vessels
        - Fine truncated vessels
    - Blue-gray pigmentation
    - Leaf-like or digit-like structures
    - Blue-gray globules: Large, ovoid, or small and multiple
    - Spoke-wheel areas
    - Ulcerations
4. Criteria for vascular lesions:
    - Red or blue-red lagoons
5. Vascular structures associated with nonmelanocytic lesions
6. Vascular structures associated with melanocytic lesions
7. Absence of the above criteria: Rule out melanocytic lesion without the classical criteria

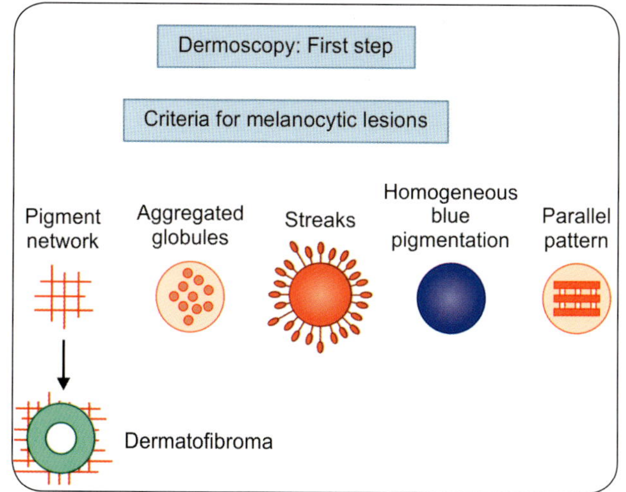

Fig. 4.1: First step: Melanocytic lesions.

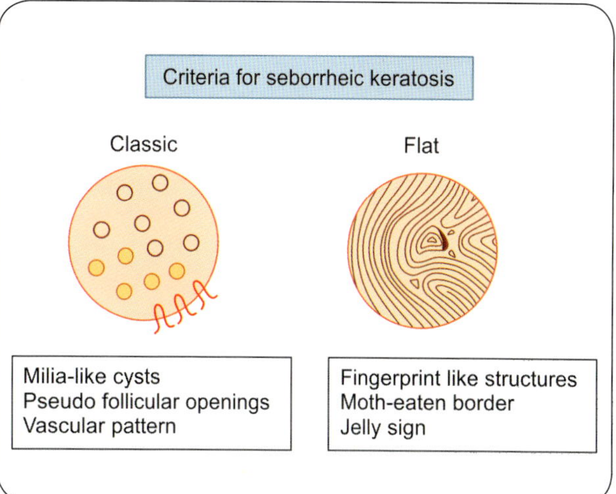

Fig. 4.2: Second step: Seborrheic keratosis.

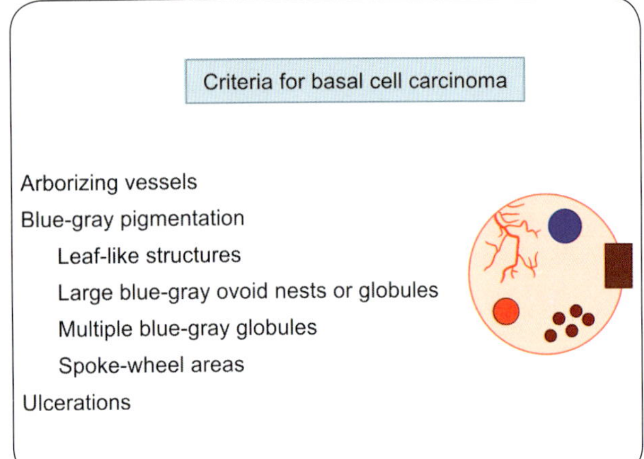

Fig. 4.3: Third step: Basal cell carcinoma.

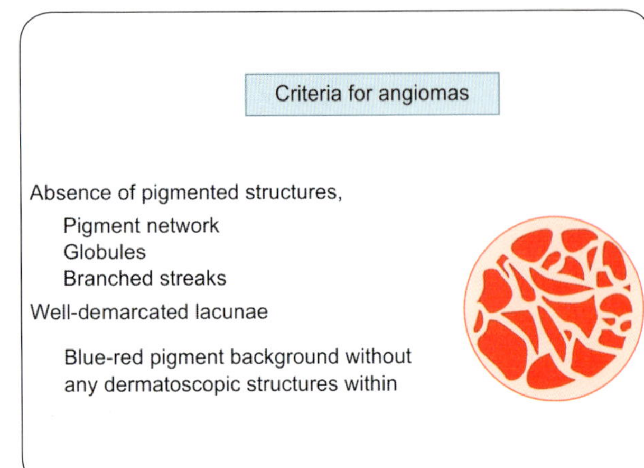

Fig. 4.4: Fourth step: Hemangiomas.

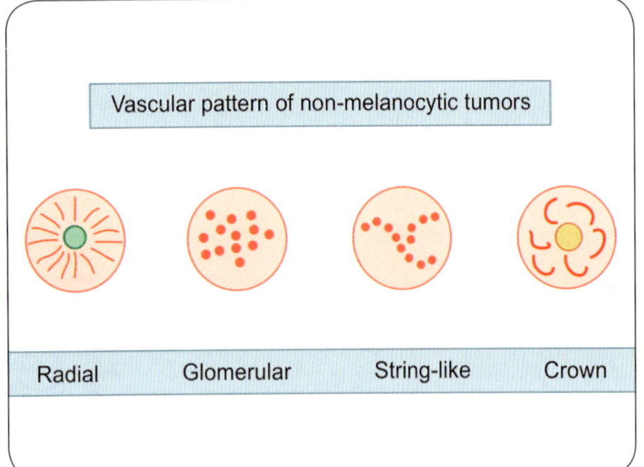

Fig. 4.5: Fifth step: Vascular patterns for nonmelanocytic lesions.

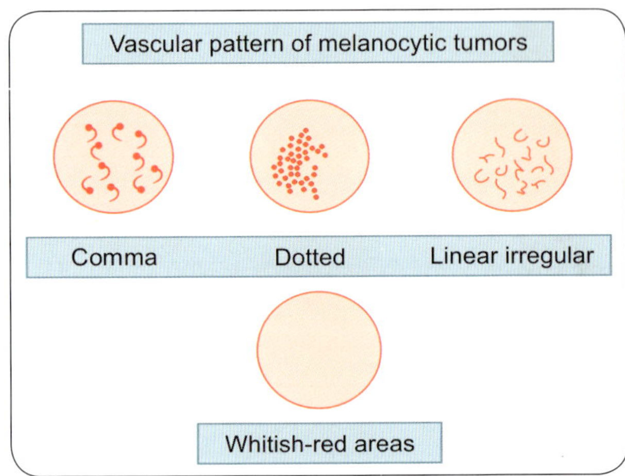

Fig. 4.6: Sixth step: Vascular patterns for melanocytic lesions.

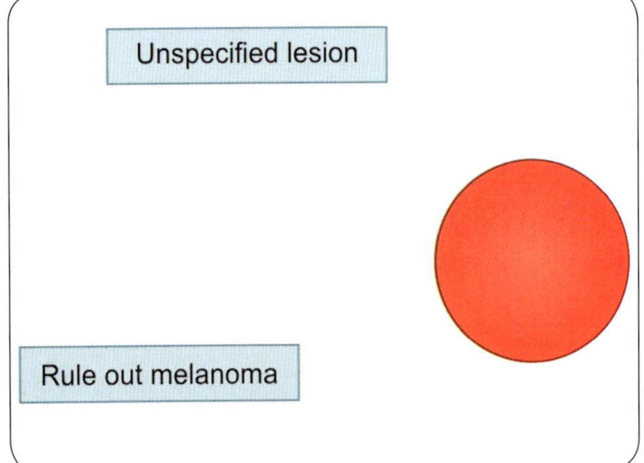

Fig. 4.7: Seventh step: In the absence of all the previous criteria, rule out a melanocytic lesion.

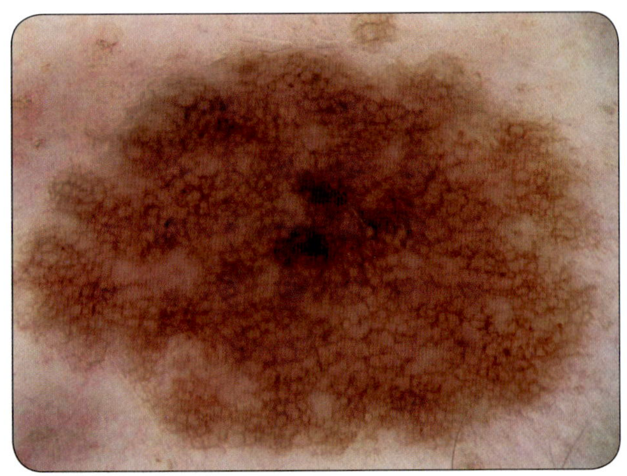

Fig. 4.8: Pigment network—junction nevus.

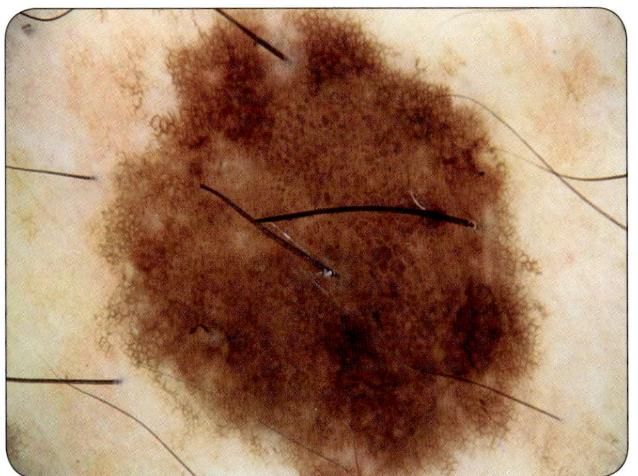

Fig. 4.9: Brown globules—compound nevus.

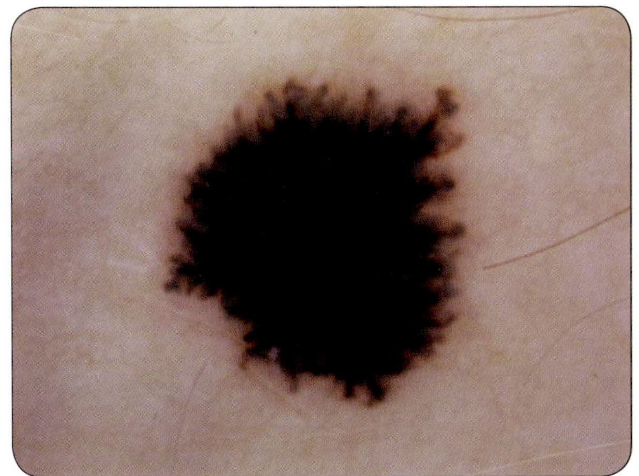

Fig. 4.10: Streaks and projections—Spitz nevus.

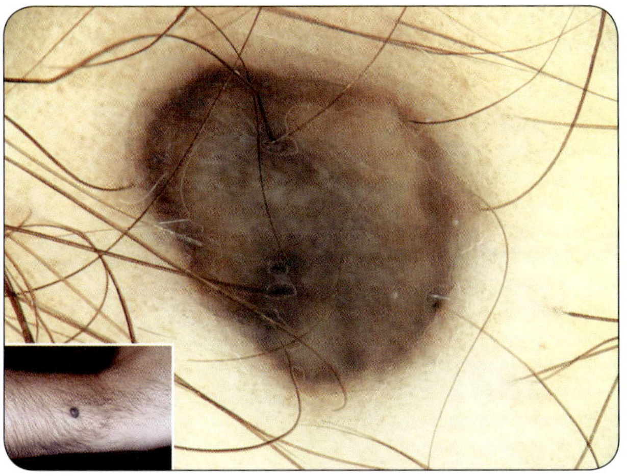

Fig. 4.11: Homogeneous blue pigmentation—blue nevus.

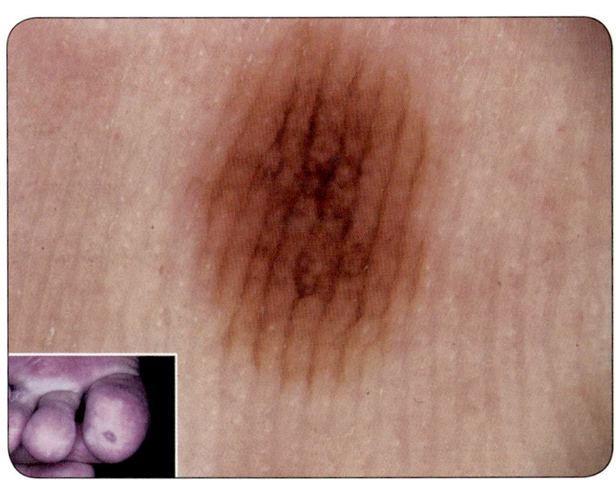

Fig. 4.12: Parallel pattern—acral nevus.

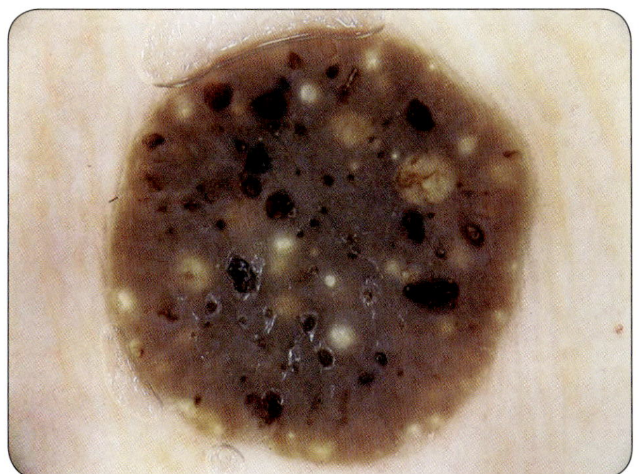

Fig. 4.13: Follicular pseudocysts and pseudo-openings—seborrheic keratosis.

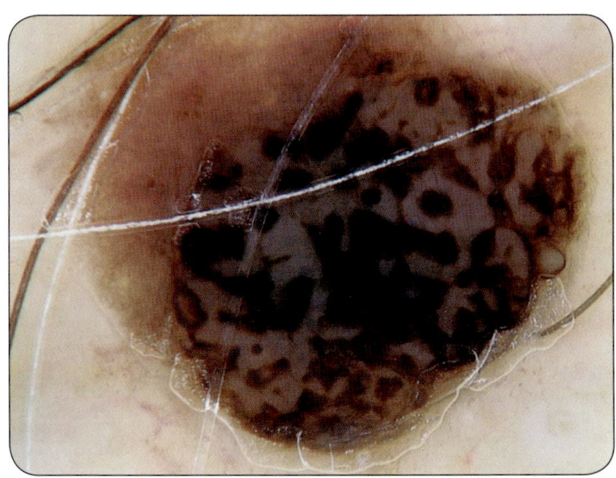

Fig. 4.14: Fissures and ridges (brain-like patterns)—seborrheic keratosis.

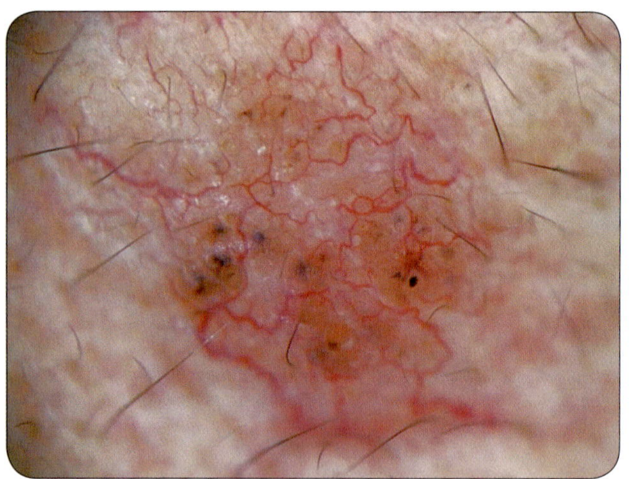

Fig. 4.15: Arborizing vessels—basal cell carcinoma.

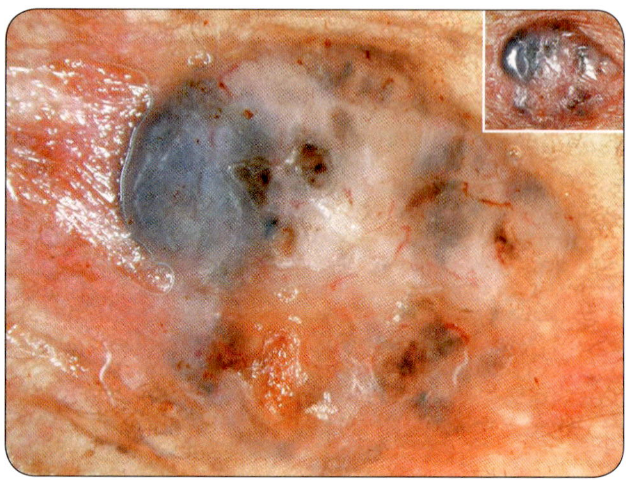

Fig. 4.16: Blue-gray globules—basal cell carcinoma.

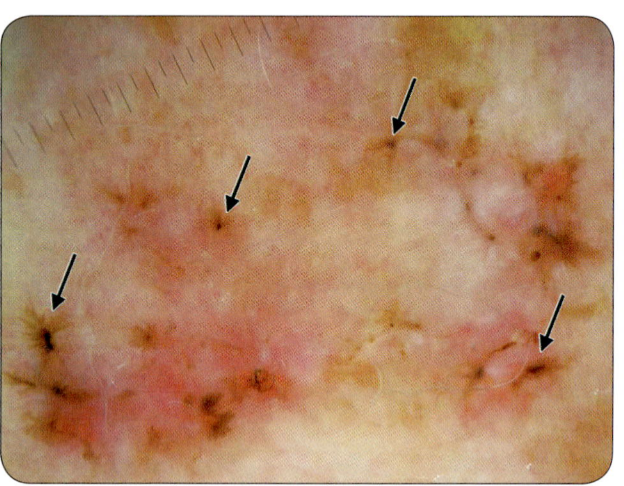

Fig. 4.17: Spoke-wheel areas (arrows)—basal cell carcinoma.

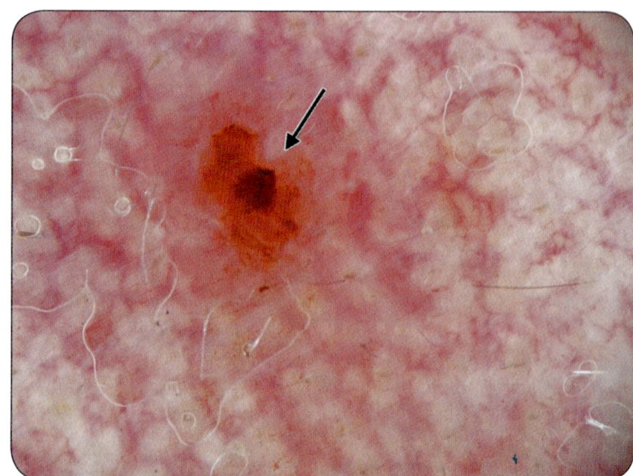

Fig. 4.18: Ulcerations (arrow)—basal cell carcinoma.

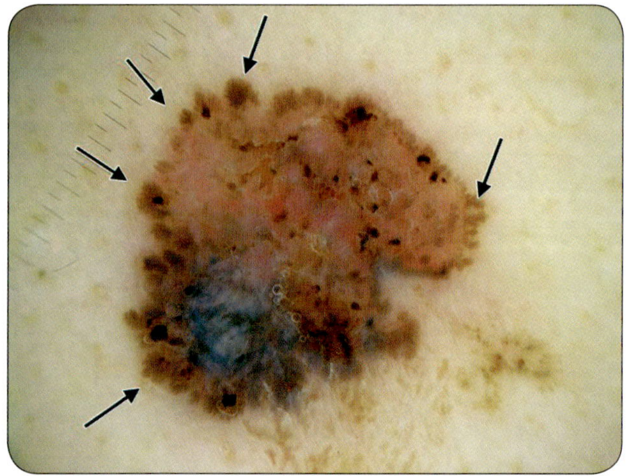

Fig. 4.19: Leaf-like structures (arrows)—basal cell carcinoma.

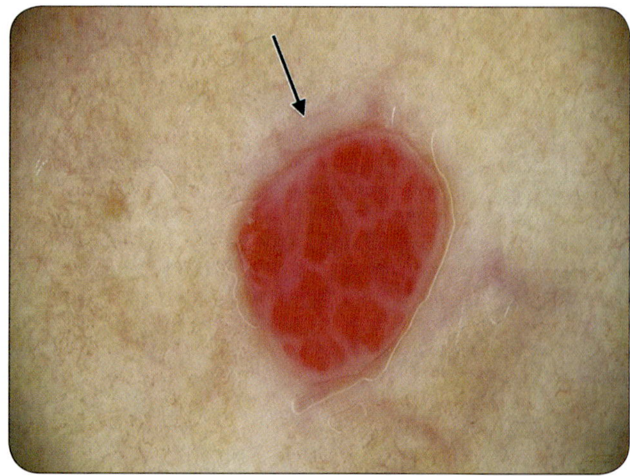

Fig. 4.20: Red-blue lagoons (arrow)—hemangioma.

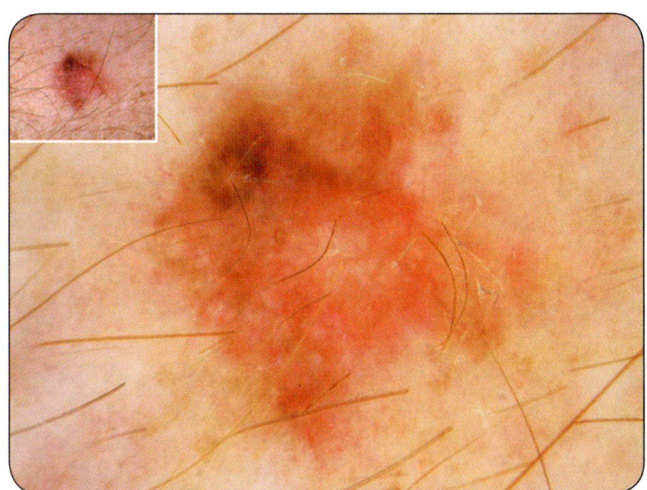

Fig. 4.21: Unspecific lesion—melanoma.

Table 4.2: Diagnostic methods for melanocytic lesions.
Pattern analysis (Pehamberger)
ABCD rule (Stolz)
11-point checklist method (Menzies)
7-point checklist method (Argenziano)
3-point checklist (Soyer)

SUGGESTED READING

Argenziano G, Soyer P, De Giorgio V, et al. Interactive Atlas of Dermoscopy. Milán: EDRA Medical Publishing & New Media; 2000.

Cabo H. Dermatoscopia. Buenos Aires, Argentina: Weber Ferro; 2000.

Cabo H. Dermatoscopia, 2nd edition. Buenos Aires, Argentina: Ediciones Journal; 2012.

Johr R, Stolz W. Dermoscopy: An Illustrated Self-Assessment Guide, 2nd edition. New York: McGraw-Hill Education; 2015.

Jorh R, Soyer P, Argenziano G, et al. Dermoscopy. The Essentials (MOABT). New York: Elsevier Ltd; 2004.

Kittler H. Dermatoscopy. An Algorithmic Method Based on Pattern Analysis 2011 Facultas Verlags- und Buchhandels AG facultas wuv Universitätsverlag, Austria www.facultas.wuv.at

Malvhey J, Puig S. Principles of Dermoscopy. Barcelona: Creaciones Gráficas; 2009.

Marghoob A, Braun R, Kopf A. Atlas of Dermoscopy. London: Taylor & Francis; 2005.

Marghoob A, Braun R. Proposal for a revised 2-step algorithm for the classification of lesions of the skin using dermoscopy. Arch Dermatol. 2010;146:426-8.

Menzies S, Crotty K, Ingvar C, et al. An Atlas of Surface Microscopy of Pigmented Skin Lesions. Sydney: McGraw-Hill Book Company; 1996.

Rabinovitz H, Kopf A. Dermoscopy: A Practical Guide. Miami: American Academy of Dermatology; 1999.

Soyer P, Argenziano G, Chimenti S, et al. Dermoscopy of Pigmented Skin Lesions. An Atlas Based on the Consensus Net Meeting on Dermoscopy. Milán: EDRA Medical Publishing & New Media; 2001.

Stolz W, Braun-Falco O, Bilek P, et al. Color Atlas of Dermatoscopy. USA: Blackwell Science; 1994.

Zalaudek I, Argenziano G, Giacomel J. Dermoscopy of Non-Pigmented Skin Tumors. Boca Raton, FL: CRC Press; 2016.

NONMELANOCYTIC LESIONS

5

Horacio A Cabo

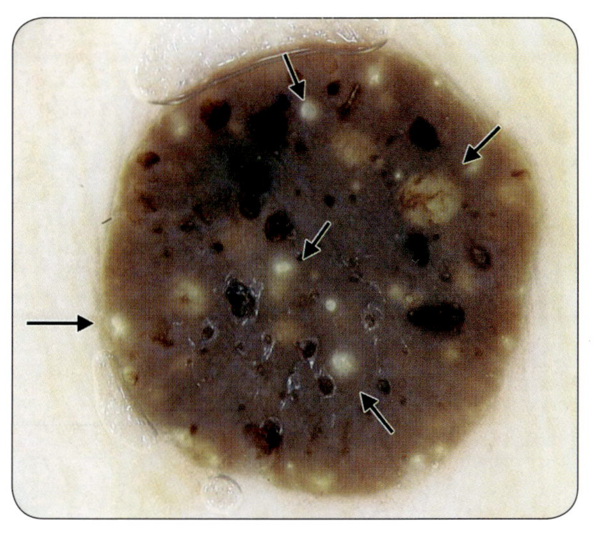

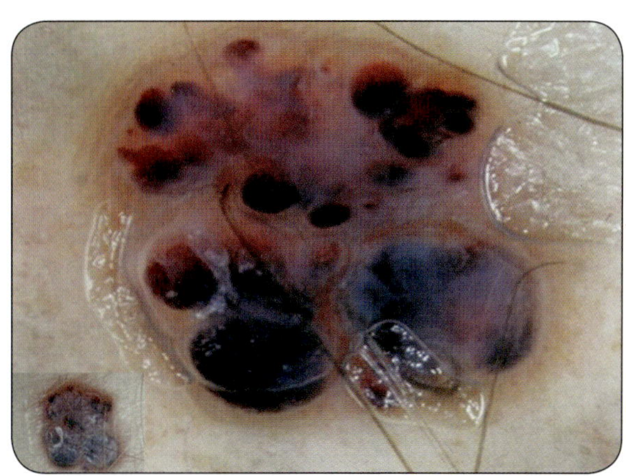

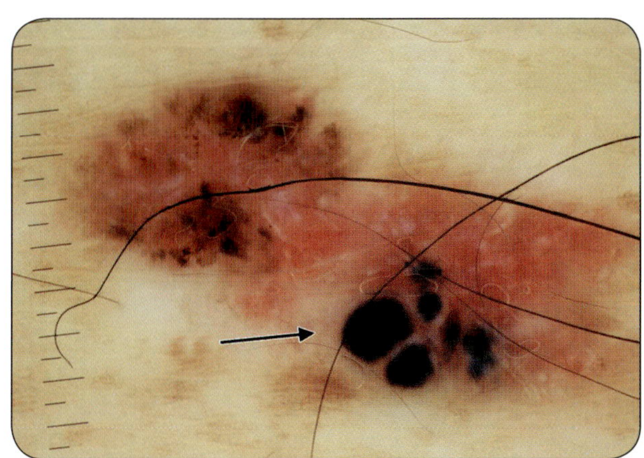

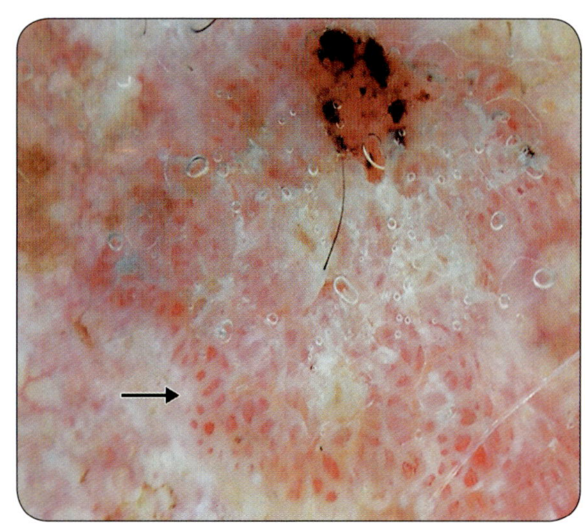

"The dermoscopic image of SK is rather different when using
polarized-light or nonpolarized-light dermoscopes.
The latter allow a better visualization of milia-like cysts.
Basal cell carcinomas are pink but sometimes BCCs are pigmented, due to melanocyte hyperplasia.
In these cases, BCC can be considered a melanoma simulator.
Squamous cell carcinoma show hyperkeratosis usually located in the central part
and also white circles surrounding the dilated infundibulum."

5.1 SEBORRHEIC KERATOSIS

Horacio A Cabo

Seborrheic keratoses (SKs) are benign skin tumors that appear toward middle aged and occasionally in young people. They are very frequent and show preferably on the face and trunk. However, it is not uncommon to find them in different areas of the cutaneous surface, except palms and soles. Generally, they are multiple and their size is variable—between a few millimeters and some centimeters. The color is not defined; it can be light brown, yellowish brown, dark brown, or black.

Initially, SKs are flat with well-demarcated edges. As they evolve, they rise and acquire a warty appearance, which is a characteristic (stuck-on appearance). In general, clinical diagnosis of SK is not difficult. Nevertheless, it is necessary to distinguish the pigmented superficial variety from lentigo malignant melanoma, while the raised variants can be taken for atypical nevi and melanoma. The irritated forms of SK can also prove difficult for the clinical diagnosis. In doubtful cases, dermoscopy optimizes clinical diagnosis more than for any other pigmented lesion, except hemangioma.

In highly verrucous varieties, it is impossible to identify characteristic structures for SK due to the high orthokeratosis present in these lesions.

The two typical criteria and characteristics of SK are milia-like cysts and follicular openings, although other less specific criteria can also be observed. All of these criteria are described hereunder.

DERMOSCOPIC CRITERIA

- Milia-like cysts
- Pseudofollicular openings (irregular ridges)
- Fissures and ridges (brain-like appearance)
- Vascular pattern

Milia-like Cysts (Fig. 5.1)

They are circular structures, white-yellow in color and small in size (0.1–1 mm). In very big or verrucous SKs, the size can be larger, while the shape may not be circular. From a histopathological point of view, we can observe horny pseudocysts in the epidermis that do not communicate with the cutaneous surface (Fig. 5.2).

Pseudofollicular Openings (Irregular Ridges) (Figs. 5.3 and 5.4)

These structures are yellowish, light brown, dark brown, or black, circular in shape, and of small size, presenting the typical appearance of a pore or a comedo. In large SKs, their size can be even bigger and the shape is irregular. From a histopathological point of view, they are horny pseudocysts that reach the cutaneous surface and communicate with it.

Fissures and Ridges (Brain-Like Appearance) (Figs. 5.5 and 5.6)

These are variants in size and shape of follicular pseudo-openings and their appearance resembles the surface of the brain.

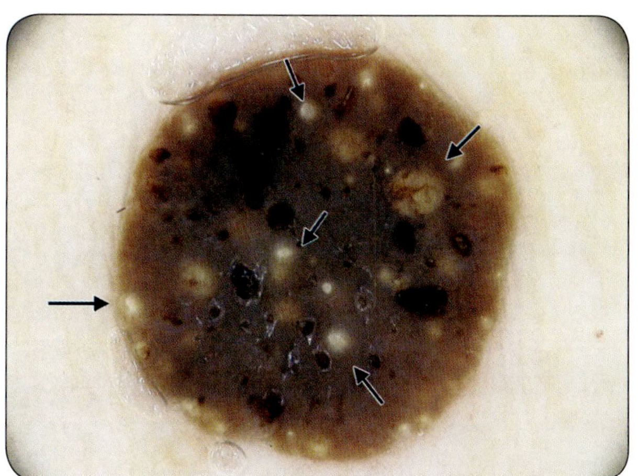

Fig. 5.1: Seborrheic keratosis. The arrows show the millia-like cysts.

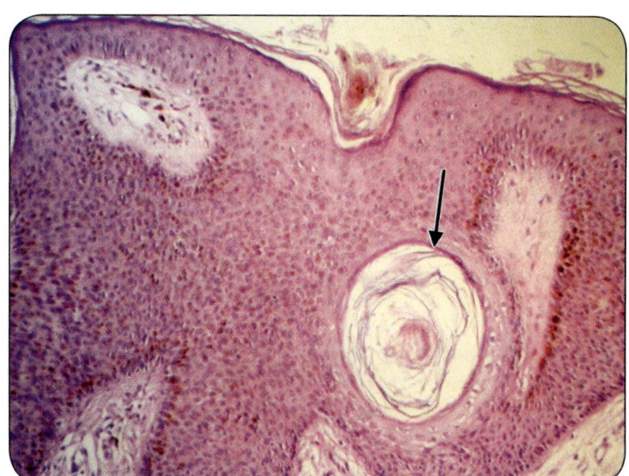

Fig. 5.2: Seborrheic keratosis. Histological image, showing the horny pseudocysts without communication with the cutaneous surface (arrow).

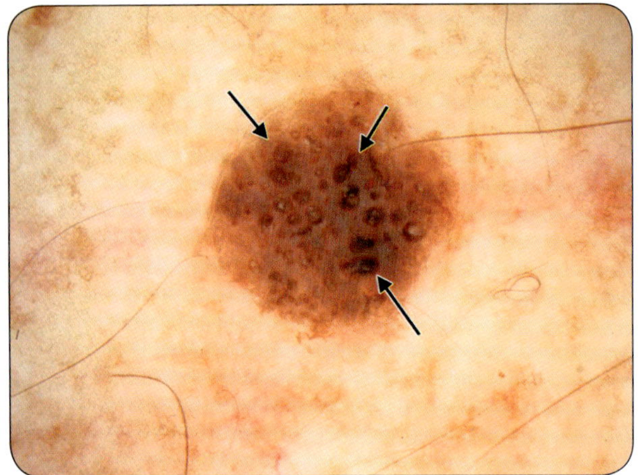

Fig. 5.3: Seborrheic keratosis. The arrows show pseudofollicular openings.

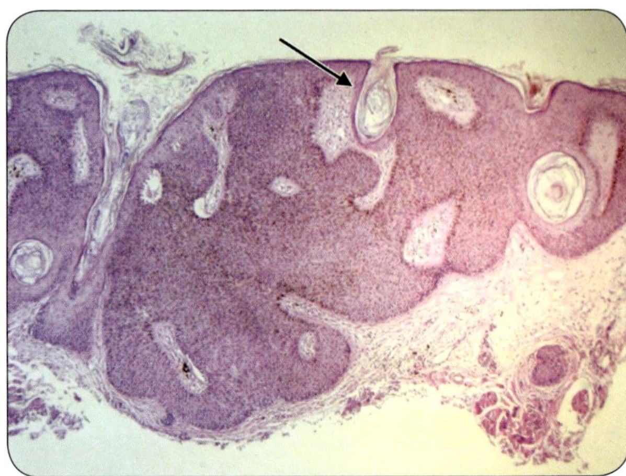

Fig. 5.4: Seborrheic keratosis. Histological images showing the horny pseudocysts with communication with the cutaneous surface (arrow).

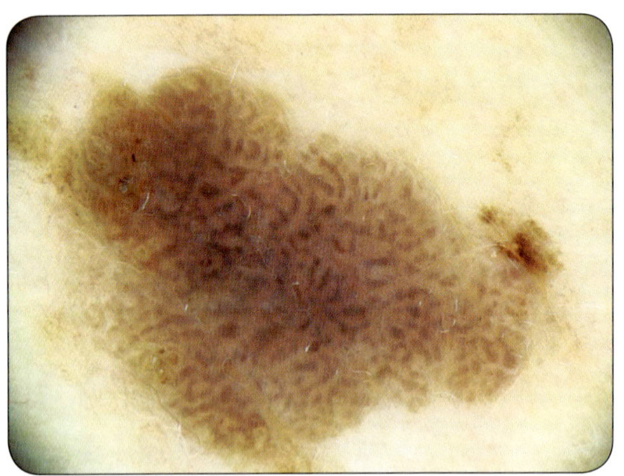

Fig. 5.5: Seborrheic keratosis. Brain-like appearance.

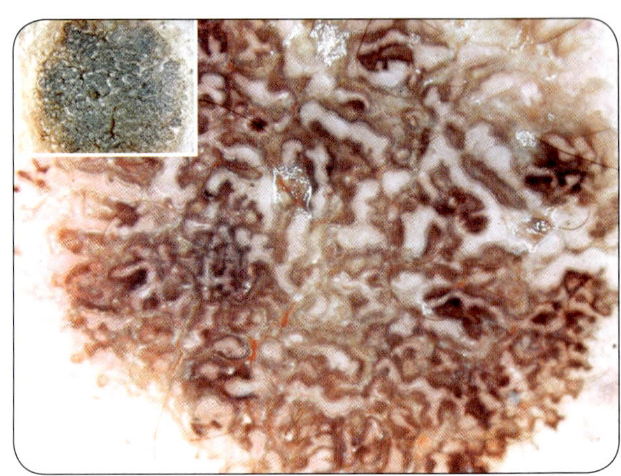

Fig. 5.6: Seborrheic keratosis. Brain-like appearance.

Vascular Pattern (Figs. 5.7 to 5.12)

Hairpin vessels in the periphery of the lesions.

HISTOPATHOLOGY

From a histopathological point of view, SKs are epidermal lesions composed of little basaloid cells, pigmented or not, with an excess keratin production that tends to form horny cysts.

Some communicate with the cutaneous surface (follicular pseudo-openings) and others do not (milia-like cysts).

Irregular ridges and fissures are variants in size and shape of the follicular pseudo-openings (Figs. 5.2 to 5.4).

ADDITIONAL OBSERVATION CRITERIA

Additionally, the following criteria can be observed:

- *Pigmented network* (exceptionally, it is possible to observe a fine delicate pigment network on the periphery of the lesion (Figs. 5.13 to 5.15).
- *Blue-white veil*: This appears in lesions with heightened orthokeratosis (Fig. 5.16).
- *Fat fingers*: These are thick digitate linear, curvilinear, branched, or oval/circular dermoscopic structures at the periphery of the lesion. They represent the gyri of their cerebriform surfaces (Figs. 5.17 and 5.18).
- *Regression:* Some SKs may show signs of regression, usually after traumas (Figs. 5.19 to 5.21).
- *Blue globular pattern:* Some SKs can show this pattern (acanthotic SKs) (*see* Fig. 5.39).

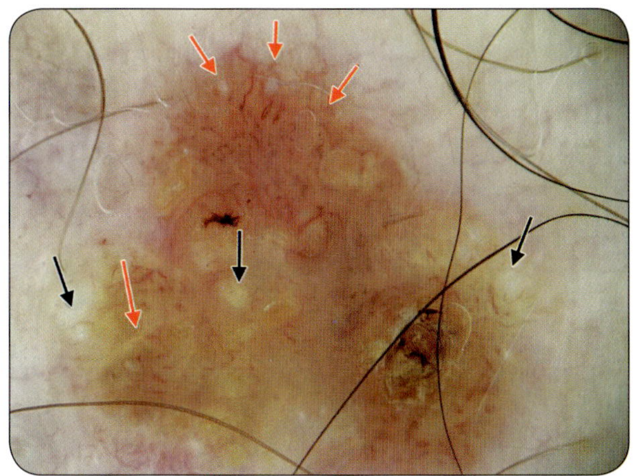

Fig. 5.7: Seborrheic keratosis. Hairpin vessels (red arrows); millia-like cysts (black arrows).

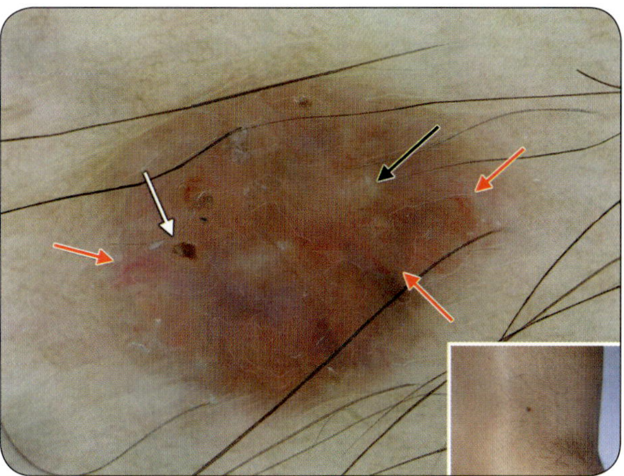

Fig. 5.8: Seborrheic keratosis. Hairpin vessels (red arrows), millia-like cysts (black arrow), pseudofollicular openings (white arrow).

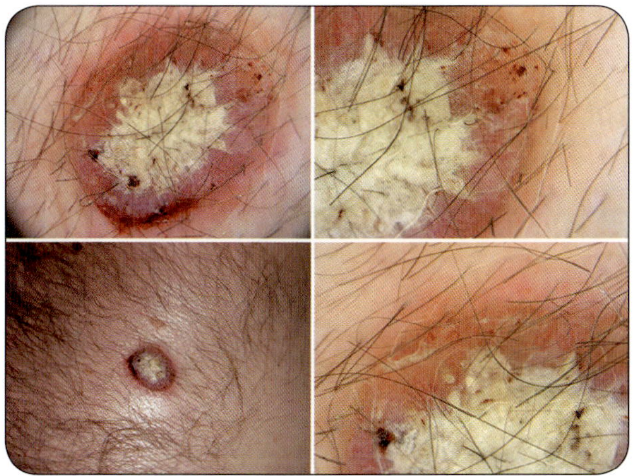

Fig. 5.9: Seborrheic keratosis. Hairpin vessels.

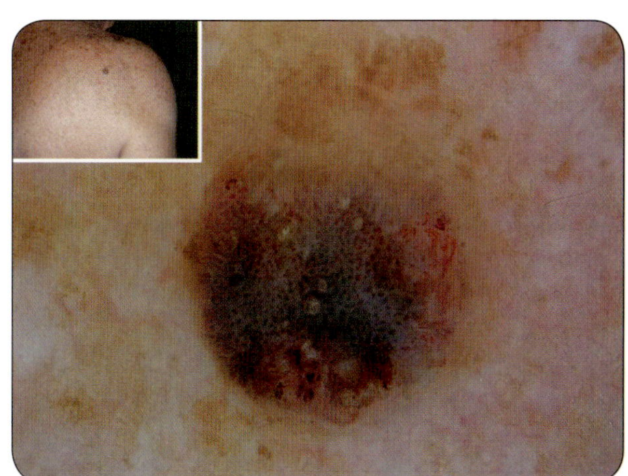

Fig. 5.10: Seborrheic keratosis. Hairpin vessels.

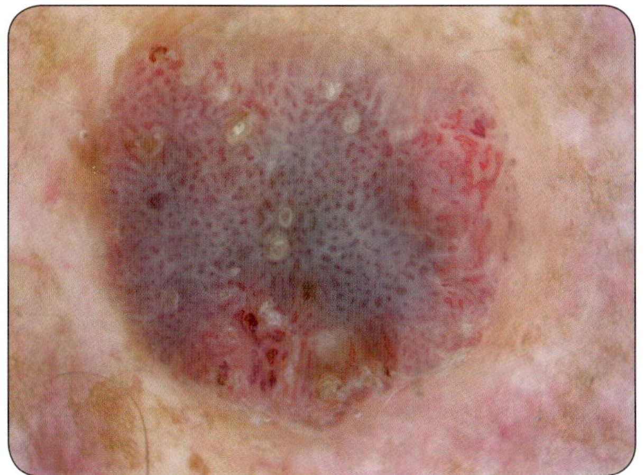

Fig. 5.11: Seborrheic keratosis. Hairpin vessels; close-up view of Figure 5.10.

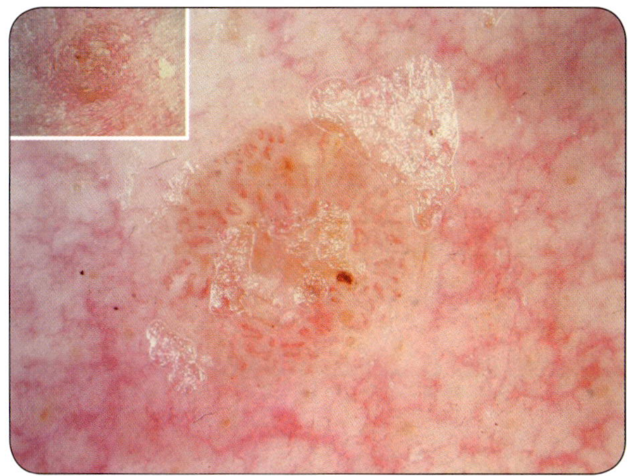

Fig. 5.12: Seborrheic keratosis. Hairpin vessels.

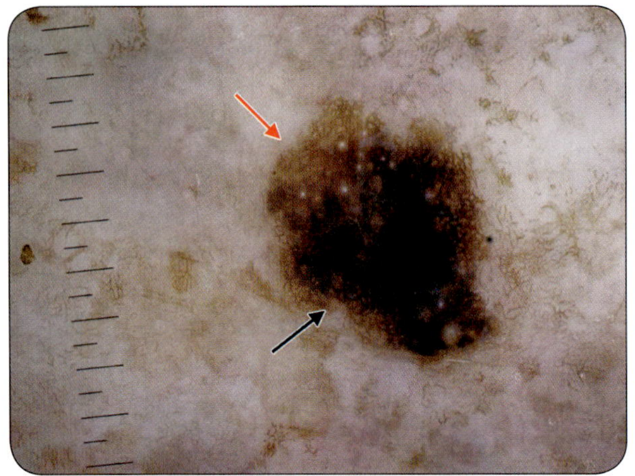

Fig. 5.13: Seborrheic keratosis with pigment network (black arrow) and millia-like cysts (red arrow).

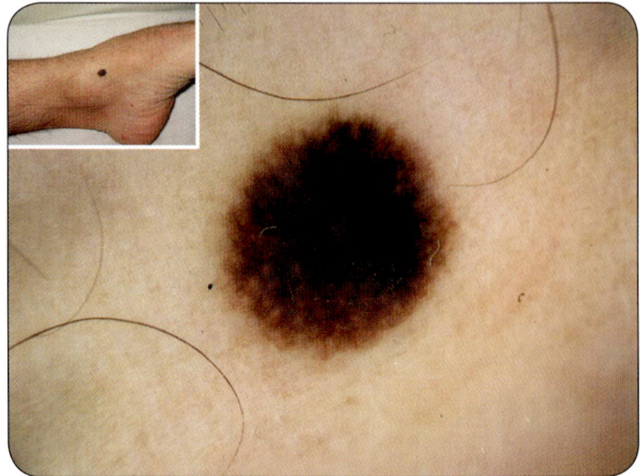

Fig. 5.14: Seborrheic keratosis with pigment network.

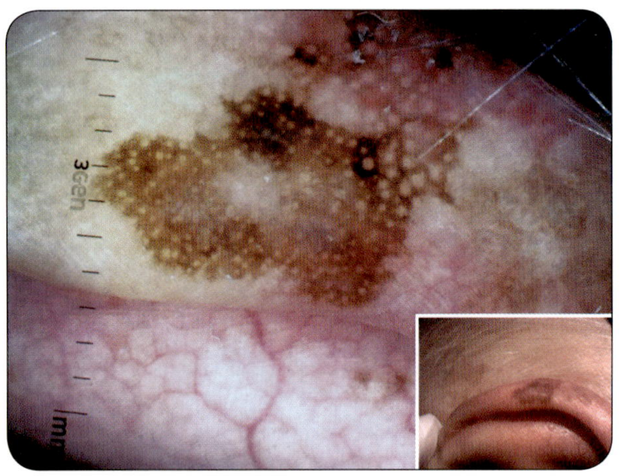

Fig. 5.15: Seborrheic keratosis with pigment network.

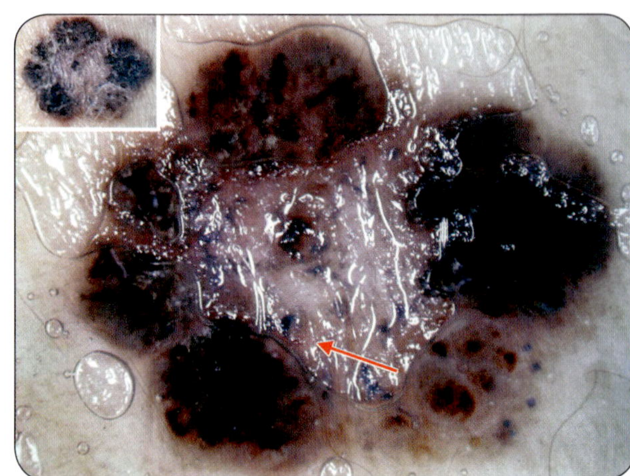

Fig. 5.16: Seborrheic keratosis with blue veil (arrow).

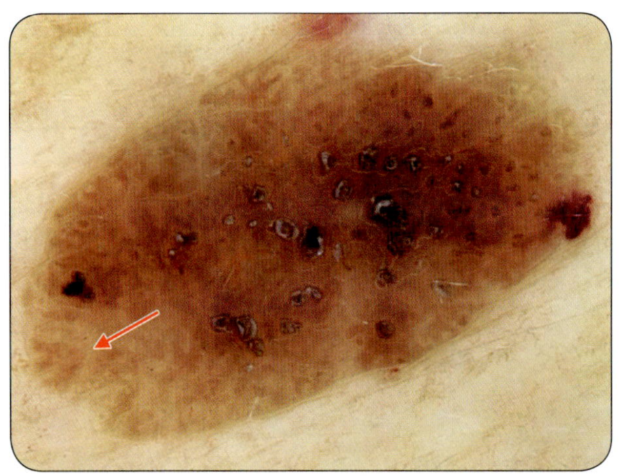

Fig. 5.17: Seborrheic keratosis. The arrow shows the fat fingers.

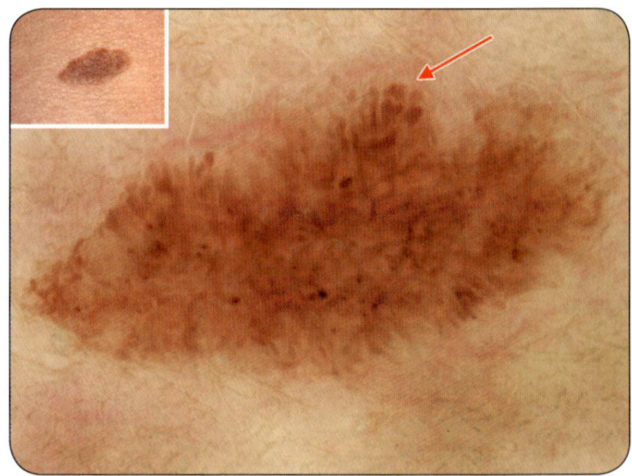

Fig. 5.18: Seborrheic keratosis. The arrow shows the fat fingers.

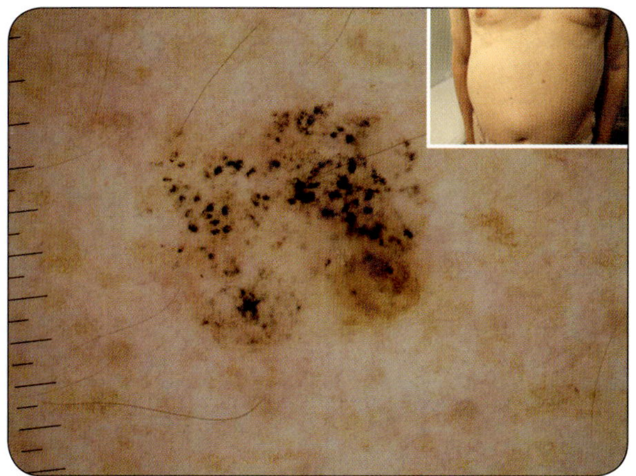

Fig. 5.19: Seborrheic keratosis with regression.

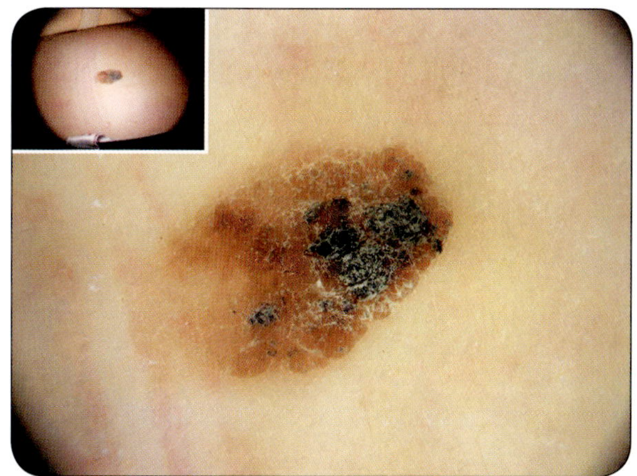

Fig. 5.20: Seborrheic keratosis with regression.

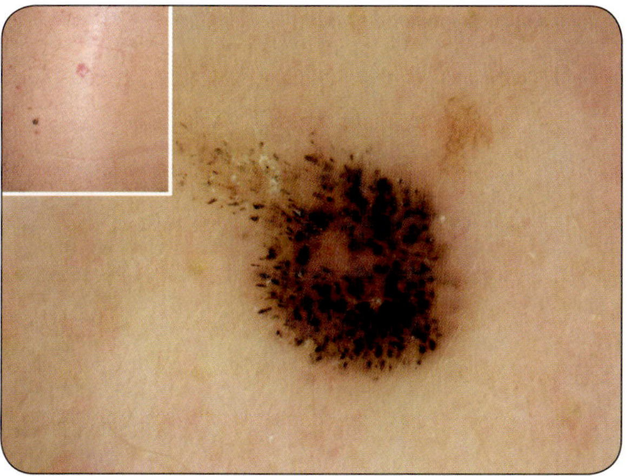

Fig. 5.21: Seborrheic keratosis with regression.

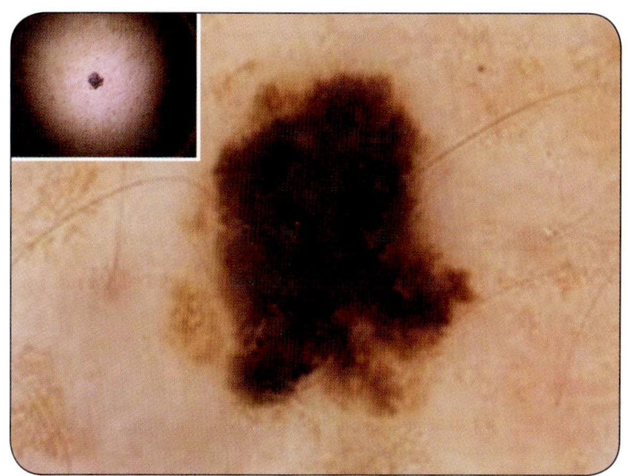

Fig. 5.22: Seborrheic keratosis—polarized light.

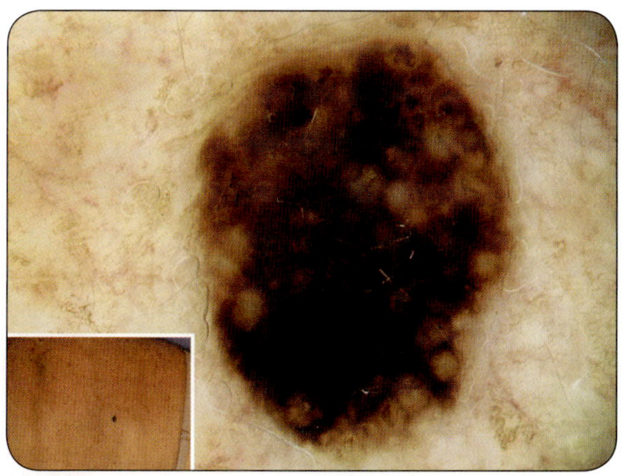

Fig. 5.23: Seborrheic keratosis—polarized light.

Polarized Light Versus Nonpolarized Light

The dermoscopic image of SK is rather different when using polarized-light or non polarized-light dermoscopes. The latter allow a better visualization of milia-like cysts (Figs. 5.22 to 5.38).

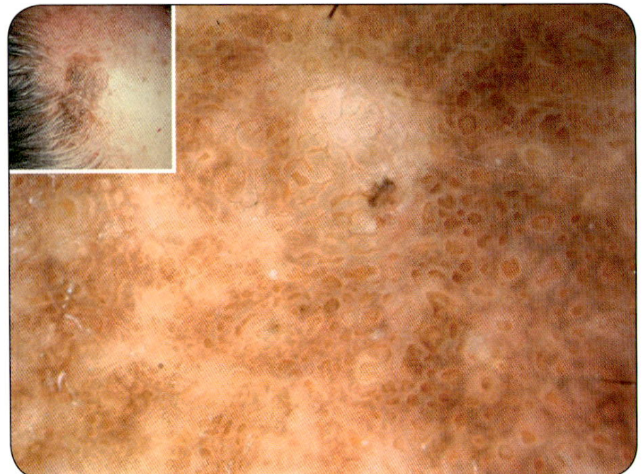

Fig. 5.24: Seborrheic keratosis—polarized light.

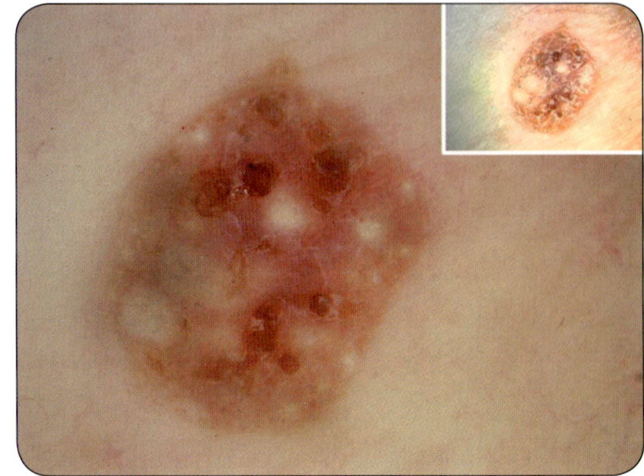

Fig. 5.25: Seborrheic keratosis—nonpolarized light.

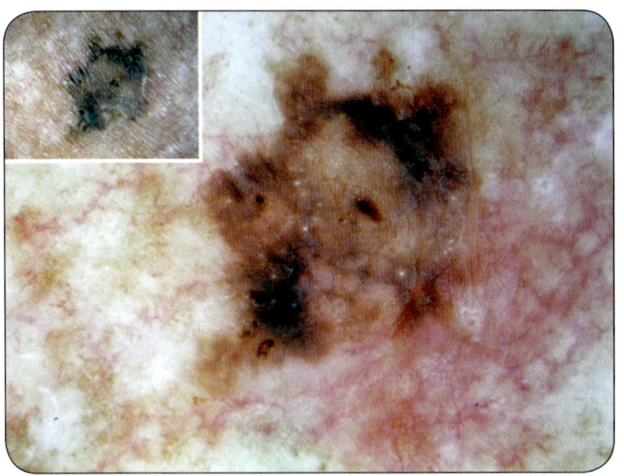

Fig. 5.26: Seborrheic keratosis—nonpolarized light.

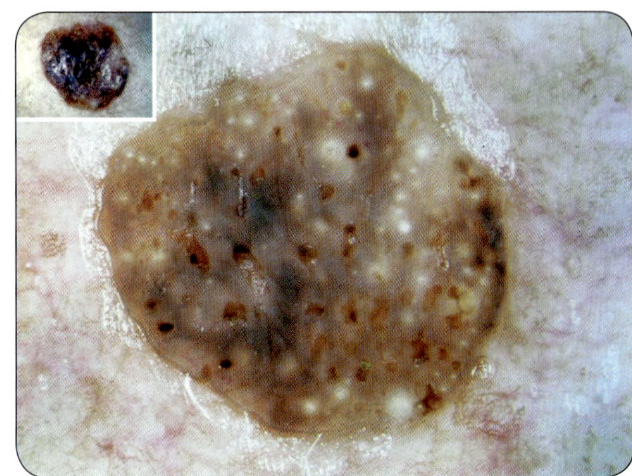

Fig. 5.27: Seborrheic keratosis—nonpolarized light.

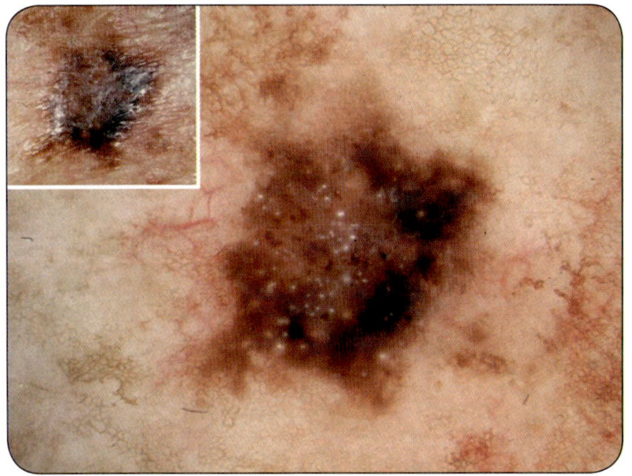

Fig. 5.28: Seborrheic keratosis—nonpolarized light.

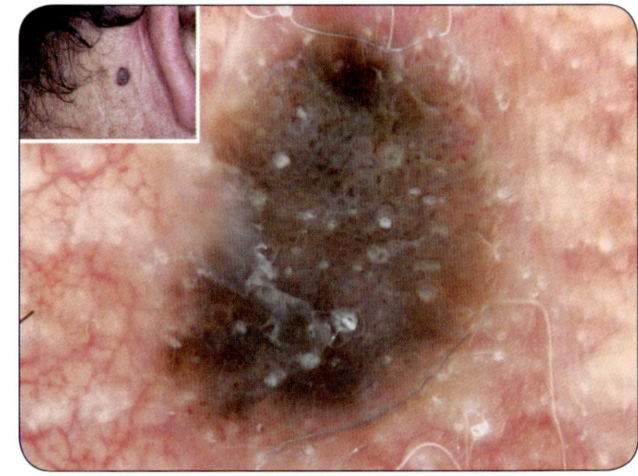

Fig. 5.29: Seborrheic keratosis—nonpolarized light.

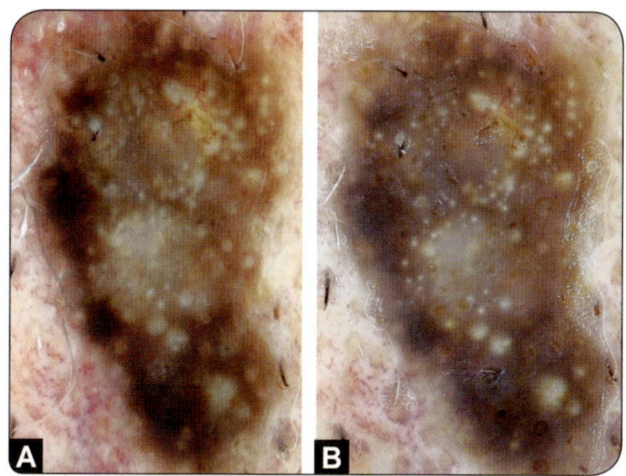

Figs. 5.30A and B: Seborrheic keratosis. (A) The image captured with a polarized light dermoscope and (B) the image captured with a nonpolarized light dermoscope.

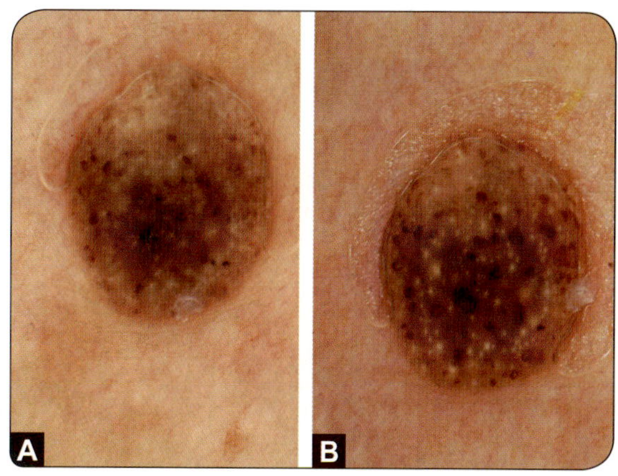

Figs. 5.31A and B: Seborrheic keratosis. (A) The image captured with a polarized light dermoscope; (B) the image captured with a nonpolarized light dermoscope.

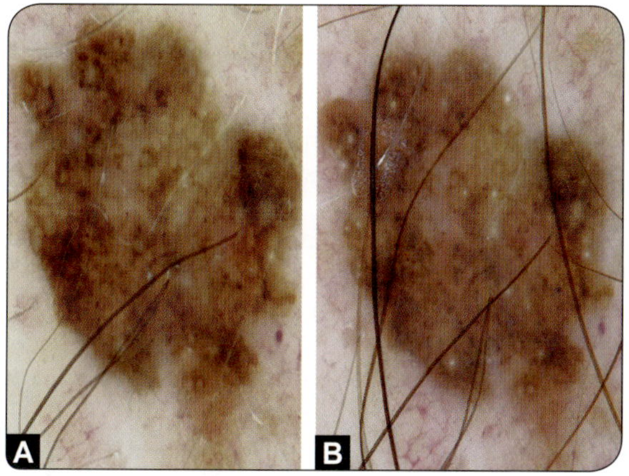

Figs. 5.32A and B: Seborrheic keratosis. (A) The image captured with a polarized light dermoscope and (B) the image captured with a nonpolarized light dermoscope.

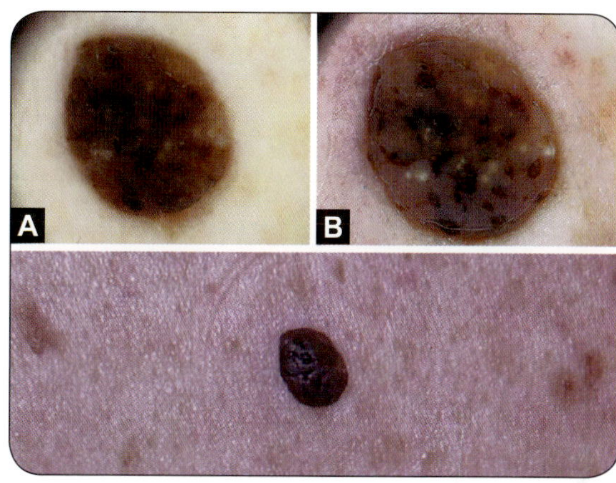

Figs. 5.33A and B: Seborrheic keratosis. (A) The image captured with a polarized light dermoscope; (B) the image captured with a nonpolarized light dermoscope.

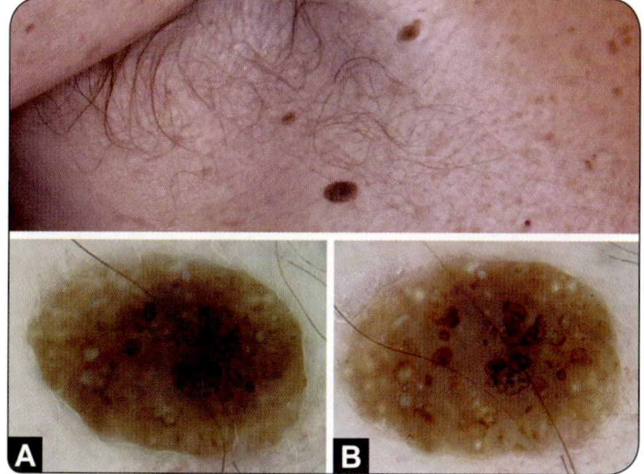

Figs. 5.34A and B: Seborrheic keratosis. (A) The image captured with a polarized light dermoscope; (B) image captured with a nonpolarized light dermoscope.

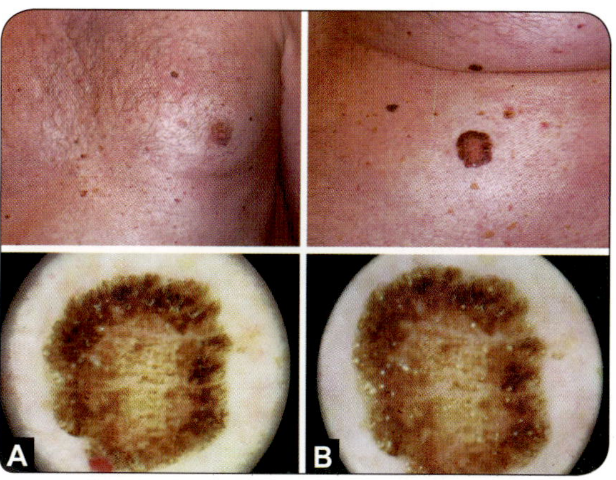

Figs. 5.35A and B: Seborrheic keratosis. (A) The image captured with a polarized light dermoscope; (B) the image captured with a nonpolarized light dermoscope.

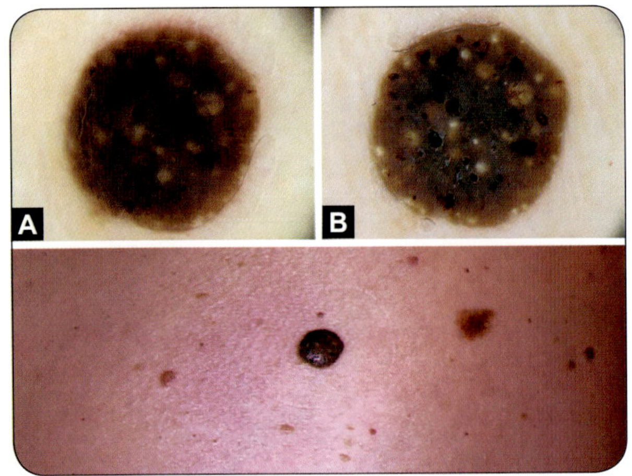

Figs. 5.36A and B: Seborrheic keratosis. (A) The image captured with a polarized light dermoscope; (B) the image captured with a nonpolarized light dermoscope.

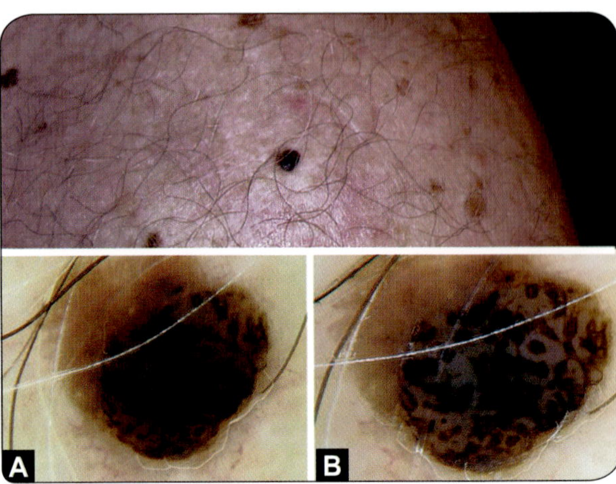

Figs. 5.37A and B: Seborrheic keratosis. (A) The image captured with a polarized light dermoscope; (B) the image captured with a nonpolarized light dermoscope.

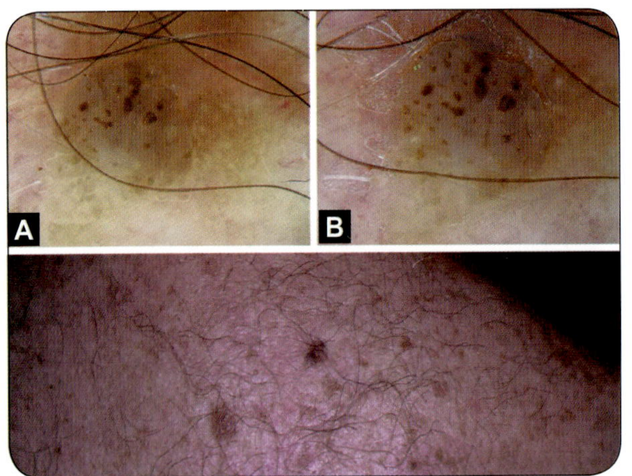

Figs. 5.38A and B: Seborrheic keratosis. (A) The image captured with a polarized light dermoscope; (B) the image captured with a nonpolarized light dermoscope.

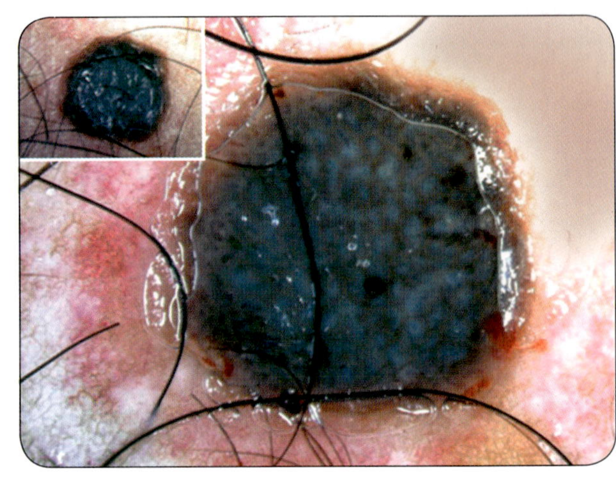

Fig. 5.39: Blue globular pattern.

SUGGESTED READING

Argenziano G, Soyer P, De Giorgio V, et al. Interactive Atlas of Dermoscopy. Milán: EDRA Medical Publishing & New Media; 2000.

Cabo H. Dermatoscopia. Buenos Aires, Argentina: Weber Ferro; 2000.

Cabo H. Dermatoscopia, 2nd edition. Buenos Aires, Argentina: Ediciones Journal; 2012.

Jorh R, Soyer P, Argenziano G, et al. Dermoscopy. The Essentials (MOABT). New York: Elsevier Ltd; 2004.

Johr R, Stolz W. Dermoscopy: An Illustrated Self-Assessment Guide, 2nd edition. New York: McGraw-Hill Education; 2015.

Kittler H. Dermatoscopy. An Algorithmic Method Based on Pattern Analysis. Vienna, Austria: facultas.wuv; 2011.

Malvhey J, Puig S. Principles of Dermoscopy. Barcelona: Creaciones Gráficas; 2009.

Marghoob A, Braun R, Kopf A. Atlas of Dermoscopy. London: Taylor & Francis; 2005.

Menzies S, Crotty K, Ingvar C, et al. An Atlas of Surface Microscopy of Pigmented Skin Lesions. Sydney: McGraw-Hill Book Company; 1996.

Rabinovitz H, Kopf A. Dermoscopy: a practical guide. Miami: American Academy of Dermatology; 1999.

Roberti V, Devirgiliis V, Curzio M, et al. The blue globular pattern in dermoscopy. Dermatology. 2013;226:260-6.

Soyer P, Argenziano G, Chimenti S, et al. Dermoscopy of Pigmented Skin Lesions. An Atlas Based on the Consensus Net Meeting on Dermoscopy. Milán: EDRA Medical Publishing & New Media; 2001.

Stolz W, Braun-Falco O, Bilek P, et al. Color Atlas of Dermatoscopy. Berlin, Germany: Blackwell Science; 1994.

Zalaudek I, Argenziano G, Giacomel J. Dermoscopy of Non-Pigmented Skin Tumors. Boca Raton, FL: CRC Press; 2016.

5.2 SOLAR LENTIGO

Horacio A Cabo

Solar lentigo and flat seborrheic keratosis (SK) are considered the same lesion.

DERMOSCOPIC CRITERIA FOR SOLAR LENTIGO (FLAT SK)

Fingerprint-Like Structures (Figs. 5.40 to 5.43)

These are brown structures, made up of fine parallel lines in fingerprint fashion. They are usually found in the peripheral part of the lesion.

Moth-Eaten Border (Figs. 5.43 to 5.45)

Concave edge of the lesion resembling the bite of a moth.

Jelly Sign (Figs. 5.46 to 5.49)

Light brown or yellowish in color, it resembles a very thin layer of jelly which has dried or a film covering the surface of the skin.

INKSPOT LENTIGO

Inkspot lentigo deserves special attention due to its clinical and dermoscopic characteristics.

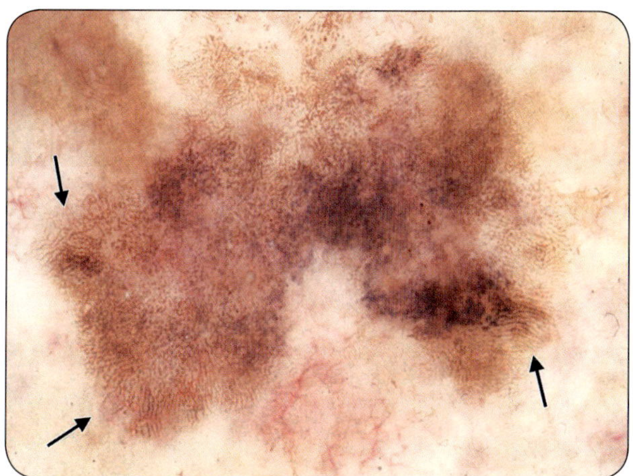

Fig. 5.40: Solar lentigo. The arrows show the fingerprint-like structures.

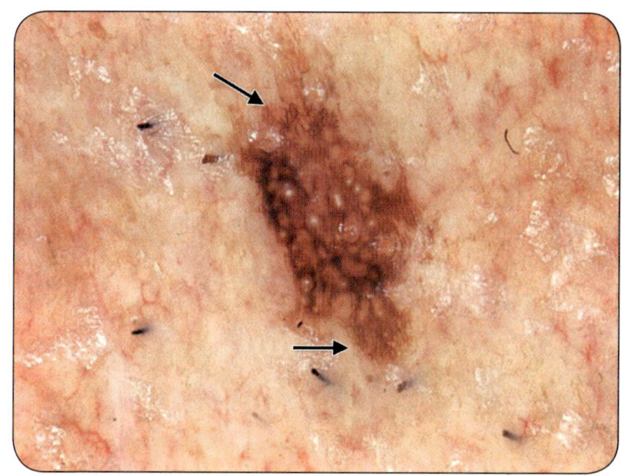

Fig. 5.41: Solar lentigo. The arrows show the fingerprint-like structures.

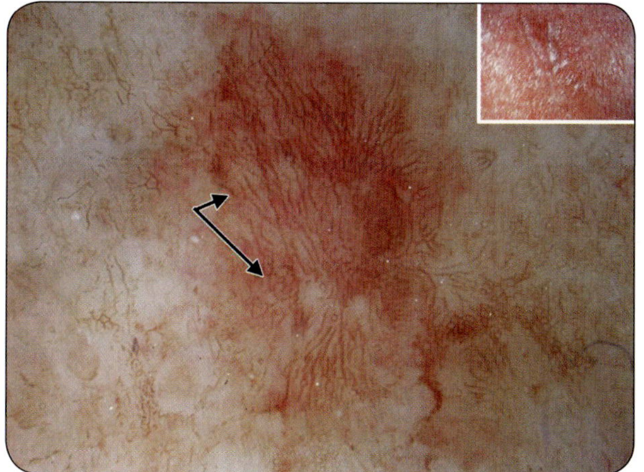

Fig. 5.42: Solar lentigo. The arrows show the fingerprint-like structures.

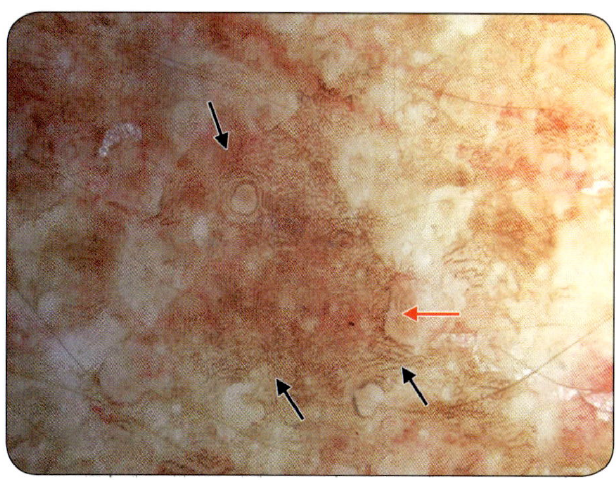

Fig. 5.43: Solar lentigo. Red arrow: moth-eaten border. Black arrows: fingerprint-like structures.

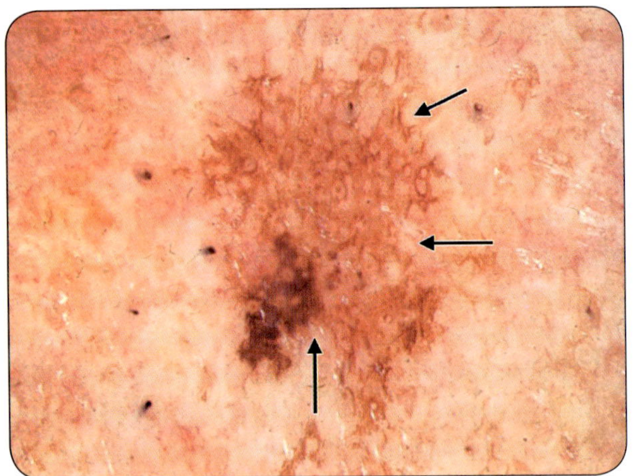

Fig. 5.44: Solar lentigo. The arrows show the moth-eaten border.

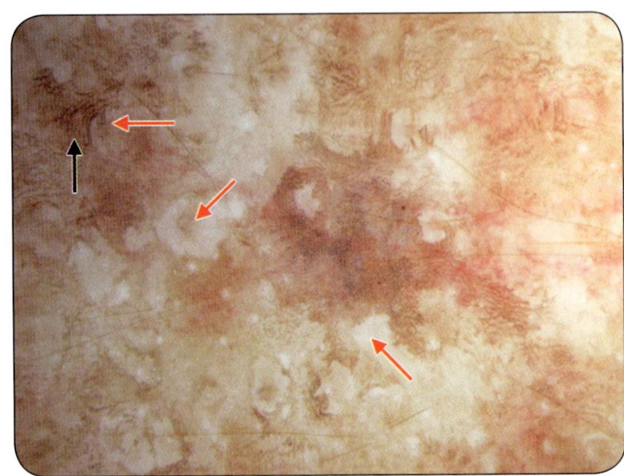

Fig. 5.45: Solar lentigo. Red arrows: moth-eaten border. Black arrow: fingerprint-like structures.

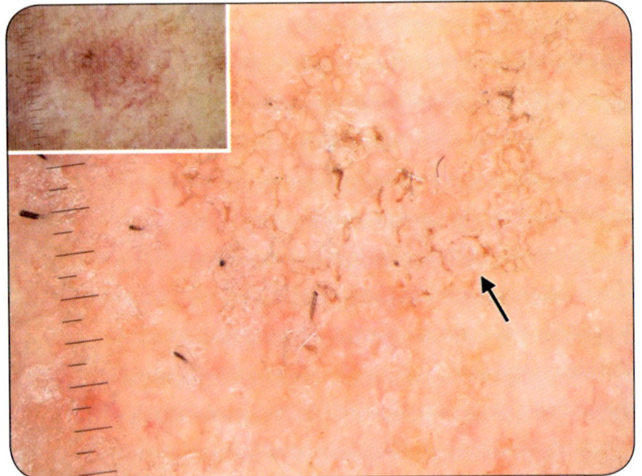

Fig. 5.46: Solar lentigo. The arrow shows the jelly sign.

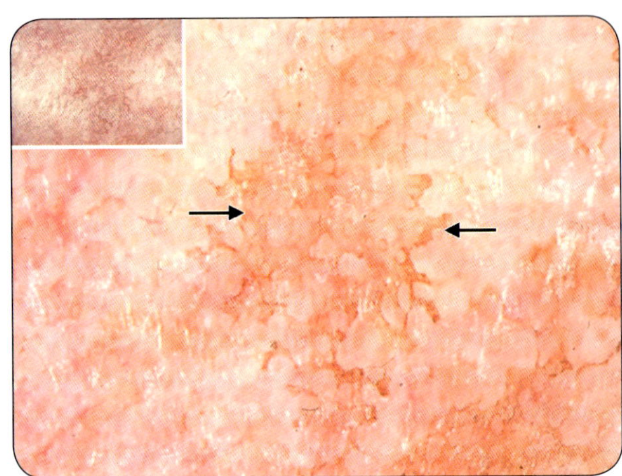

Fig. 5.47: Solar lentigo. The arrows show the jelly sign.

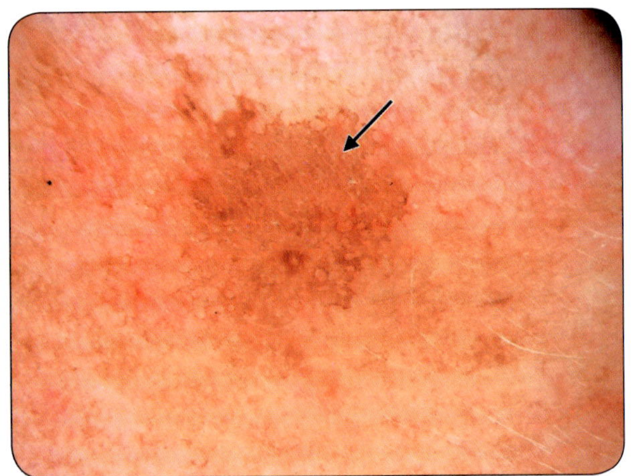

Fig. 5.48: Solar lentigo. The arrow shows the jelly sign.

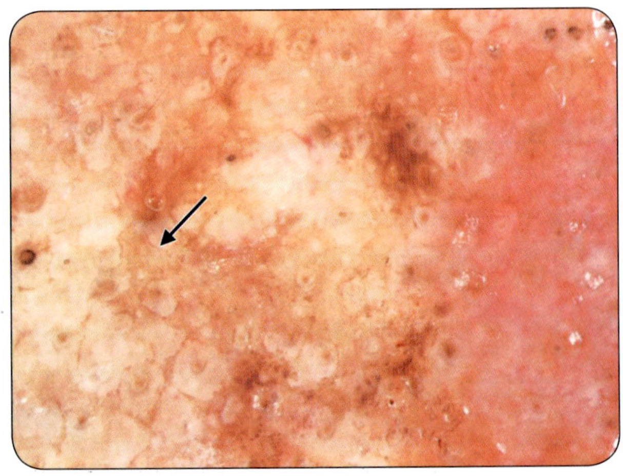

Fig. 5.49: Solar lentigo. The arrow shows the jelly sign.

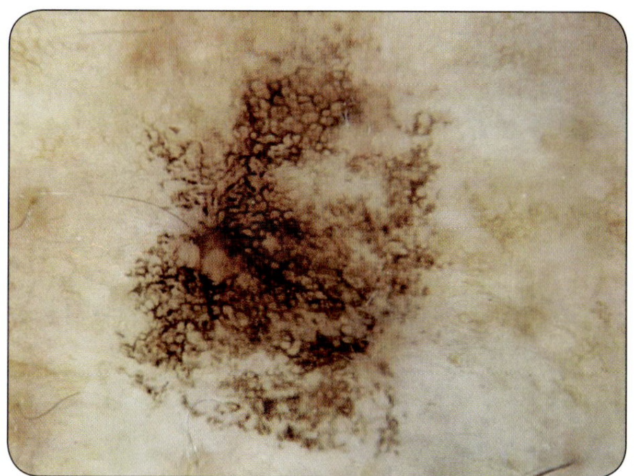

Fig. 5.50: Solar lentigo. Inkspot lentigo.

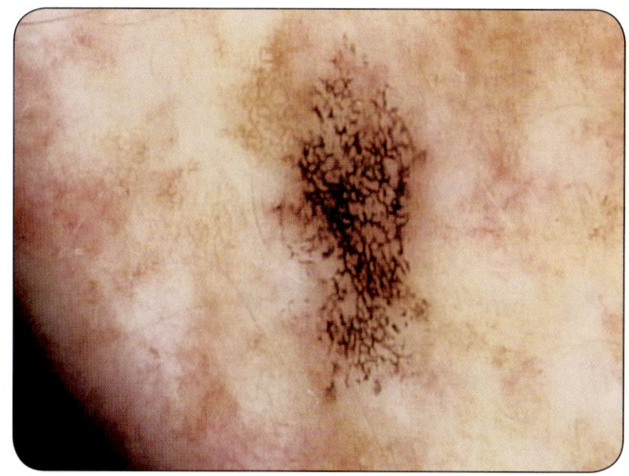

Fig. 5.51: Solar lentigo. Inkspot lentigo.

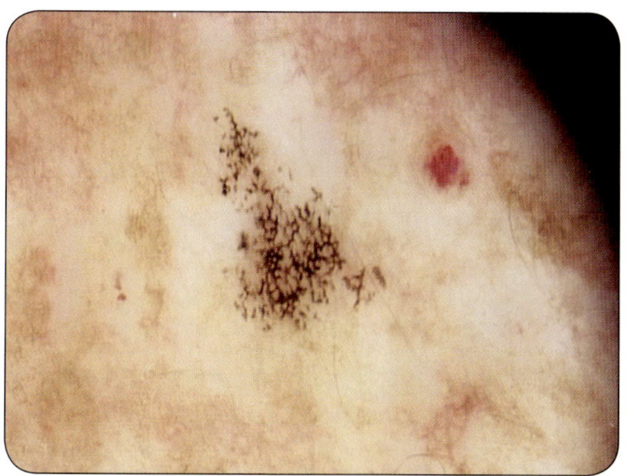

Fig. 5.52: Solar lentigo. Inkspot lentigo.

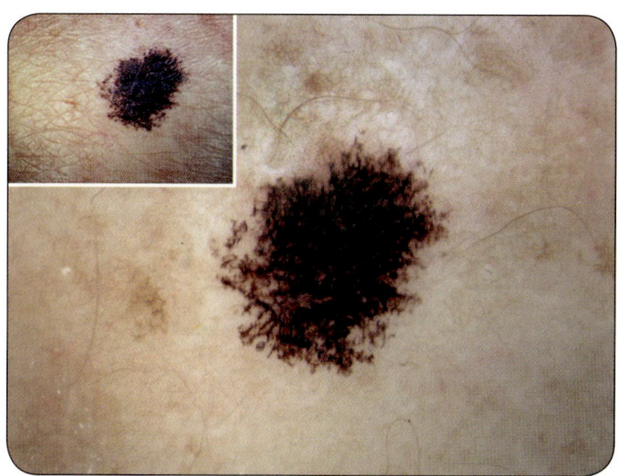

Fig. 5.53: Solar lentigo. Inkspot lentigo.

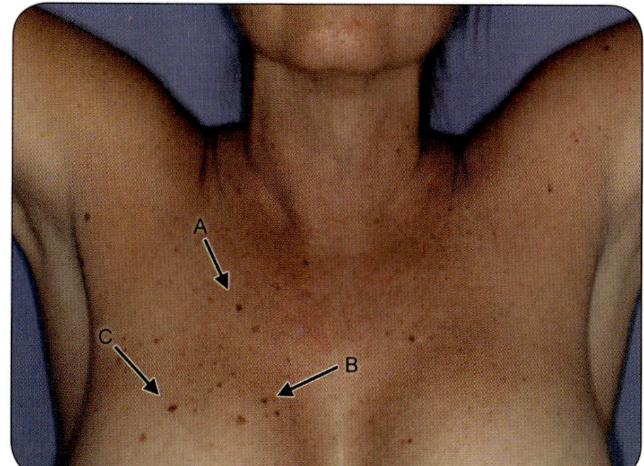

Fig. 5.54: A 52-year-old female patient with sun damage and multiple lentigos on chest (A-B-C).

It generally appears in highly photodamaged skin, as a small lesion, with flat smooth surface and black color (resembling an inkspot, hence its name).

Under dermoscopic examination, we can observe a black pigment network, thickened and irregular, which may lead the less-experienced observers to a misdiagnosis of melanoma (Figs. 5.50 and 5.51).

On occasion, solar lentigo can show pigment network and make it difficult to reach a differential diagnosis from melanocytic lesions (Figs. 5.52 to 5.55).

Also, solar lentigo may occasionally show pigmentation of the follicular opening, sometimes asymmetric, and two brown concentric circles, which may render it difficult to make the differential diagnosis from malignant lentigo and pigmented actinic keratosis (Figs. 5.56 to 5.62).

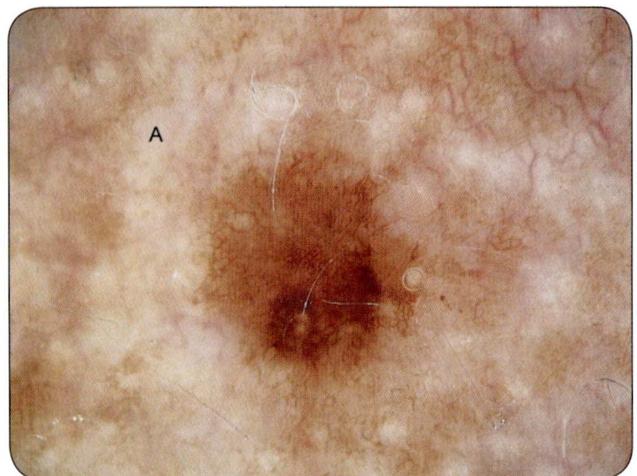

Fig. 5.55: Solar lentigo with reticular pattern (A).

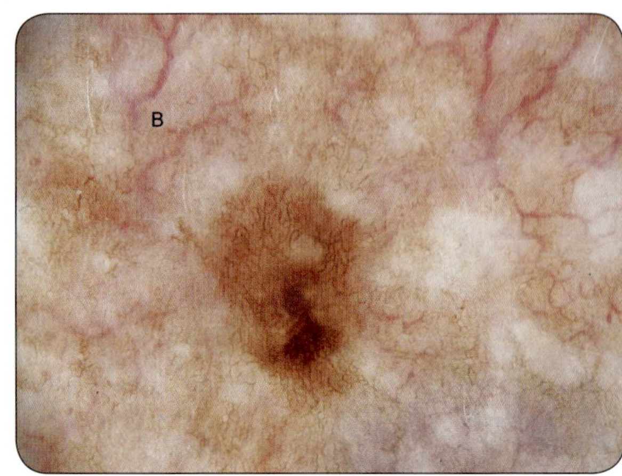

Fig. 5.56: Solar lentigo with reticular pattern (B).

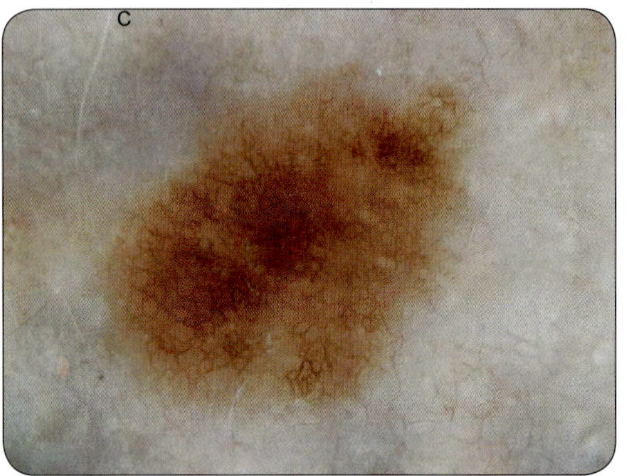

Fig. 5.57: Solar lentigo with reticular pattern (C).

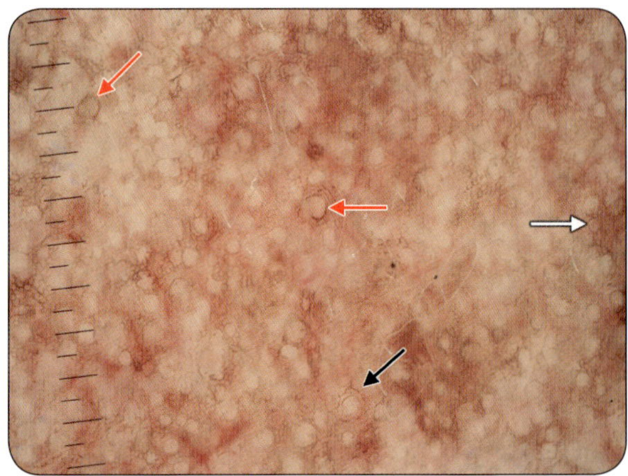

Fig. 5.58: Solar lentigo: red arrows: asymmetric pigmentation of the follicular openings; black arrow: circle within a circle; white arrow: brown pigmentation of the follicular openings.

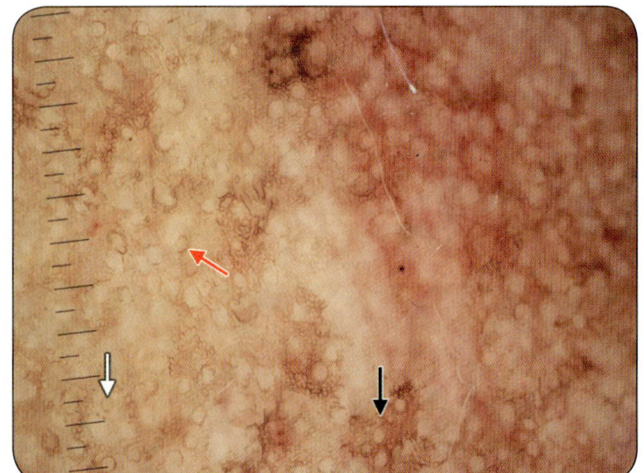

Fig. 5.59: Solar lentigo: red arrow: asymmetric pigmentation of the follicular openings; black arrow: circle within a circle; white arrow: brown pigmentation of the follicular openings.

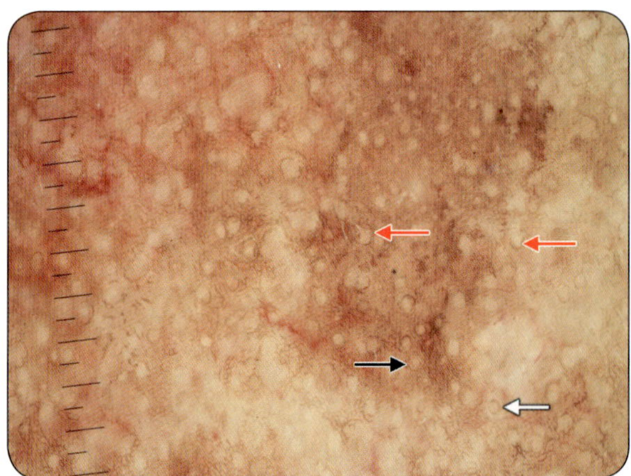

Fig. 5.60: Solar lentigo: red arrows: asymmetric pigmentation of the follicular openings; black arrow: circle within a circle; white arrow: brown pigmentation of the follicular openings.

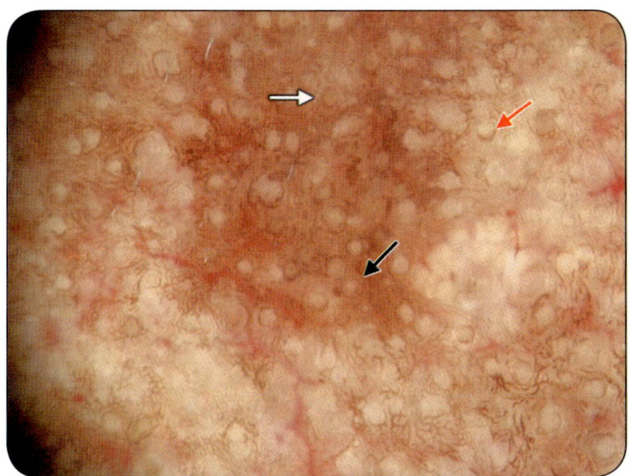

Fig. 5.61: Solar lentigo: red arrow: asymmetric pigmentation of the follicular openings; black arrow: circle within a circle; white arrow: brown pigmentation of the follicular openings.

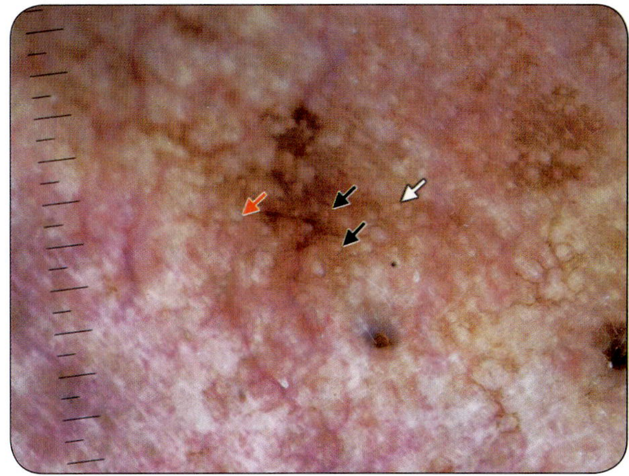

Fig. 5.62: Solar lentigo: red arrow: asymmetric pigmentation of the follicular openings; black arrows: circle within a circle; white arrow: brown pigmentation of the follicular openings.

SUGGESTED READING

Argenziano G, Soyer P, De Giorgio V, et al. Interactive Atlas of Dermoscopy. Milán: EDRA Medical Publishing & New Media; 2000.

Cabo H. Dermatoscopia. Buenos Aires, Argentina: Weber Ferro; 2000.

Cabo H. Dermatoscopia, 2nd edition. Buenos Aires, Argentina: Ediciones Journal; 2012.

Jorh R, Soyer P, Argenziano G, et al. Dermoscopy. The Essentials (MOABT). New York: Elsevier Ltd.; 2004.

Johr R, Stolz W. Dermoscopy: An Illustrated Self-Assessment Guide, 2nd edition. New York: McGraw-Hill Education; 2015.

Kittler H. Dermatoscopy. An Algorithmic Method Based on Pattern Analysis. Vienna, Austria: facultas.wuv; 2011.

Lallas A. Dermoscopy in general dermatology, Dermatol Clin. 2013;31:679-694.

Malvhey J, Puig S. Principles of Dermoscopy. Barcelona: Creaciones Gráficas; 2009.

Marghoob A, Braun R, Kopf A. Atlas of Dermoscopy. London: Taylor & Francis; 2005.

Menzies S, Crotty K, Ingvar C, et al. An Atlas of Surface Microscopy of Pigmented Skin Lesions. Sydney: McGraw-Hill Book Company; 1996.

Rabinovitz H, Kopf A. Dermoscopy: A Practical Guide. Miami: American Academy of Dermatology; 1999.

Soyer P, Argenziano G, Chimenti S, et al. Dermoscopy of Pigmented Skin Lesions. An Atlas Based on the Consensus Net Meeting on Dermoscopy. Milán: EDRA Medical Publishing & New Media; 2001.

Stolz W, Braun-Falco O, Bilek P, et al. Color Atlas of Dermatoscopy. Berlin, Germany: Blackwell Science; 1994.

Zalaudek I, Argenziano G, Giacomel J. Dermoscopy of Non-Pigmented Skin Tumors. Boca Raton, FL: CRC Press; 2016.

5.3 BASAL CELL CARCINOMA

Horacio A Cabo

Basal cell carcinoma (BCC) is the most frequent of all malignant skin tumors and cancers that may affect human beings. This malignant tumor does not generally metastasize and its incidence increases with sun exposure and over the age of 40. It is more frequent in men and less common in dark complexions. In general, the lesions are pink but sometimes BCCs are pigmented, due to melanocyte hyperplasia. In these cases, BCC can be considered a melanoma simulator (Figs. 5.63 and 5.64).

From a histologic point of view, we can observe globules or basaloid cell strings distributed in the periphery forming a palisade. In general, it is possible to visualize fibrovascular stroma with abundant mucin surrounding the tumor (Fig. 5.65).

DERMOSCOPIC CRITERIA FOR BASAL CELL CARCINOMA

Basal cell carcinoma can present classical criteria, non-classical criteria (generally the onset of classical criteria) and, on occasion, highly pigmented BCCs can show criteria similar to those of melanocytic lesions.

Classical Criteria

Basal cell carcinoma typically presents three well-defined criteria: arborizing vessels, blue-gray pigmentation, and ulcerations (Figs. 5.66 to 5.68).

Since BCC is not a melanocytic lesion, we rarely observe pigment network (Figs. 5.69 and 5.70); nevertheless, its absence does not rule BCC out. In consequence, besides the lack of pigment network, it is necessary to detect some of the following criteria:

- *Vascular pattern*: This can be the only criterion present in nonpigmented BCC. It is characterized by the presence of two vessel types.
  - Thick vessels with numerous branching, or arborizing vessels (Figs. 5.71 to 5.73)
  - Narrow truncated vessels (Figs. 5.74 to 5.78)

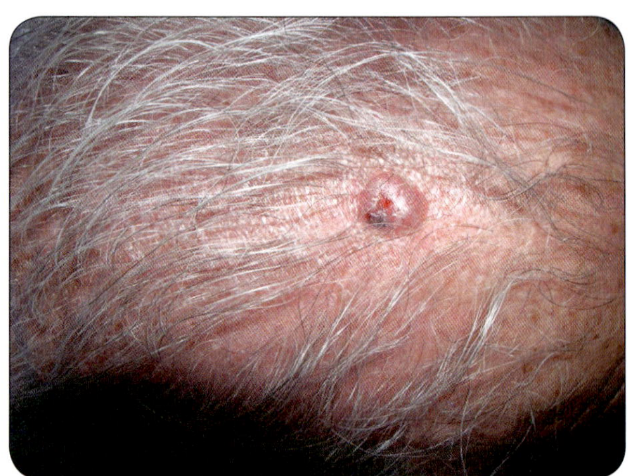

Fig. 5.63: Basal cell carcinoma clinical image.

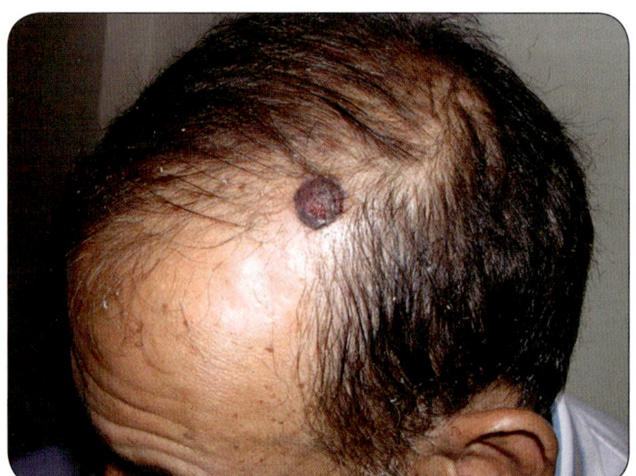

Fig. 5.64: Clinical image of a pigmented basal cell carcinoma.

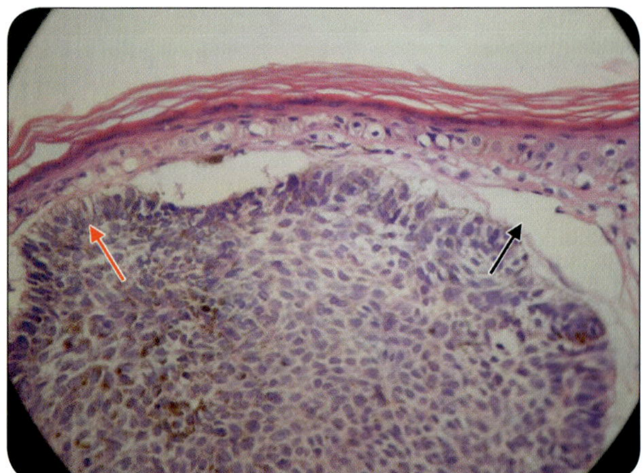

Fig. 5.65: Histological image showing the basaloid cell strings distributed in the periphery forming a palisade (red arrow) and fibrovascular stroma with abundant mucin surrounding the tumor (black arrow).

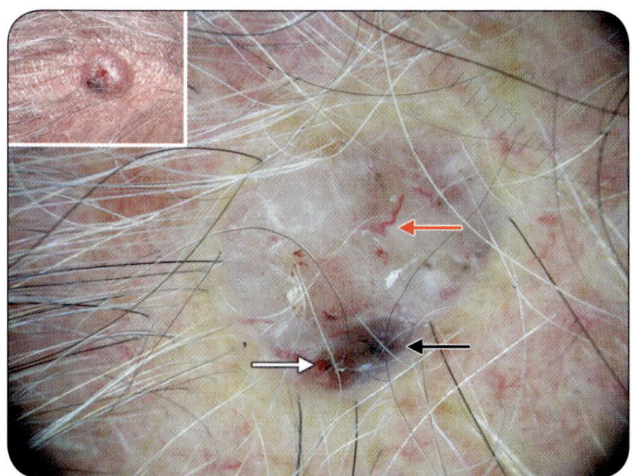

Fig. 5.66: Basal cell carcinoma with the three major criteria: arborizing vessels (red arrow), blue-gray pigmentation (black arrow), ulceration (white arrow).

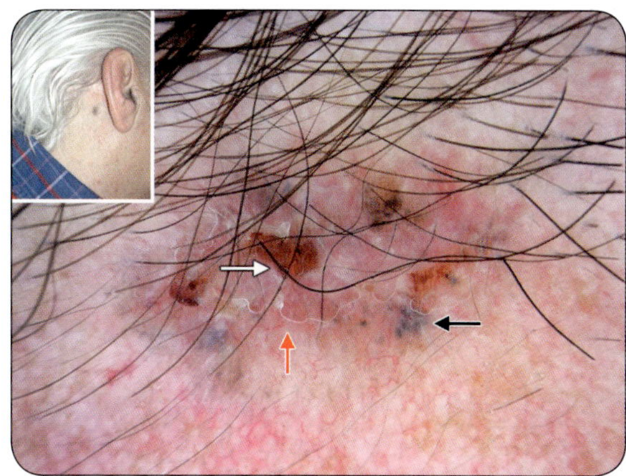

Fig. 5.67: Basal cell carcinoma with the three major criteria: arborizing vessels (red arrow), blue-gray pigmentation (black arrow), ulceration (white arrow).

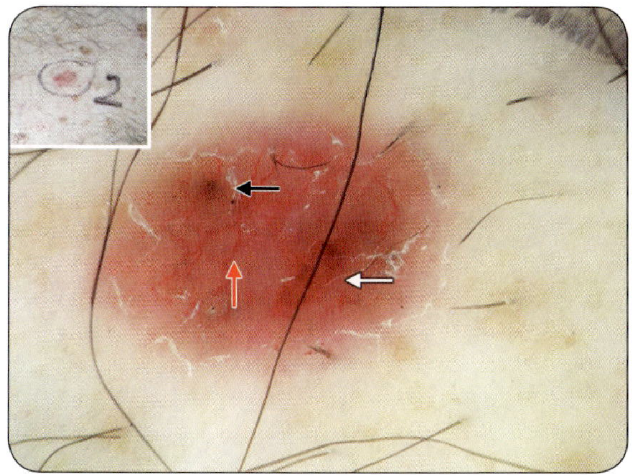

Fig. 5.68: Basal cell carcinoma with the three major criteria: arborizing vessels (red arrow), blue-gray pigmentation (black arrow), ulceration (white arrow).

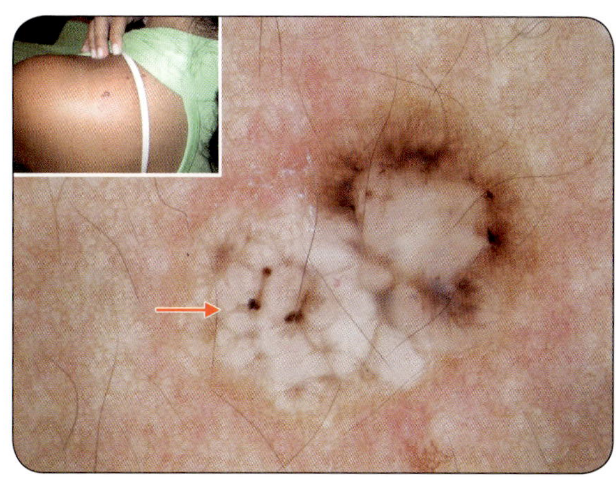

Fig. 5.69: Basal cell carcinoma with pigment network (arrow).

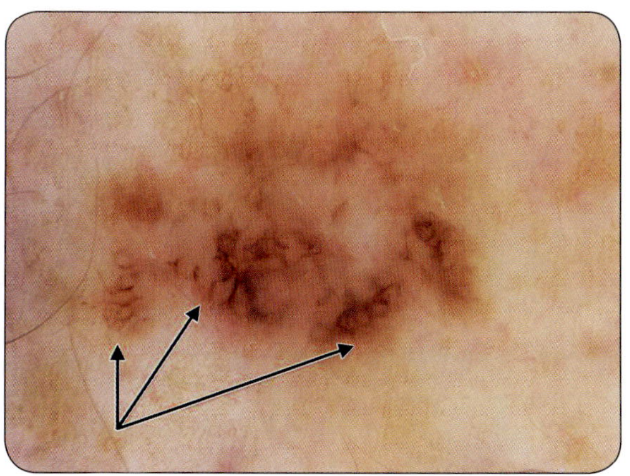

Fig. 5.70: Basal cell carcinoma with pigment network (arrows).

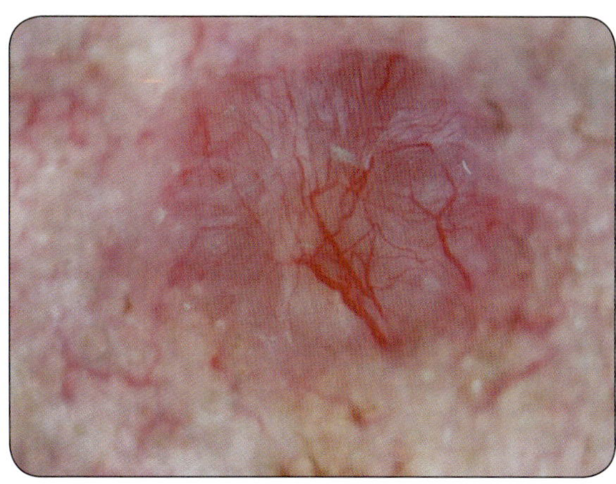

Fig. 5.71: Basal cell carcinoma. Arborizing vessels.

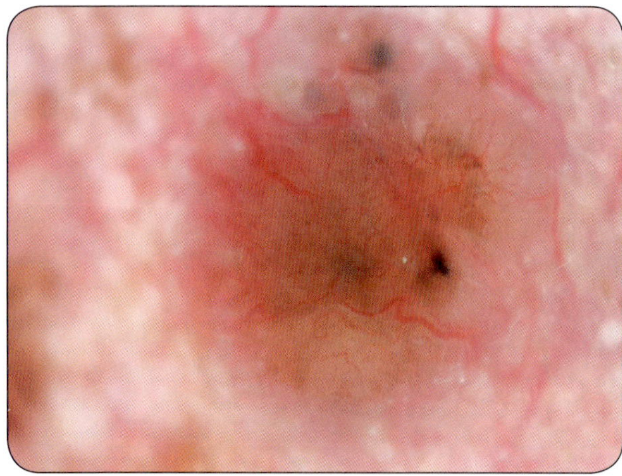

Fig. 5.72: Basal cell carcinoma. Arborizing vessels.

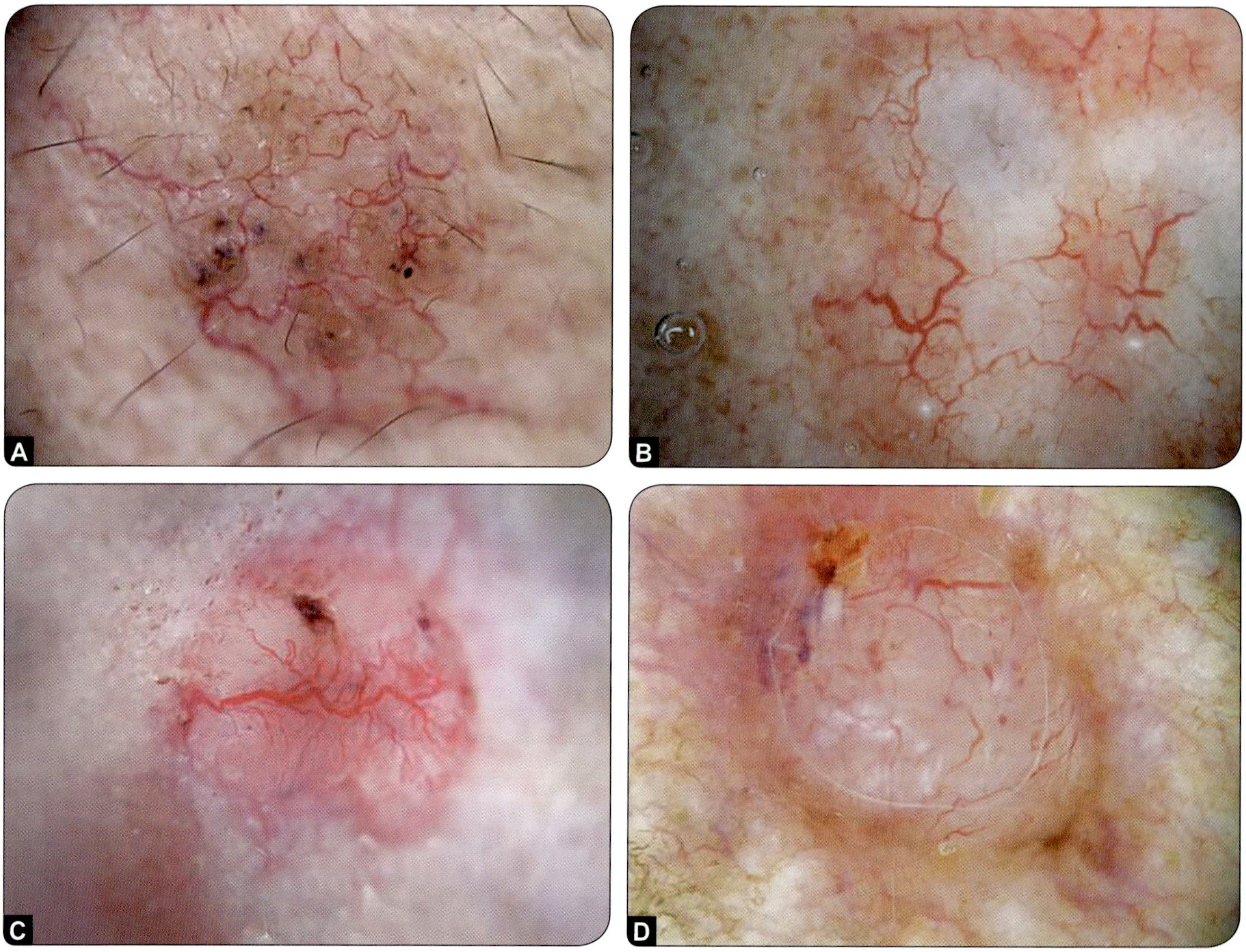

Figs. 5.73A to D: Basal cell carcinoma. Arborizing vessels.

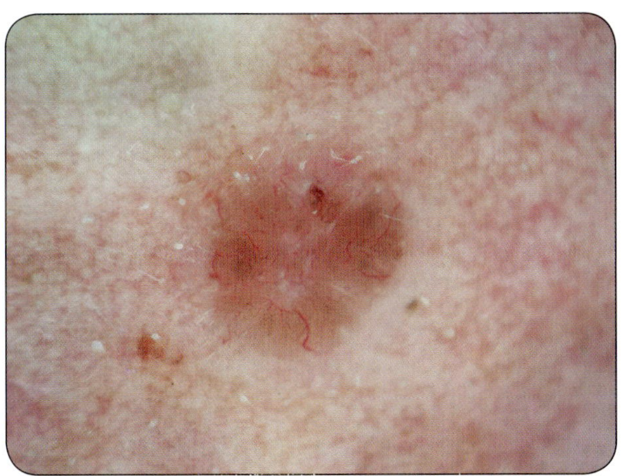

Fig. 5.74: Basal cell carcinoma. Narrow truncated vessels or narrow short telangiectasia.

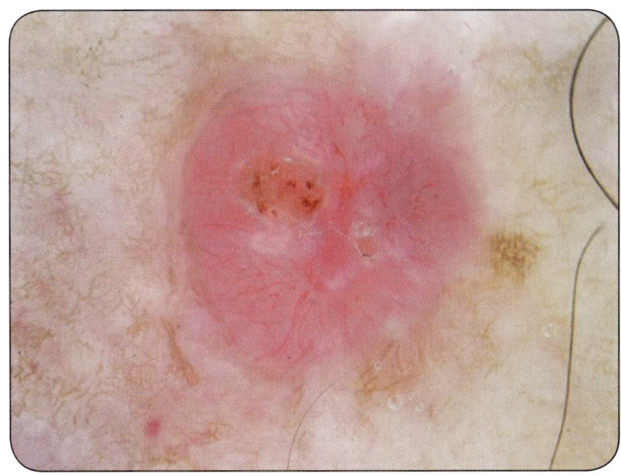

Fig. 5.75: Basal cell carcinoma. Narrow truncated vessels or narrow short telangiectasia.

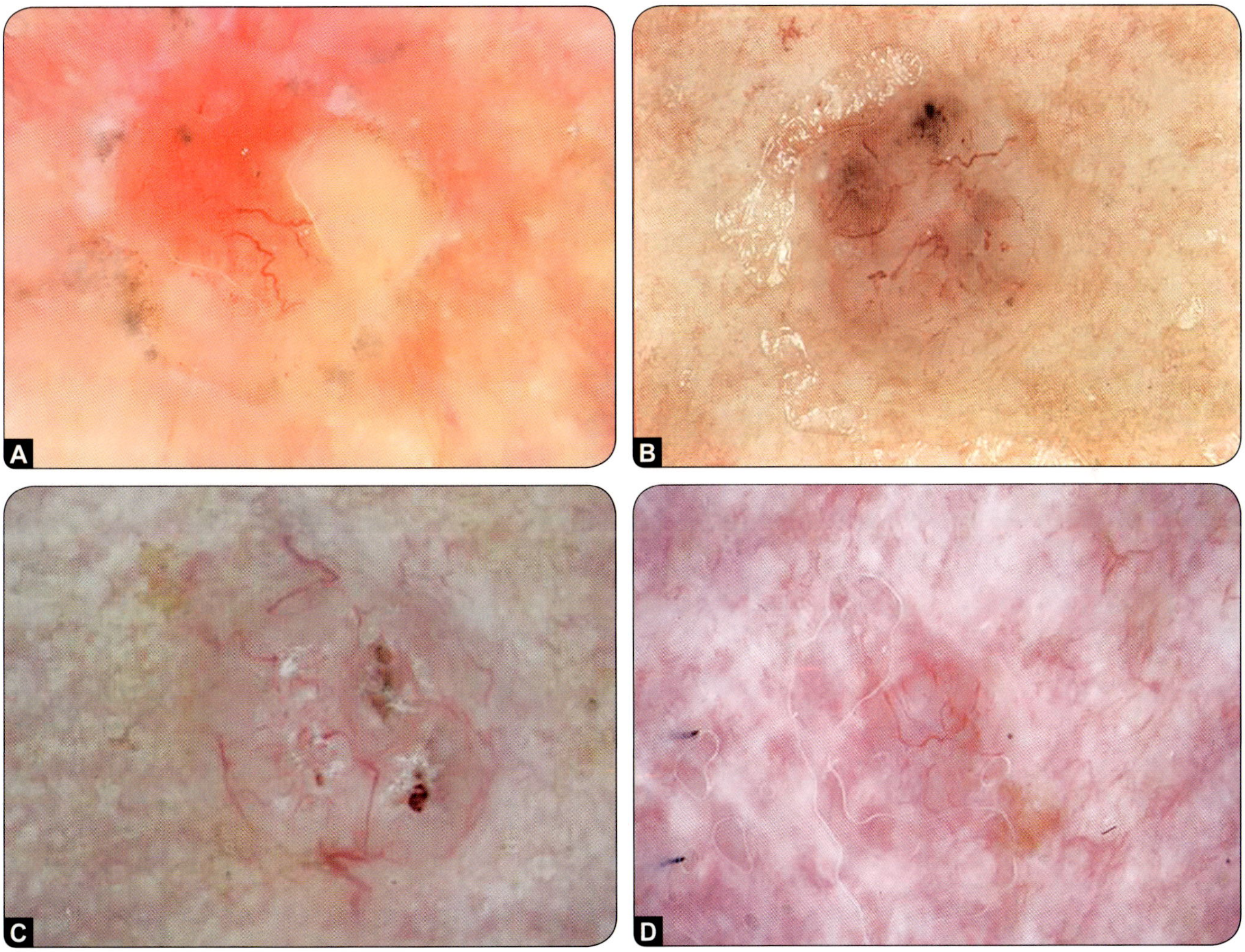

Figs. 5.76A to D: Basal cell carcinoma. Narrow truncated vessels or narrow short telangiectasia.

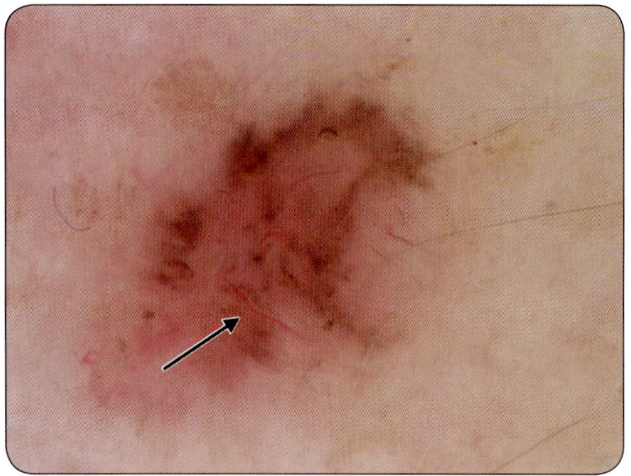

Fig. 5.77: Basal cell carcinoma. Narrow truncated vessels or narrow short telangiectasia (arrow).

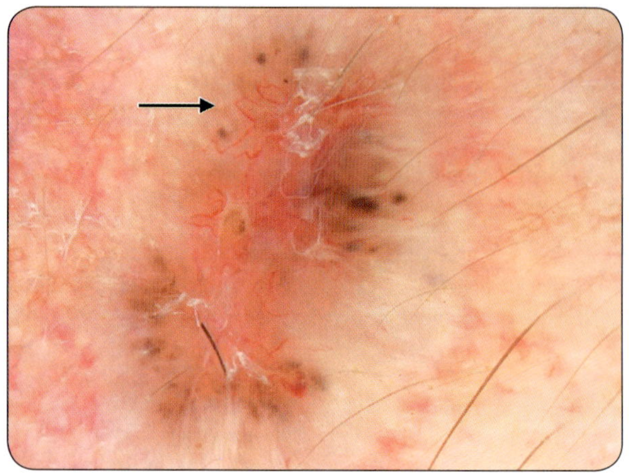

Fig. 5.78: Basal cell carcinoma. Narrow truncated vessels or narrow short telangiectasia (arrow).

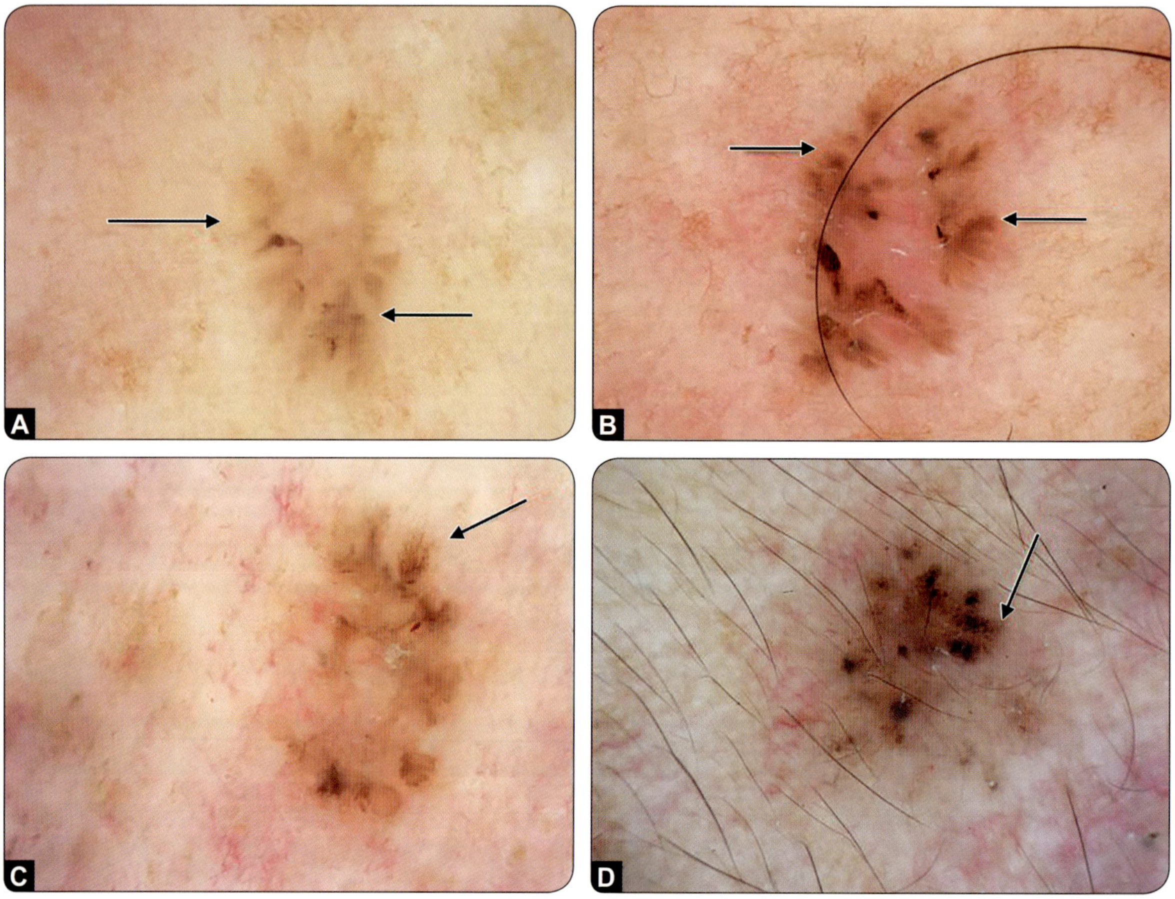

Figs. 5.79A to D: Basal cell carcinoma. Leaf-like structures (arrows).

- *Blue-gray pigmentation:* Depending on the pigment distribution in the lesion, we can observe the following structures:
  - *Leaf-like structures* (Figs. 5.79 to 5.83): Also known as maple-leaf structures. They are usually located in the periphery of the lesion, blue-gray in color and observable in pigmented BCCs.

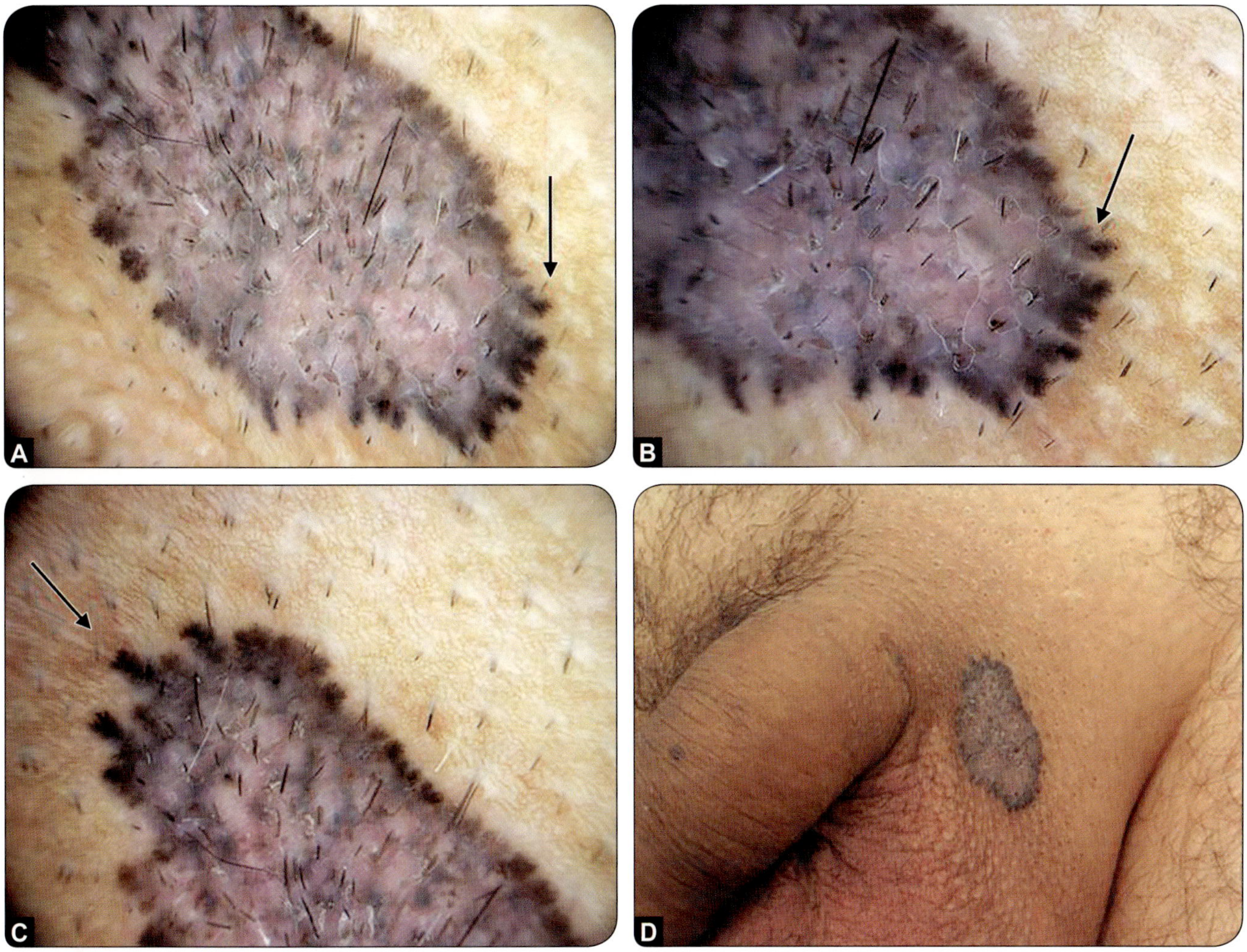

Figs. 5.80A to D: Basal cell carcinoma. Leaf-like structures (arrows).

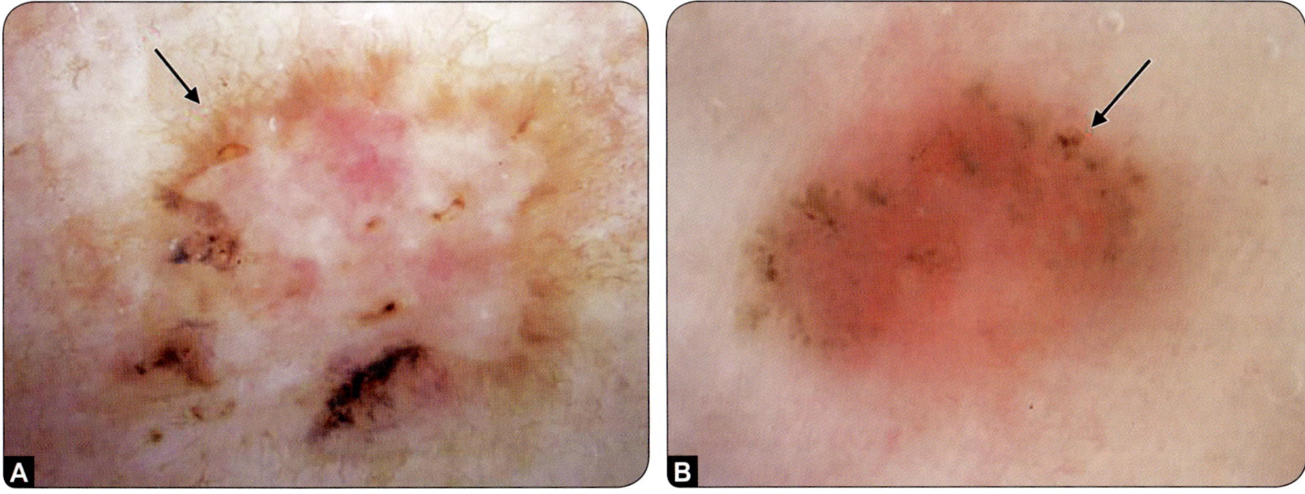

Figs. 5.81A and B

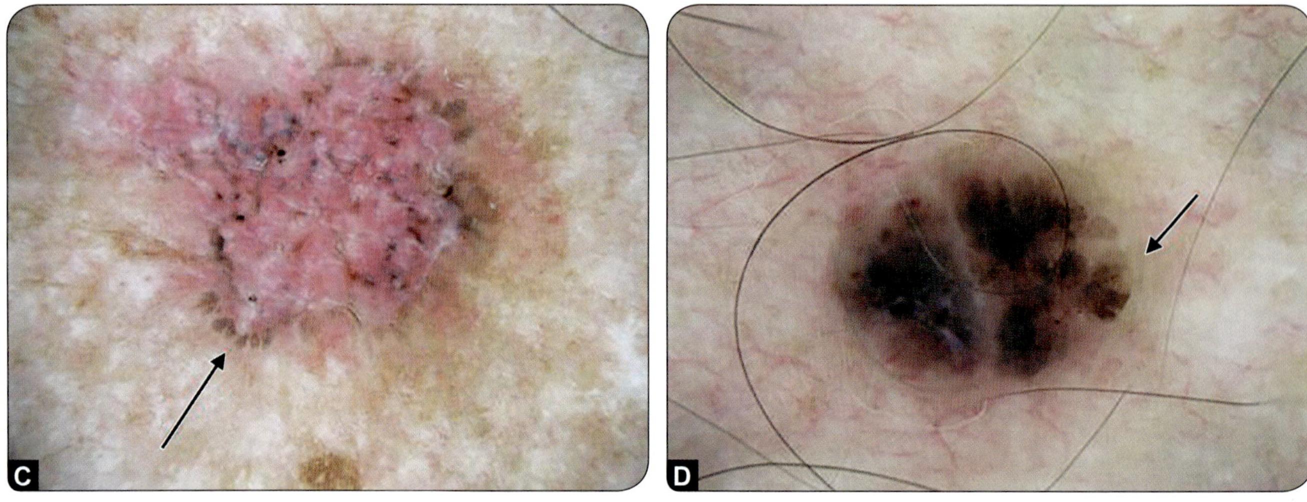

Figs. 5.81A to D: Basal cell carcinoma. Leaf-like structures (arrows).

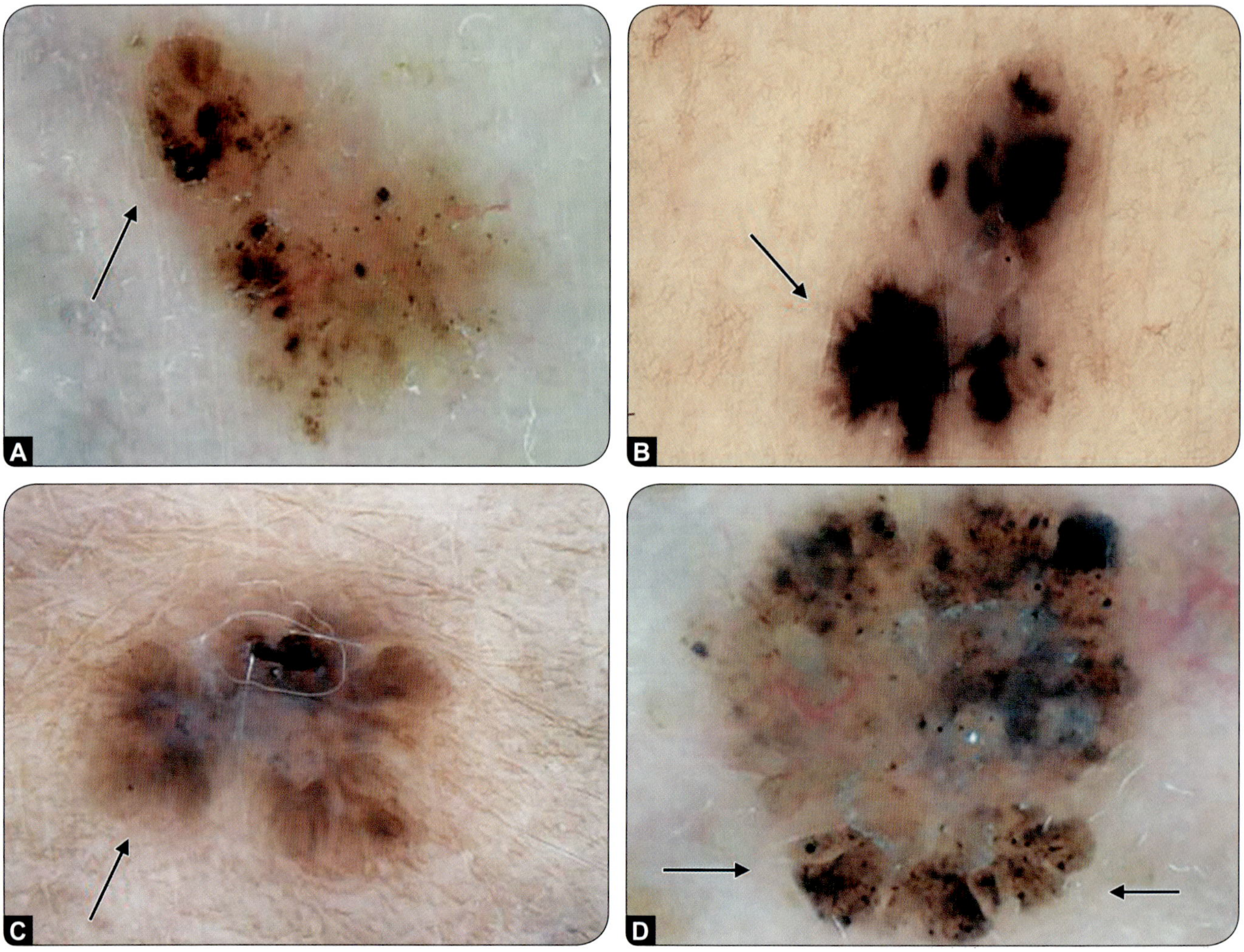

Figs. 5.82A to D: Basal cell carcinoma. Leaf-like structures (arrows).

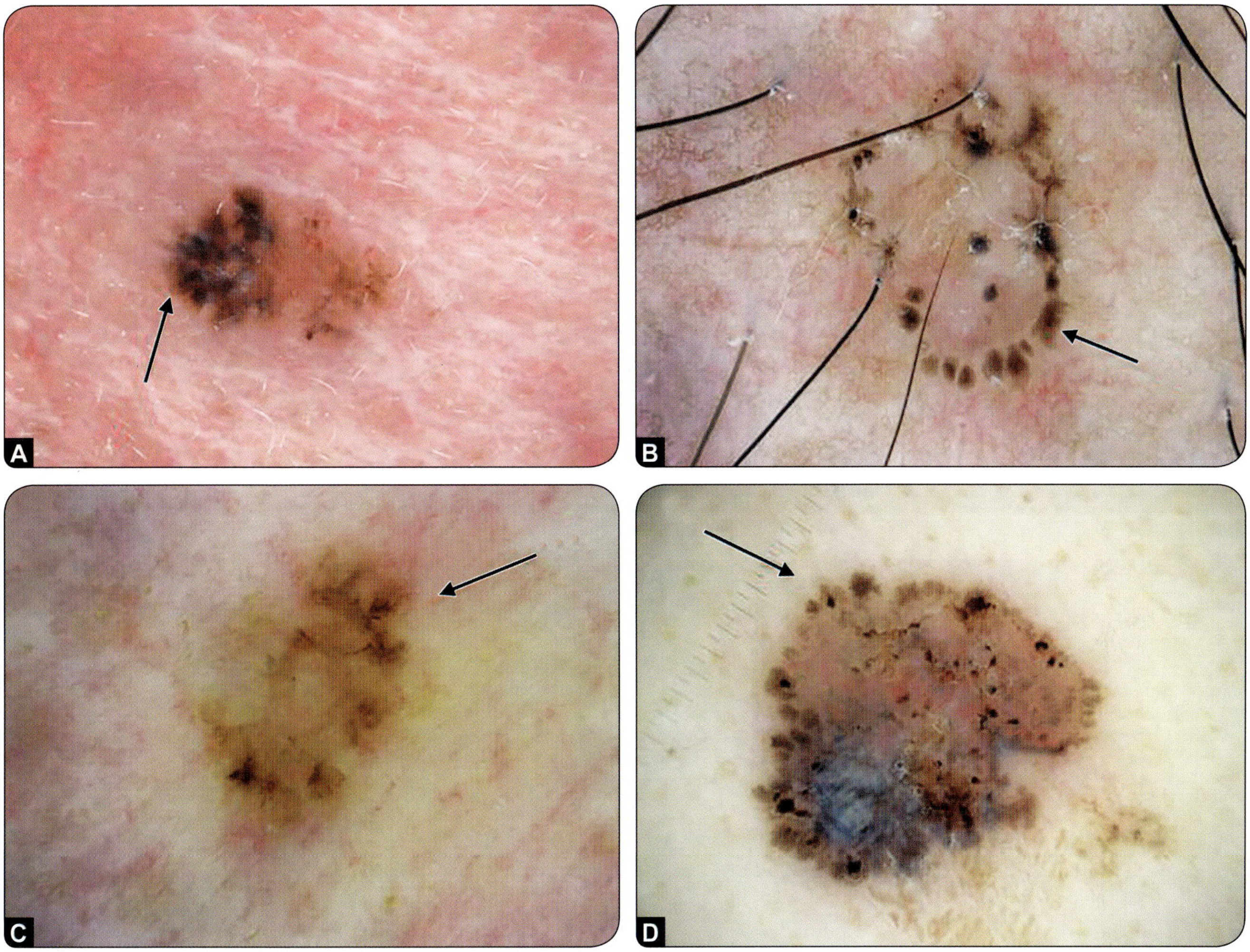

Figs. 5.83A to D: Basal cell carcinoma. Leaf-like structures (arrows).

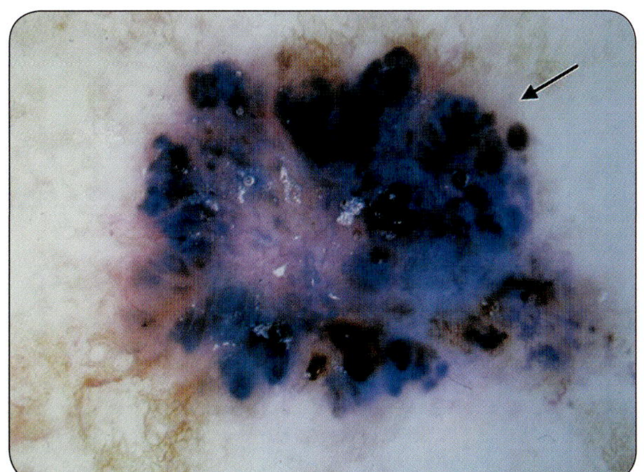

Fig. 5.84: Basal cell carcinoma. Large blue-gray ovoid nests or globules (arrow).

Histologically they are the result of melanin pigment due to hyperplastic melanocytes.

- *Large blue-gray ovoid nests or globules*: These are also due to an increase in melanin and to hyperplastic melanocytes. They are globular or ovoid formations with sharp edges and homogeneous coloration (Figs. 5.84 to 5.88).
- *Multiple blue-gray globules*: These have the same origin as the structures previously mentioned, but are smaller in size (Figs. 5.89 and 5.90).
- *Spoke-wheel areas or radial areas*: These are well-circumscribed radial projections, brown, blue, or gray in color, projecting from a central axis, generally darker (Figs. 5.91 to 5.94).

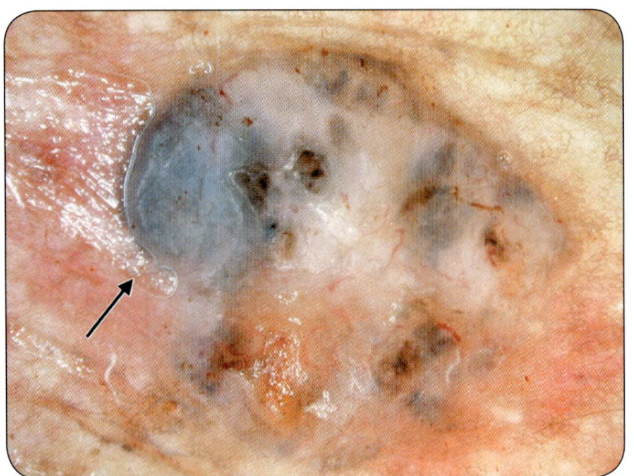

Fig. 5.85: Basal cell carcinoma. Large blue-gray ovoid nests or globules (arrow).

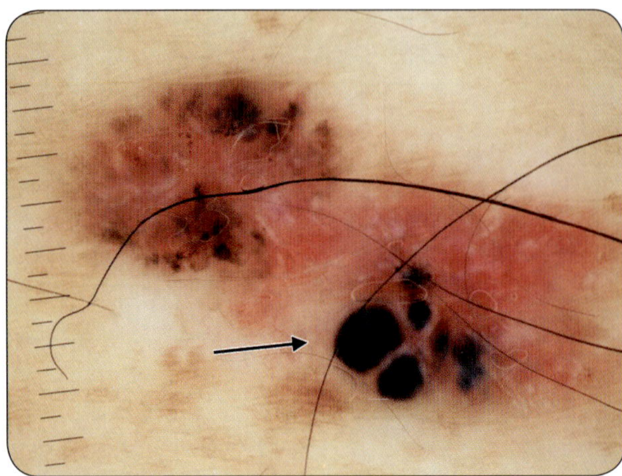

Fig. 5.86: Basal cell carcinoma. Large blue-gray ovoid nests or globules (arrow).

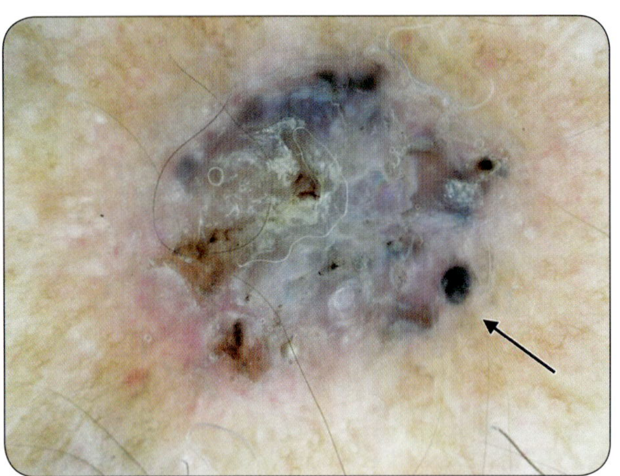

Fig. 5.87: Basal cell carcinoma. Large blue-gray ovoid nests or globules (arrow).

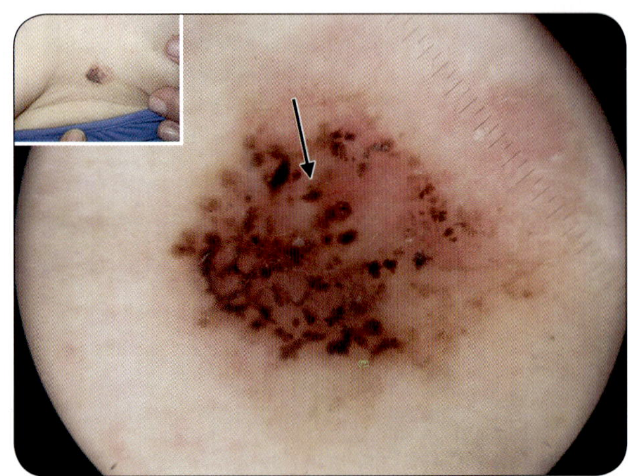

Fig. 5.88: Basal cell carcinoma. Large blue-gray ovoid nests or globules (arrow).

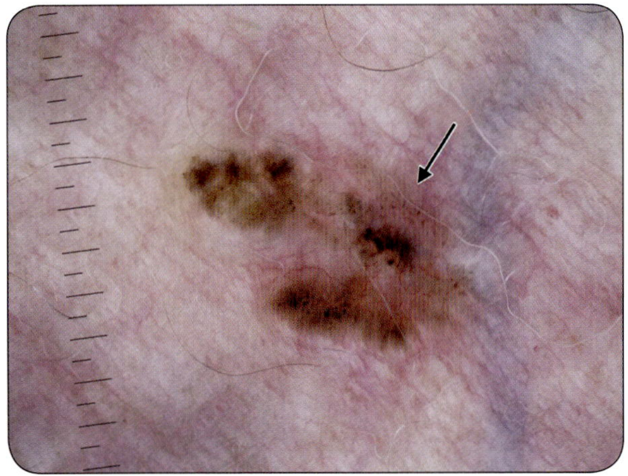

Fig. 5.89: Basal cell carcinoma. Multiple blue-gray globules (arrow).

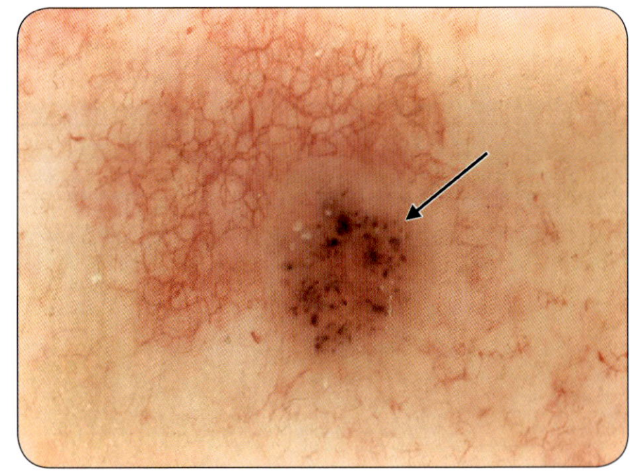

Fig. 5.90: Basal cell carcinoma. Multiple blue-gray globules (arrow).

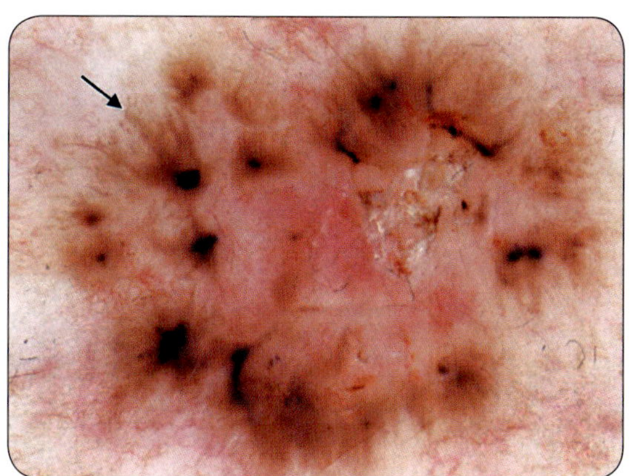

Fig. 5.91: Basal cell carcinoma. Spoke-wheel areas (arrow).

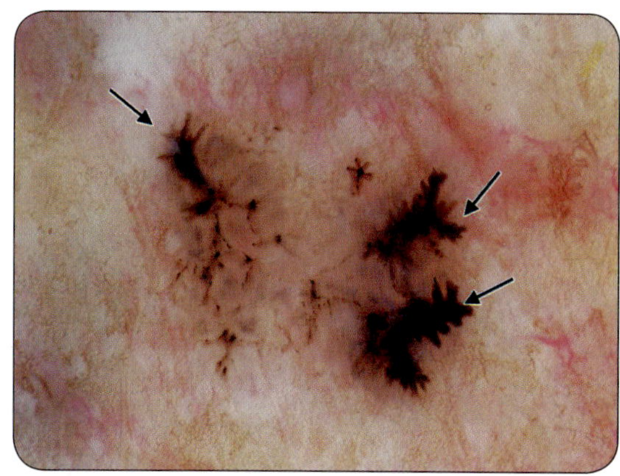

Fig. 5.92: Basal cell carcinoma. Spoke-wheel areas (arrows).

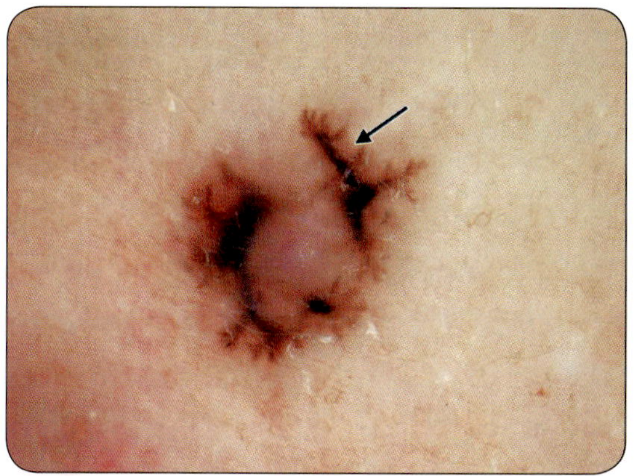

Fig. 5.93: Basal cell carcinoma. Spoke-wheel areas (arrow).

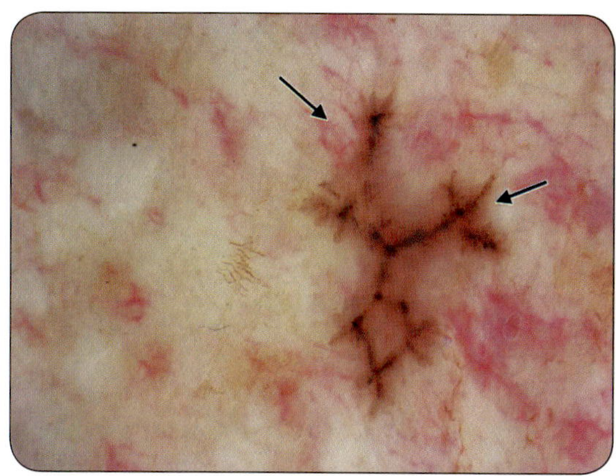

Fig. 5.94: Basal cell carcinoma. Spoke-wheel areas (arrows).

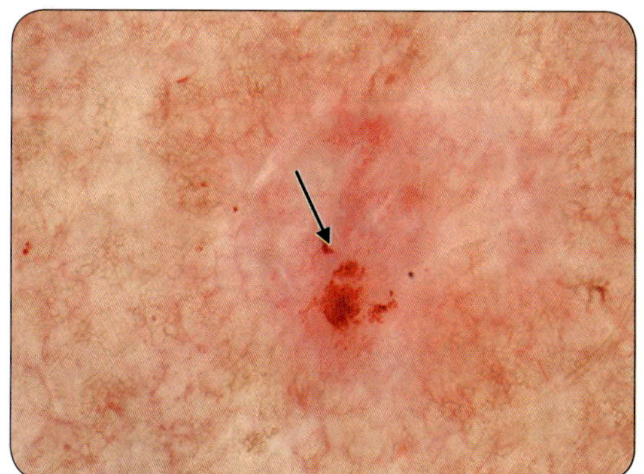

Fig. 5.95: Basal cell carcinoma. Ulceration (arrow).

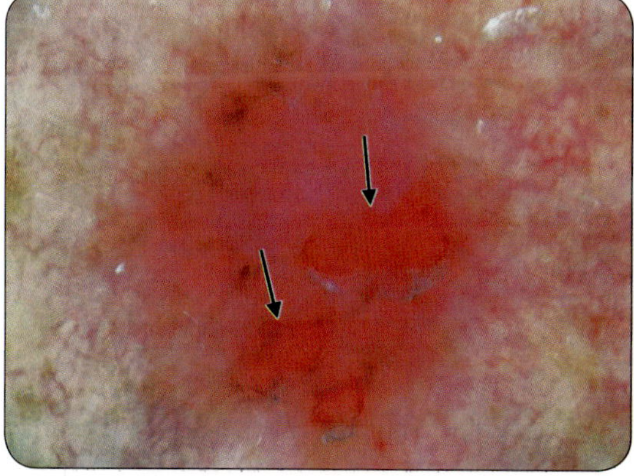

Fig. 5.96: Basal cell carcinoma. Ulceration (arrows).

- *Ulcerations*: These can be single or multiple and in different sizes. Their coloration can be red, blue, or black, depending on tumor pigmentation (Figs. 5.95 to 5.99).

If the aforementioned criteria are employed in the course of the elaboration of the BCC dermoscopic diagnosis, the sensitivity of the method is 93%, while the specificity is 89%.

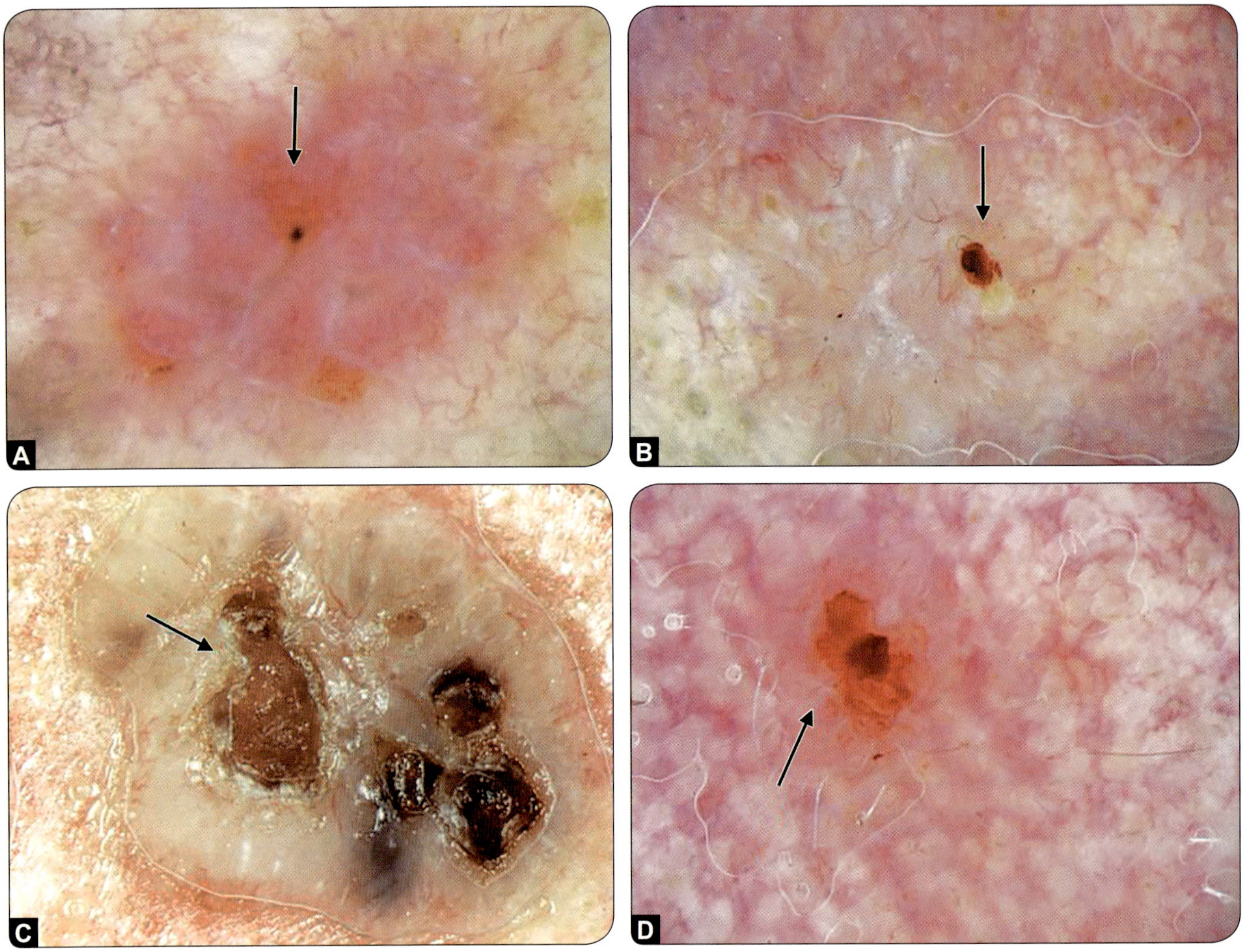

Figs. 5.97A to D: Basal cell carcinoma. Ulceration (arrows).

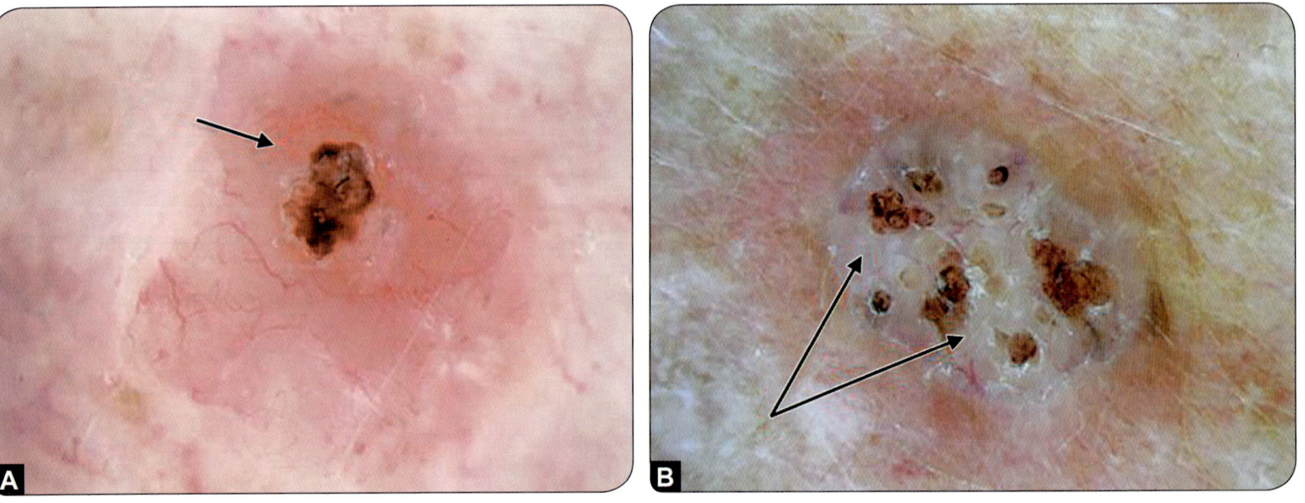

Figs. 5.98A and B

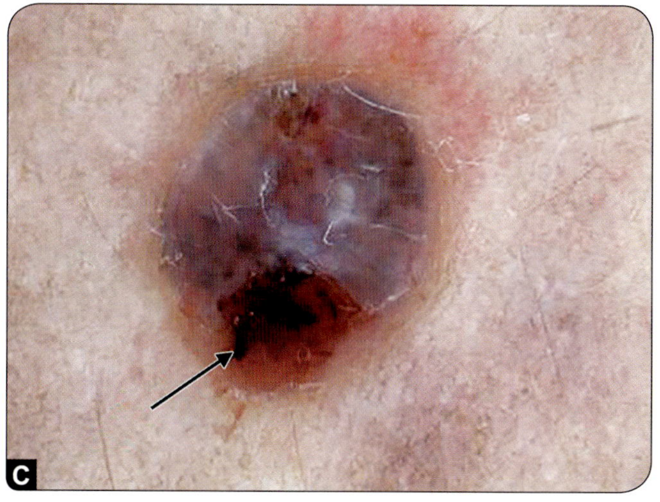

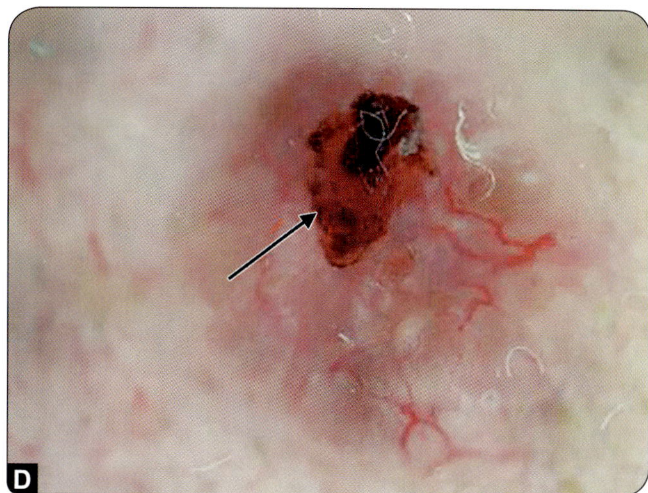

Figs. 5.98A to D: Basal cell carcinoma. Ulceration (arrows).

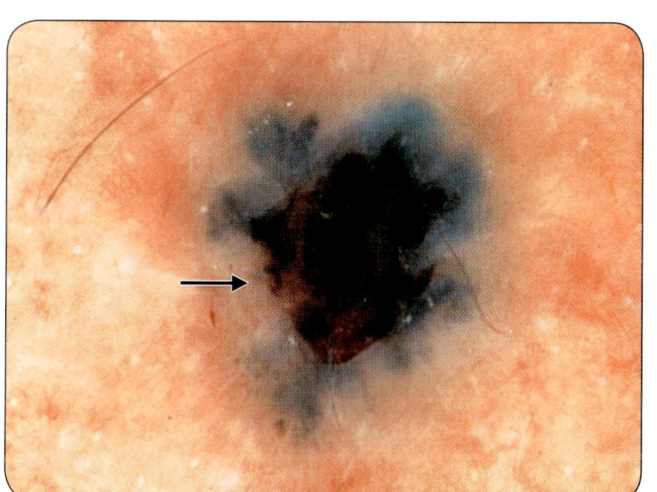

Fig. 5.99: Basal cell carcinoma. Ulceration (arrow).

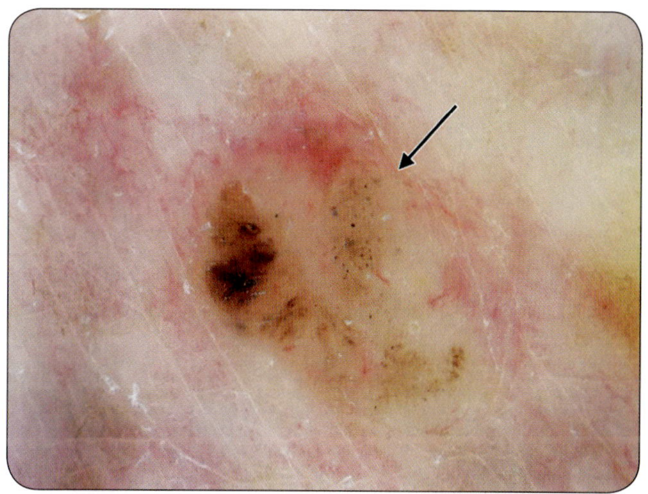

Fig. 5.100: Basal cell carcinoma multiple blue-gray dots (arrow).

Nonclassic Criteria

These criteria, like the classic ones, are related to pigmentation, vessels, and the loss of cutaneous surface.

- Blue-gray pigmentation
  - *Multiple focalized blue-gray dots*: Very small areas with blue-gray pigment (Figs. 5.100 and 5.101).
  - *Concentric structures*: Round areas with a darker center (Figs. 5.102 to 5.106).
- Narrow short telangiectasia (*see* Figs. 5.74 to 5.78)
- Small multiple erosions (Figs. 5.107 and 5.108) (Table 5.1)

Criteria Similar to those of Melanocytic Lesions

Highly pigmented BCCs, or those observed in people of very dark skin, may present dermoscopic characteristics similar to the dermoscopy criteria of melanocytic lesions. These true melanoma simulators often force us to perform a histopathologic study (Fig. 5.109; Table 5.2):

- Multiple dots/brown-black globules (Fig. 5.110)
- Structures similar to blue-white veil (*see* Fig. 5.84)
- Nonarborizing vessels (Fig. 5.111)
- Pigment network (*see* Figs. 5.69 and 5.70)

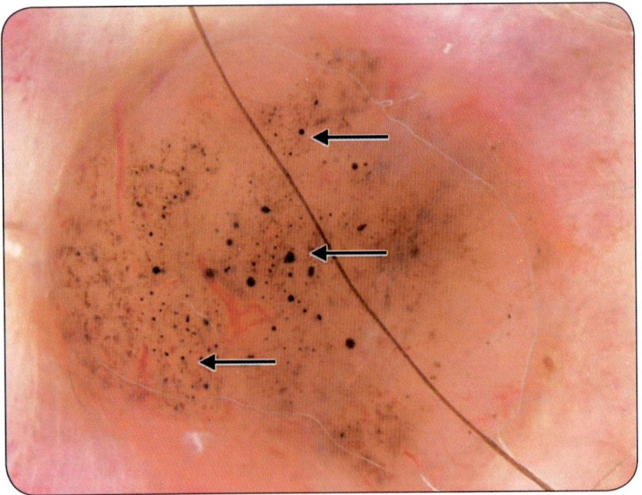

Fig. 5.101: Basal cell carcinoma multiple blue-gray dots (arrows).

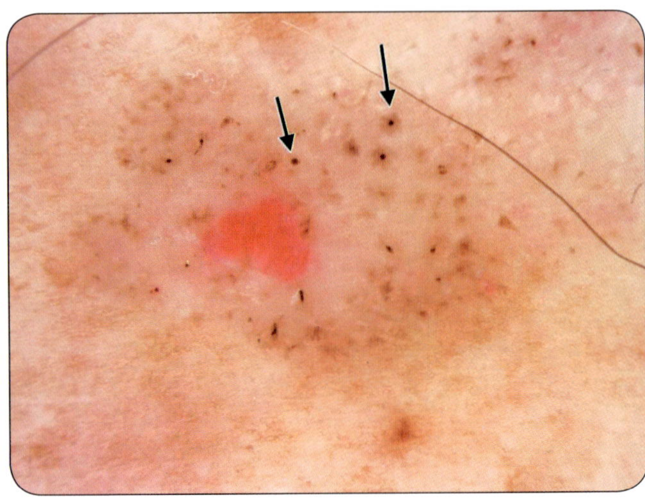

Fig. 5.102: Basal cell carcinoma concentric structures (arrows).

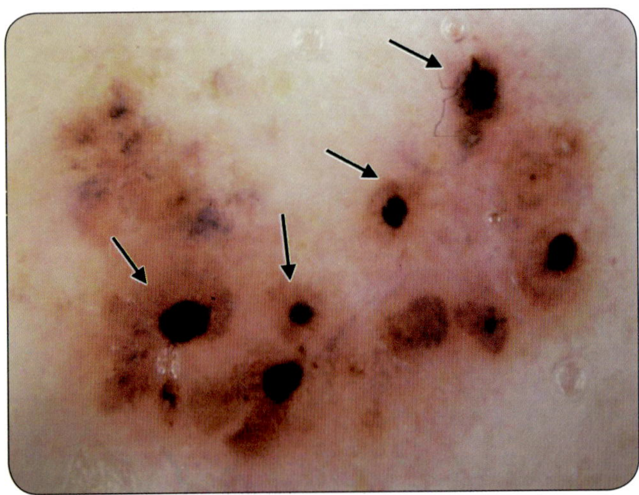

Fig. 5.103: Basal cell carcinoma concentric structures (arrows).

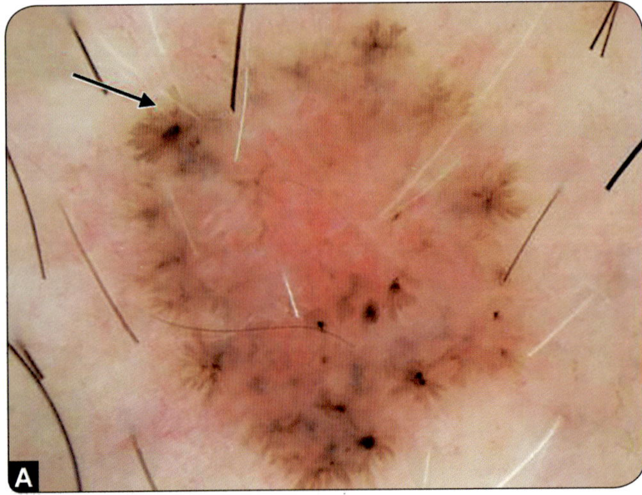

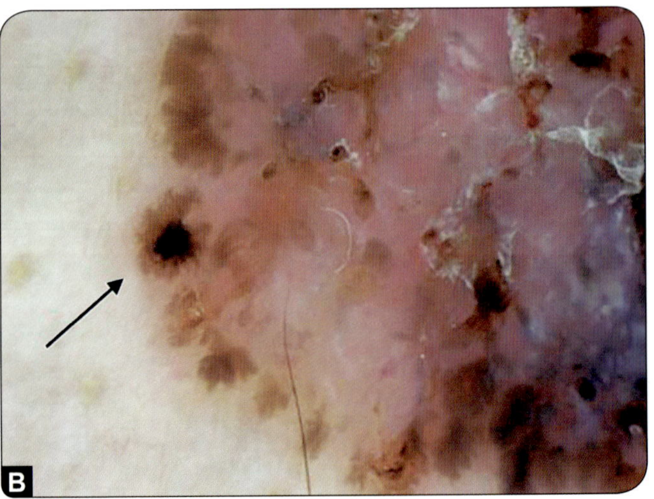

Figs. 5.104A and B

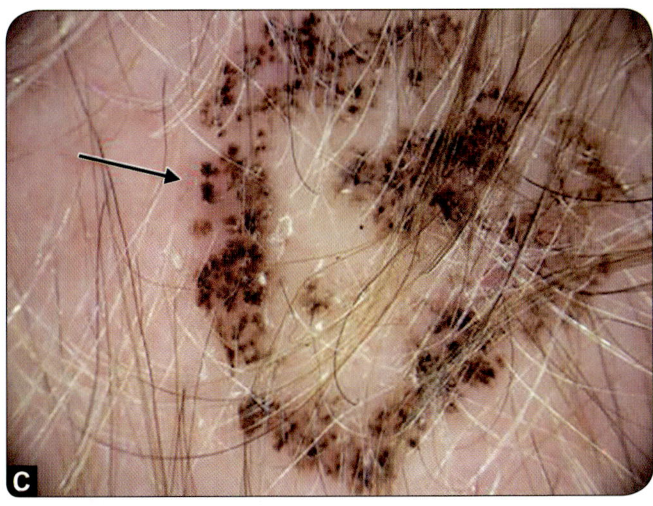

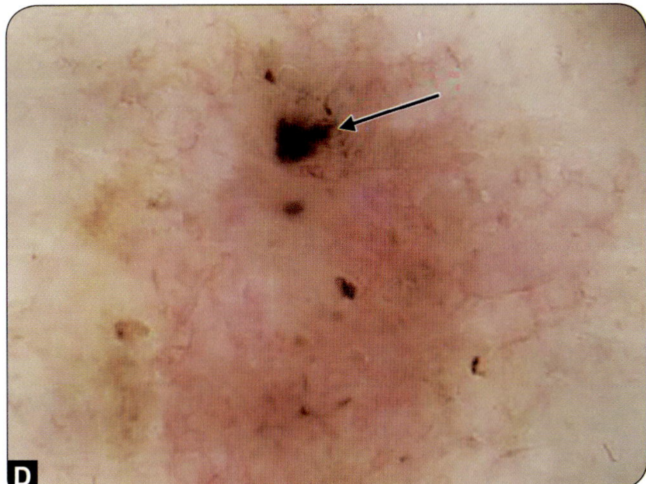

Figs. 5.104A to D: Basal cell carcinoma concentric structures (arrows).

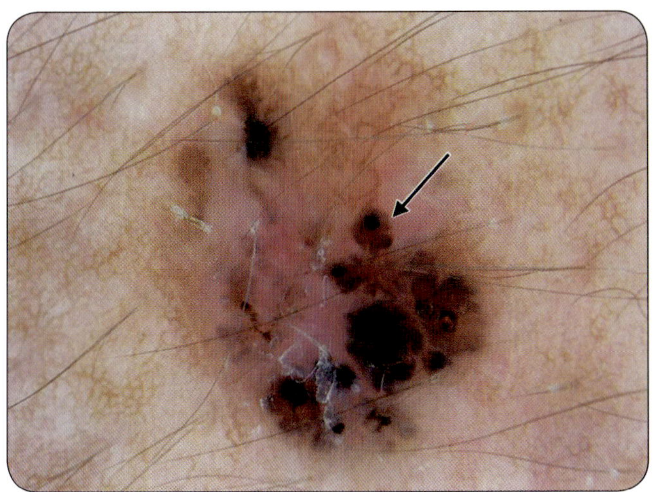

Fig. 5.105: Basal cell carcinoma concentric structures (arrow).

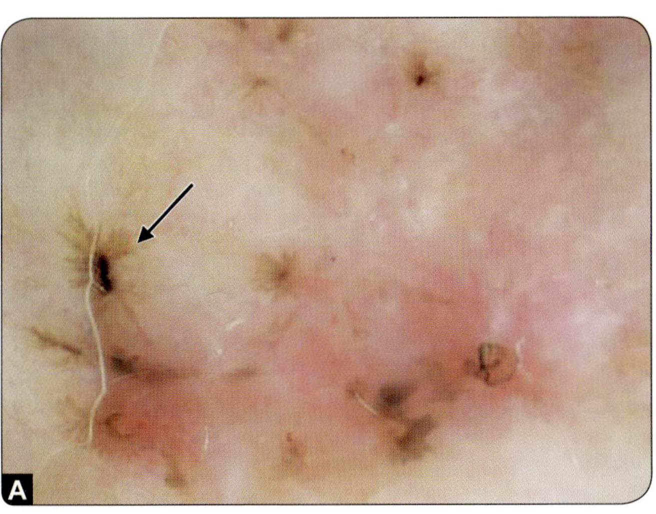

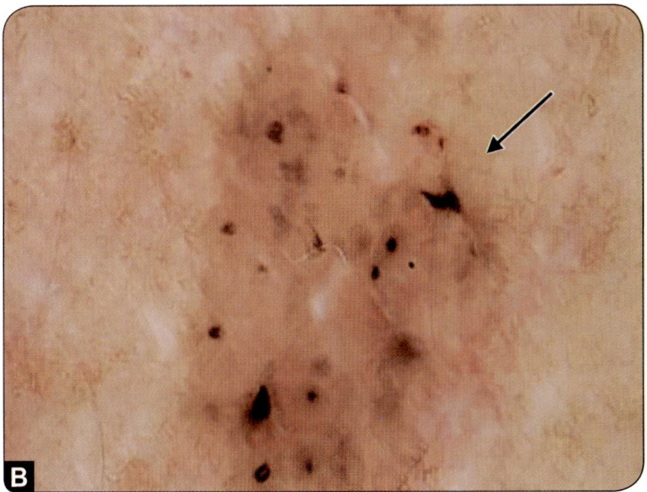

Figs. 5.106A and B

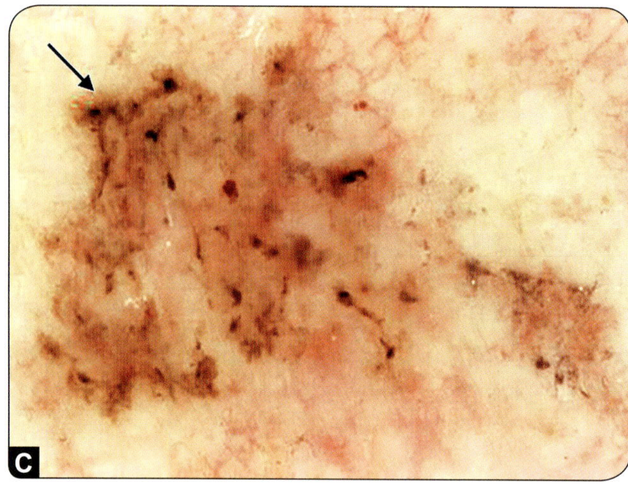

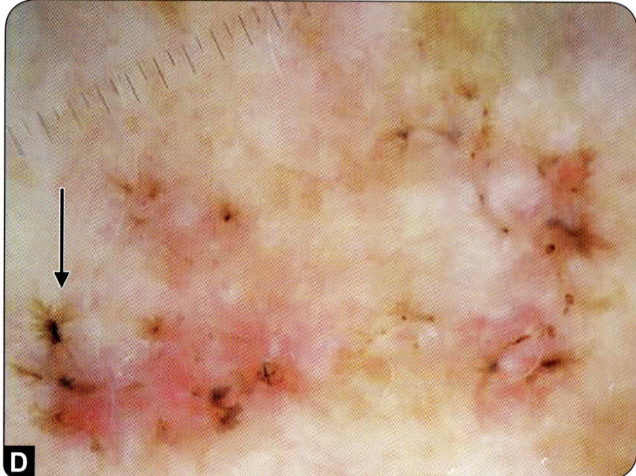

Figs. 5.106A to D: Basal cell carcinoma concentric structures (arrows).

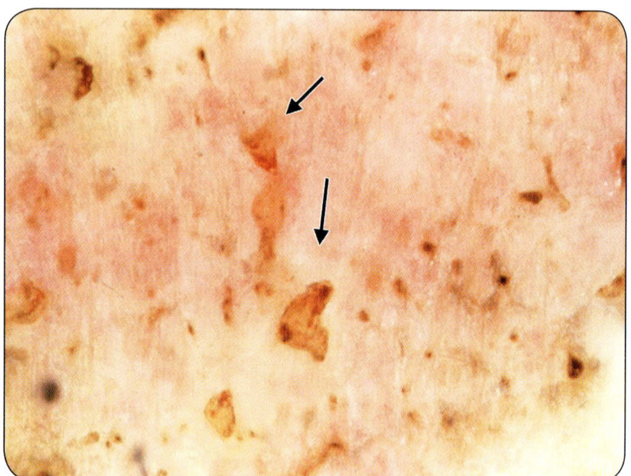

Fig. 5.107: Basal cell carcinoma small multiple erosions (arrows).

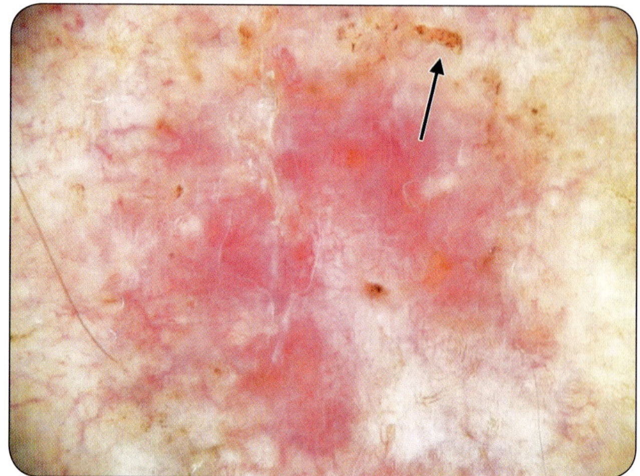

Fig. 5.108: Basal cell carcinoma small multiple erosions (arrow).

Table 5.1: Basal cell carcinoma.

Classic patterns	*Nonclassic patterns*
Blue-gray pigmentation	Blue-gray pigmentation
• Leaf-like structures	• Multiple focalized blue-gray dots
• Large blue-gray ovoid nests	• Concentric structures
• Multiple blue-gray globules	
• Spoke-wheel areas	
Arborizing vessels	Narrow short telangiectasia
Ulceration	Multiple small erosions

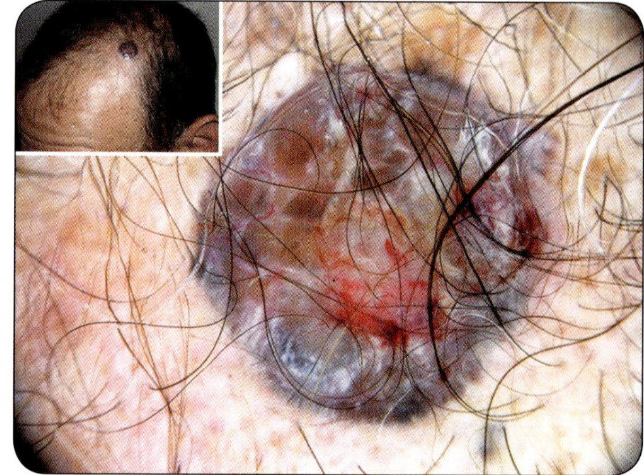

Fig. 5.109: Clinical and dermoscopic images of a pigmented basal cell carcinoma simulating a melanoma.

Table 5.2: Basal cell carcinoma.
Criteria similar to those of melanocytic lesions
• Multiple Brown-black dots/globules
• Structures resembling blue-white veil
• Nonarborizing vessels
• Pigment network
• Multiple blue-gray dots (pepper-like)
• Radial projections or pseudopods

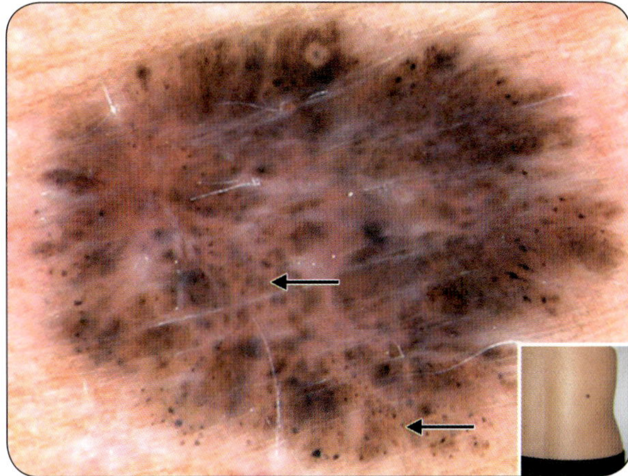

Fig. 5.110: Basal cell carcinoma: multiple dots/brown-black globules (arrows).

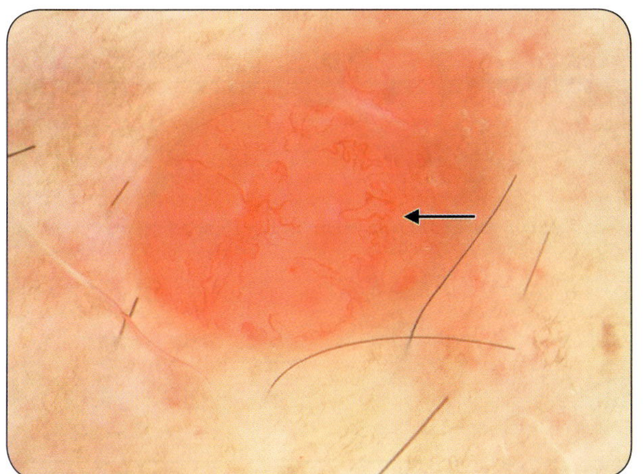

Fig. 5.111: Basal cell carcinoma with nonarborizing vessels (arrow).

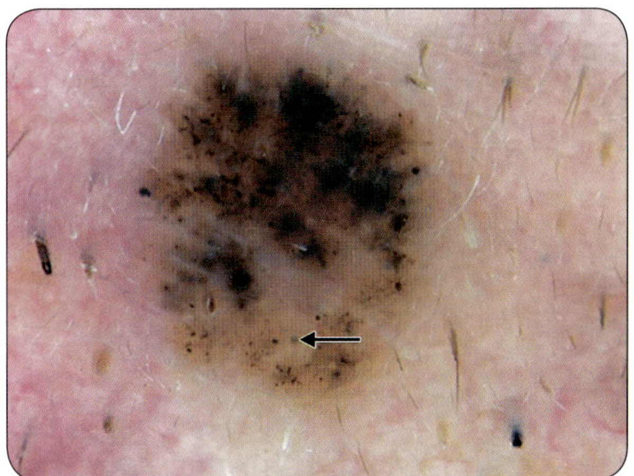

Fig. 5.112: Basal cell carcinoma with multiple blue-gray dots (pepper-like) (arrow).

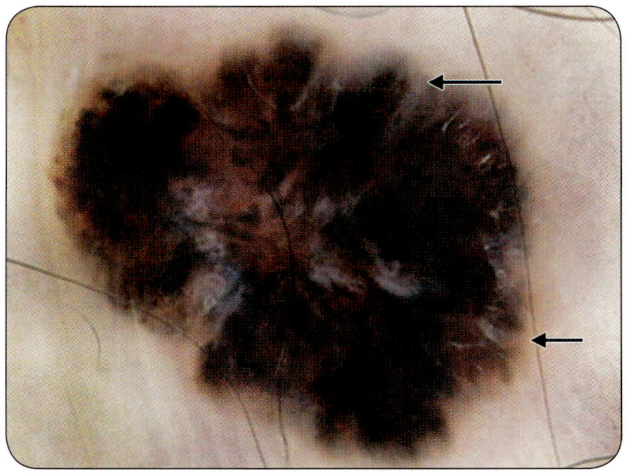

Fig. 5.113: Basal cell carcinoma with radial projections or pseudopods (arrows).

- Multiple blue-gray dots (pepper-like) (Fig. 5.112)
- Radial projections or pseudopods (Fig. 5.113 and Table 5.2)

White shiny or crystalline structures: These have been described in recent years (Figs. 5.114 to 5.116):

- They are bright lineal streaks of pearly white color.
- They are invisible to the naked eye or the nonpolarized light of the dermatoscope.
- Observable in lesions with an increased amount of collagen. The collagen streaks are birefringent, causing a quick randomization of the polarized light.
- It is a dynamic polarized dermoscopy:
  - By rotating the dermoscope but keeping it in contact with the cutaneous surface, the direction of the crystalline structures can be changed.

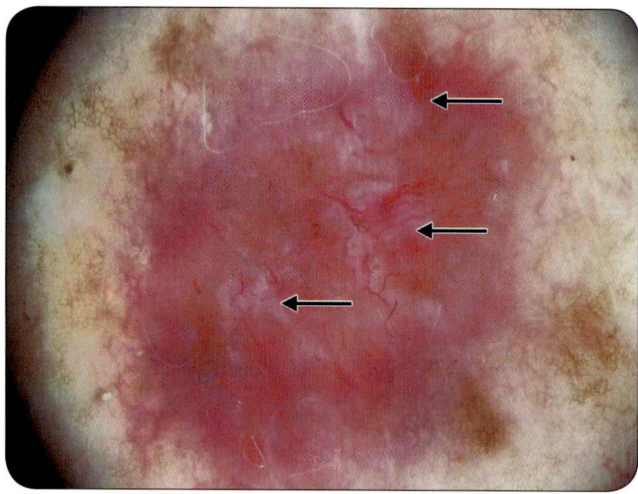

Fig. 5.114: Basal cell carcinoma with white shiny or crystalline structures (arrows).

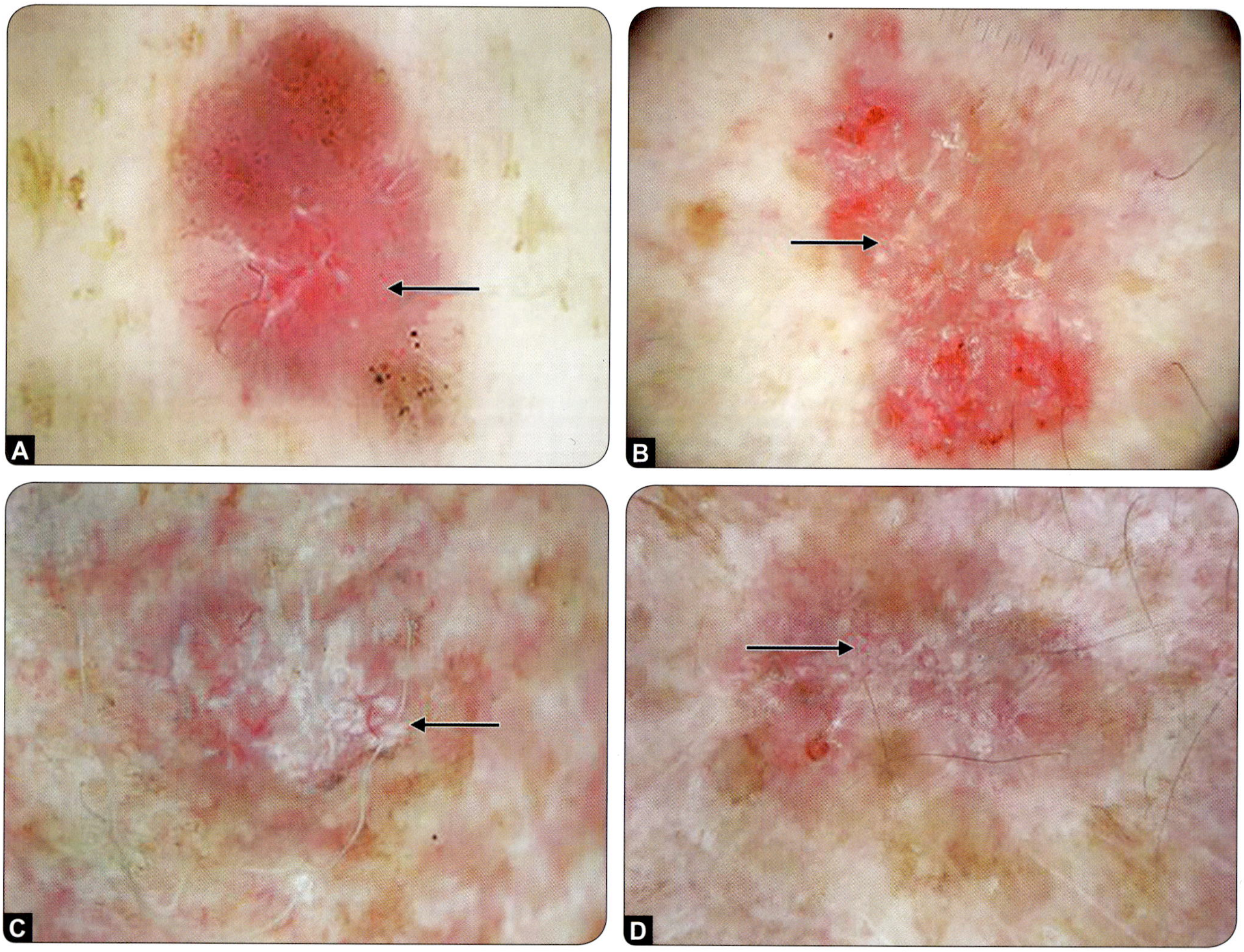

Figs. 5.115A to D: Basal cell carcinoma with white shiny or crystalline structures (arrows).

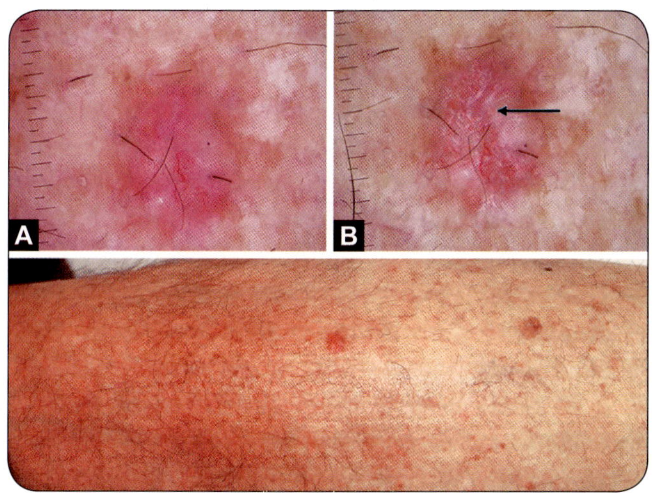

Figs. 5.116A and B: Basal cell carcinoma: (A) image captured with nonpolarized light—no crystalline structures are observed; (B) image captured with polarized light where crystalline structures are observed (arrow).

- Because of the angular dependence of the polarized light, reflecting the nonrandom distribution of the collagen fibers in the dermis.

- They can be found in any type of BCC and also in dermatofibroma, melanoma, Spitz nevus, and scars.

SUGGESTED READING

Argenziano G, Soyer P, De Giorgio V, et al. Interactive Atlas of Dermoscopy. Milán: EDRA Medical Publishing & New Media; 2000.

Altamura D, Menzies S, Argenziano G, et al. Dermatoscopy of basal cell carcinoma: Morphologic variability of global and local features and accuracy of diagnosis. J Am Acad Dermatol. 2010;62:67-75.

Balagula Y, Braun RP, Rabinovitz HS, et al. The significance of crystalline/chrysalis structures in the diagnosis of melanocytic and nonmelanocytic lesions. J Am Acad Dermatol. 2012;67:194.e1-8.

Cabo H. Dermatoscopia. Buenos Aires, Argentina: Weber Ferro; 2000.

Cabo H. Dermatoscopia, 2nd edition. Buenos Aires, Argentina: Ediciones Journal; 2012.

Felder S, Rabinovitz H, Oliviero M, et al. Dermoscopic pattern of pigmented basal cell carcinoma, blue-white variant. Dermatol Surg. 2006;32:569-70.

Giacomel J, Zalaudek I. Dermoscopy of superficial basal cell carcinoma. Dermatol Surg. 2005;31:1710-3.

Jorh R, Soyer P, Argenziano G, et al. Dermoscopy. The Essentials (MOABT). New York: Elsevier Ltd; 2004.

Johr R, Stolz W. Dermoscopy: An Illustrated Self-Assessment Guide, 2nd edition. New York: McGraw-Hill Education; 2015.

Kittler H. Dermatoscopy. An Algorithmic Method Based on Pattern Analysis 2011 Facultas Verlags- und Buchhandels AG facultas wuv Universitätsverlag, Austria www.facultas.wuv.at.

Lallas A. Dermoscopy in general dermatology. Dermatol Clin. 2013;3:679-94.

Lallas A, Tzellos T, Kyrgidis A, et al. Accuracy of dermoscopic criteria for discriminating superficial from other subtypes of basal cell carcinoma. J Am Acad Dermatol. 2014;70:303-11.

Malvhey J, Puig S. Principles of Dermoscopy. Barcelona: Creaciones Gráficas; 2009.

Marghoob A, Braun R, Kopf A. Atlas of Dermoscopy. London: Taylor & Francis; 2005.

Menzies S, Crotty K, Ingvar C, et al. An Atlas of Surface Microscopy of Pigmented Skin Lesions. Sydney: McGraw-Hill Book Company; 1996.

Menzies S, Westerhoff K, Rabinivitz H, et al. Surface microscopy of pigmented basal cell carcinoma. Arch Dermatol. 2000;136:1012-6.

Menzies SW. Dermoscopy of pigmented basal cell carcinoma. Clin Dermatol. 2002;20:268-9.

Rabinovitz H, Kopf A. Dermoscopy: A Practical Guide. Miami: American Academy of Dermatology; 1999.

Soyer P, Argenziano G, Chimenti S, et al. Dermoscopy of Pigmented Skin Lesions. An Atlas Based on the Consensus Net Meeting on Dermoscopy. Milán: EDRA Medical Publishing & New Media; 2001.

Stolz W, Braun-Falco O, Bilek P, et al. Color Atlas of Dermatoscopy. Germany: Blackwell Science; 1994.

Tschandl P, Rosendahl C, Kittler H. Dermoscopy of flat pigmented facial lesion. J Eur Acad Dermatol Venereol. 2015;29(1):120-7.

Zalaudek I, Argenziano G, Giacomel J. Dermoscopy of Non-Pigmented Skin Tumors. Boca Raton, FL: CRC Press; 2016.

Zalaudek I, Cabo H, Ferrara G, et al. Dermoscopic-pathologic correlation in an unusual case of pigmented basal cell carcinoma. Dermatol Surg. 2006;32:1509-12.

5.4 ANGIOMAS AND ANGIOKERATOMAS

Horacio A Cabo

ANGIOMAS

In general, a clinical diagnosis is enough for the majority of hemagiomas and vascular malformations, although in some cases they can be misdiagnosed as other lesions or even suspected of being melanomas. It is here that dermoscopy plays a very important role.

The most frequent dermoscopic criterion is the presence of well-demarcated areas, red or blue-red, blue-black or brown, which almost always correspond histologically to dilated blood vessels in the dermis. Their metaphoric name is "lacunae" and they may vary in size and color within the same lesion (Figs. 5.117 to 5.126).

If there are thrombosed vessels, we can observe black areas (Figs. 5.127 and 5.128).

The dermoscopic criteria for the diagnosis of hemangioma are as follows:

- Absence of pigmented structures, such as pigment network, globules and/or branched streaks.

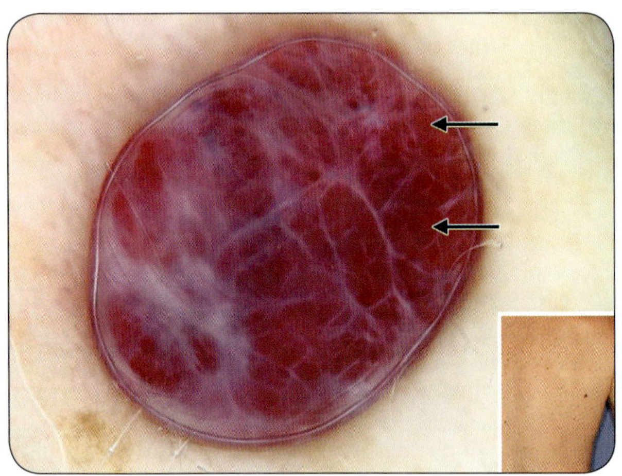

Fig. 5.117: Angioma: well-demarcated lacunae on a blue–red pigment background (arrows).

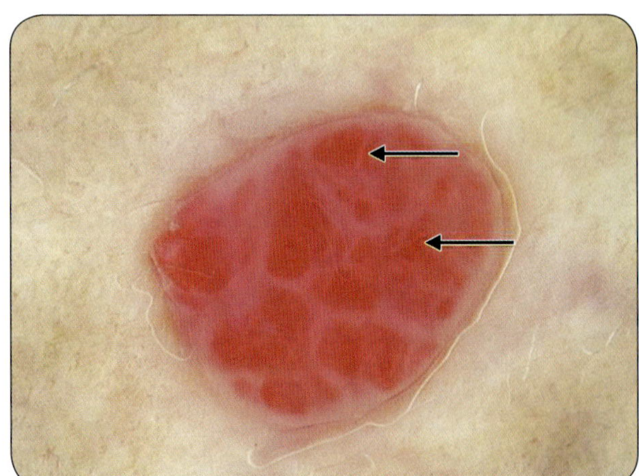

Fig. 5.118: Angioma: well-demarcated lacunae on a blue–red pigment background without any dermoscopic structures within (arrows).

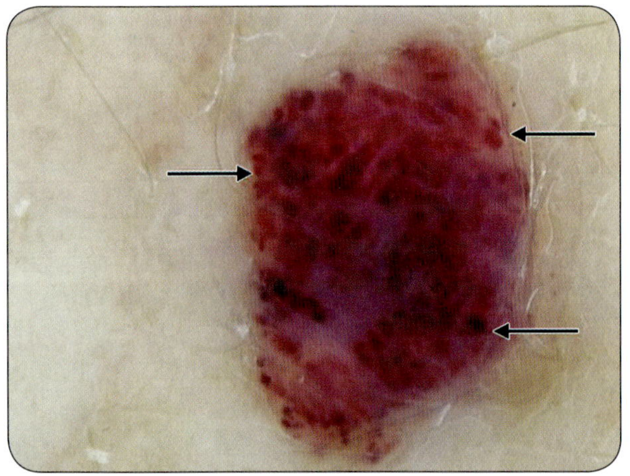

Fig. 5.119: Angioma: well-demarcated lacunae on a blue–red pigment background without any dermoscopic structures within (arrows).

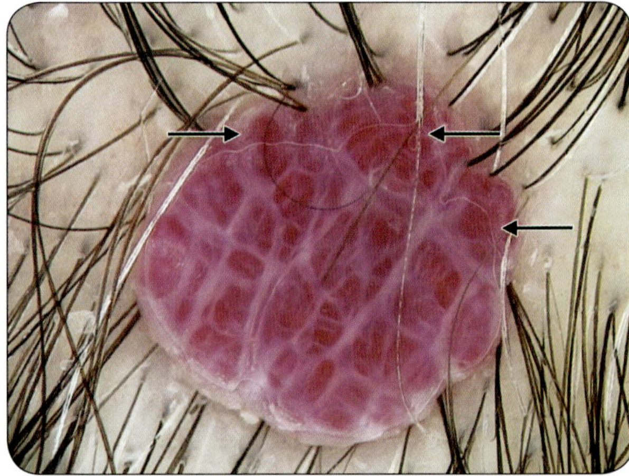

Fig. 5.120: Angioma: well-demarcated lacunae on a blue–red pigment background without any dermoscopic structures within (arrows).

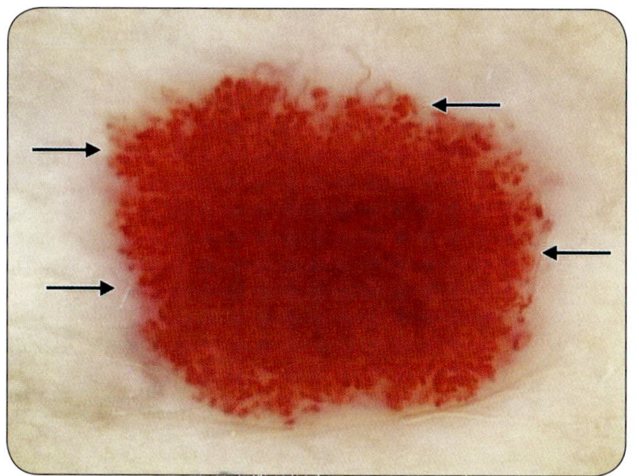

Fig. 5.121: Angioma: well-demarcated lacunae on a blue–red pigment background without any dermoscopic structures within (arrows).

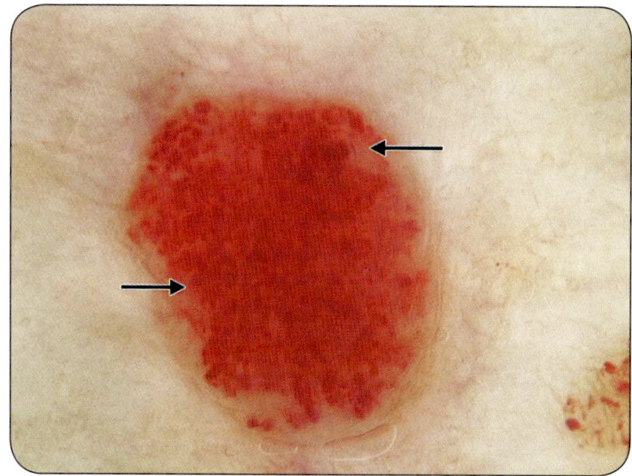

Fig. 5.122: Angioma: well-demarcated lacunae on a blue–red pigment background without any dermoscopic structures within (arrows).

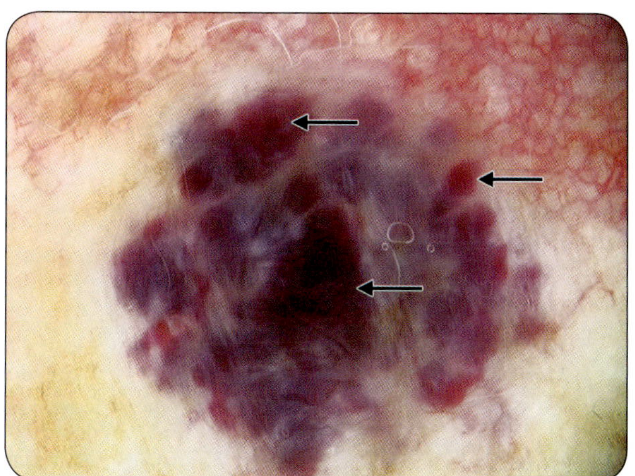

Fig. 5.123: Angioma: well-demarcated lacunae on a blue–red pigment background without any dermoscopic structures within (arrows).

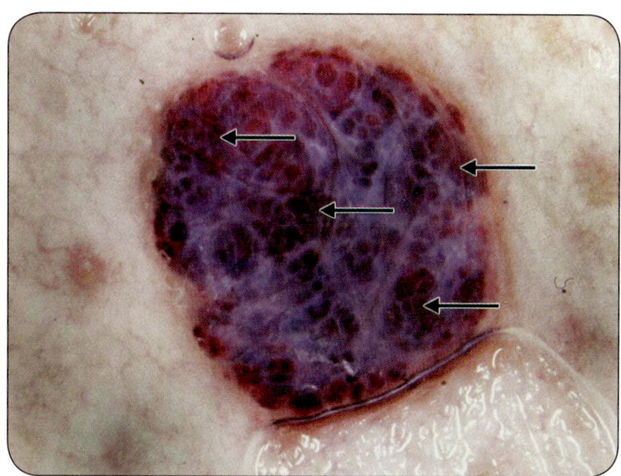

Fig. 5.124: Angioma: well-demarcated lacunae on a blue–red pigment background without any dermoscopic structures within (arrows).

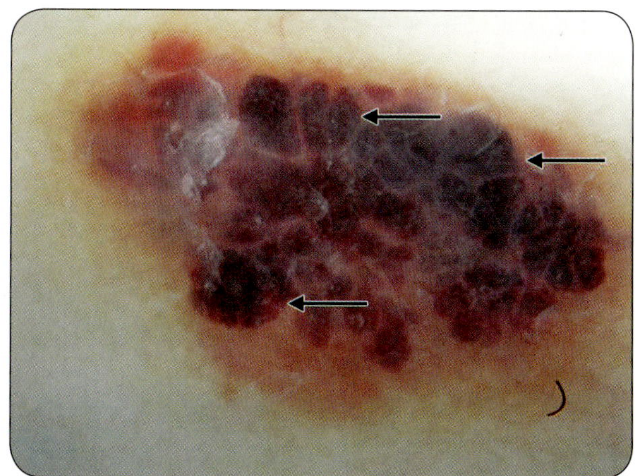

Fig. 5.125: Angioma: well-demarcated lacunae on a blue–red pigment background without any dermoscopic structures within (arrows).

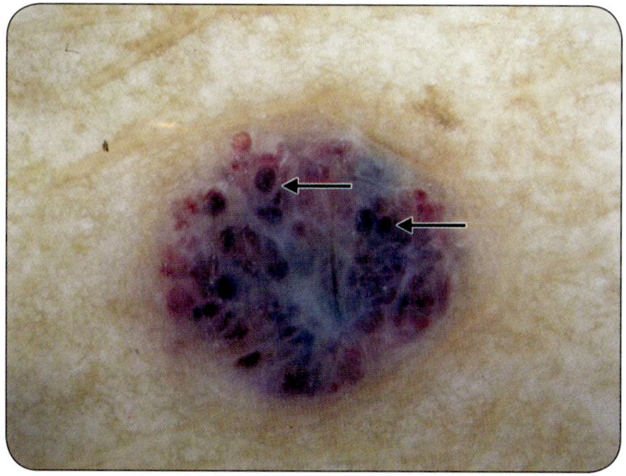

Fig. 5.126: Angioma: well-demarcated lacunae on a blue–red pigment background without any dermoscopic structures within (arrows).

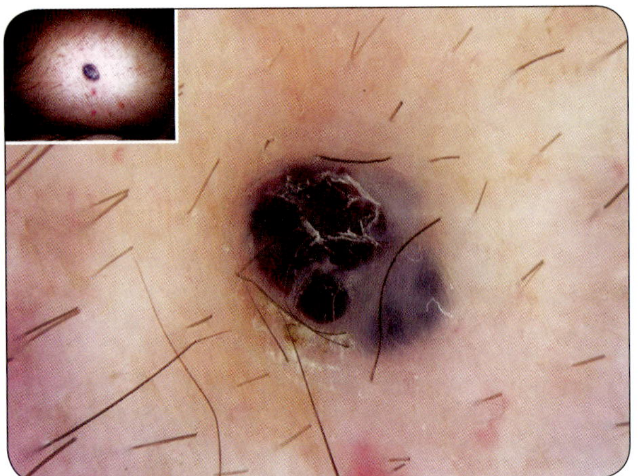

Fig. 5.127: Thrombosed or traumatized angioma.

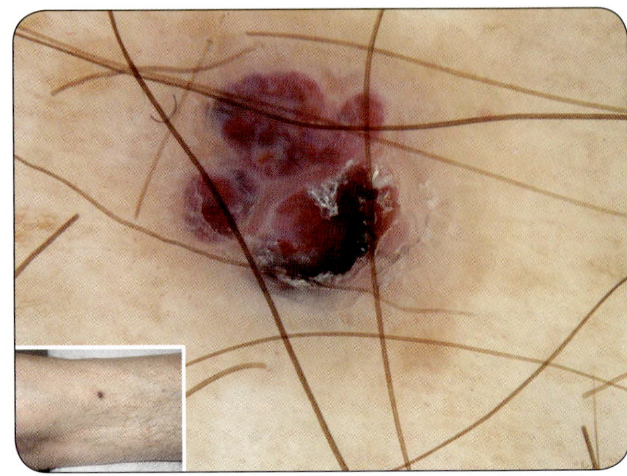

Fig. 5.128: Thrombosed or traumatized angioma.

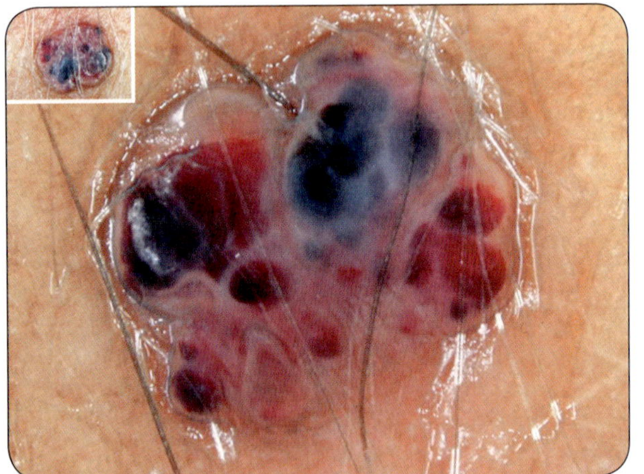

Fig. 5.129: Angiokeratoma.

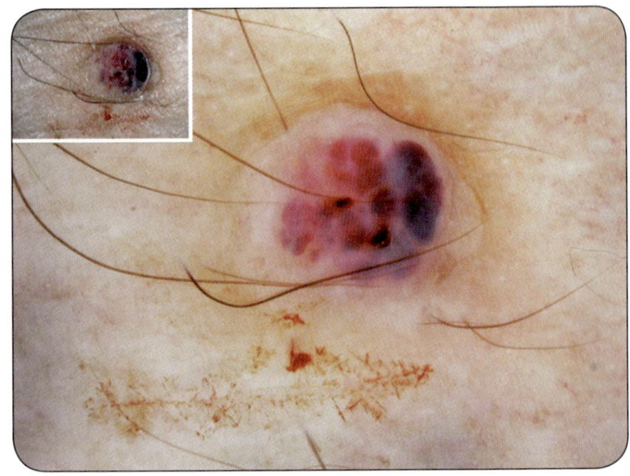

Fig. 5.130: Angiokeratoma.

- Well-demarcated lacunae on a blue-red pigment background without any dermoscopic structures within.

Angiokeratomas

The solitary angiokeratoma may clinically be a melanoma simulator. It develops by superficial telangiectasia in the papillary dermis, and is generally due to traumatism with reactive hyperkeratosis. It appears in youngsters and adults, more frequently in the lower extremities, although it can also manifest in the upper limbs and trunk.

At an early stage, the lesions are elevated, small and dark red or purple. As they evolve, they acquire a blue-black color with hyperkeratosis. They are asymptomatic but may bleed and crust if traumatized or thrombosed.

Their dermoscopic appearance also varies depending on their time of evolution and the presence or absence of thrombosis. Early lesions have minimal hyperkeratosis and consist of round or oval lacunae, well demarcated, red or blue-red; therefore, they are very similar to, and on occasion indistinguishable from, hemangiomas (Figs. 5.129 to 5.132).

Later-stage angiokeratomas contain multiple lacunae with the characteristic blue-red or blue-black color, though darker. However, these lacunae are not well demarcated and often lie on a white-yellowish background, due to epidermal acanthosis and hyperkeratosis.

When thrombosed or traumatized, there are homogeneous and confluent areas of blue-black pigment that simulate a melanoma (Fig. 5.133).

Dermoscopic criteria for angiokeratoma can be synthesized as follows:

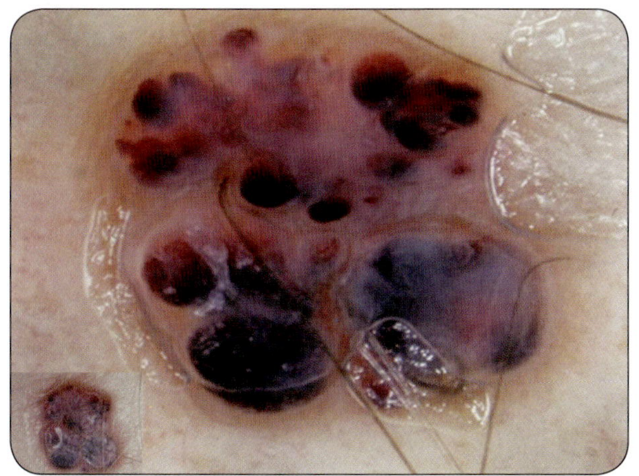

Fig. 5.131: Angiokeratoma.

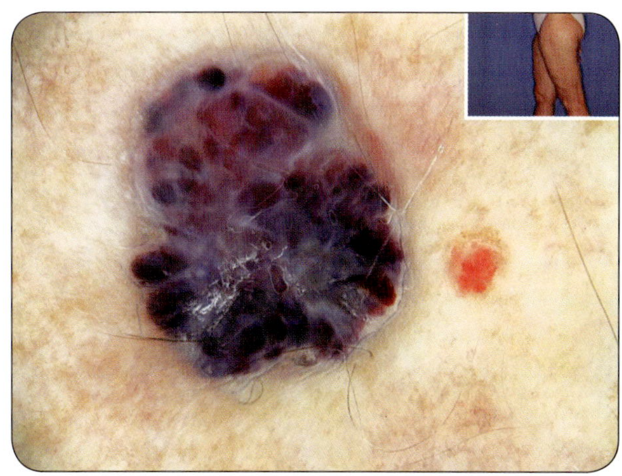

Fig. 5.132: Angiokeratoma.

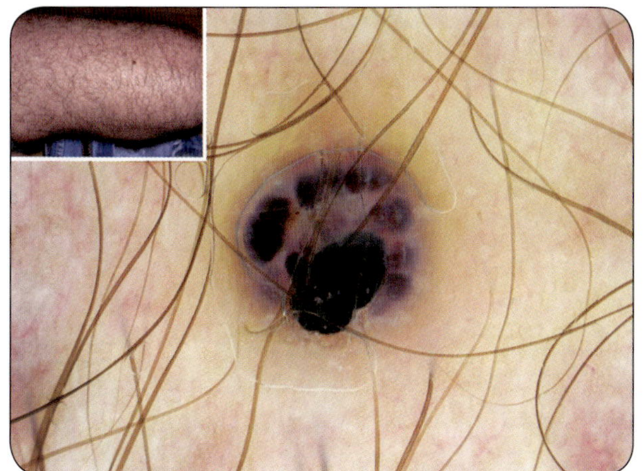

Fig. 5.133: Angiokeratoma.

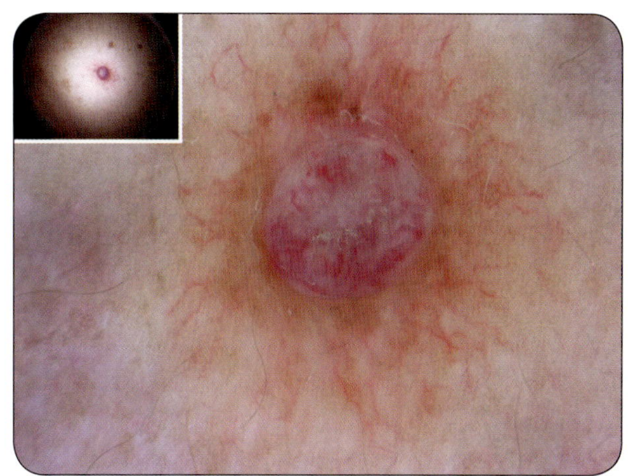

Fig. 5.134: Targetoid hemosiderotic hemangioma.

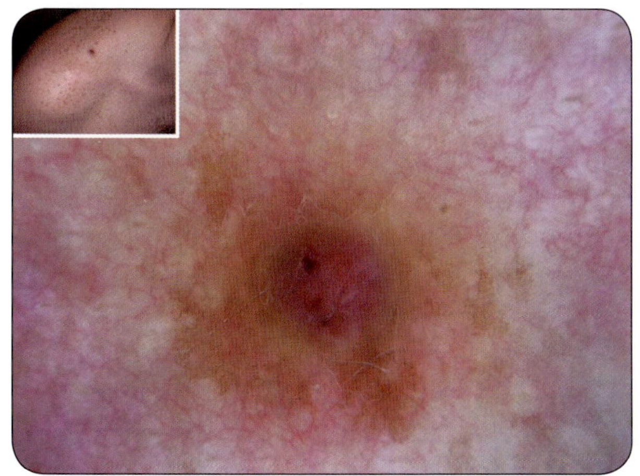

Fig. 5.135: Targetoid hemosiderotic hemangioma.

- Absence of pigmented structures (pigmented network, globules, or branched streaks)
- Lacunae less demarcated than in hemangiomas
- Acanthosis and hyperkeratosis may show white-yellowish areas.

Targetoid Hemosiderotic Hemangioma

It is an uncommon, vascular, benign solitary lesion that can be misdiagnosed as other tumors including melanomas.

Dermoscopy features: Red or dark lacunae and a peripheral circular reddish violaceous or brown homogeneous area (Figs. 5.134 and 5.135).

SUGGESTED READING

Argenziano G, Soyer P, De Giorgio V, et al. Interactive Atlas of Dermoscopy. Milán: EDRA Medical Publishing & New Media; 2000.

Argenziano G, Zalaudek I, Corona R, et al. Vascular structures in skin tumors. A dermoscopy study. Arch Dermatol. 2004;140:1485-9.

Cabo H. Dermatoscopia. Buenos Aires, Argentina: Weber Ferro; 2000.

Cabo H. Dermatoscopia, 2nd edition. Buenos Aires, Argentina: Ediciones Journal; 2012.

Jorh R, Soyer P, Argenziano G, et al. Dermoscopy. The Essentials (MOABT). New York: Elsevier Ltd.; 2004.

Johr R, Stolz W. Dermoscopy: An Illustrated Self-Assessment Guide, 2nd edition. New York: McGraw-Hill Education; 2015.

Kittler H. Dermatoscopy. An Algorithmic Method Based on Pattern Analysis 2011 Facultas Verlags- und Buchhandels AG facultas wuv Universitätsverlag, Austria www.facultas.wuv.at.

Kreusch J. Vascular patterns in skin tumors. Clin Dermatol. 2002;20:248-54.

Lallas A. Dermoscopy in general dermatology. Dermatol Clin. 2013;3:679-94.

Malvhey J, Puig S. Principles of Dermoscopy. Barcelona: Creaciones Gráficas; 2009.

Marghoob A, Braun R, Kopf A. Atlas of Dermoscopy. London: Taylor & Francis; 2005.

Menzies S, Crotty K, Ingvar C, et al. An Atlas of Surface Microscopy of Pigmented Skin Lesions. Sydney: McGraw-Hill Book Company; 1996.

Rabinovitz H, Kopf A. Dermoscopy: A Practical Guide. Miami: American Academy of Dermatology; 1999.

Schiller PI. Angiokeratomas: an update. Dermatology. 1996;193: 275-82.

Soyer P, Argenziano G, Chimenti S, et al. Dermoscopy of Pigmented Skin Lesions. An Atlas Based on the Consensus Net Meeting on Dermoscopy. Milán: EDRA Medical Publishing & New Media; 2001.

Stolz W, Braun-Falco O, Bilek P, et al. Color Atlas of Dermatoscopy. Germany: Blackwell Science, 1994.

Zaballos P, Daufí C, Puig S, et al. Dermoscopy of solitary angiokeratomas: a morphological study. Arch Dermatol. 2007; 143(3):318-25.

Zalaudek I, Argenziano G, Giacomel J. Dermoscopy of Non-Pigmented Skin Tumors. Boca Raton, FL: CRC Press; 2016.

5.5 DERMATOFIBROMA

Horacio A Cabo

Dermatofibroma is a frequent benign fibrohistiocytic tumor, which usually manifests clinically as an elevated nodule, firm, of variable coloration (from pinkish to brownish) localized preferably in the lower extremities of young adults. Under lateral compression, a depression appears called "dimple sign."

Histology shows a dermal nodular proliferation of fibroblasts and histiocytes accompanied by an increase in the number and the thickness of the collagen fibers. The epidermis covering the lesion is usually hyperplastic, with elongated epidermal ridges and hyperpigmentation in the basal layer.

Clinical diagnosis of dermatofibroma is simple and dermoscopy helps with the more uncommon forms.

Dermoscopic pattern (Figs. 5.136 to 5.143):

- Delicate peripheral pigment network
- Central white patch

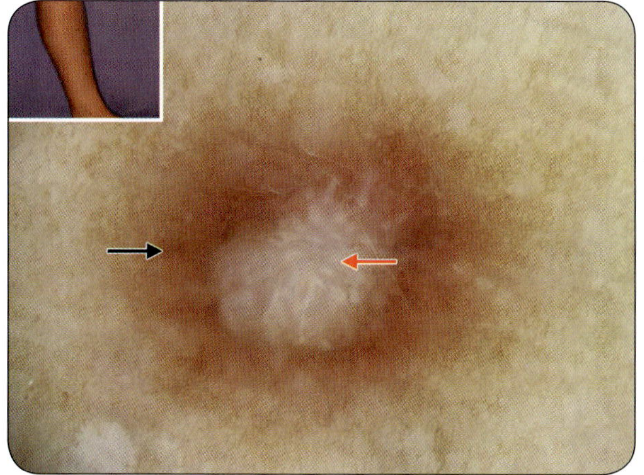

Fig. 5.136: Dermatofibroma: delicate peripheral pigment network (black arrow) and central white patch (red arrow).

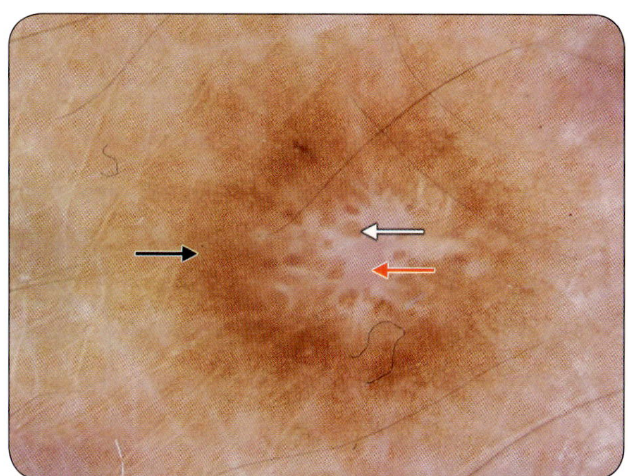

Fig. 5.137: Dermatofibroma: delicate peripheral pigment network (black arrow) and central white patch (red arrow). Round grayish or brown (globule-like) areas in the central part (white arrow).

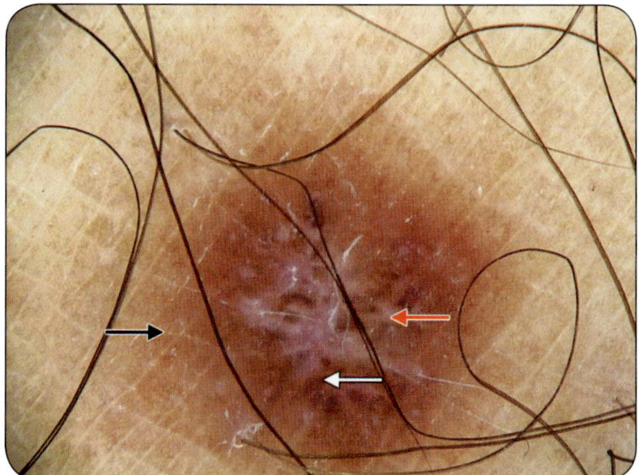

Fig. 5.138: Dermatofibroma: delicate peripheral pigment network (black arrow) and central white patch (red arrow). Round grayish or brown (globule-like) areas in the central part (white arrow).

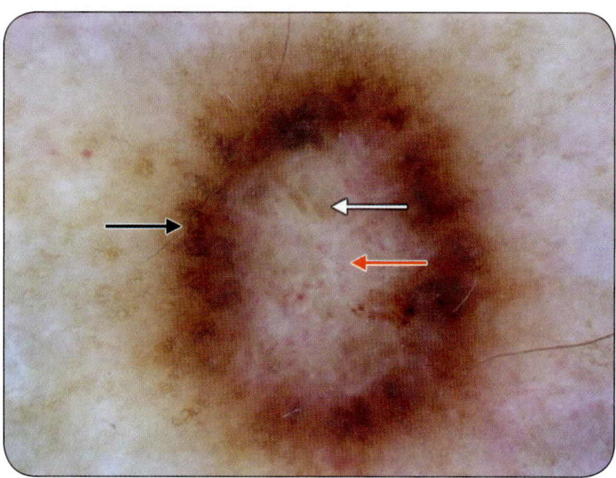

Fig. 5.139: Dermatofibroma: delicate peripheral pigment network (black arrow) and central white patch (red arrow). Round grayish or brown (globule-like) areas in the central part (white arrow).

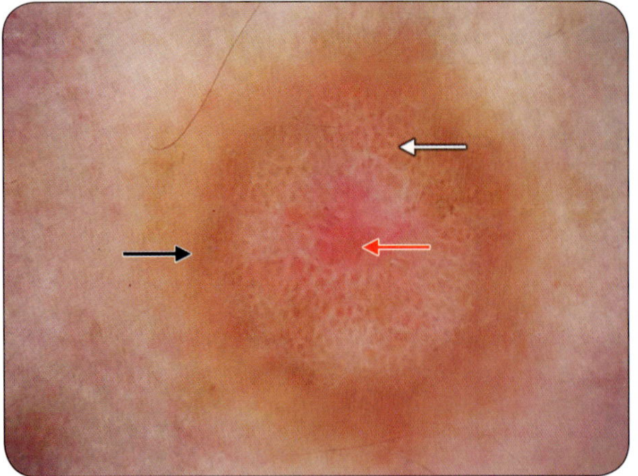

Fig. 5.140: Dermatofibroma: delicate peripheral pigment network (black arrow) and central white patch (red arrow). Round grayish or brown (globule-like) areas in the central part (white arrow).

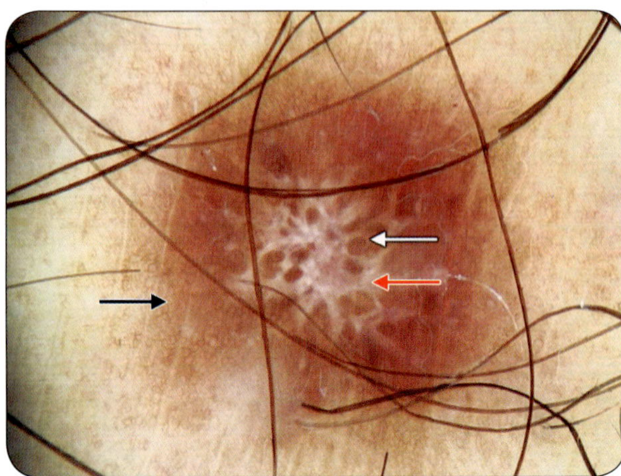

Fig. 5.141: Dermatofibroma: delicate peripheral pigment network (black arrow) and central white patch (red arrow). Round grayish or brown (globule-like) areas in the central part (white arrow).

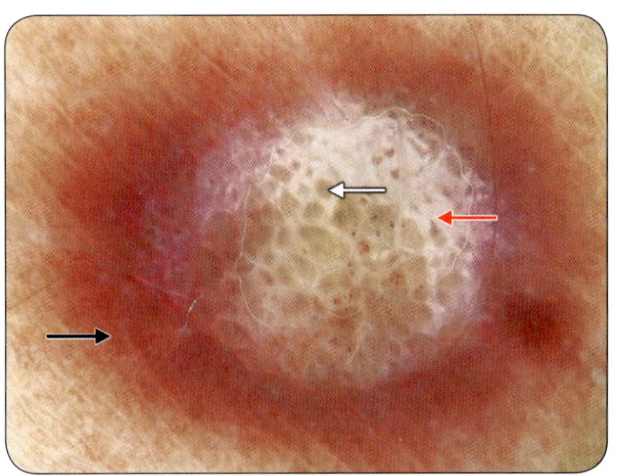

Fig. 5.142: Dermatofibroma: delicate peripheral pigment network (black arrow) and central white patch (red arrow). Round grayish or brown (globule-like) areas in the central part (white arrow).

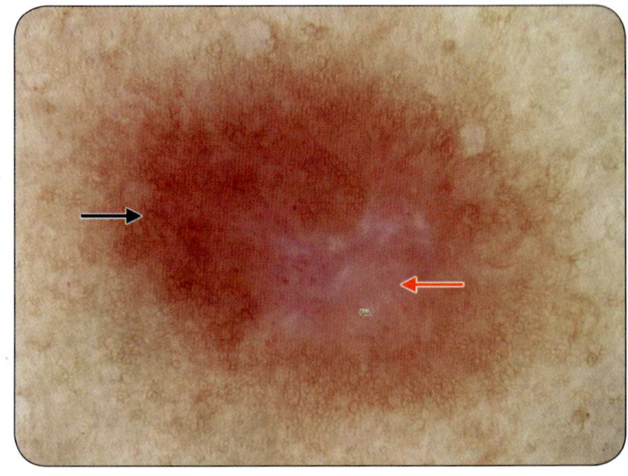

Fig. 5.143: Dermatofibroma: delicate peripheral pigment network (black arrow) and central white patch (red arrow).

Delicate peripheral pigment network: It is not a true pigment network since it is due to melanic rather than melanocytic pigmentation.

Central white pach or area: It has a scar-like appearance and is due to the superficial dermic fibrosis of this tumor.

It is usually in this central zone where the most dermoscopic variations are observed:

- Central white patches covering an important area of the lesion (Figs. 5.144 to 5.146)
- Round grayish or brown (globule-like) areas in the central part (Figs. 5.137 to 142, 144, and 5.147)
- Presence of linear vessels, occasionally with reticular appearance (Figs. 5.148 to 5.150)
- Blue or red areas (hemosiderotic dermatofibroma) (Fig. 5.151)
- Absence of white patch in highly pigmented lesions (Figs. 5.152 to 5.155)

White shiny linear streaks or crystal structures (Figs. 5.156 to 5.160):

- White shiny linear streaks not visible to the naked eye or with the dermoscope with nonpolarized light. They are visible in lesions with an increased amount of collagen (melanoma, dermatofibroma, scars, and basal cell

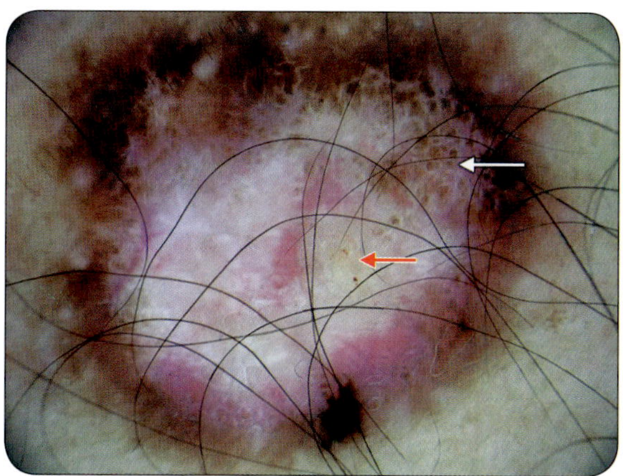

Fig. 5.144: Dermatofibroma: central white patches covering an important area of the lesion (red arrow). Round grayish or brown areas in the central part (globule-like) (white arrow).

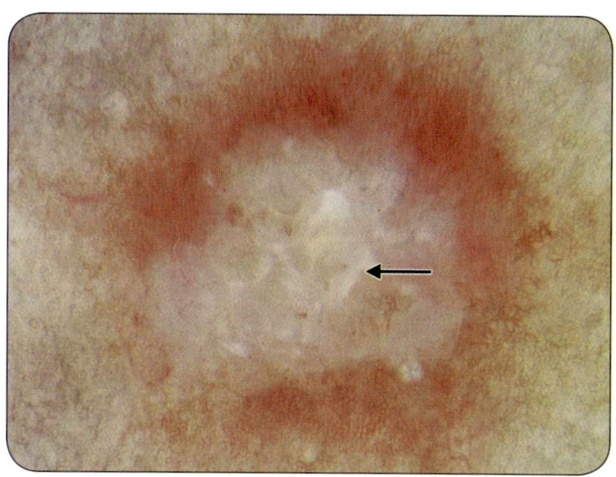

Fig. 5.145: Dermatofibroma: central white patches covering an important area of the lesion (arrow).

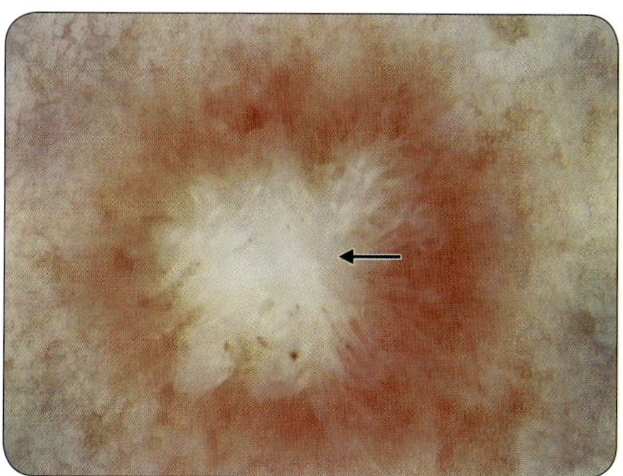

Fig. 5.146: Dermatofibroma: central white patches covering an important area of the lesion (arrow).

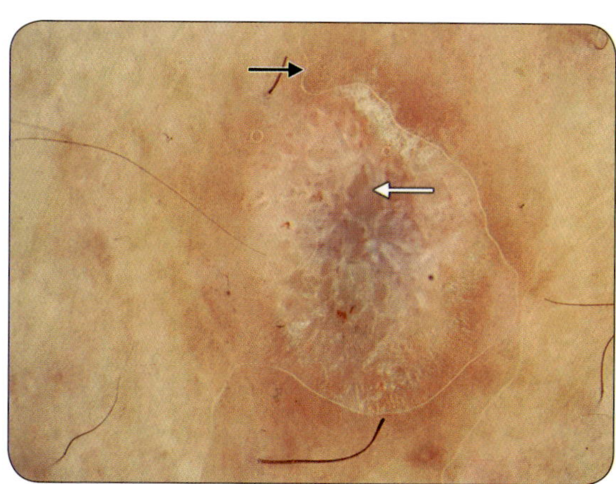

Fig. 5.147: Dermatofibroma: round grayish or brown areas in the central part (globule-like) (white arrow). Delicate peripheral pigment network (black arrow).

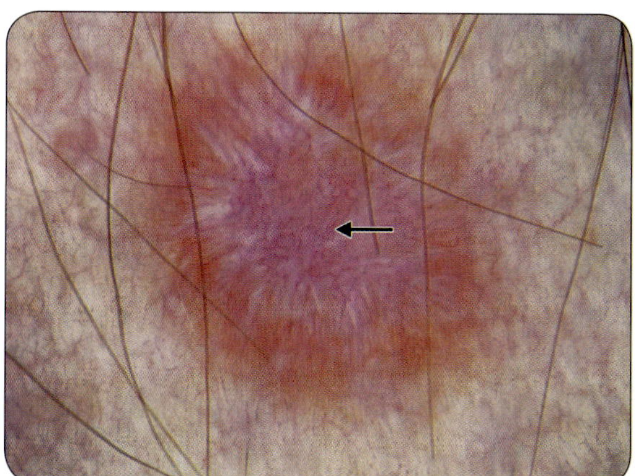

Fig. 5.148: Dermatofibroma: presence of linear vessels, occasionally with reticular appearance (arrow).

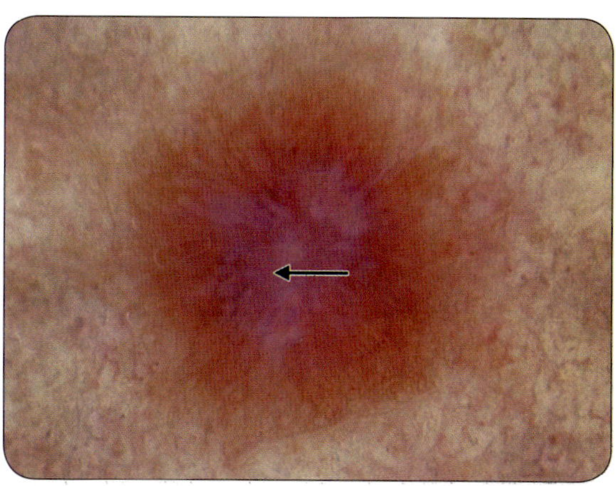

Fig. 5.149: Dermatofibroma: presence of linear vessels, occasionally with reticular appearance (arrow).

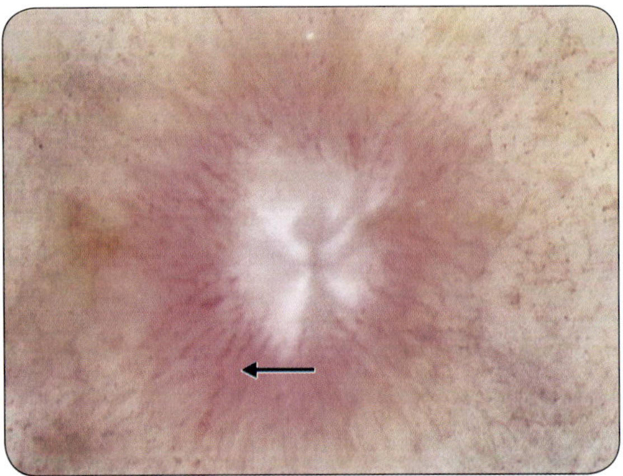

Fig. 5.150: Dermatofibroma: presence of linear vessels, occasionally with reticular appearance (arrow).

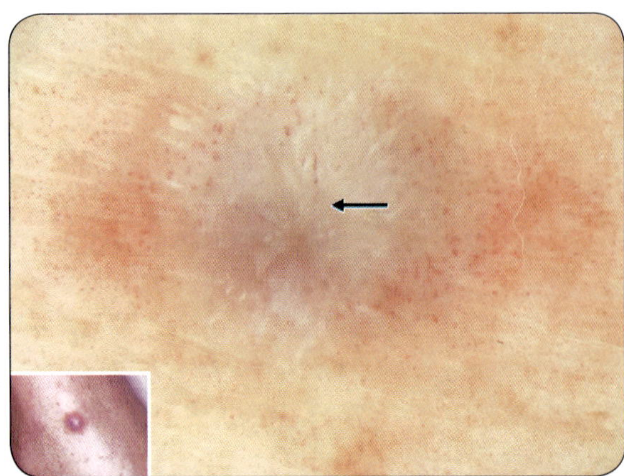

Fig. 5.151: Dermatofibroma: blue or red areas (hemosiderotic dermatofibroma) (arrow).

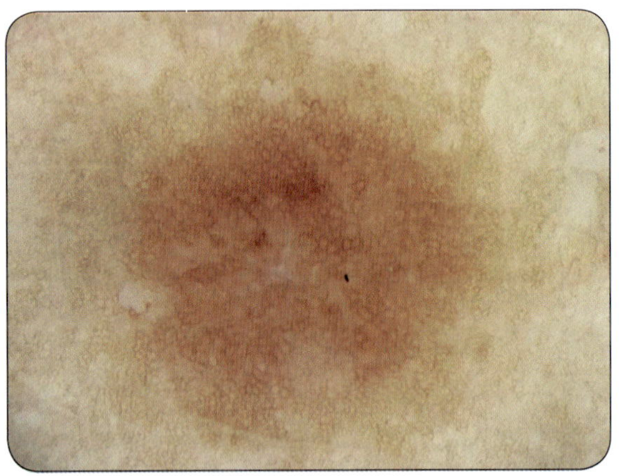

Fig. 5.152: Dermatofibroma. Absence or irregular distribution of white patch in highly pigmented lesions

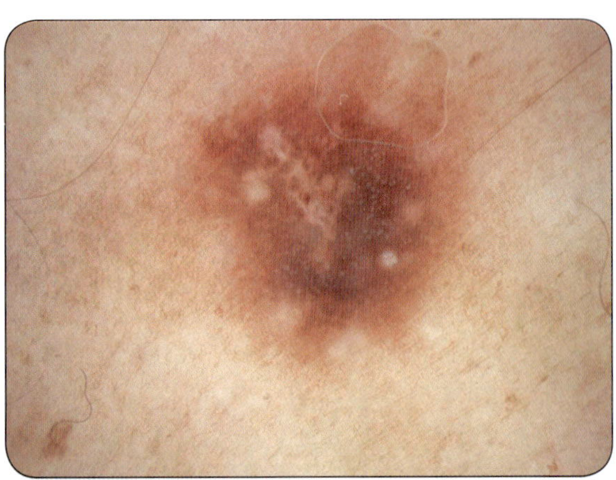

Fig. 5.153: Dermatofibroma: absence or irregular distribution of white patch in highly pigmented lesions.

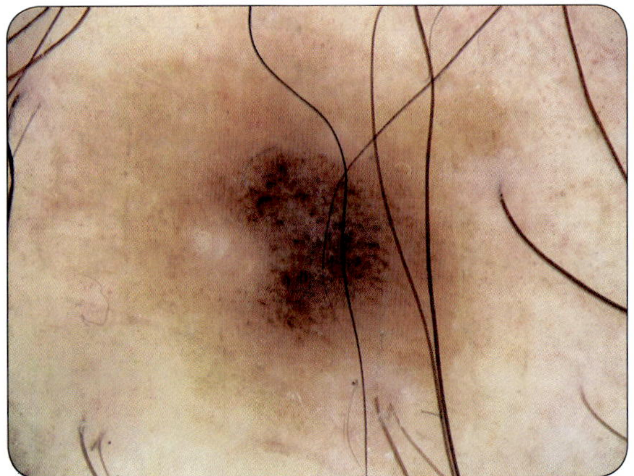

Fig. 5.154: Dermatofibroma: absence or irregular distribution of white patch in highly pigmented lesions.

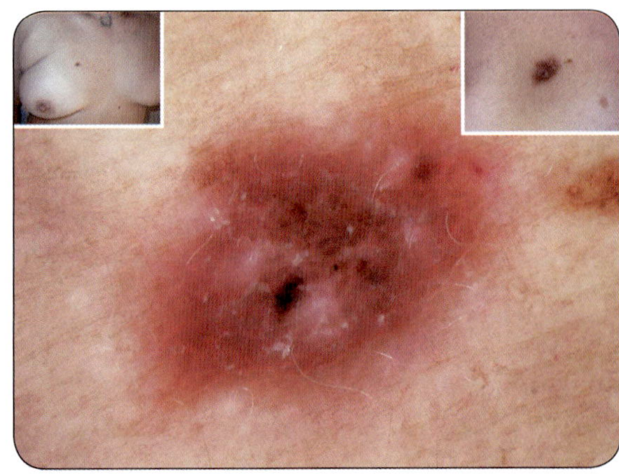

Fig. 5.155: Dermatofibroma: absence or irregular distribution of white patch in highly pigmented lesions.

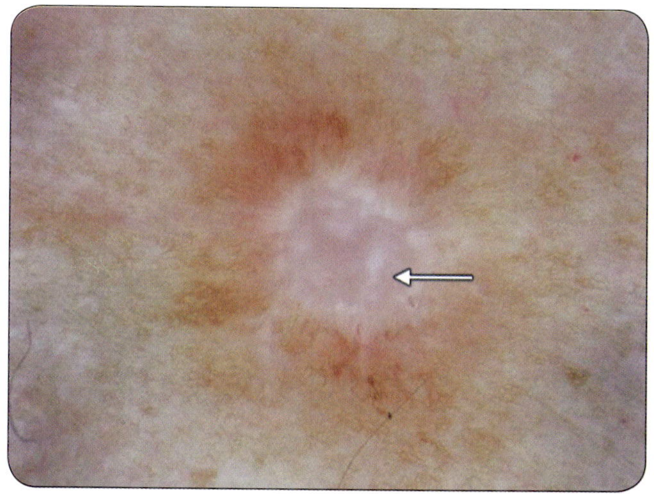

Fig. 5.156: White shiny linear streaks or crystal structures (arrow).

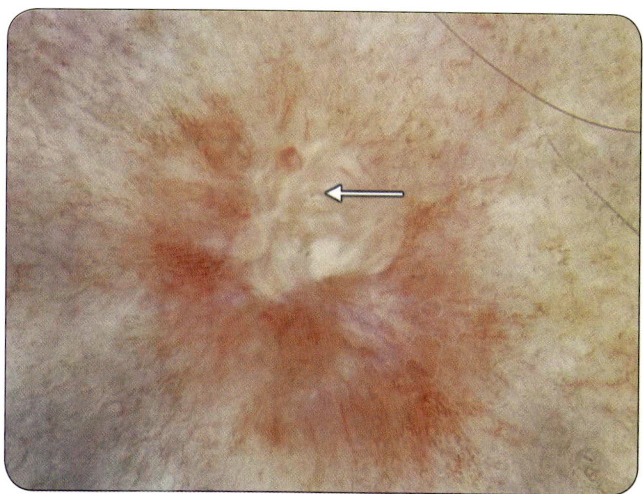

Fig. 5.157: White shiny linear streaks or crystal structures (arrow).

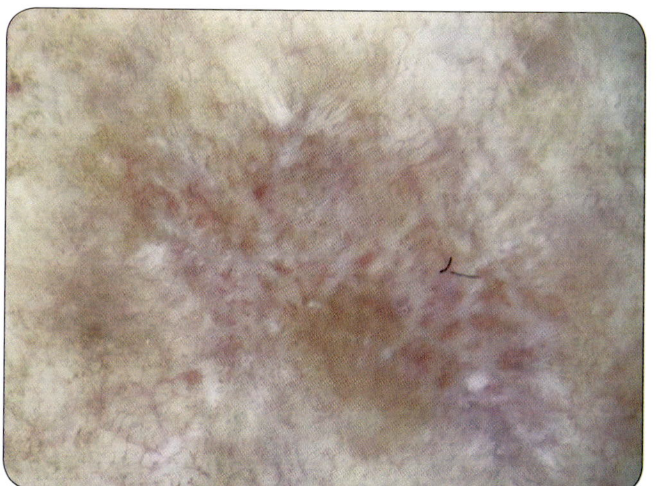

Fig. 5.158: White shiny linear streaks or crystal structures.

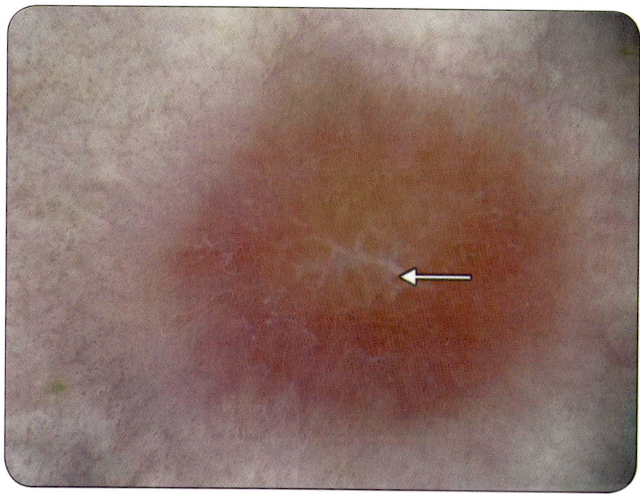

Fig. 5.159: White shiny linear streaks or crystal structures (arrow).

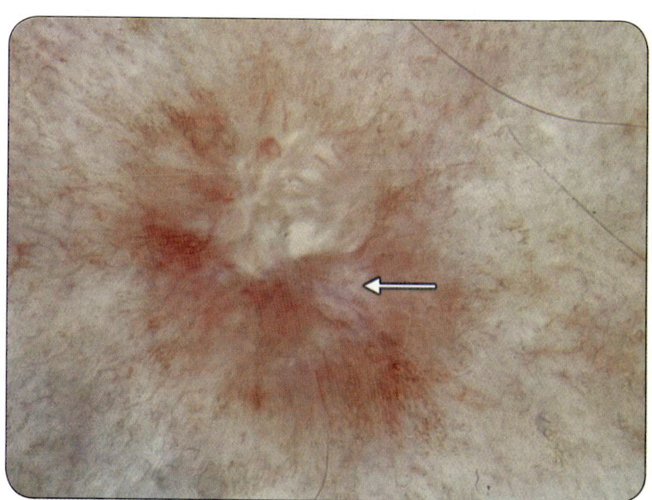

Fig. 5.160: White shiny linear streaks or crystal structures (arrow).

carcinoma). The collagen fasciae are birefringent and these give rise to a rapid randomization of the polarized light.

- It is a dynamic polarized dermoscopy since by rotating the dermoscope while keeping it in contact with the cutaneous surface, the orientation of the crystalline structures changes. This is owing to the angular dependence of the polarized light, reflecting the non-randomized distribution of the collagen fibers in the dermis.

SUGGESTED READING

Argenziano G, Soyer HP, Chimenti S, et al. Dermoscopy of pigmented skin lesions: results of a consensus meeting via the internet. J Am Acad Dermatol. 2003;48:679-93.

Argenziano G, Zalaudek I, Corona R, et al. Vascular structures in skin tumors: a dermoscopy study. Arch Dermatol. 2004;140:1485-9.

Arpaia N, Cassano N, Vena GA. Dermoscopic patterns of dermatofibroma. Dermatol Surg. 2005;31:1336-9.

Cabo H. Dermatoscopia, 2nd edition. Buenos Aires, Argentina: Ediciones Journal; 2012.

Johr R, Stolz W. Dermoscopy: An Illustrated Self-Assessment Guide, 2nd edition. New York: McGraw-Hill Education; 2015.

Ferrari A, Soyer HP, Peris K, et al. Central white scarlike patch: a dermoscopic clue for the diagnosis of dermatofibroma. J Am Acad Dermatol. 2000;43:1123-5.

Kilinc Karaarslan I, Gencoglan G, Akalin T, et al. Different dermoscopic faces of dermatofibromas. J Am Acad Dermatol. 2007;57:401-6.

Zaballos P, Guionnet N, Puig S, et al. Central white network: an additional dermoscopic feature for the diagnosis of dermatofibroma. Dermatol Surg. 2005;31:960-2.

Zaballos P, Llambrich A, Ara M, et al. Dermoscopic findings of haemosiderotic and aneurysmal dermatofibroma: report of six patients. Br J Dermatol. 2006;154:244-50.

Zaballos P, Puig S, Llambrich A, et al. Dermoscopy of dermatofibromas: a prospective morphological study of 412 cases. Arch Dermatol. 2008;144:75-83.

5.6 ACTINIC KERATOSES

Rosario Peralta, Horacio A Cabo

Actinic or solar keratoses (AKs) are the most frequent among solar-exposure-related cutaneous tumors.

They are considered premalignant lesions, since between 10 and 20% of them may evolve into a squamous cell carcinoma (SCC). Bowen's disease is considered an SCC in situ.

These lesions are more frequent in fair-skinned, light-eyed, and blond-haired people.

Nevertheless, they can manifest in any kind of skin, depending on the level of solar exposure. The most affected areas are the exposed ones.

Clinical diagnosis is made on pink-colored lesions with scaly surface. Actinic keratosis may become pigmented as well.

The main differential diagnoses are as follows (Figs. 5.161 to 5.164):

- *Nonpigmented forms*: Nonpigmented superficial basal cell carcinoma and early or flat seborrheic keratosis (solar lentigo)
- *Pigmented forms*: Lentigo maligna (LM) and solar lentigo

In all hyperkeratotic AK with increased erythema and induration, we should perform a biopsy to discard SCC.

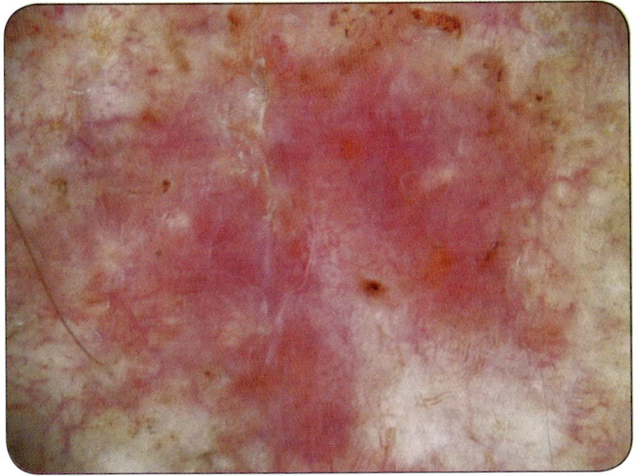

Fig. 5.161: Superficial basal cell carcinoma. Pink lesion with differential diagnosis of actinic keratosis.

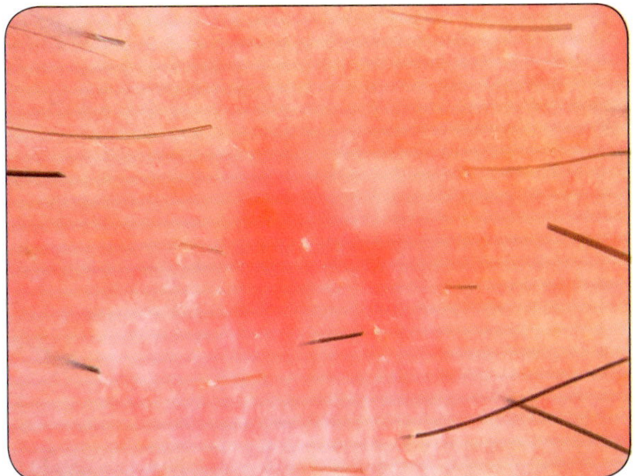

Fig. 5.162: Superficial basal cell carcinoma. Pink lesion with differential diagnosis of actinic keratosis.

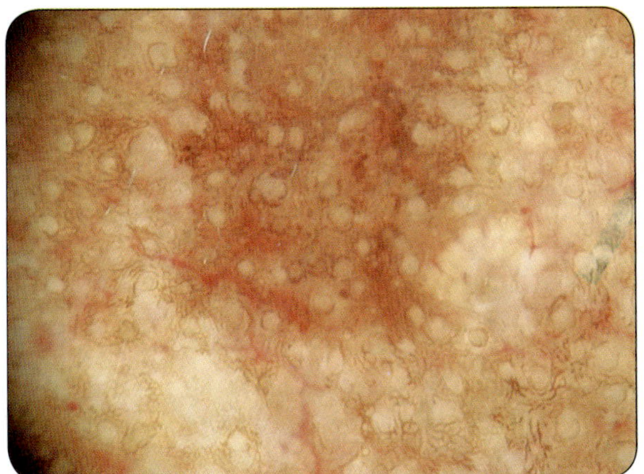

Fig. 5.163: Solar lentigo. Differential diagnosis of pigmented actinic keratosis.

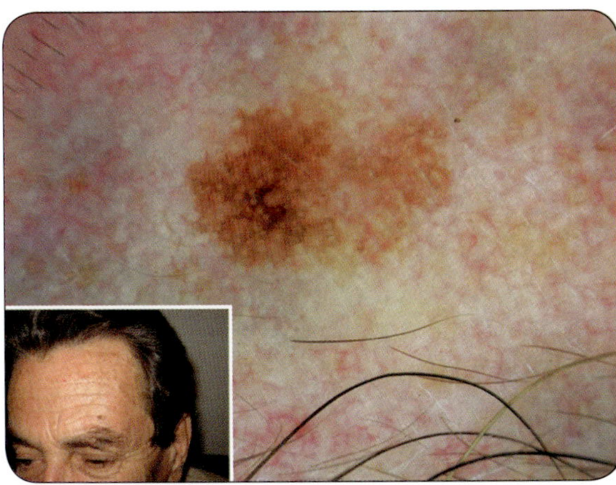

Fig. 5.164: Solar lentigo. Differential diagnosis of pigmented actinic keratosis.

DERMOSCOPIC CRITERIA

Nonpigmented Actinic Keratosis

- *Strawberry-like pattern*: It is possible to observe white or white-yellow follicular openings in a reddish background with the appearance of the surface of a strawberry (Figs. 5.165 to 5.168).
- Vascular pattern with fine undulated vessels surrounding the hair follicle, dot-like vessels, and spiral-like vessels (Figs. 5.168 to 5.170).
- Superficial yellowish-white scales (Figs. 5.167 and 5.171)
- Hyperkeratotic follicles (Fig. 5.168)
- *Rosettes*: They are observable with polarized light and correspond to four grouped white dots, resembling a four-leafed clover, located mainly within the follicular opening. They are nonspecific, and observable also in other tumors, specially keratinizing ones (Figs. 5.171 to 5.174).

Pigmented Actinic Keratosis (Fig. 5.175)

They may be very difficult to distinguish from LM since they present almost the same criteria, except for the homogeneous blue-gray areas, which may spread or not into the follicular openings (Figs. 5.168, 5.174, 5.176 to 5.178).

- Superficial brown color with the appearance of broken pseudonetwork
- Hyperkeratotic follicles
- *Inner gray halo*: Subtle homogeneous gray or light brown halo surrounding the follicular openings in

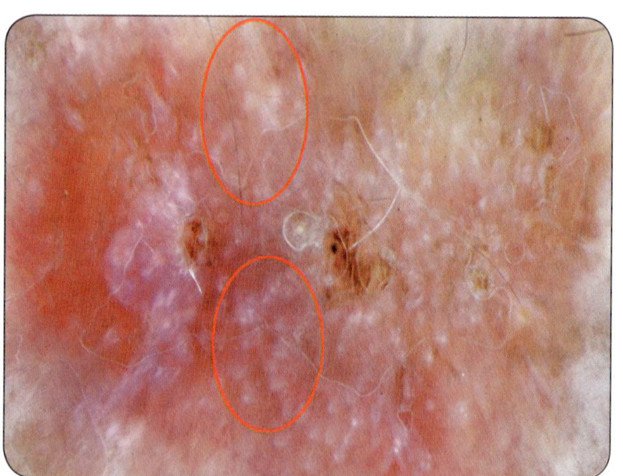

Fig. 5.165: Actinic keratosis: strawberry pattern (red circles).

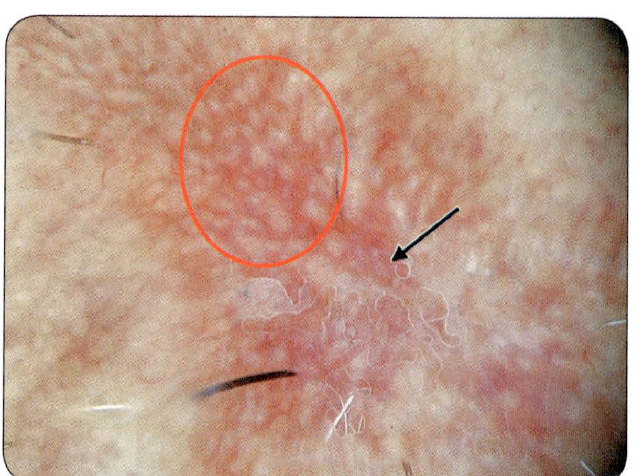

Fig. 5.166: Actinic keratosis: strawberry pattern (red circle). Rosette-like structures (black arrow).

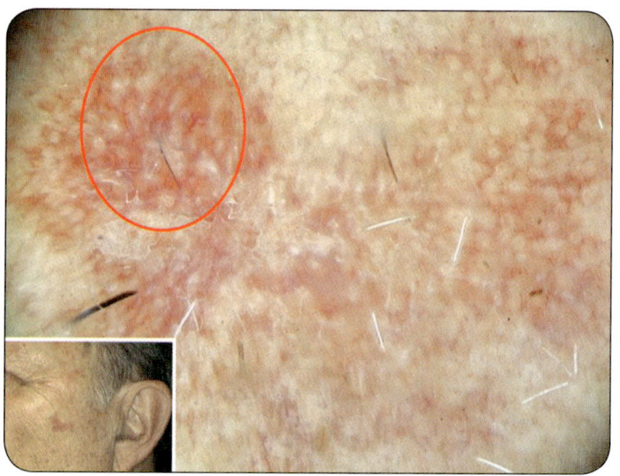

Fig. 5.167: Actinic keratosis: strawberry pattern (red circle).

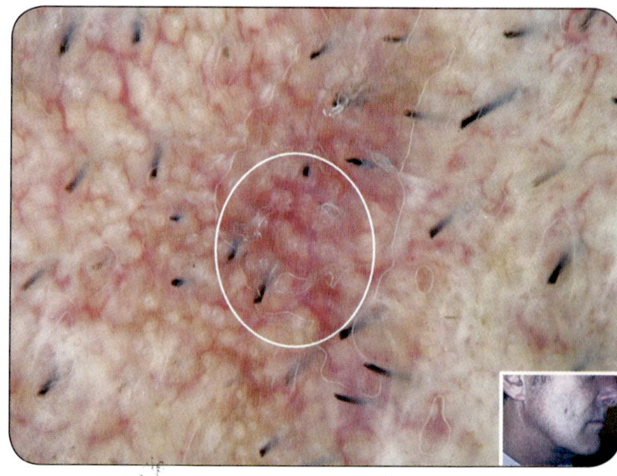

Fig. 5.168: Undulated vessels surrounding the hair follicle (white circle).

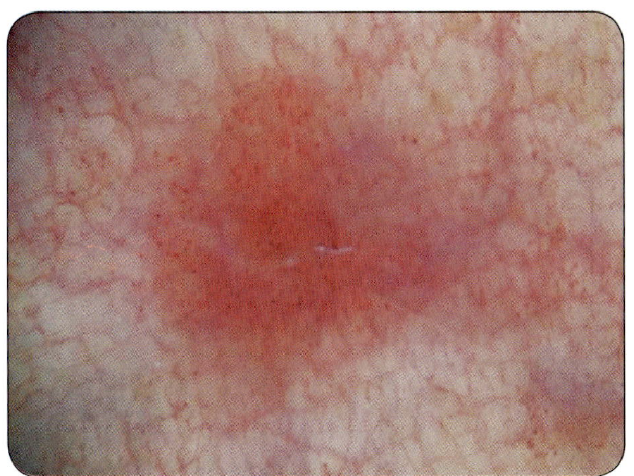

Fig. 5.169: Actinic keratosis: dot-like vessels.

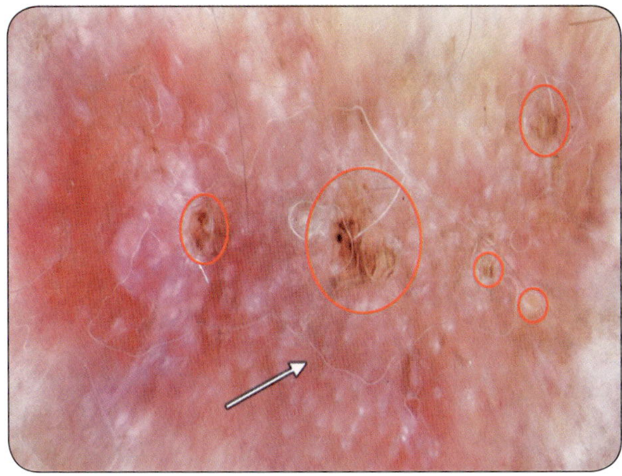

Fig. 5.170: Actinic keratosis: strawberry pattern (white arrow); white-to-yellow surface scale (red circles).

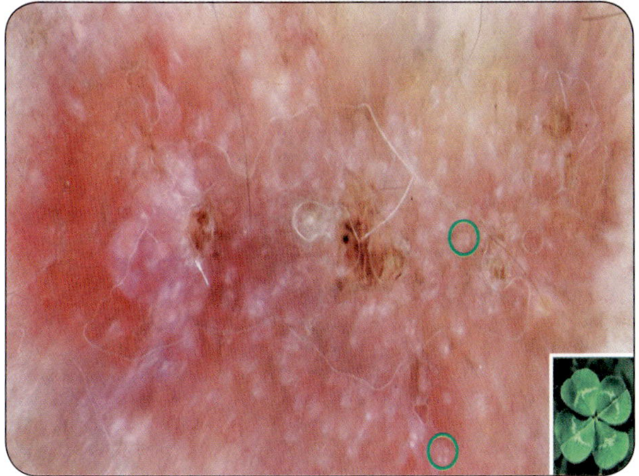

Fig. 5.171: Actinic keratosis: rosette-like structures (green circles).

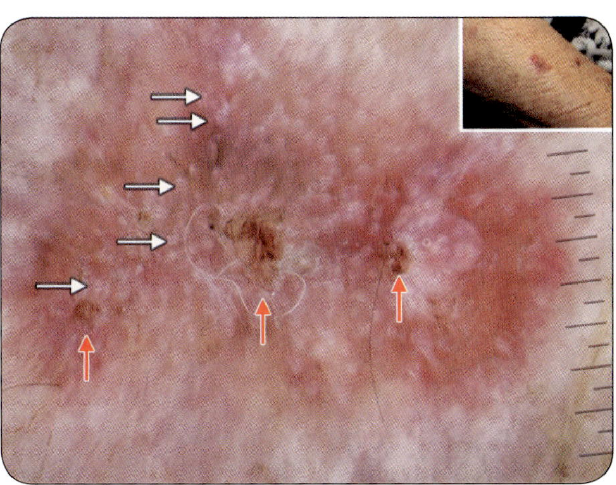

Fig. 5.172: Actinic keratosis: rosette-like structures (white arrows); white-to-yellow surface scale and small erosion (red arrows).

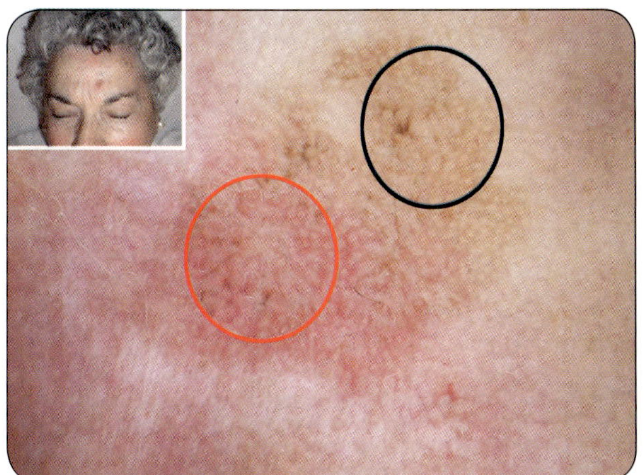

Fig. 5.173: Pigmented (black circle) and nonpigmented (red circle) actinic keratosis in the same lesion.

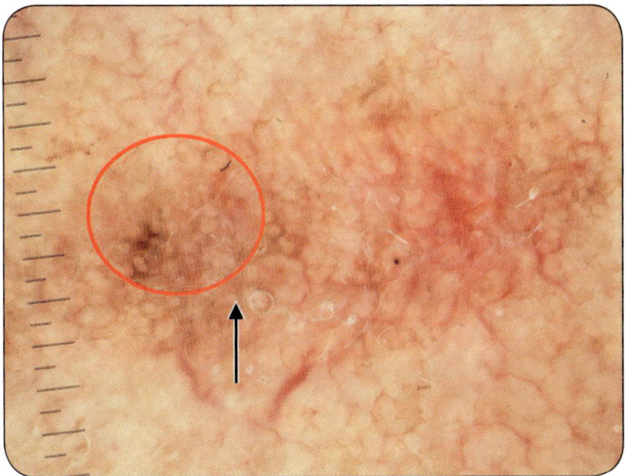

Fig. 5.174: Pigmented actinic keratosis: pigmentation of the follicular openings (red circle); rosette-like structures (black arrow).

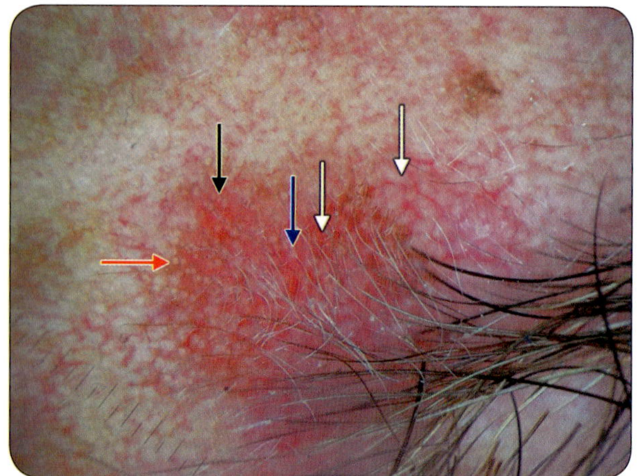

Fig. 5.175: Actinic keratosis: pigmentation of the follicular openings (red arrow); strawberry pattern (black arrow); undulated vessels surrounding the hair follicle (white arrows); and hyperkeratotic follicles (blue arrow).

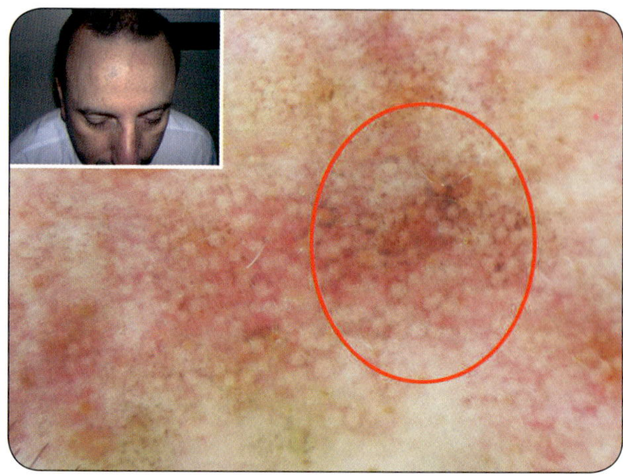

Fig. 5.176: Pigmented actinic keratosis; annular–granular pattern with symmetric and asymmetric slate-gray pigmentation of the follicular openings (red circle).

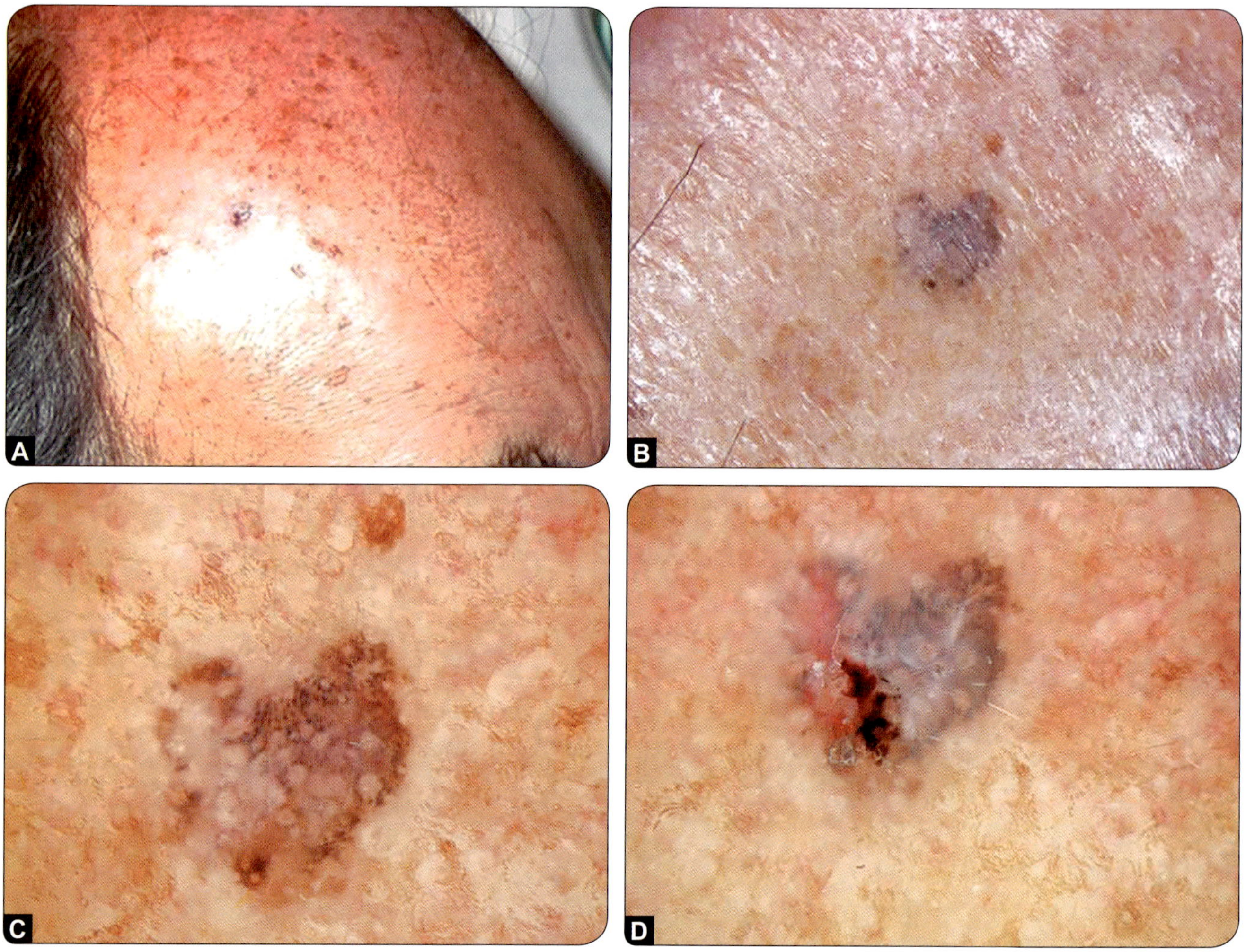

Figs. 5.177A to D: Pigmented actinic keratosis; clinical and dermoscopy images.

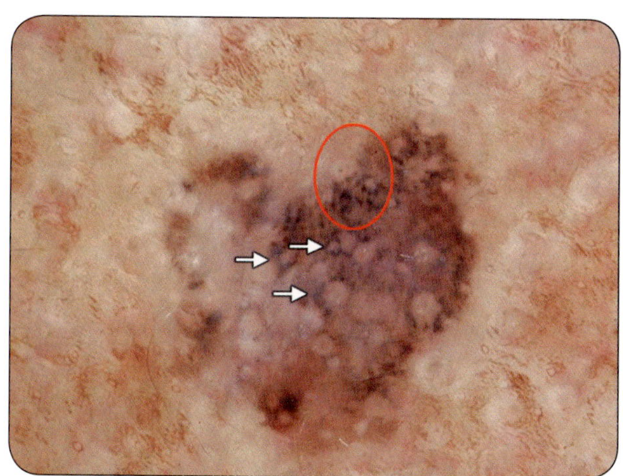

Fig. 5.178: Pigmented actinic keratosis (closeup view of Figures 5.177C): slate gray to black dots and slate gray to black globules as part of an annular–granular pattern (red circle). Rhomboidal structures (white arrows).

the manner of an inner ring within the mesh of the brown pseudonetwork. It is the result of the pigmentation of the basal keranocytes surrounding the hair follicle.

- Asymmetric pigmentation of the follicular opening (which can also be found in LM)
- Rhomboidal structures (also found in LM)

Histopathological examination can be difficult, since on occasion it is hard to differentiate pigmented keranocytes from melanocytes.

SUGGESTED READING

Argenziano G, Soyer P, De Giorgio V, et al. Interactive Atlas of Dermoscopy. Milán: EDRA Medical Publishing & New Media; 2000.

Cabo H. Dermatoscopia. Buenos Aires, Argentina: Weber Ferro; 2000.

Cabo H. Dermatoscopia, 2nd edition. Buenos Aires, Argentina: Ediciones Journal; 2012.

Cuellar F, Vilalta A, Puig S, et al. New dermoscopic pattern in actinic keratosis and related conditions. Arch Dermatol. 2009;145:732.

Jorh R, Soyer P, Argenziano G, et al. Dermoscopy. The Essentials (MOABT). New York: Elsevier Ltd.; 2004.

Johr R, Stolz W. Dermoscopy: An Illustrated Self-Assessment Guide, 2nd edition. New York: McGraw-Hill Education; 2015.

Kittler H. Dermatoscopy. An Algorithmic Method Based on Pattern Analysis 2011 Facultas Verlags- und Buchhandels AG facultas wuv Universitätsverlag, Austria www.facultas.wuv.at.

Lallas A. Dermoscopy in general dermatology, Dermatol Clin. 2013;3:679-94.

Lallas A, Argenziano G, Moscarella E, et al. Diagnosis and management of facial pigmented macules. Clin Dermatol. 2014; 32:94-100.

Malvhey J, Puig S. Principles of Dermoscopy. Barcelona: Creaciones Gráficas; 2009.

Marghoob A, Braun R, Kopf A. Atlas of Dermoscopy. London: Taylor & Francis; 2005.

Menzies S, Crotty K, Ingvar C, et al. An Atlas of Surface Microscopy of Pigmented Skin Lesions. Sydney: McGraw-Hill Book Company; 1996.

Nascimento M, Shitara D, Enokihara M, et al. Inner gray halo, a novel dermoscopic feature for the diagnosis of pigmented actinic keratosis: Clues for the differential diagnosis with lentigo maligna. J Am Acad Dermatol. 2014;71:708-15.

Rabinovitz H, Kopf A. Dermoscopy: A Practical Guide. Miami: American Academy of Dermatology; 1999.

Soyer P, Argenziano G, Chimenti S, et al. Dermoscopy of Pigmented Skin Lesions. An Atlas Based on the Consensus Net Meeting on Dermoscopy. Milán: EDRA Medical Publishing & New Media; 2001.

Stolz W, Braun-Falco O, Bilek P, et al. Color Atlas of Dermatoscopy. Germany: Blackwell Science; 1994.

Tschandl P. Dermoscopy of flat pigmented facial lesion. J Eur Acad Dermatol Venereol. 2015:29:120-7.

Zalaudek I. Morphologic grading and treatment of facial actinic keratosis. Clin Dermatol. 2014;32(1):80-7.

Zalaudek I, Argenziano G, Giacomel J. Dermoscopy of Non-Pigmented Skin Tumors. Boca Raton, FL: CRC Press; 2016.

Zalaudek I, Ferrara G, Leinweber B, et al. Pitfalls in the clinical and dermoscopic diagnosis of pigmented actinic keratosis. J Am Acad Dermatol. 2005;53:1071-4.

Zalaudek I, Giacomel J, Argenziano G, et al. Dermatoscopy of facial non-pigmented actinic keratosis. Br J Dermatol. 2006; 155:951-6.

5.7 KERATOACANTHOMA, BOWEN'S DISEASE AND SQUAMOUS CELL CARCINOMA

Rosario Peralta, Horacio A Cabo

KERATOACANTHOMA

Keratoacanthoma (KA) is a keratinizing tumor presenting a central crater or hyperkeratosis (Fig. 5.179).

Dermoscopically, it is characterized by the presence of mainly thick hairpin vessels with peripheral distribution and central hyperkeratosis. It is also frequent to observe irregular linear vessels (Fig. 5.180).

It is worth mentioning that both in KA and in squamous cell carcinoma (SCC), it is possible to find keratin structures, blood spots, and white areas and circles. The presence of these dermoscopic characteristics makes it feasible to differentiate KA and SCC from other nonpigmented tumorous lesions.

Central hyperkeratosis is more frequent in KA than in SCC. The blood spots are distributed in the keratin. The white circles are located around the dilated infundibulum filled with a central keratin plug (yellowish keratotic plug) and observable as a yellow or an orange area (clods); these structures do not correspond to keratin pearls. Histopathologically, they present acantholysis and epidermal infundibular hypergranulosis (Figs. 5.181 to 5.184).

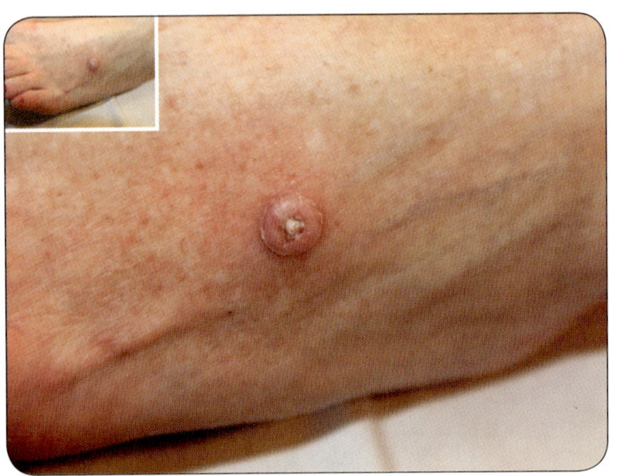

Fig. 5.179: Keratoacanthoma.

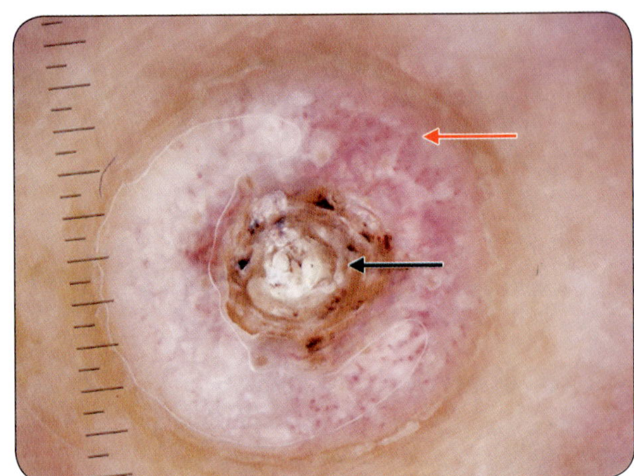

Fig. 5.180: Keratoacanthoma: central hyperkeratosis (black arrow); peripheral vessels (red arrow).

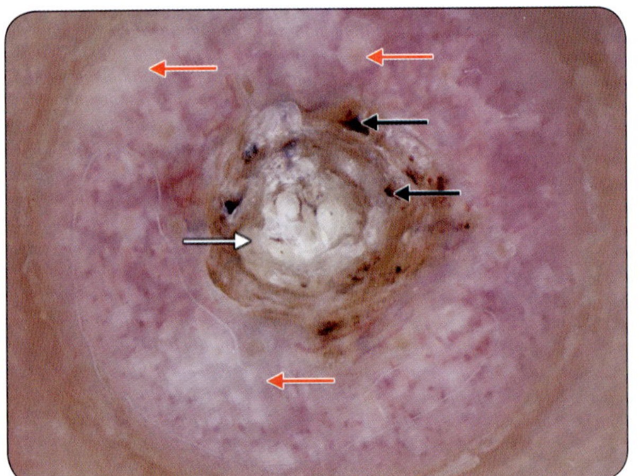

Fig. 5.181: Keratoacanthoma: central hyperkeratosis (white arrow); blood spots in the central crater or hyperkeratosis (black arrows); white circles or areas (red arrows).

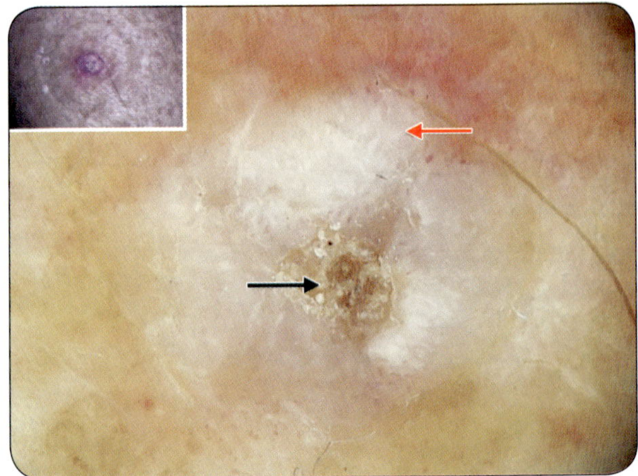

Fig. 5.182: Keratoacanthoma: central hyperkeratosis (black arrow); white circles or areas (red arrow).

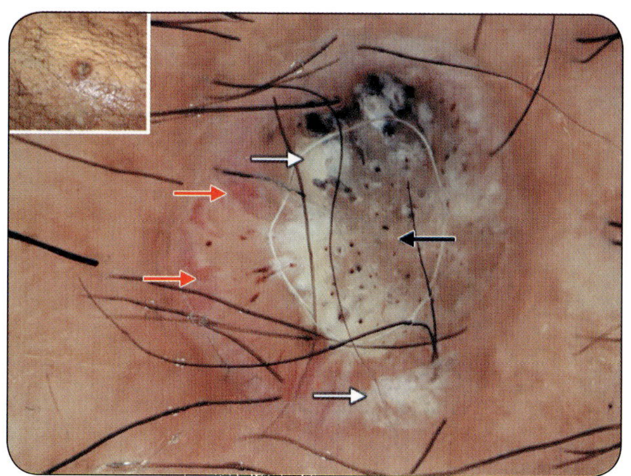

Fig. 5.183: Keratoacanthoma: central hyperkeratosis (black arrow); peripheral hairpin vessels (red arrows); white, yellow, or orange areas (white arrows).

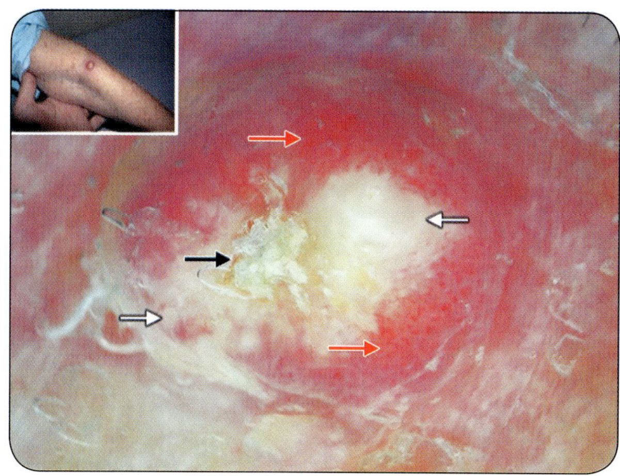

Fig. 5.184: Keratoacanthoma: central hyperkeratosis (black arrow); peripheral hairpin vessels (red arrows); white, yellow, or orange areas or circles (white arrows).

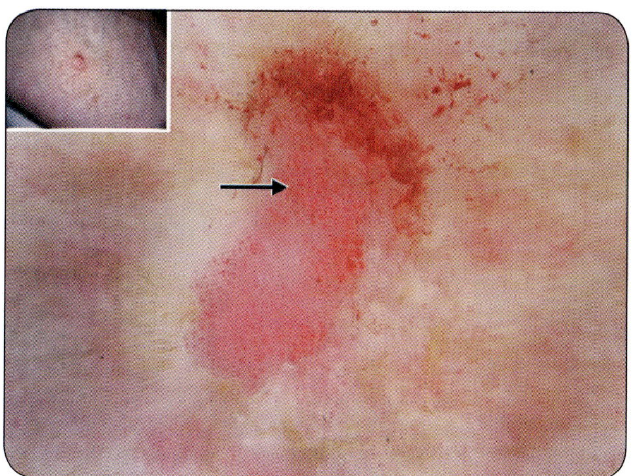

Fig. 5.185: Squamous cell carcinoma in situ—nonpigmented Bowen's disease: glomerular or spiral vessels, monomorphic pattern, focal distribution (arrow).

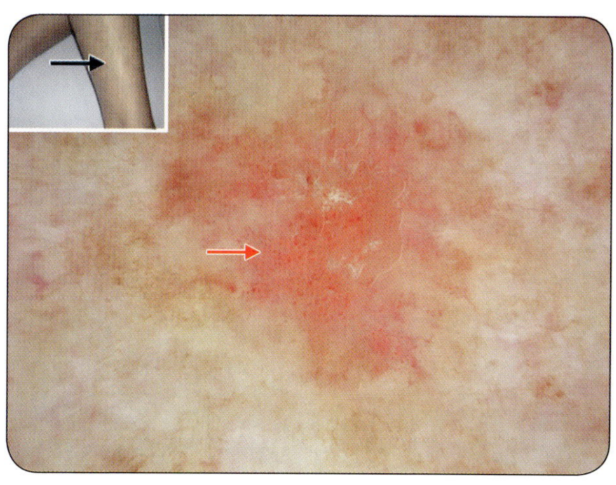

Fig. 5.186: Squamous cell carcinoma in situ—nonpigmented Bowen's disease: glomerular or spiral vessels, monomorphic pattern, focal distribution (red arrow) (clinical view black arrow).

Dermoscopic Criteria

- Central hyperkeratosis
- Vessels
  - Thick hairpin vessels with peripheral distribution
  - Linear irregular vessels
- Blood spots
- White areas and circles

Bowen's Disease

Squamous Cell Carcinoma In Situ—Nonpigmented Bowen's Disease

Dermoscopy is useful in the diagnosis of SCC in situ or Bowen's disease (BD). The most frequent variant is the nonpigmented form.

In most cases, its clinical manifestation is a well-demarcated pink and scaly (squamous) plaque. Differential diagnosis includes actinic keratosis, eczema, psoriasis, seborrheic dermatitis, Paget's disease, and superficial basal cell carcinoma.

The dermoscopic key in nonpigmented BD is the monomorphic vascular pattern with focal distribution, whose morphology is spiral or glomerular (tight spiral vessels, which may resemble areas or globules at small magnification) (Figs. 5.185 to 5.196).

Dermoscopic Criteria

- Vessels
  - Glomerular or spiral vessels

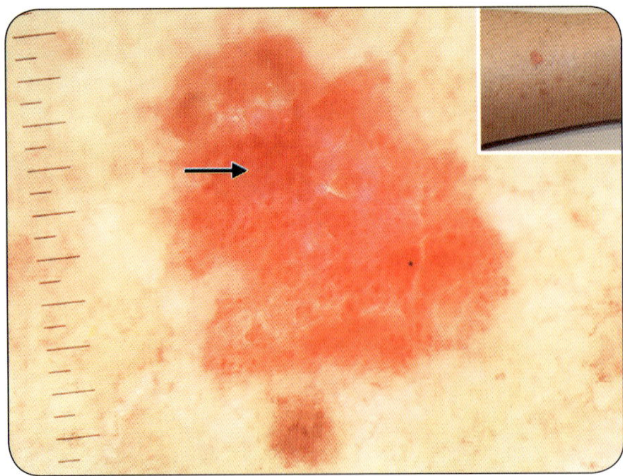

Fig. 5.187: Squamous cell carcinoma in situ—nonpigmented Bowen's disease: glomerular or spiral vessels, monomorphic pattern, focal distribution (arrow).

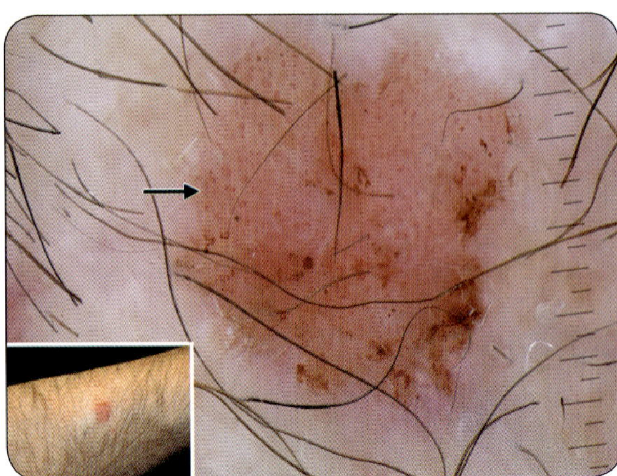

Fig. 5.188: Squamous cell carcinoma in situ—nonpigmented Bowen's disease: glomerular or spiral vessels, monomorphic pattern, focal distribution (arrow).

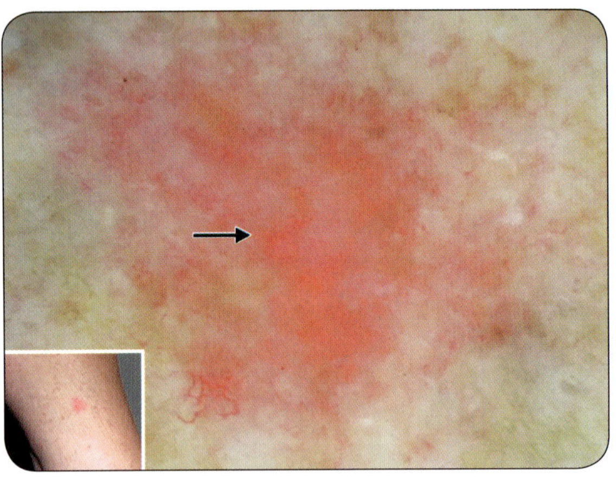

Fig. 5.189: Squamous cell carcinoma in situ—nonpigmented Bowen's disease: glomerular or spiral vessels, monomorphic pattern, focal distribution (arrow).

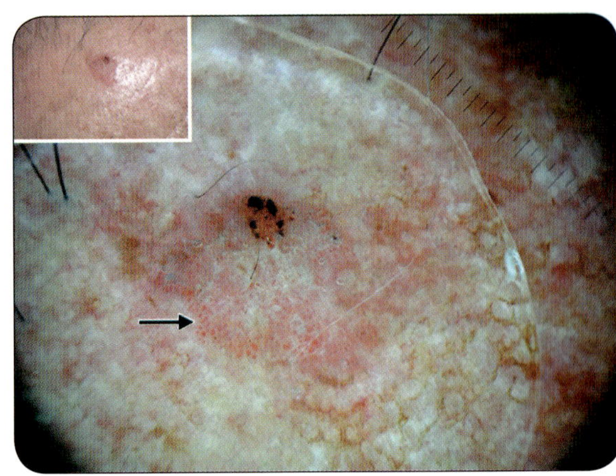

Fig. 5.190: Squamous cell carcinoma in situ—nonpigmented Bowen's disease: glomerular or spiral vessels, monomorphic pattern, focal distribution (arrow).

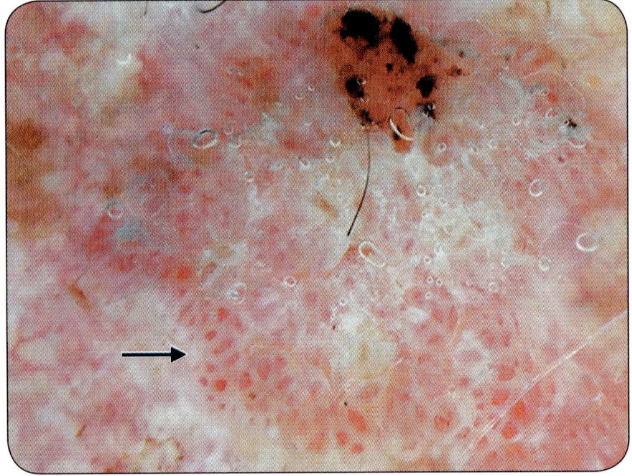

Fig. 5.191: Squamous cell carcinoma in situ—nonpigmented Bowen's disease: (close up of Fig. 5.190) glomerular or spiral vessels, monomorphic pattern, focal distribution (arrow).

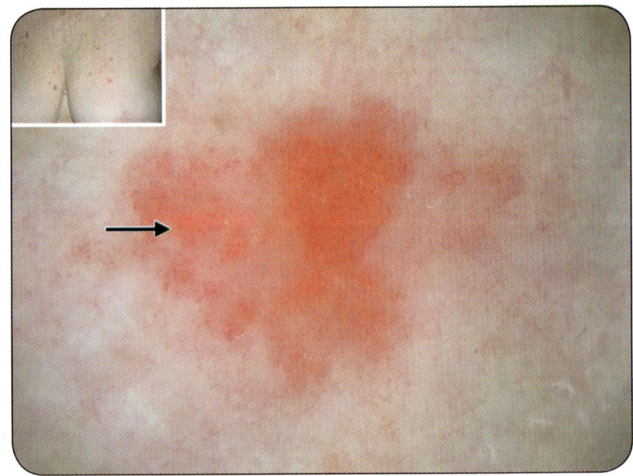

Fig. 5.192: Squamous cell carcinoma in situ—nonpigmented Bowen's disease: glomerular or spiral vessels, monomorphic pattern, focal distribution (arrow).

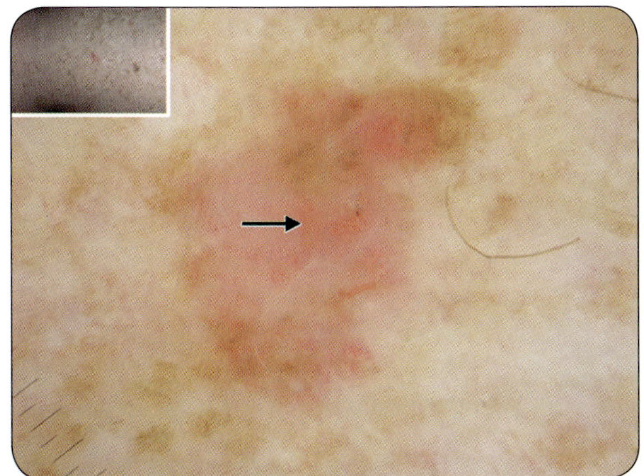

Fig. 5.193: Squamous cell carcinoma in situ—nonpigmented Bowen's disease: glomerular or spiral vessels, monomorphic pattern, focal distribution (arrow).

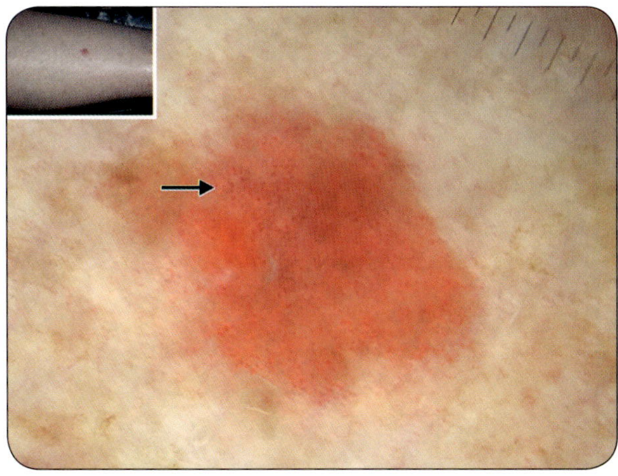

Fig. 5.194: Squamous cell carcinoma in situ–nonpigmented Bowen's disease: glomerular or spiral vessels, monomorphic pattern, focal distribution (arrow).

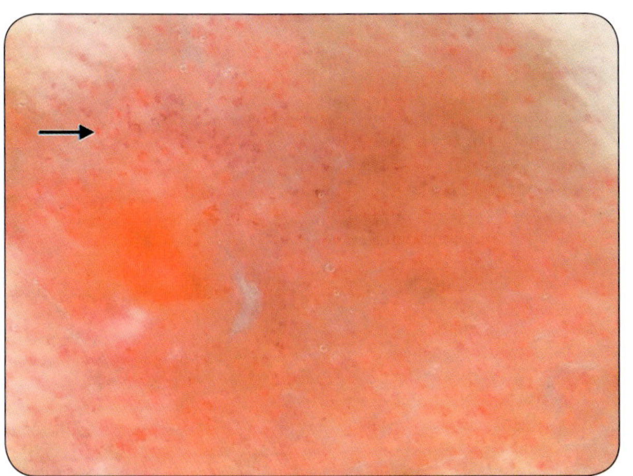

Fig. 5.195: Squamous cell carcinoma in situ—nonpigmented Bowen's disease: (close up Fig. 5.194) glomerular or spiral vessels, monomorphic pattern, focal distribution (arrow).

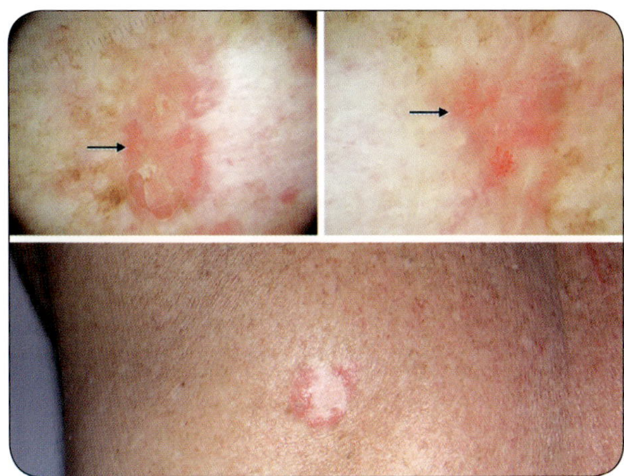

Fig. 5.196: Squamous cell carcinoma in situ—nonpigmented Bowen's disease: glomerular or spiral vessels, monomorphic pattern, focal distribution (arrows marking left and right side of the lesion).

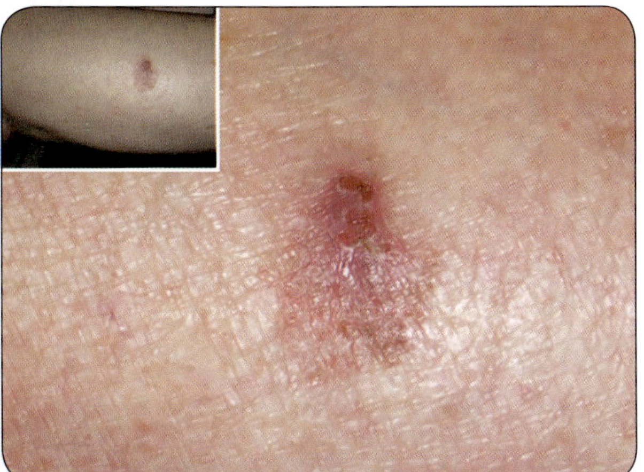

Fig. 5.197: Squamous cell carcinoma. (Pigmented Bowen's disease) clinical view.

  - Monomorphic pattern
  - Focal distribution
- Rough surface

Squamous Cell Carcinoma In Situ—Pigmented Bowen's Disease

Pigmented Bowen's disease (PBD) is a rare variant of BD (Fig. 5.197).

Its clinical manifestation is a well-demarcated pink or brownish macula or squamous plaque. The differential diagnosis includes pigmented actinic keratosis, solar lentigo, seborrheic keratosis, lichen planus-like keratosis, pigmented basal cell carcinoma, nevi, and melanomas.

Pigmented Brown's disease presents a characteristic dermoscopic pattern, prominently a pattern of structureless

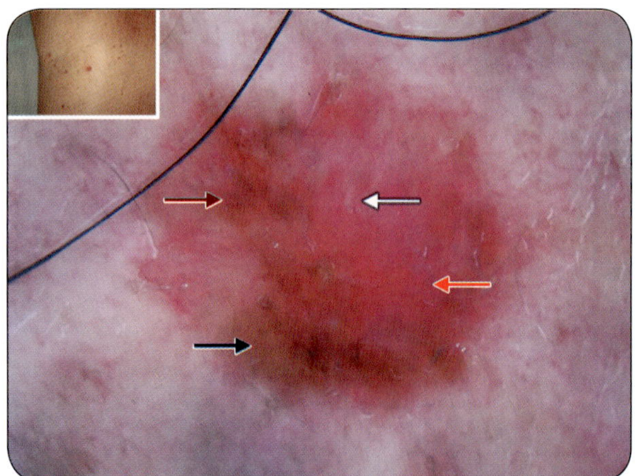

Fig. 5.198: Squamous cell carcinoma in situ—pigmented Bowen's disease: brown color (brown arrow); structureless areas (hypopigmented: pink, skin colored, or white) (white arrow); linear arrangement of brown or gray dots (black arrow); coiled vessels: arranged in linear fashion or in clusters (red arrow).

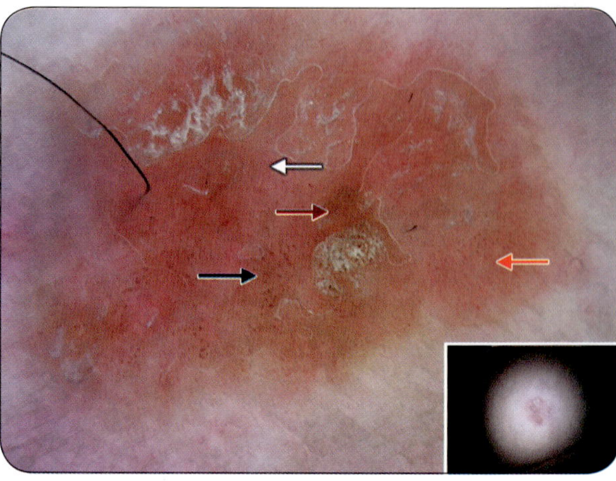

Fig. 5.199: Squamous cell carcinoma in situ—pigmented Bowen's disease: brown color (brown arrow); structureless areas (hypopigmented: pink, skin colored, or white) (white arrow); linear arrangement of brown or gray dots (black arrow); coiled vessels: arranged in linear fashion or in clusters (red arrow).

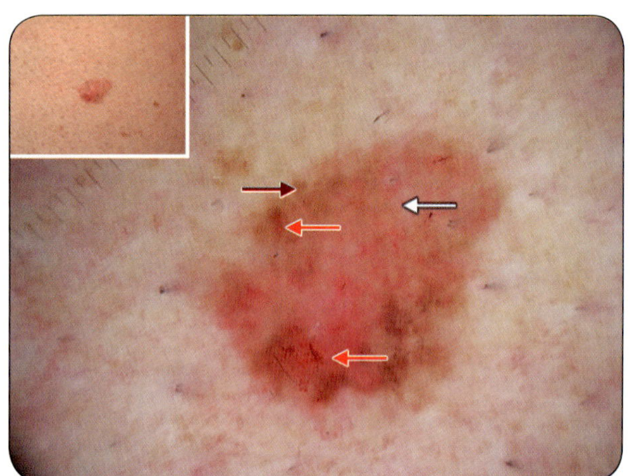

Fig. 5.200: Squamous cell carcinoma in situ—pigmented Bowen's disease: brown color (brown arrow); structureless areas (hypopigmented: pink, skin colored, or white) (white arrow); coiled vessels: arranged in linear fashion or in clusters (red arrows).

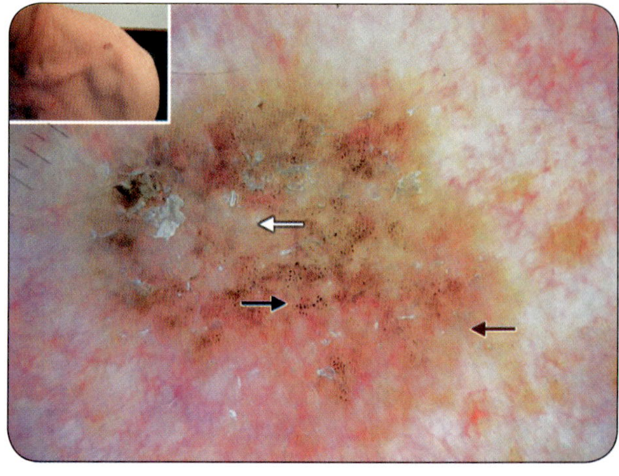

Fig. 5.201: Squamous cell carcinoma in situ—pigmented Bowen's disease: brown color (brown arrow); structureless areas (hypopigmented: pink, skin colored, or white) (white arrow); linear arrangement of brown or gray dots (black arrow).

areas, as well as a combination of brown or gray dots. The most common color in these lesions is brown in its chromatic variants. The vessels, spiral or loop-like, are arranged in linear fashion in the periphery of the lesion or in clusters or groups. On occasion, PBD may not present any of these dermoscopic clues (Figs. 5.198 to 5.206).

Dermoscopic Criteria

Linear arrangement of brown or gray dots

This feature lies most frequently in the periphery of the lesion with the lines radially arranged.

- Brown color
- Structureless areas
- Hypopigmented—pink skin colored, or white.
  - Vessels
- Spiral or loop-like vessels
- Linear arrangement
- In clusters or groups
  - Without dermoscopic clues

Squamous Cell Carcinoma

In its progression, infiltrating SCC invades the underlying tissue. The typical lesion is a firm and pink raised plaque

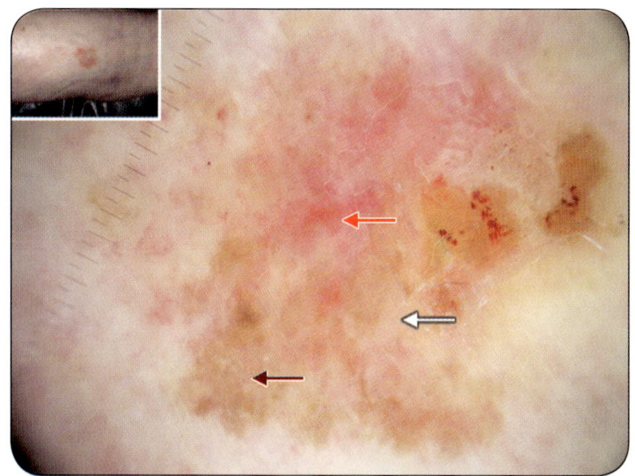

Fig. 5.202: Squamous cell carcinoma in situ—pigmented Bowen's disease: brown color (brown arrow); structureless areas (hypopigmented: pink, skin colored, or white) (white arrow); coiled vessels: arranged clusters (red arrow).

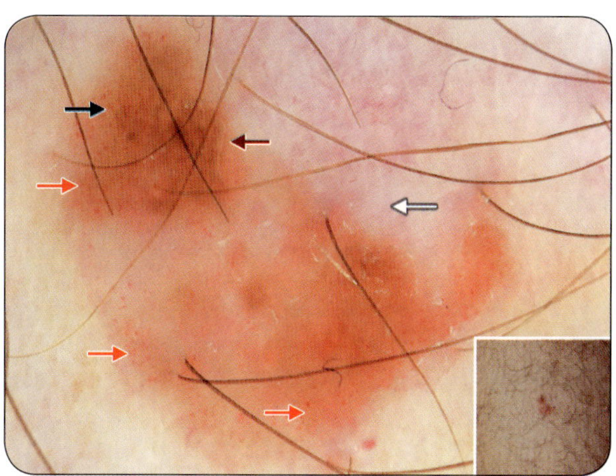

Fig. 5.203: Squamous cell carcinoma in situ—pigmented Bowen's disease: brown color (brown arrow); structureless areas (hypopigmented: pink, skin colored, or white) (white arrow); linear arrangement of brown or gray dots (black arrow); coiled vessels: arranged in linear fashion or in clusters (red arrows).

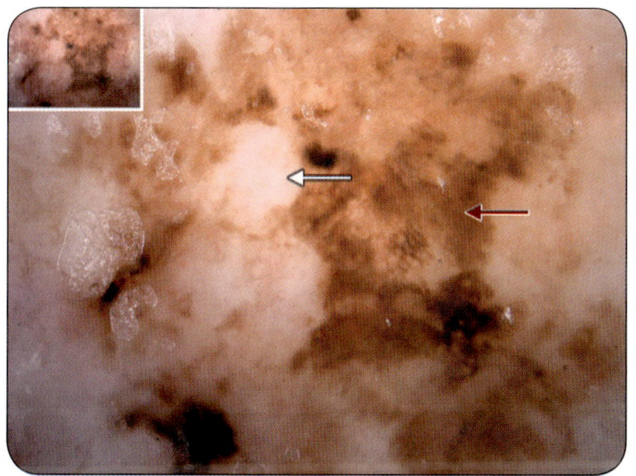

Fig. 5.204: Squamous cell carcinoma in situ—pigmented Bowen's disease: brown color (brown arrow); structureless areas (hypopigmented: pink, skin colored, or white) (white arrow).

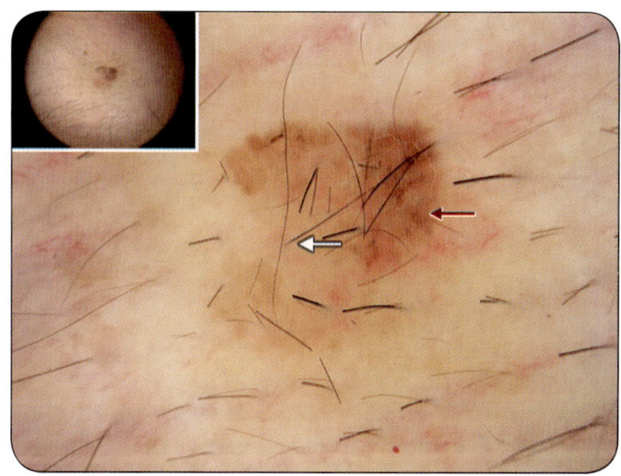

Fig. 5.205: Squamous cell carcinoma in situ—pigmented Bowen's disease: brown color (brown arrow); structureless areas (hypopigmented: pink, skin colored, or white) (white arrow).

or tumor on photodamaged skin. The surface may be covered in crusts or ulcerated. Differential diagnosis must be made, especially, with KA, ulcerated BCC, and amelanotic melanoma (Fig. 5.207).

Dermoscopically, it is possible to observe, in the center of the lesion, areas without structure, white, yellow, or light brown in color, and amorphous areas corresponding to hyperkeratosis usually located in the central part; also blood spots distributed in the keratin and white circles surrounding the dilated infundibulum filled with a central keratin plug resembling yellow or orange clods. The vessels can be glomerular, although these tumors typically present mostly hairpin vessels or irregular linear vessels, arranged in the periphery of the lesion; it may be associated with variable ulceration areas and scales (Figs. 5.208 to 5.211).

Dermoscopic Criteria

- Hyperkeratosis usually located in the central part of the lesion
- Blood spots in the hyperkeratosis areas
- White, yellow, or light brown structureless areas
- White circles
- *Vessels*: glomerular, hairpin, or irregular linear vessels
- Ulceration
- Scales

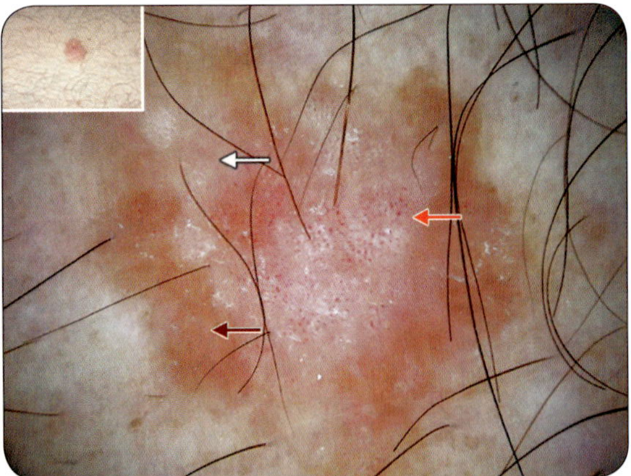

Fig. 5.206: Squamous cell carcinoma in situ—pigmented Bowen's disease: brown color (brown arrow); structureless areas (hypopigmented: pink, skin colored, or white) (white arrow); coiled vessels: arranged in clusters (red arrow).

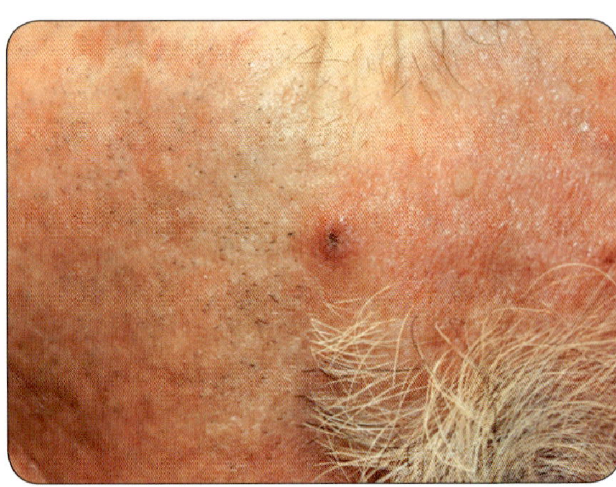

Fig. 5.207: Squamous cell carcinoma (Clinical view).

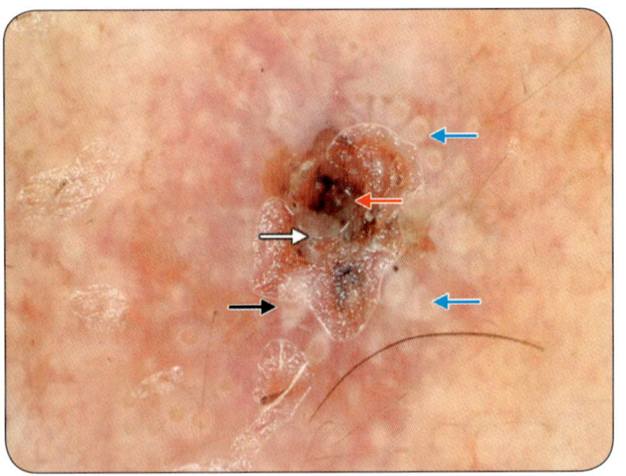

Fig. 5.208: Squamous cell carcinoma: hyperkeratosis (white arrow); blood spots and ulceration (red arrow); white structureless areas (black arrow); white circles (blue arrows); glomerular, hairpin, or irregular linear vessels.

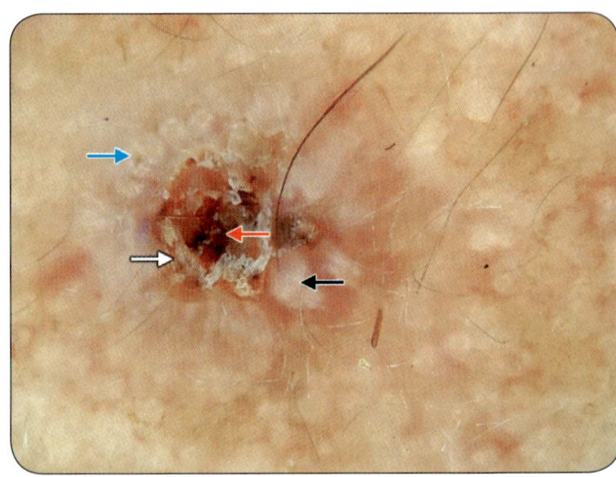

Fig. 5.209: Squamous cell carcinoma: hyperkeratosis (white arrow); blood spots and ulceration (red arrow); white structureless areas (black arrow); white circles (blue arrow).

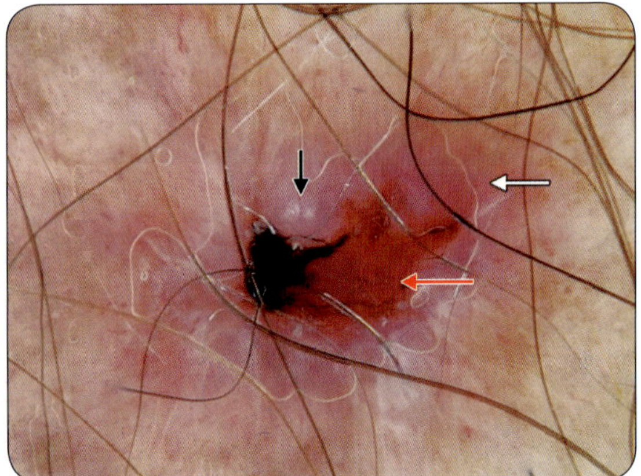

Fig. 5.210: Squamous cell carcinoma: blood spots and ulceration (red arrow); white structureless areas (black arrow); hairpin and linear irregular vessels (white arrow).

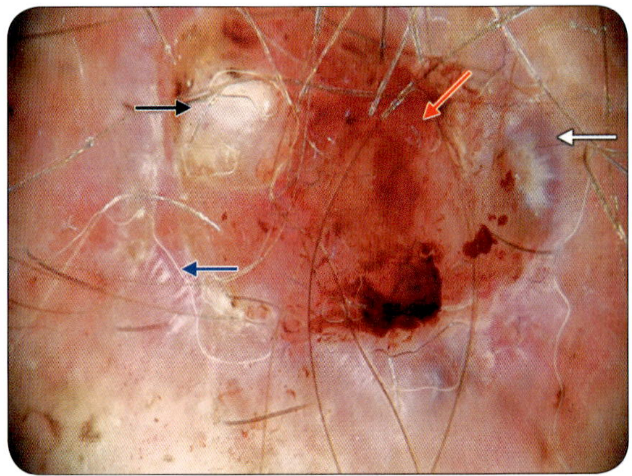

Fig. 5.211: Squamous cell carcinoma: blood spots and ulceration (red arrow); white structureless areas (black arrow); white circles (blue arrow); hairpin and linear irregular vessels (white arrow).

SUGGESTED READING

Argenziano G, Soyer P, De Giorgio V, et al. Interactive Atlas of Dermoscopy. Milán: EDRA Medical Publishing & New Media; 2000.

Cabo H. Dermatoscopia. Buenos Aires, Argentina: Weber Ferro; 2000.

Cabo H. Dermatoscopia, 2nd edition. Buenos Aires, Argentina: Ediciones Journal; 2012.

Cameron A, Rosendahl C, Tschandl P, et al. Dermatoscopy of pigmented Bowen's disease. J Am Acad Dermatol. 2010;62: 597-604.

Jorh R, Soyer P, Argenziano G, et al. Dermoscopy. The Essentials (MOABT). New York: Elsevier Ltd.; 2004.

Johr R, Stolz W. Dermoscopy: An Illustrated Self-Assessment Guide, 2nd edition. New York: McGraw-Hill Education; 2015.

Kim C, Ko CJ, Leffell DJ. Cutaneous squamous cell carcinomas of the lower extremity: a distinct subset of squamous cell carcinomas. J Am Acad Dermatol. 2014;70:70-4.

Kittler H. Dermatoscopy. An Algorithmic Method Based on Pattern Analysis 2011 Facultas Verlags- und Buchhandels AG facultas wuv Universitätsverlag, Austria www.facultas.wuv.at.

Lallas A. Dermoscopy in general dermatology. Dermatol Clin. 2013;3:679-94.

Lin MJ, Pan Y, Jalilian C, et al. Dermoscopic characteristics of nodular squamous cell carcinoma and keratoacanthoma. Dermatol Pract Concept. 2014;4(2):9-15.

Malvhey J, Puig S. Principles of Dermoscopy. Barcelona: Creaciones Gráficas; 2009.

Marghoob A, Braun R, Kopf A. Atlas of Dermoscopy. London: Taylor & Francis; 2005.

Menzies S, Crotty K, Ingvar C, et al. An Atlas of Surface Microscopy of Pigmented Skin Lesions. Sydney: McGraw-Hill Book Company; 1996.

Rabinovitz H, Kopf A. Dermoscopy: A Practical Guide. Miami: American Academy of Dermatology; 1999.

Rosendahl C, Cameron A, Argenziano G, et al. Dermoscopy of squamous cell carcinoma and keratoacanthoma. Arch Dermatol. 2012;148(12):1386-92.

Soyer P, Argenziano G, Chimenti S, et al. Dermoscopy of Pigmented Skin Lesions. An Atlas Based on the Consensus Net Meeting on Dermoscopy. Milán: EDRA Medical Publishing & New Media; 2001.

Stolz W, Braun-Falco O, Bilek P, et al. Color Atlas of Dermatoscopy. Germany: Blackwell Science; 1994.

Vazquez-Lopez F, Manjon-Haces JA, Maldonado-Seral C, et al. Dermoscopy of Bowen's disease. Br J Dermatol. 2004; 150: 1112-6.

Zalaudek I, Argenziano G, Giacomel J. Dermoscopy of Non-Pigmented Skin Tumors. Boca Raton, FL: CRC Press; 2016.

Zalaudek I, Citarella L, Soyer HP, et al., Dermoscopy features of pigmented squamous cell carcinoma: a case report. Dermatol Surg. 2004;30:539-40.

Zalaudek I, Di Stefani A, Argenziano G. The specific dermoscopic criteria of Bowen's disease. J Eur Acad Dermatol Venereol. 2006;20:361-2.

Zalaudek I, Giacomel J, Schmid K, et al. Dermatoscopy of actinic keratosis, intraepidermal carcinoma and invasive squamous cell carcinoma: a progression model. J Am Acad Dermatol. 2012;66(4):589-97.

5.8 OTHER NONMELANOCYTIC LESIONS

5.8.1 Eccrine Poroma

Carolina Marcucci, Horacio A Cabo

Eccrine poroma (EP) is a benign adnexal tumor derived from the acrosyringium and the intraepidermal part of the eccrine sweat glands excretory duct. Clinically, it appears as a solitary pink nodule, generally located at acral level (palms and soles) in adults. Differential diagnosis must be performed with benign tumorous lesions (mainly pyogenic granuloma and seborrheic keratosis) and malignant lesions [basal cell carcinoma (BCC) and melanoma].

Eccrine poroma has two variants: Pigmented (less frequent) and nonpigmented. Dermoscopy has proved to be especially useful since it enables the evaluation of vascular structures showing a *polymorphic vascular pattern*, with hairpin vessels, dotted vessels, irregular linear vessels, and pink lacunae surrounded by a whitish halo looking like *"frog eggs."* There have also been descriptions of arborizing vessels, typically with a *flower-like* or *grail-like appearance* (Figs. 5.212 to 5.218).

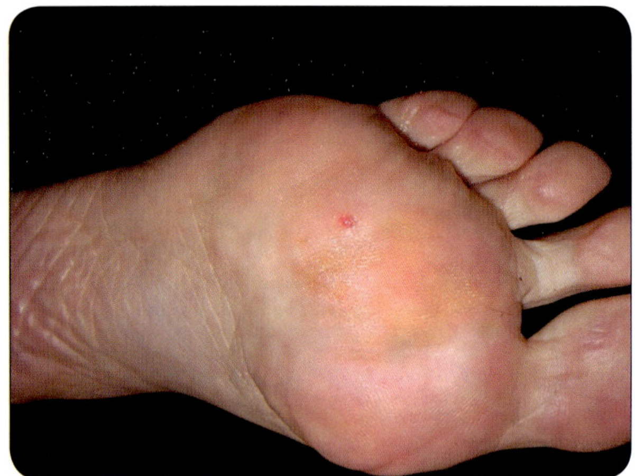

Fig. 5.212: Eccrine poroma (nonpigmented form).

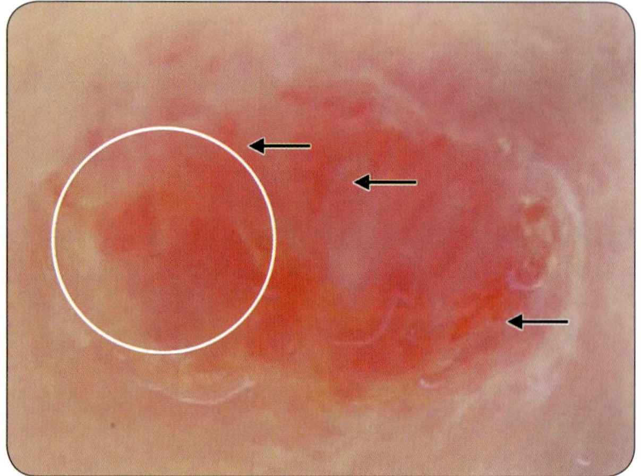

Fig. 5.213: Eccrine poroma: flower-like appearance (black arrows); frog eggs like appearance (white circle).

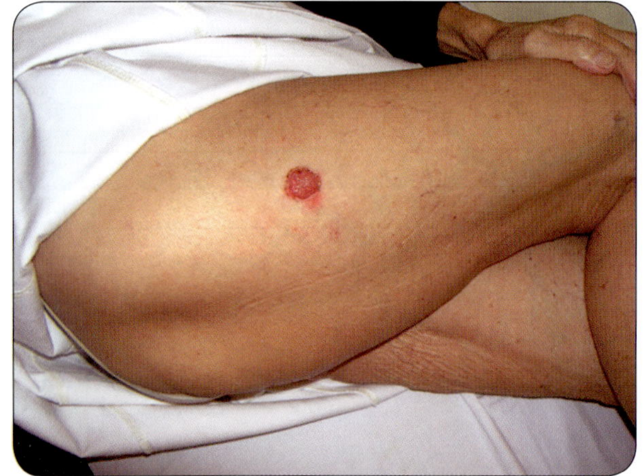

Fig. 5.214: Eccrine poroma (nonpigmented form).

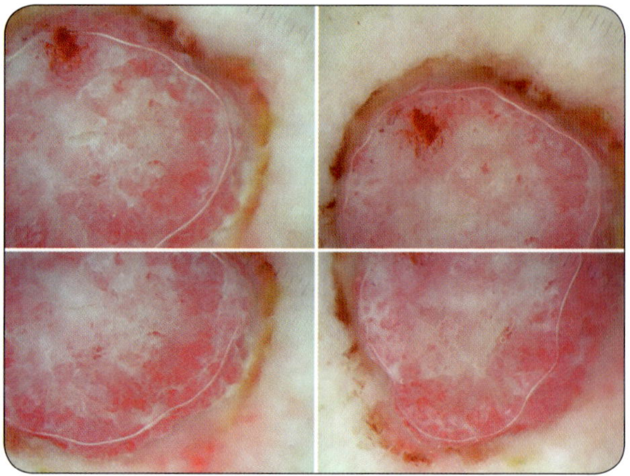

Fig. 5.215: Eccrine poroma: different views of the same lesion showing the typical frog eggs' aggregation.

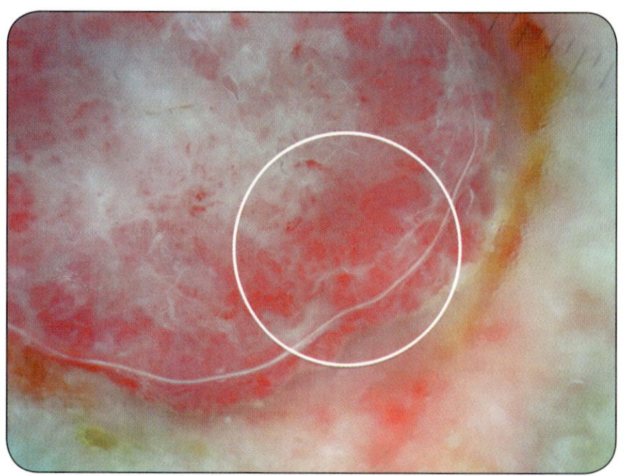

Fig. 5.216: Eccrine poroma: frog eggs like appearance (white circle).

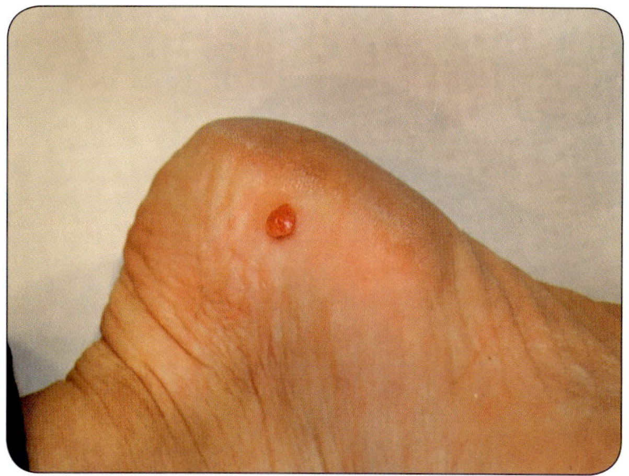

Fig. 5.217: Eccrine poroma (nonpigmented form).

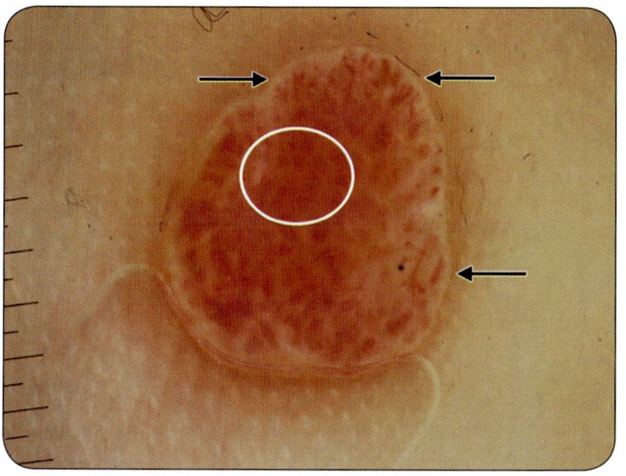

Fig. 5.218: Eccrine poroma: flower-like appearance (black arrows); frog eggs like appearance (white circle).

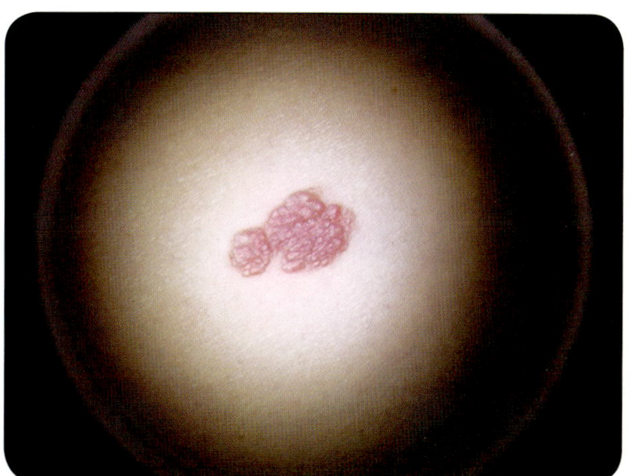

Fig. 5.219: Eccrine poroma (pigmented form).

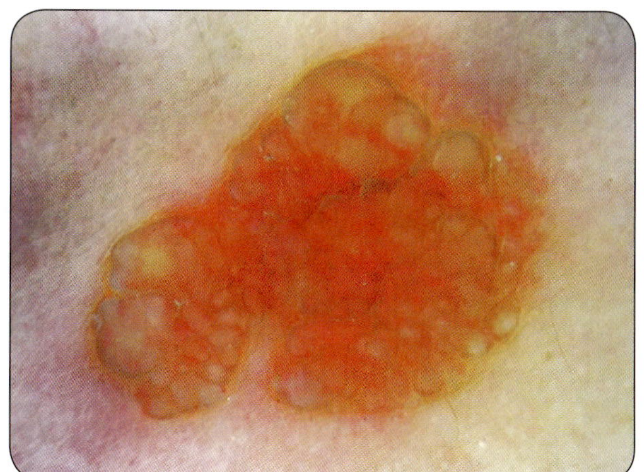

Fig. 5.220: Eccrine poroma (pigmented form): round light-brown areas divided by a darker colored partition. Pseudo-red appearance.

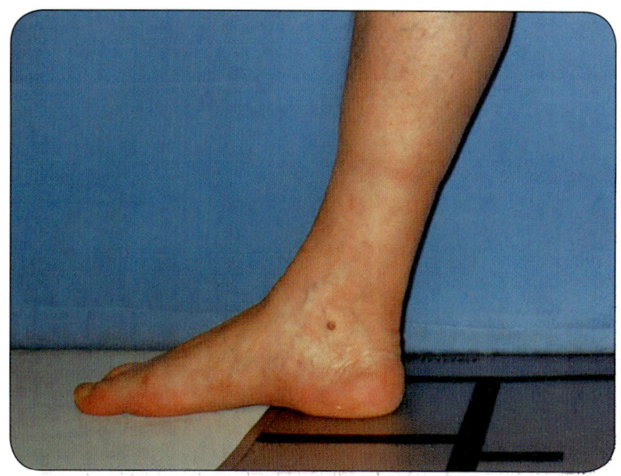

Fig. 5.221: Eccrine poroma (pigmented form).

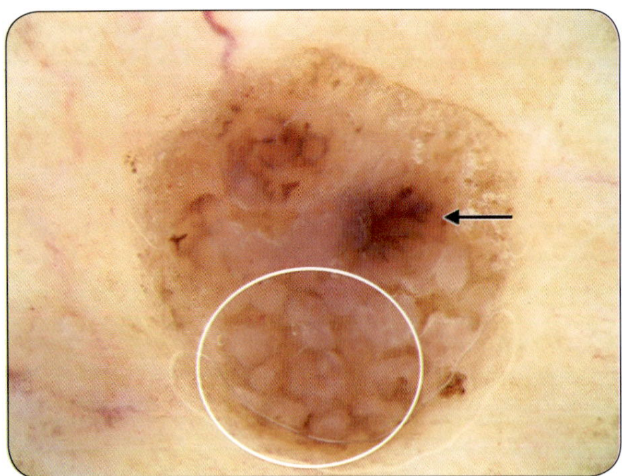

Fig. 5.222: Eccrine poroma (pigmented form): round light-brown areas or nests divided by darker brown partitions. Pseudo-network image (white circle); flower-like appearance (black arrow).

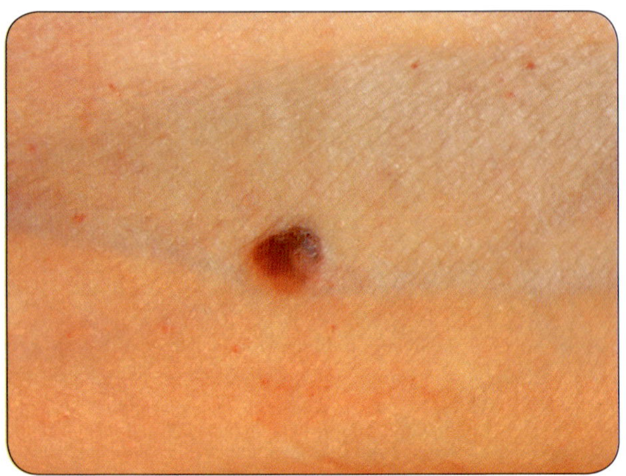

Fig. 5.223: Eccrine poroma (pigmented form).

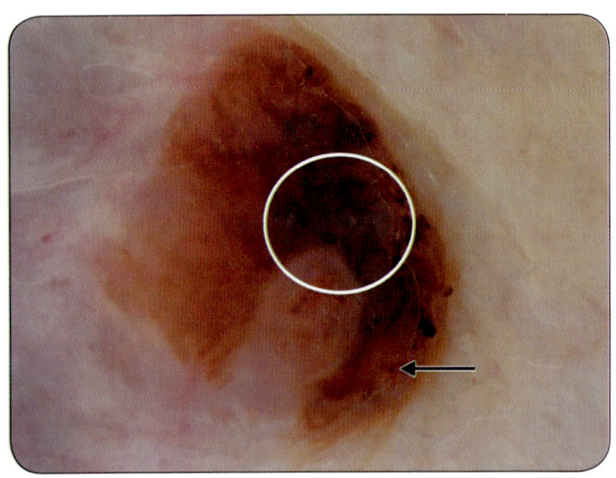

Fig. 5.224: Eccrine poroma (pigmented form): round blue–gray areas or nests (white circle); flower-like appearance (black arrow).

Besides the vascular structures, the pigmented variant presents nests and brown or blue-gray dots; as a result, it must be differentiated from pigmented BCC. However, EP lacks other criteria that are present in BCC (Figs. 5.219 to 5.224).

SUGGESTED READING

Ferrari A, Buccini P, Silipo V, et al. Eccrine poroma: a clinical-dermoscopic study of seven cases. Acta Derm Venereol. 2009;89:160-4.

Minagawa A, Koga H. Dermatology. Dermoscopy of pigmented poromas. Dermatology. 2010;221:78-83.

Minagawa A, Koga H, Takahashi M, et al. Dermoscopic features of nonpigmented eccrine poromas in association with their histopathological features. Br J Dermatol. 2010;163:1264-8.

5.8.2 Clear Cell Acanthoma

Carolina Marcucci, Horacio A Cabo

Clear cell acanthoma is a rare benign tumor that appears as a pink papuloid lesion localized in the lower limb of adults.

Under dermoscopic examination, it is possible to observe dotted or globular vessels with linear arrangement, like a "string of pearls." Although dotted vessels are typical of melanocytic tumors, they are evenly distributed over the whole lesion. On the other hand, in clear cell acanthoma the dotted vessels are surrounded by a whitish halo, typical of keratinizing tumors (Figs. 5.225 to 5.227).

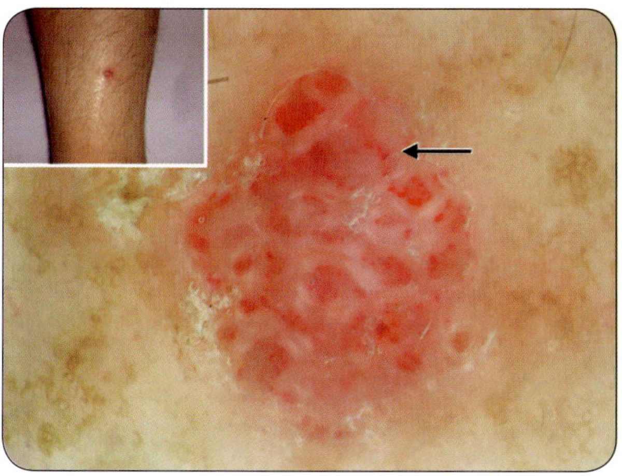

Fig. 5.225: Clear cell acanthoma: dotted or globular vessels in linear arrangement, like a "string of pearls" (arrow).

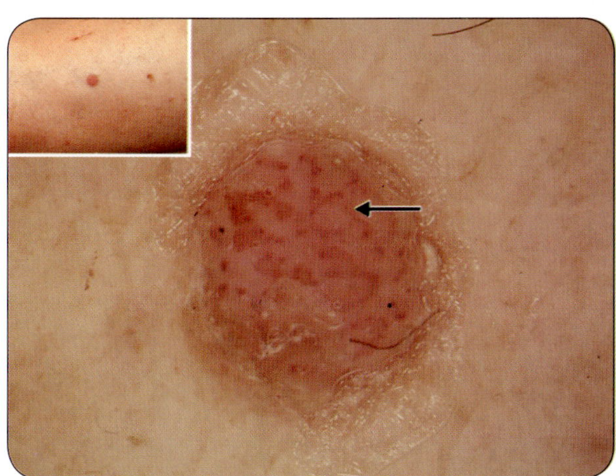

Fig. 5.226: Clear cell acanthoma: dotted or globular vessels in linear arrangement, like a "string of pearls" (arrow).

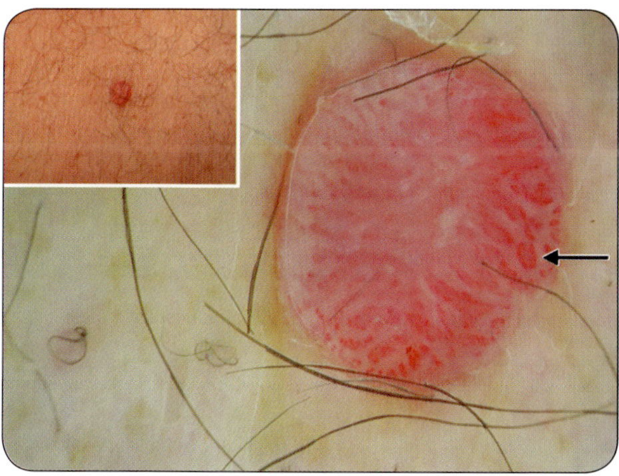

Fig. 5.227: Clear cell acanthoma: dotted or globular vessels in linear arrangement, like a "string of pearls" (arrow).

SUGGESTED READING

Blum A, Metzler G, Bauer J, et al. The dermoscopic pattern of clear-cell acanthoma resembles psoriasis vulgaris. Dermatology. 2001;203:50-2.

Cabo H. Dermatoscopia, 2nd edition. Buenos Aires, Argentina: Ediciones Journal; 2012.

Johr R, Stolz W. Dermoscopy: An Illustrated Self-Assessment Guide, 2nd edition. New York: McGraw-Hill Education; 2015.

Malvhey J, Puig S. Principles of Dermoscopy. Barcelona: Creaciones Gráficas; 2009.

Marghoob A, Braun R, Kopf A. Atlas of Dermoscopy. London: Taylor & Francis; 2005.

5.8.3 Cylindroma

Carolina Marcucci, Horacio A Cabo

Cylindromas are benign tumors derived from the apocrine glands. They appear as dome-shaped erythematous nodules, solitary or multiple, and generally localized in the head and neck, although they can also appear in the upper trunk.

In dermoscopy, it is possible to observe pink areas, arborizing vessels, blue dots or globules, and ulceration, all of which make the cylindroma a basal cell carcinoma simulator, as both tumors share the same dermoscopic criteria (Fig. 5.228).

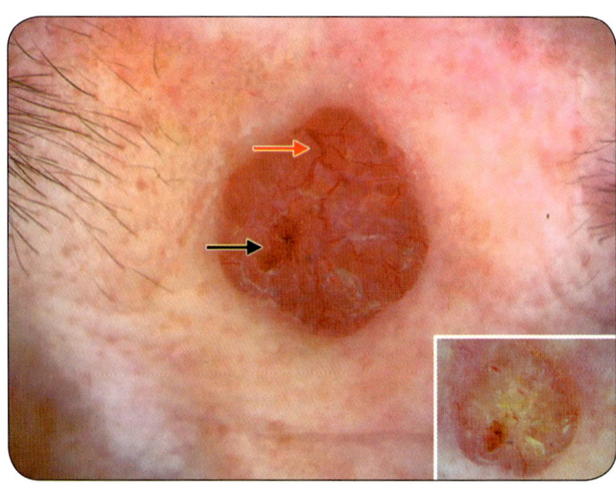

Fig. 5.228: Cylindroma: arborizing vessels (red arrow) and ulceration (black arrow).

SUGGESTED READING

Cabo H, Pedrini F, Cohen Sabban E. Dermoscopy of cylindroma. Dermatol Res Pract. 2010;2010:285392.

Cohen Y, Elpern D. Dermoscopic pattern of a cylindroma. Dermatol Pract Concept. 2013;4(1):10.

Lallas A, Apalla Z, Tzellos T, et al. Dermoscopy of solitary cylindroma. Eur J Dermatol. 2011;21(4):645-6.

5.8.4 Trichoepithelioma

Carolina Marcucci, Horacio A Cabo

Trichoepithelioma (TE) is a benign adnexal tumor derived from the germinal matrix of the hair follicle. Most frequently, there is a solitary lesion, although there are also multiple forms, and a desmoplastic TE variant. Clinically, it appears as a pink papule or nodule, usually occurring on the face in young individuals. Its main differential diagnosis is basal cell carcinoma (BCC).

In dermoscopy, solitary tumors present arborizing telangiectasia and white shiny or crystalline structures, similar to BCC. However, TE usually lacks the other dermoscopic criteria of BCC, namely blue-gray globules and nests, and maple-leaf structures (Fig. 5.229).

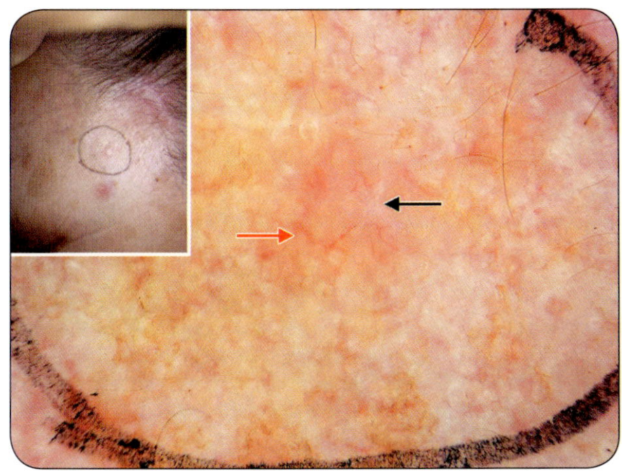

Fig. 5.229: Trichoepithelioma with arborizing vessels (red arrow); white shiny or crystalline structures (black arrow).

SUGGESTED READING

Lazaridou E, Fotiadou C, Patsatsi A, et al. Solitary trichoepithelioma in an 8-year-old child: clinical, dermoscopic and histopathologic findings. Dermatol Pract Concept. 2014; 4(2): 55-8.

5.8.5 Verrucae Vulgaris

Paula Friedman, Horacio A Cabo

Verrucae vulgaris (VV) are caused by some types of human papilloma virus. They appear as hyperkeratotic papules, scaly, and rough, solitary or multiple. They are more frequent in children and young adults, occurring in hands, feet, and limbs.

Dermoscopically, VV is characterized by the following (Figs. 5.230 to 5.232):

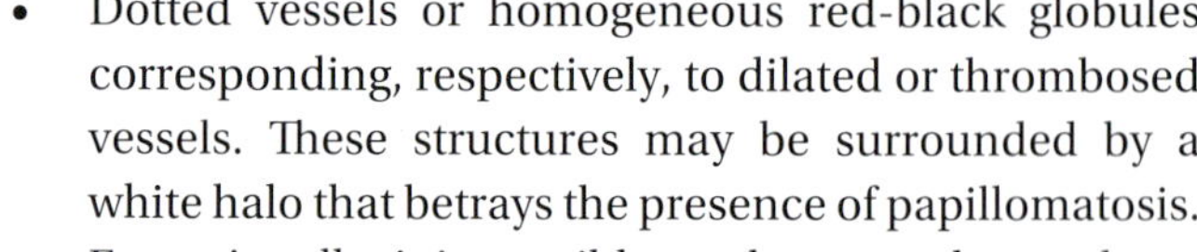

- Dotted vessels or homogeneous red-black globules corresponding, respectively, to dilated or thrombosed vessels. These structures may be surrounded by a white halo that betrays the presence of papillomatosis.
- Exceptionally, it is possible to observe polymorphous vessels (hairpin, dotted, spiral, or irregular linear vessels) and ulceration areas.

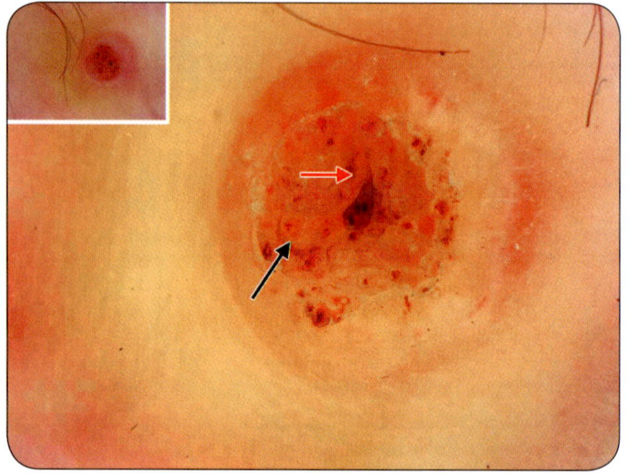

Fig. 5.230: Verrucae vulgaris: thrombotic or dilated vessels (red arrow) in multiple round or oval areas (black arrow).

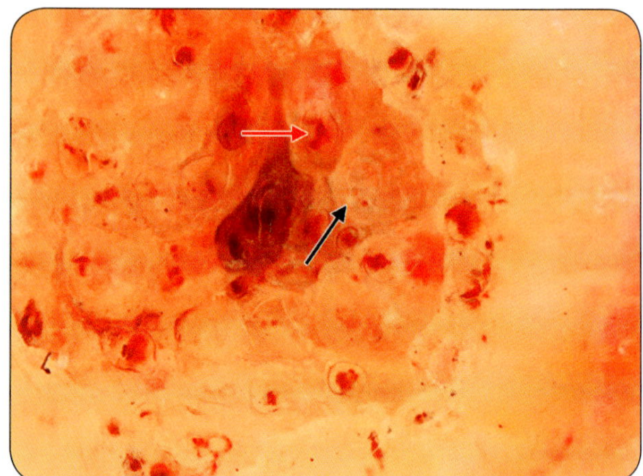

Fig. 5.231: Verrucae vulgaris: thrombotic or dilated vessels (red arrow) in multiple round or oval areas (black arrow) (closeup view of Figure 5.230).

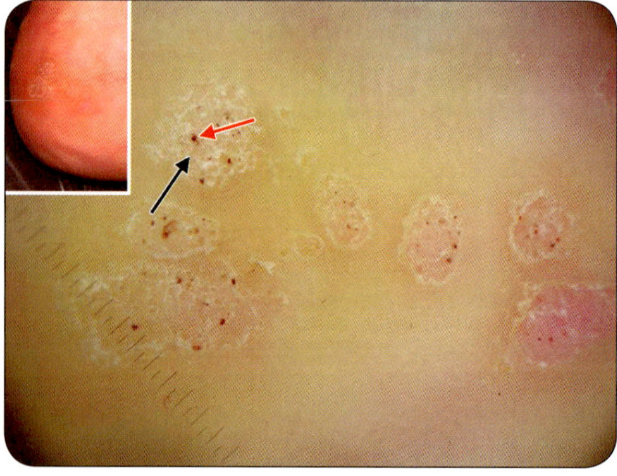

Fig. 5.232: Verrucae vulgaris: thrombotic or dilated vessels (red arrow) in multiple round or oval areas (black arrow).

SUGGESTED READING

Cabo H. Dermatoscopia, 2nd edition. Buenos Aires, Argentina: Ediciones Journal; 2012.

Malvhey J, Puig S. Principles of Dermoscopy. Barcelona: Creaciones Gráficas; 2009.

Marghoob A, Braun R, Kopf A. Atlas of Dermoscopy. London: Taylor & Francis; 2005.

5.8.6 Molluscum Contagiosum

Paula Friedman, Horacio A Cabo

Disease is occurring worldwide. Its etiologic agent is the molluscum contagiosum (MC) virus, which belongs to the poxvirus family. It is more frequent in children, but can also appear in adults, in which case it is considered a sexually transmitted infection. Clinically, it appears as round dome-shaped papules, umbilicated, translucent and firm, 2–5 mm, pink, pearly white, or skin colored (Fig. 5.233).

Dermoscopically, MC presents the following patterns (Fig. 5.234):

- "Fried egg" pattern, due to the presence of round structures with a central pore
- Polylobular amorphous white–yellow structure
- *Orifice*: The growth of viral matter may cause a break in the skin.
- Peripheral hairpin vessels in "red crown" arrangement not crossing the central lobules
- Linear (radial) vessels arranged perpendicularly without crossing the central pore
- Dotted vessels

Most frequently, the central pore has radial and crown vessels. When these vessels surround the lesion completely, the lesion is called "mixed flower-like pattern." This recently described pattern appears to be MC specific.

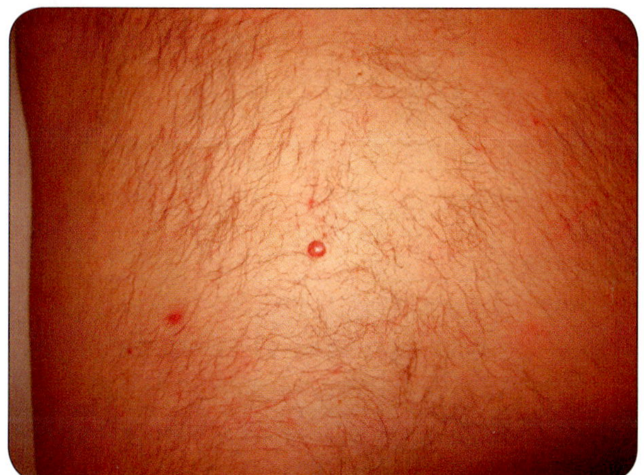

Fig. 5.233: Molluscum contagiosum.

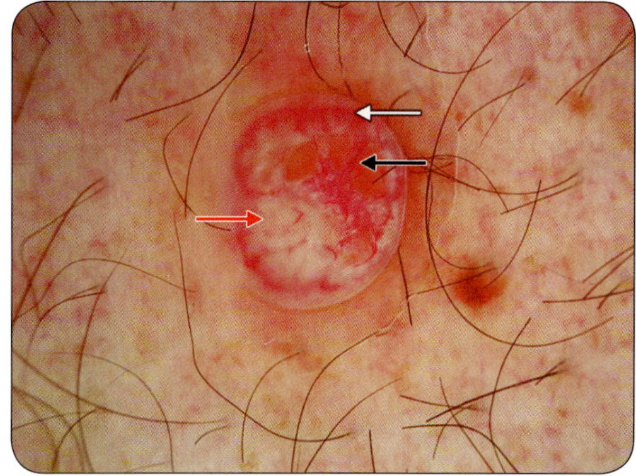

Fig. 5.234: Molluscum contagiosum: polylobular amorphous white–yellow structure (red arrow); peripheral hairpin vessels in "red crown" arrangement (white arrow); linear (radial) vessels arranged perpendicularly without crossing the central pore (black arrow).

SUGGESTED READING

Cabo H. Dermatoscopia, 2nd edition. Buenos Aires, Argentina: Ediciones Journal; 2012.

Malvhey J, Puig S. Principles of Dermoscopy. Barcelona: Creaciones Gráficas; 2009.

Marghoob A, Braun R, Kopf A. Atlas of Dermoscopy. London: Taylor & Francis; 2005.

Zaballos P, Ara M, Puig S, et al. Dermoscopy of molluscum contagiosum: a useful tool for clinical diagnosis in adulthood. J Eur Acad Dermatol Venereol. 2006;20:482-3.

5.8.7 Sebaceous Hyperplasia

Paula Friedman, Horacio A Cabo

Sebaceous hyperplasia (SH) is a common benign tumoral lesion occurring on the face of adult patients. From a clinical point of view, it presents as a white-yellowish papule, sometimes umbilicated, of <1 cm. Among its differential diagnoses, we find molluscum contagiosum, basal cell carcinoma, milia-like cysts, and fibrous papula (Figs. 5.235 and 5.236).

Dermoscopically, SH presents the following patterns (Figs. 5.237 to 5.239):

- Structureless white-yellowish aggregated areas
- Central umbilication, corresponding to the hyperplasic sebaceous gland duct
- Curved linear vessels with peripheral radial or crown arrangement, surrounding the center of the lesion but without crossing it

The sign, known as "toffee chocolate sign," has been described, corresponding to a central depression surrounded by white-yellowish aggregated globules. This

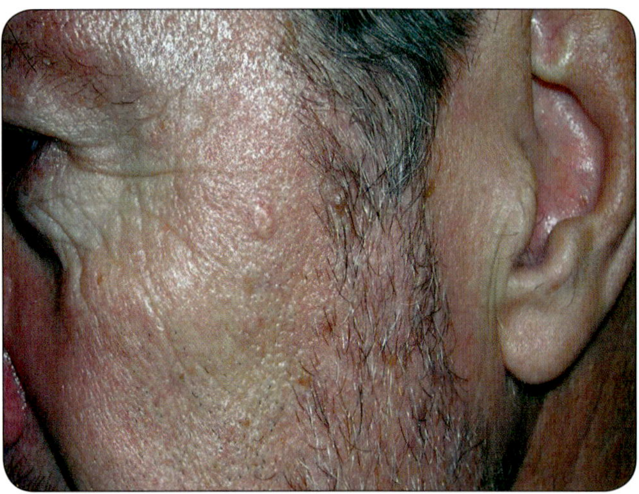

Fig. 5.235: Sebaceous hyperplasia: clinical image.

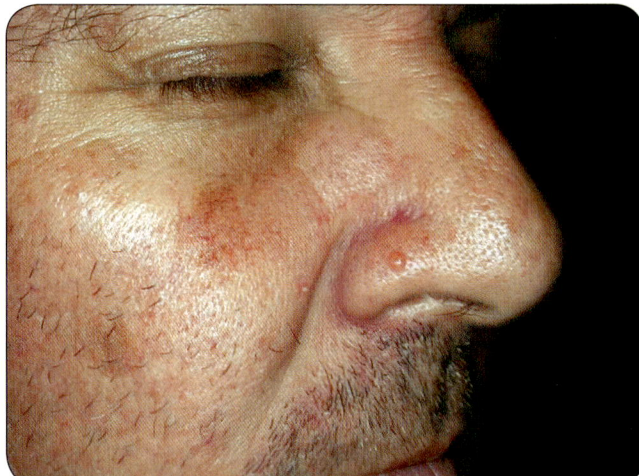

Fig. 5.236: Sebaceous hyperplasia: clinical image.

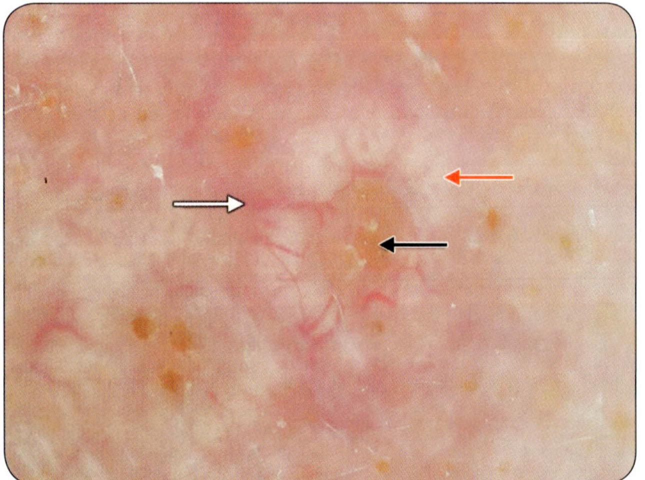

Fig. 5.237: Sebaceous hyperplasia: structureless white-yellowish aggregated areas (red arrow); central umbilication (black arrow); curved linear vessels with peripheral radial or crown arrangement (white arrow).

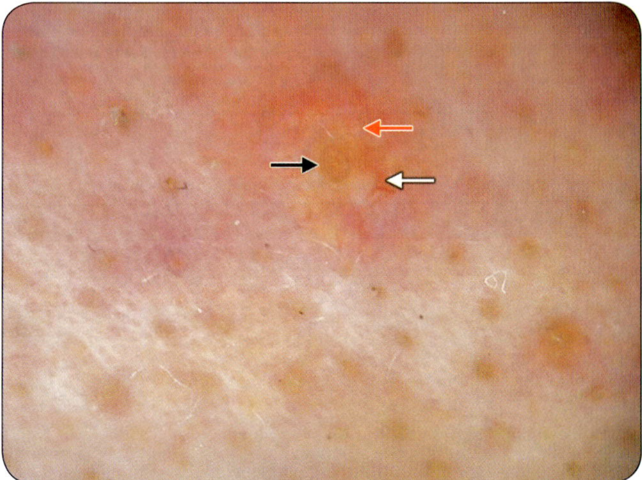

Fig. 5.238: Sebaceous hyperplasia: structureless white-yellowish aggregated areas (red arrow); central umbilication (black arrow); curved linear vessels with peripheral radial or crown arrangement (white arrow).

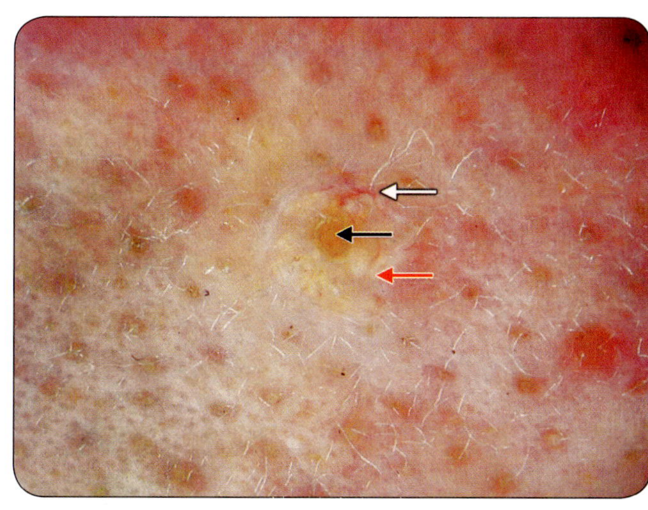

Fig. 5.239: Sebaceous hyperplasia: structureless white-yellowish aggregated areas (red arrow); central umbilication (black arrow); curved linear vessels with peripheral radial or crown arrangement (white arrow).

umbilication would correspond to the visible presence of the gland ostium.

SUGGESTED READING

Cabo H. Dermatoscopia, 2nd edition. Buenos Aires, Argentina: Ediciones Journal; 2012.

Malvhey J, Puig S. Principles of Dermoscopy. Barcelona: Creaciones Gráficas; 2009.

Marghoob A, Braun R, Kopf A. Atlas of Dermoscopy. London: Taylor & Francis; 2005.

Zaballos P, Ara M, Puig S, et al. Dermoscopy of sebaceous hyperplasia. Arch Dermatol. 2005;141:808.

5.8.8 Porokeratosis

Paula Friedman, Horacio A Cabo

Porokeratosis (PK) comprises a group of skin diseases due to a hereditary keratinization alteration. It has different clinical manifestations sharing the same histopathologic pattern: a cornoid lamella (Fig. 5.240).

Dermoscopically, PK features as follows:

- A well-demarcated annular gray or whitish peripheral border, known as "white tract." Sometimes the classical double "rail band" is present. This structure apparently corresponds to the cornoid lamella (Fig. 5.241).
- The central area may have brown pigmentation, which probably represents the longitudinal ridge of the lesion; there may also be dots, globules, and red lines due to dilated capillaries present underneath an atrophic epidermis, or a scar-like zone with scales (a scale scar-like zone) (Fig. 5.242).

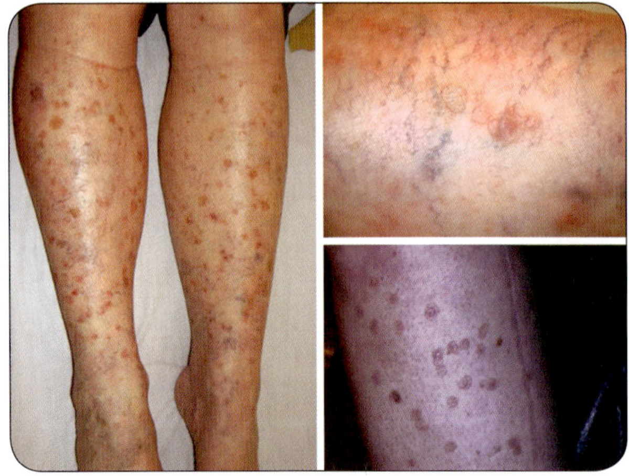

Fig. 5.240: Porokeratosis.

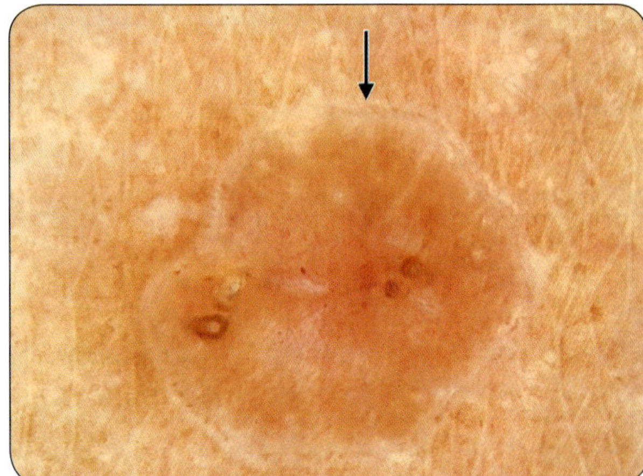

Fig. 5.241: Porokeratosis: classical double "rail band" (arrow).

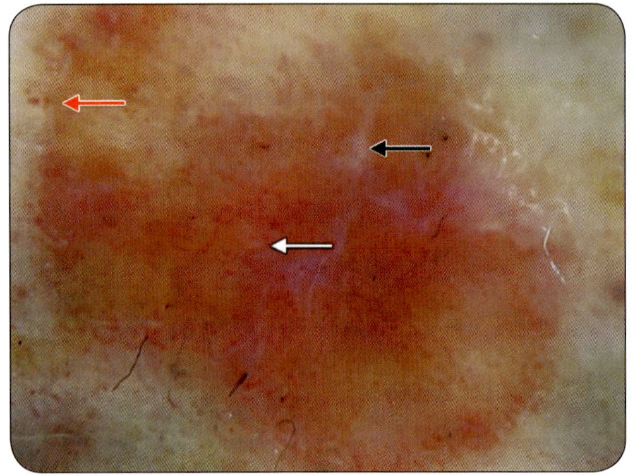

Fig. 5.242: Porokeratosis: classical double "rail band" (red arrow); dots, globules, and red lines due to dilated capillaries (white arrow); scar-like depigmentation (black arrow).

SUGGESTED READING

Cabo H. Dermatoscopia, 2nd edition. Buenos Aires, Argentina: Ediciones Journal; 2012.

Malvhey J, Puig S. Principles of Dermoscopy. Barcelona: Creaciones Gráficas; 2009.

Marghoob A, Braun R, Kopf A. Atlas of Dermoscopy. London: Taylor & Francis; 2005.

Zaballos P, Puig S, Malvehy J. Dermoscopy of disseminated superficial actinic porokeratosis. Arch Dermatol. 2004;140:1410.

5.8.9 Pyogenic Granuloma

Horacio A Cabo

Dermoscopically, pyogenic granuloma features reddish homogeneous or whitish-red areas, with white collarete and white rail lines crossing the lesion. Occasionally, there may be a hemorrhagic crust (Figs. 5.243 and 5.244).

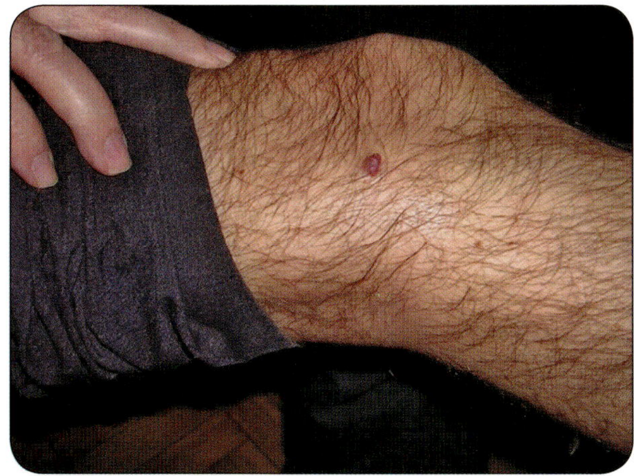

Fig. 5.243: Pyogenic granuloma (clinical image).

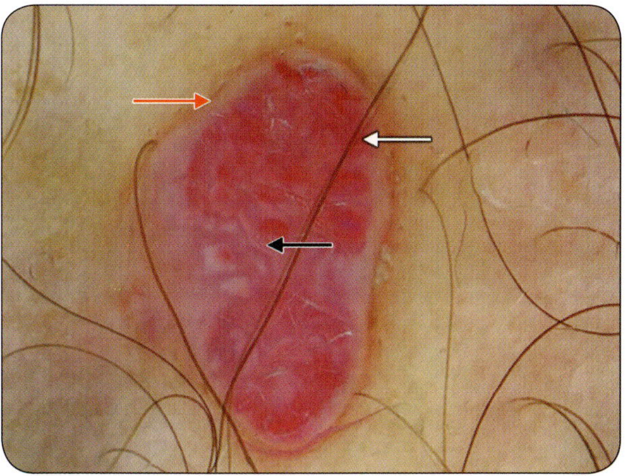

Fig. 5.244: Pyogenic granuloma: reddish homogeneous or whitish-red areas (white arrow); white collarette (red arrow); white rail lines crossing the lesion (black arrow).

SUGGESTED READING

Cabo H. Dermatoscopia, 2nd edition. Buenos Aires, Argentina: Ediciones Journal; 2012.

Malvhey J, Puig S. Principles of Dermoscopy. Barcelona: Creaciones Gráficas; 2009.

Marghoob A, Braun R, Kopf A. Atlas of Dermoscopy. London: Taylor & Francis; 2005.

Zaballos P, Llambrich A, Cuellar F, et al. Dermoscopic findings in pyogenic granuloma. Br J Dermatol. 2006;154:1108-11.

5.8.10 Lichen Planus

Paula Friedman, Horacio A Cabo

Lichen planus (LP) may affect skin, mucosa, and hair (Fig. 5.245).

The classic cutaneous lesion is a flat polygonal papule slightly erythematous or purplish, in whose upper part it is possible to observe reticular or whitish dotted formations. The surface presents reticular or white dot-like formations, known as Wickham streaks (WSs), which characterize this disease.

Dermoscopic findings consist in pearly white polymorphous structures corresponding to WS with arborizing projections, "fern-leaf-like" appearance. In the borders, there may appear linear vessels (capillary vessels) and erythematous globules. The presence of WS in the dermoscopic analysis is the diagnosis key to differentiate LP from other disorders like pityriasis rosea and psoriasis (Fig. 5.246).

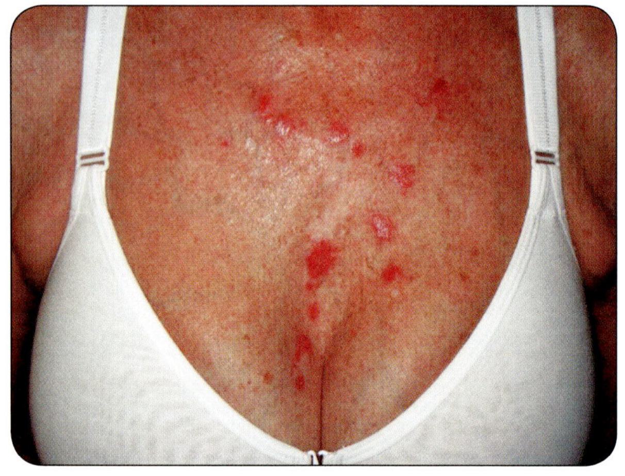

Fig. 5.245: Lichen planus clinical image.

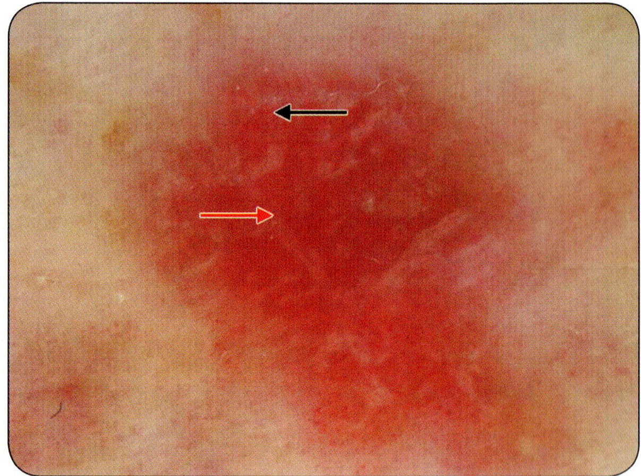

Fig. 5.246: Lichen planus: fern-leaf-like appearance (red arrow); linear vessels (black arrow).

SUGGESTED READING

Cabo H. Dermatoscopia, 2nd edition. Buenos Aires, Argentina: Ediciones Journal; 2012.

Friedman P, Cohen Sabban E, Marcucci C, et al. Dermoscopic findings in different clinical variants of lichen planus. Is dermoscopy useful? Dermatol Pract Concept. 2015;5(4):51-5.

Malvhey J, Puig S. Principles of Dermoscopy. Barcelona: Creaciones Gráficas; 2009.

Marghoob AA. Dermoscopic features of plaque psoriasis and lichen planus: new observations. Dermatology. 2003;207:151-6.

5.8.11 Bowenoid Papulosis

Carolina Marcucci, Horacio A Cabo

Bowenoid papulosis is a multifocal intraepithelial neoplasm occurring in the anogenital region. The main differential diagnosis, both clinical and dermoscopic, is the verruca genitalis (Figs. 5.247A and B).

The characteristic features of this lesion are as follows (Figs. 5.248 to 5.250):

- Dotted vessels or homogeneous red-black globules corresponding respectively to dilated or thrombosed vessels. These structures may be surrounded by a white halo that betrays the presence of papilomatosis.
- Gray-brown dots, in linear arrangement, located in the periphery of the lesion.

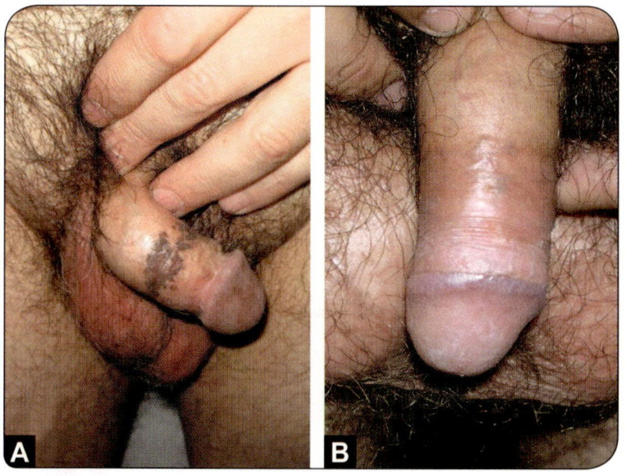

Figs. 5.247A and B: Bowenoid papulosis: clinical images (A and B).

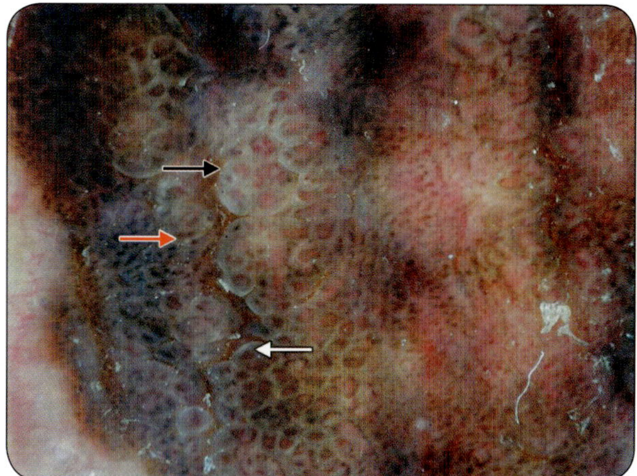

Fig. 5.248: Bowenoid papulosis: (case A) red or blue dilated vessels (red arrow) in multiple round or oval areas (black arrow). These structures are surrounded by a white halo which betrays the presence of papillomatosis (white arrow).

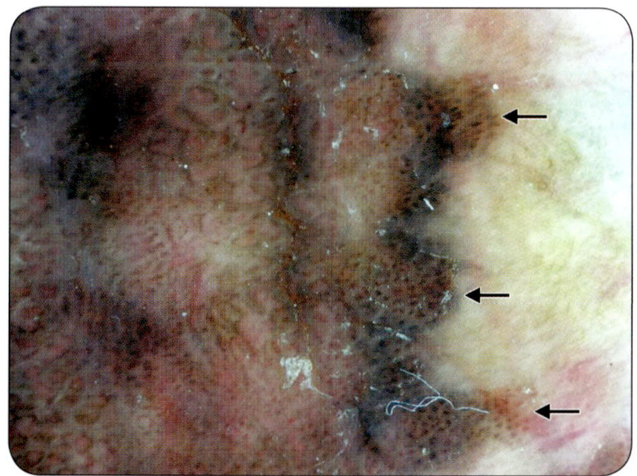

Fig. 5.249: Bowenoid papulosis: (case A) gray-brown dots, in linear arrangement, in the periphery of the lesion (arrows).

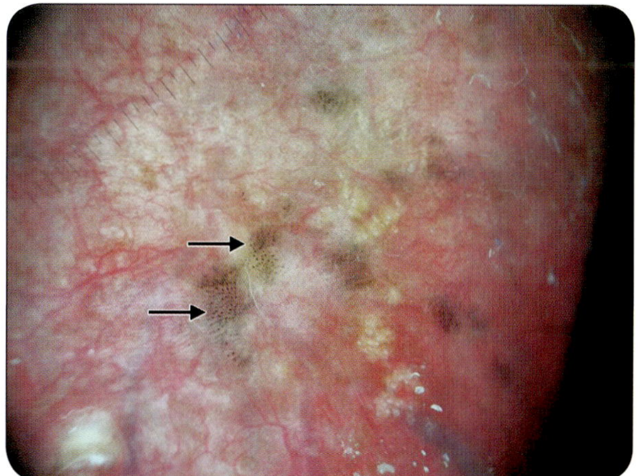

Fig. 5.250: Bowenoid papulosis: (case B) gray-brown dots, in linear arrangement, in the periphery of the lesion (arrows).

SUGGESTED READING

Marcucci C, Cohen Sabban E, Friedman P, et al. Dermoscopic findings in bowenoid papulosis: report of two cases. Dermatol Pract Concept. 2014;4(4):61-3.

MELANOCYTIC LESIONS

6

Horacio A Cabo

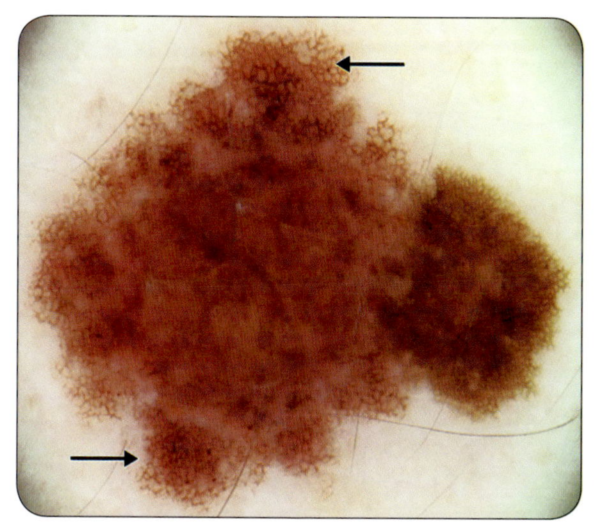

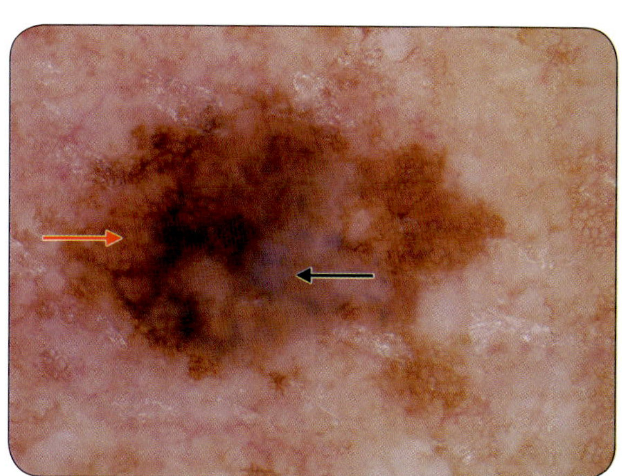

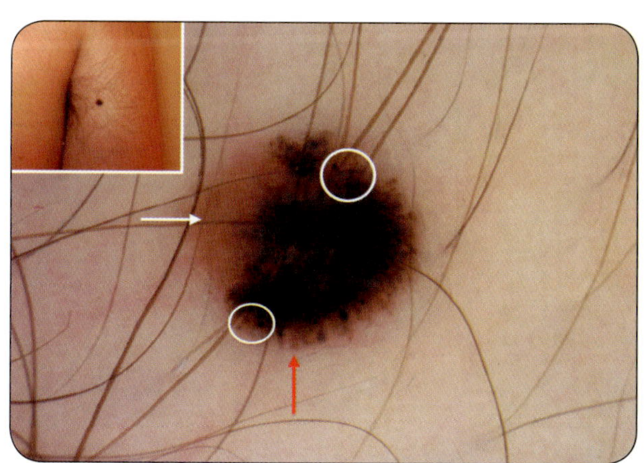

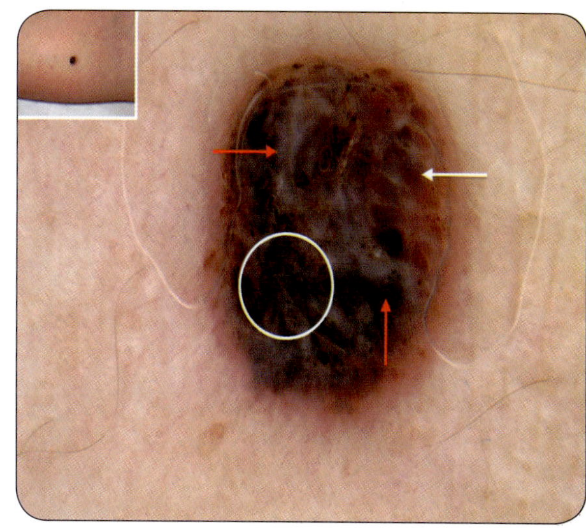

"The dermoscopic study of pigmented lesions is performed in two steps. The first step involves determining if the lesion is melanocytic or nonmelanocytic. If it is a melanocytic lesion, the physician must continue with the second step, which means differentiating a benign melanocytic lesion from a melanoma.
In this chapter, we include concepts of Nevogenesis, the different types of nevus, such as congenital, acquired, atypical, blue nevus, combined and recurrent nevus.
The different types of melanoma, superficial spreading melanoma, nodular melanoma, lentigo maligna melanoma and acral melanoma will be included as well.
Finally, we will focusing in the approach of patients with multiple nevi."

6.1 CRITERIA OF MELANOCYTIC LESIONS

Horacio A Cabo

The dermoscopic study of pigmented lesions is performed in two steps. The first step involves determining if the lesion is melanocytic or nonmelanocytic. If it is a melanocytic lesion, the physician must continue with the second step, which means differentiating a benign melanocytic lesion from a melanoma.

Therefore, in order to proceed to the second step, it is essential to know the different criteria that may be used to determine if a pigmented lesion is melanocytic or not.

These criteria are:

- Pigment network
- Aggregated globules
- Streaks or projections
- Homogeneous blue pigmentation
- Parallel pattern

Pigment Network

Pigment network consists of brown or black lines with a reticular or grid appearance on a lighter background, resembling "holes". From a histologic point of view, it represents the rete ridges of the epidermis. The holes correspond to pigmented cells in the area of the dermal papilla, while the lines correspond to the cells located in the interpapillary area. In this manner, it is possible to observe lines and holes that may be very similar to or different from each other, of different color, width and size, giving rise to a typical pigment network (in benign melanocytic lesions) or an atypical one (melanoma) (Figs. 6.1 to 6.5).

Aggregated Globules

Multiple oval or round structures, well demarcated; of different sizes, though generally over 0.1 mm; brown, gray, or black. They correlate with nests of melanocytes in the area of the dermoepidermal junction (Figs. 6.6 to 6.9).

Streaks or Projections

At present, we include branching (radial streaming) and pseudopods under this name.

Branching (radial streaming) are radial extensions in the pigment network at the periphery of the lesions.

Pseudopods are radial projections of the pigment network in the periphery of the lesion and invading apparently healthy skin. They are thicker than branching and have a bulbous end.

Both branching and pseudopods are expressions of an altered pigment network.

Histologically, they correspond to nests of melanocytes in lineal arrangement located in the dermoepidermal junction (Figs. 6.10 to 6.13).

Homogeneous Blue Pigmentation

This is a blue-gray area lacking structural components. In the histologic correlation, the melanocytes are located in the middle and deep dermis (Fig. 6.14).

Parallel Pattern

It can be seen in acral lesions. Depending on the localization of the melanocytic cells, the dermatoglyphics ridges

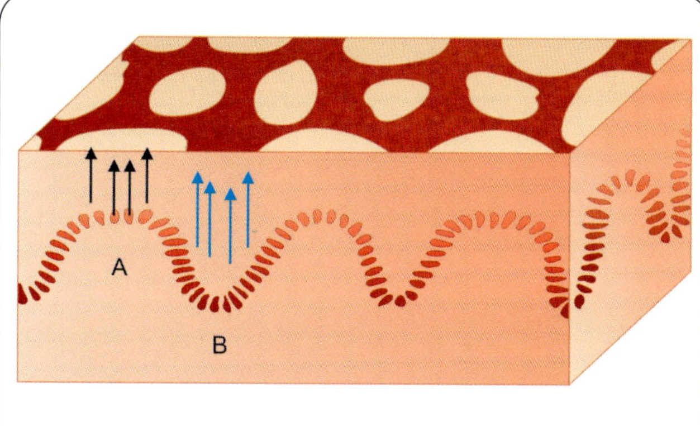

Fig. 6.1: Pigment network.

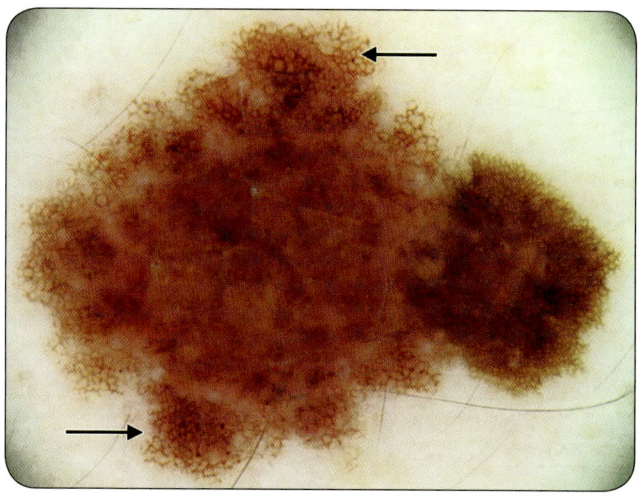

Fig. 6.2: Pigment network (arrows).

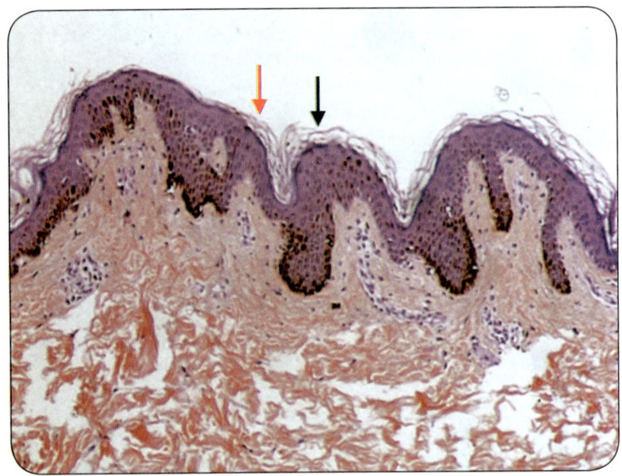

Fig. 6.3: Pigment network histopathological correlation (red arrow—holes; black arrow—lines).

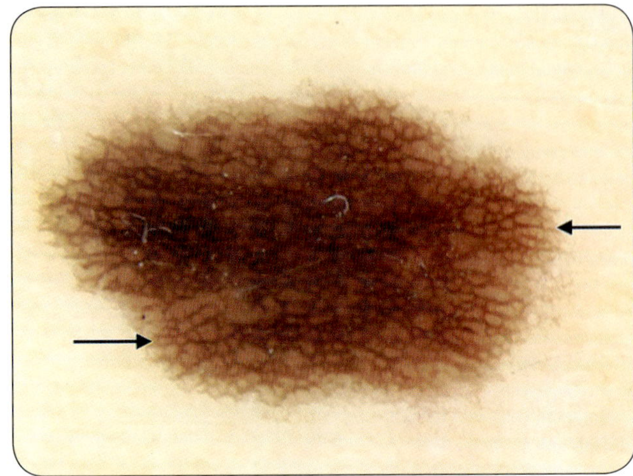

Fig. 6.4: Pigment network (arrows).

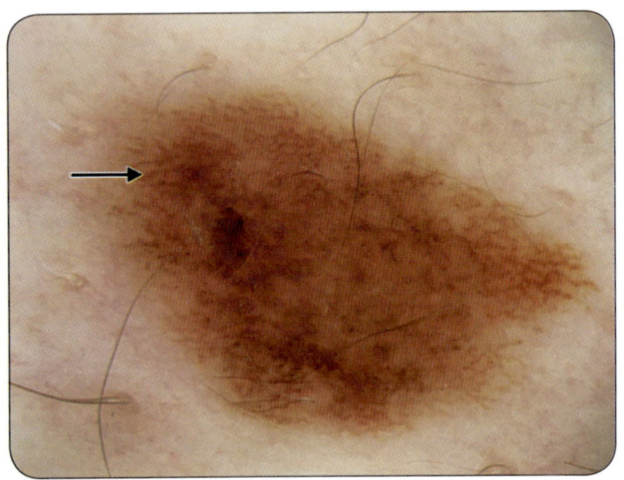

Fig. 6.5: Pigment network (arrow).

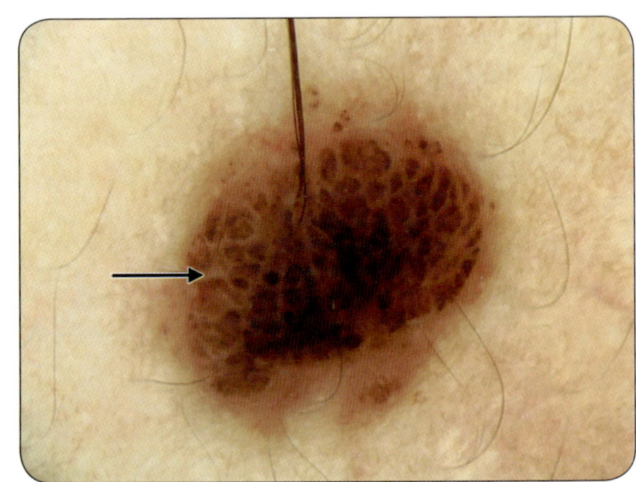

Fig. 6.6: Aggregated globules (arrow).

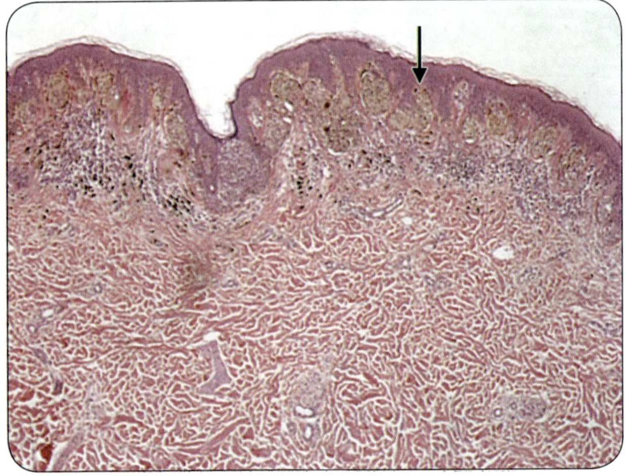

Fig. 6.7: Aggregated globules: histopathological correlation—nests of melanocytes in the area of the dermoepidermal junction (arrow).

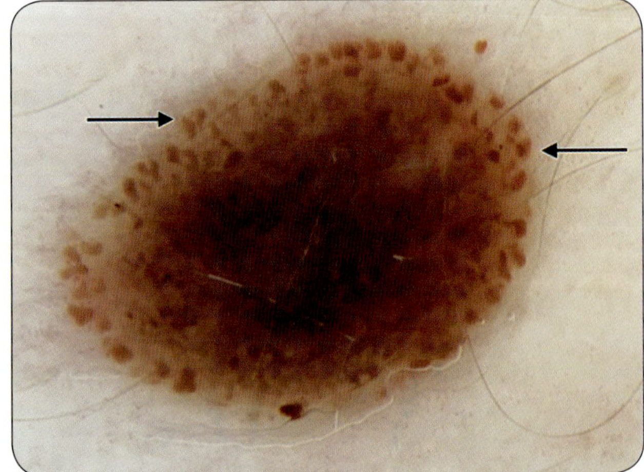

Fig. 6.8: Aggregated globules (arrows).

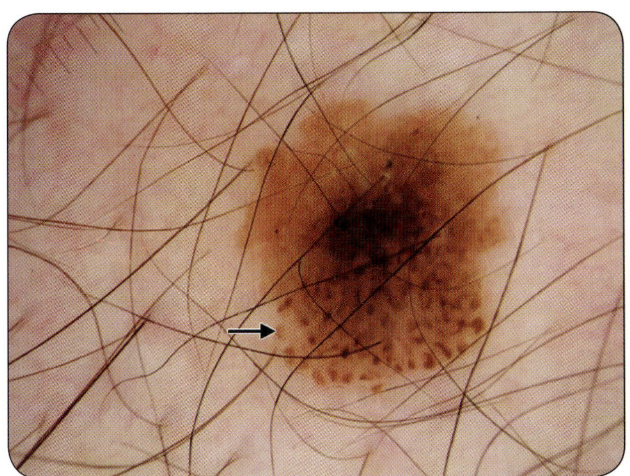

Fig. 6.9: Aggregated globules (arrow).

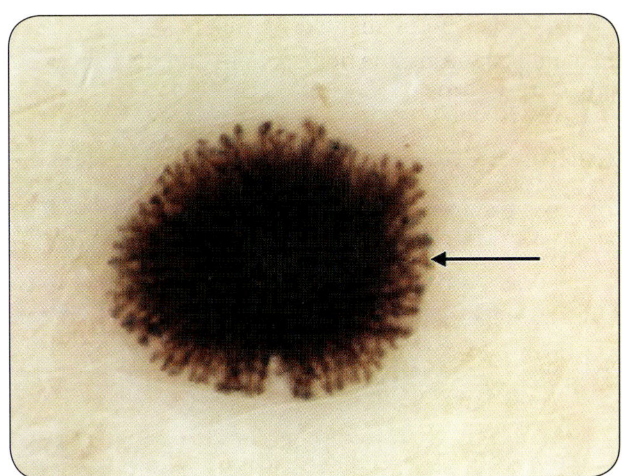

Fig. 6.10: Streaks or projections (arrow).

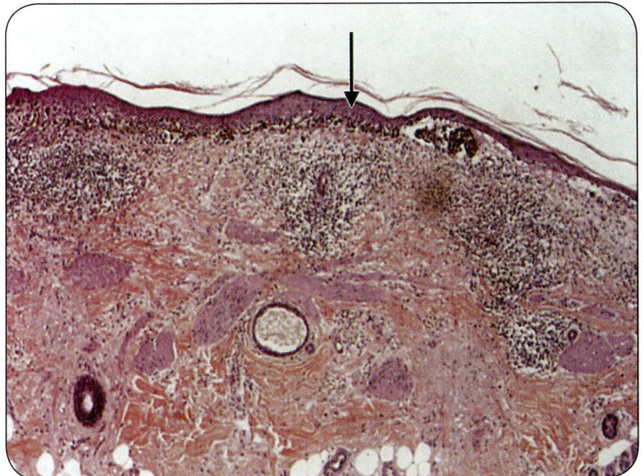

Fig. 6.11: Streaks or projections: histopathological correlation—nests of melanocytes in lineal arrangement located in the dermoepidermal junction (arrow).

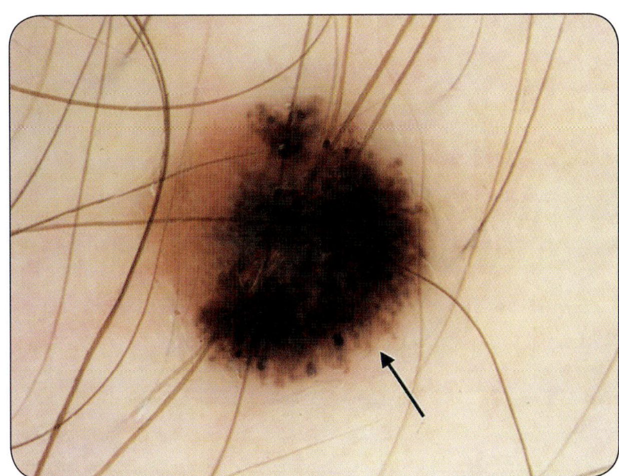

Fig. 6.12: Streaks or projections (arrow).

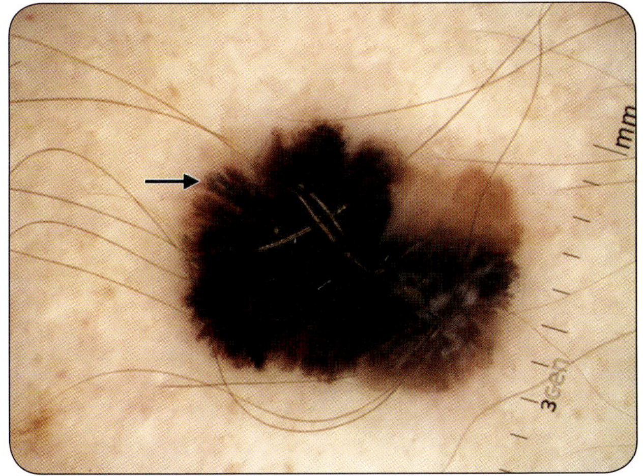

Fig. 6.13: Streaks or projections (arrow).

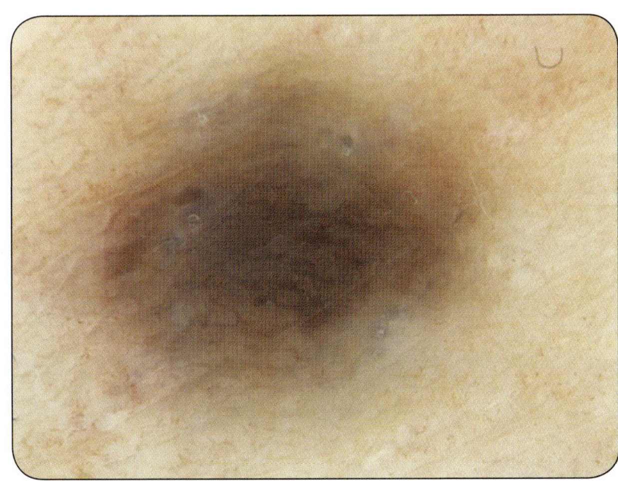

Fig. 6.14: Homogeneous blue pigmentation.

or furrows may be pigmented. In this manner, there are two parallel patterns, the ridge pattern and the furrow one (Figs. 6.15 to 6.18).

Additional Criteria for Melanocytic Lesions

It is possible to observe other criteria in melanocytic lesions, but they also occur, on occasion, in nonmelanocytic ones. Thus, they are not considered absolute criteria for melanocytic lesions. Nevertheless, when they are accompanied by the criteria previously described for melanocytic lesions, they acquire a great significance to the diagnosis.

These features are dots, regression, whitish veil, and hyperpigmented stains.

Dots

These are round structures, <0.1 mm, black, brown, or blue-gray. Color depends on the location of the pigment: stratum corneum, epidermis, or dermis (Figs. 6.19 and 6.20).

Regression

This corresponds to white areas (histologically, fibrosis) and blue areas (histologically, melanosis or melanophages). The latter may present blue peppering appearance. Clinically, they correspond to the nonelevated part of the lesion (Figs. 6.21 to 6.24).

Blue-White Veil

This is represented by areas lacking irregular structures, of color blue, blue-gray or whitish blue, with ground glass

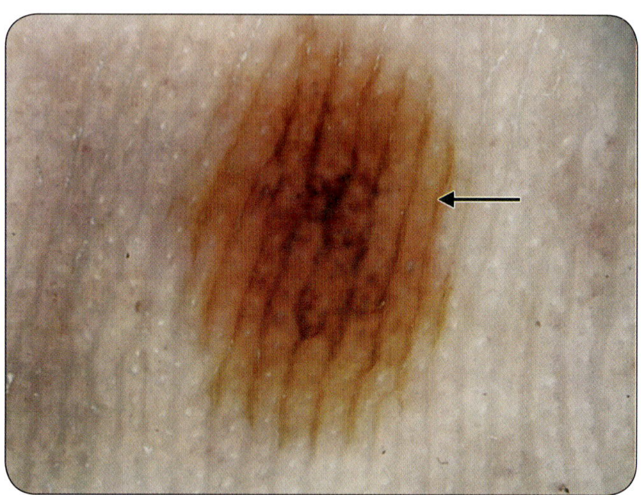

Fig. 6.15: Parallel furrow pattern (arrow).

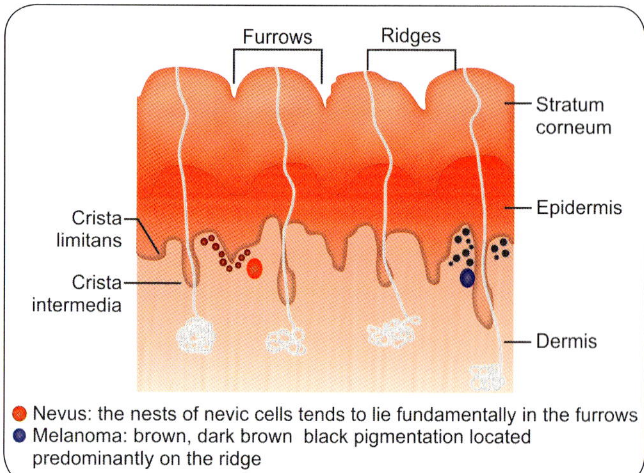

Fig. 6.16: Schematic representation of the anatomy of the skin in acral zones.

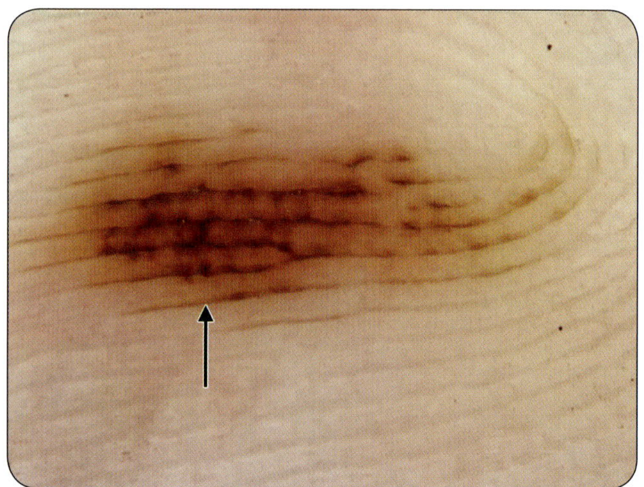

Fig. 6.17: Parallel furrow pattern (arrow).

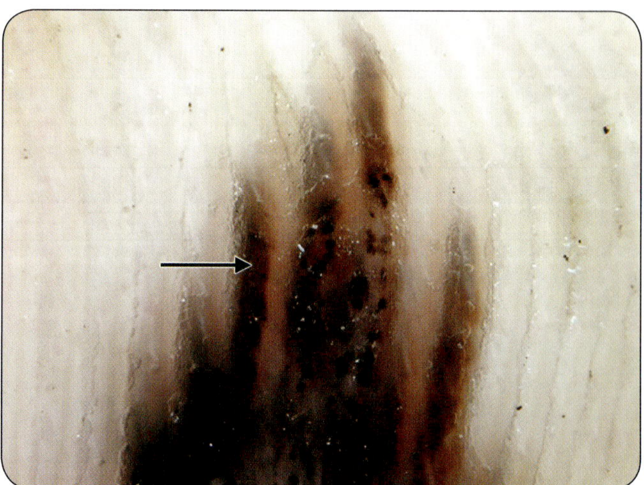

Fig. 6.18: Parallel ridge pattern (arrow).

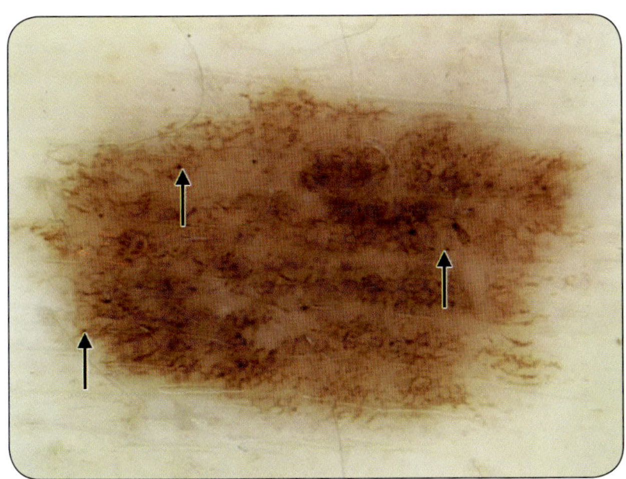

Fig. 6.19: Dots (arrows).

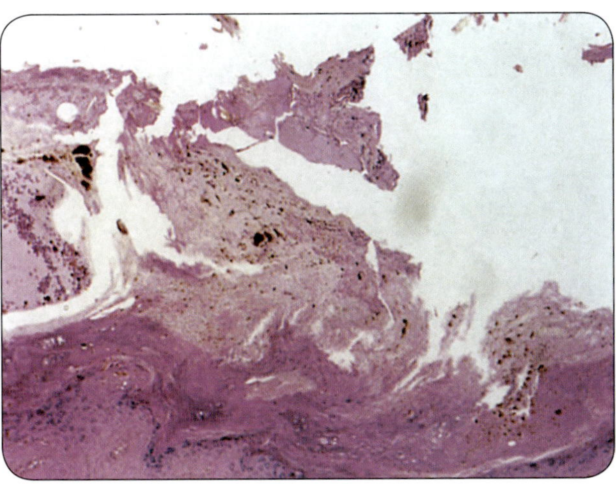

Fig. 6.20: Dots: histopathological correlation—aggregated melanocytes or granules of melanin in the stratum corneum, epidermis, or dermis.

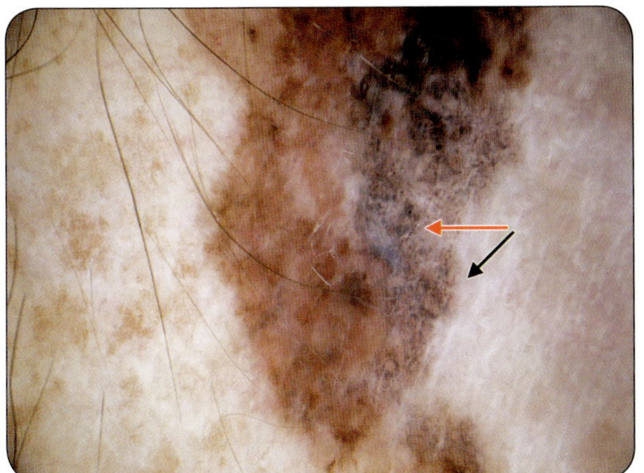

Fig. 6.21: Regression: melanosis (red arrow); fibrosis (black arrow).

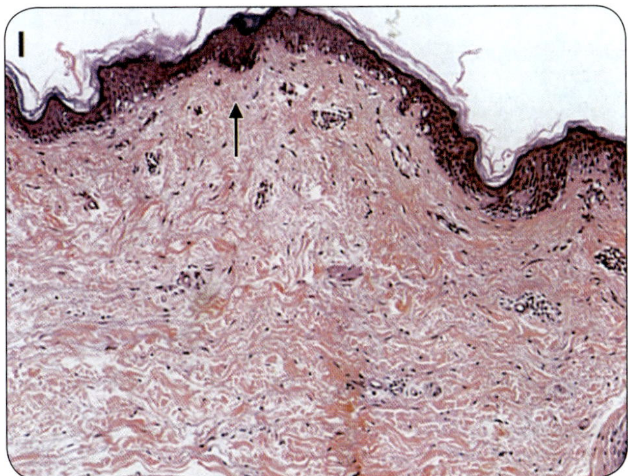

Fig. 6.22: Regression: histopathological correlation—fibrosis (white scar-like) (arrow).

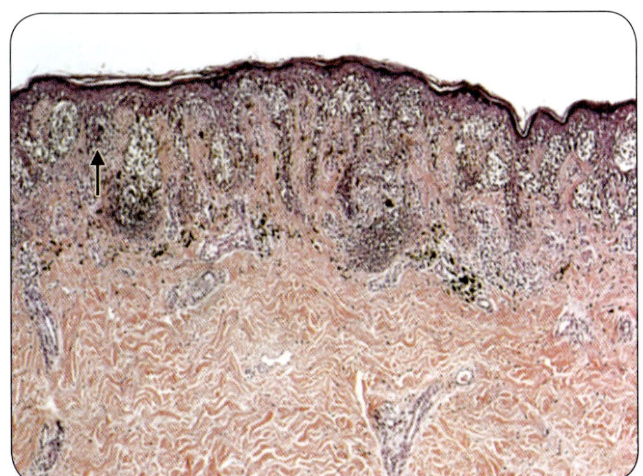

Fig. 6.23: Regression: histopathological correlation—melanosis (blue-gray areas)

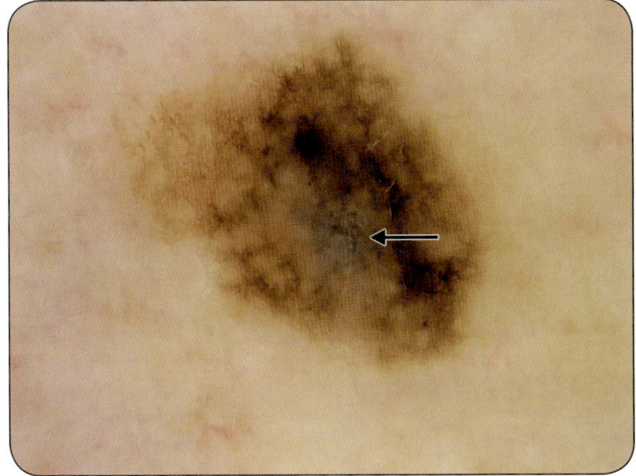

Fig. 6.24: Regression (arrow).

appearance. From a clinical point of view, blue-white veil corresponds to the raised parts of the lesion. From a histologic point of view, it is possible to observe orthokeratosis and deeply pigmented cells in the superficial dermis (Figs. 6.25 to 6.28).

Hyperpigmented Areas

These are pigment areas that do not allow the recognition of any structure within. They may be localized or diffuse; regular or irregular; and of color black, dark brown, or gray. They are due to a large concentration of melanin throughout the epidermis and/or dermis (Figs. 6.29 to 6.31).

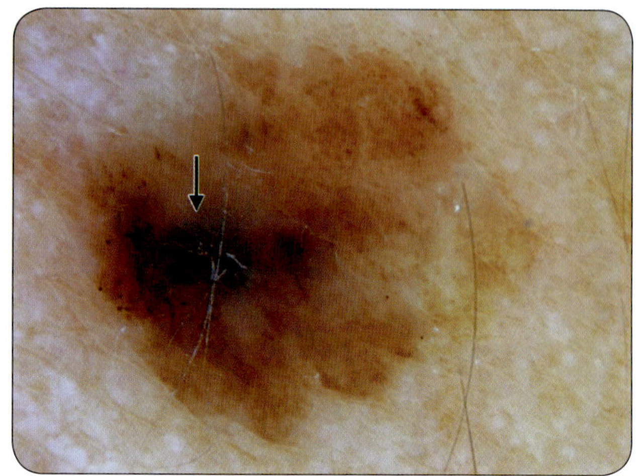

Fig. 6.25: Blue-white veil (arrow).

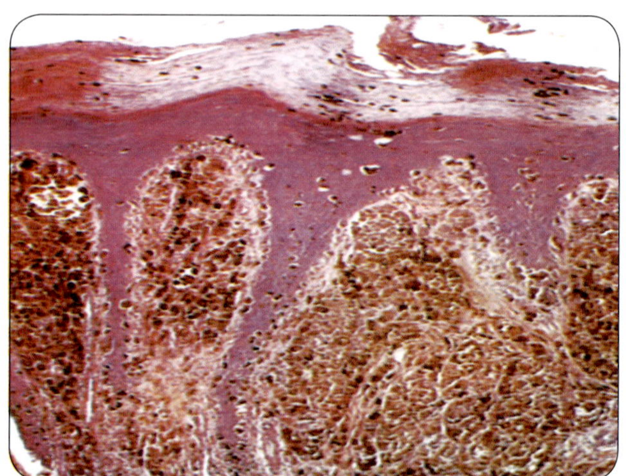

Fig. 6.26: Blue-white veil: histopathological correlation—orthokeratosis and deeply pigmented cells in the superficial dermis.

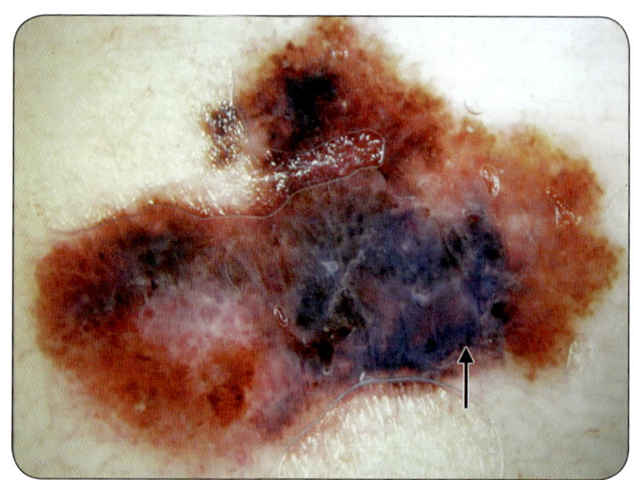

Fig. 6.27: Blue-white veil (arrow).

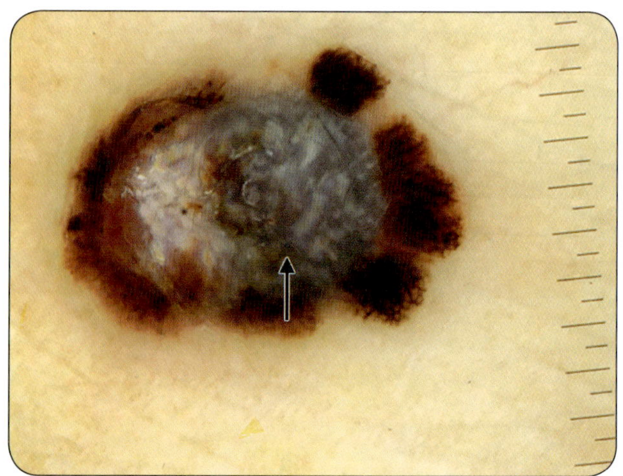

Fig. 6.28: Blue-white veil (arrow).

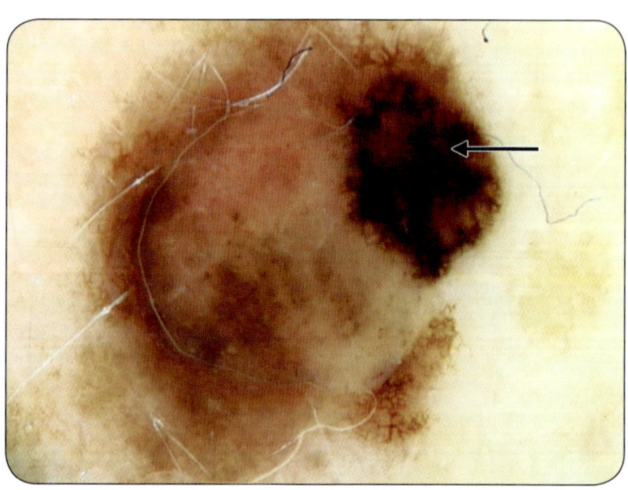

Fig. 6.29: Hyperpigmented areas (arrow).

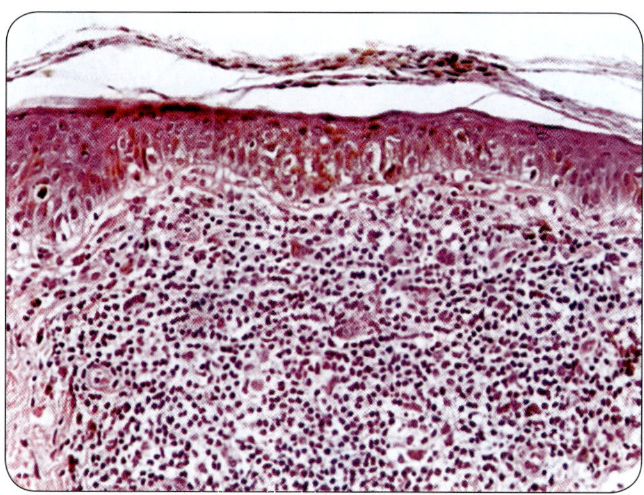

Fig. 6.30: Hyperpigmented areas: histopathological correlation—due to a large concentration of melanin throughout the epidermis and/or dermis.

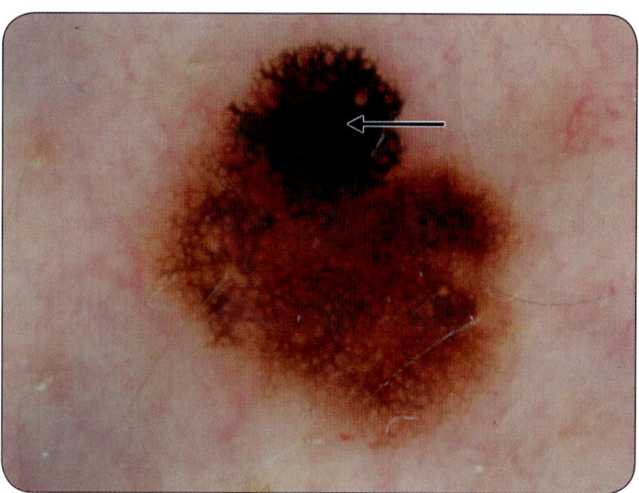

Fig. 6.31: Hyperpigmented areas (arrow).

SUGGESTED READING

Argenziano G, Soyer P, De Giorgio V, et al. Interactive Atlas of Dermoscopy. Milán: EDRA Medical Publishing & New Media; 2000.

Cabo H. Dermatoscopia. Buenos Aires, Argentina: Weber Ferro; 2000.

Cabo H. Dermatoscopia, 2nd edition. Buenos Aires, Argentina: Ediciones Journal; 2012.

Johr R, Stolz W. Dermoscopy: An Illustrated Self-Assessment Guide, 2nd edition. McGraw-Hill Education; 2015.

Johr R, Stolz W. Dermoscopy: An Illustrated Self-Assessment Guide, 2nd edition. New York: McGraw-Hill Education; 2015.

Kittler H. Dermatoscopy. An Algorithmic Method Based on Pattern Analysis 2011 Facultas Verlags- und Buchhandels AG facultas wuv Universitätsverlag, Austria www.facultas.wuv.at.

Lallas A. Dermoscopy in general dermatology. Dermatol Clin. 2013;3:679-94.

Malvhey J, Puig S. Principles of Dermoscopy. Barcelona: Creaciones Gráficas; 2009.

Marghoob A, Braun R, Kopf A. Atlas of Dermoscopy. London: Taylor & Francis; 2005.

Menzies S, Crotty K, Ingvar C, et al. An Atlas of Surface Microscopy of Pigmented Skin Lesions. Sydney: McGraw-Hill Book Company; 1996.

Rabinovitz H, Kopf A. Dermoscopy: A Practical Guide. Miami: American Academy of Dermatology; 1999.

Soyer P, Argenziano G, Chimenti S, et al. Dermoscopy of Pigmented Skin Lesions. An Atlas Based on the Consensus Net Meeting on Dermoscopy. Milán: EDRA Medical Publishing & New Media; 2001.

Stolz W, Braun-Falco O, Bilek P, et al. Color atlas of Dermatoscopy. Germany: Blackwell Science; 1994.

Zalaudek I, Argenziano G, Giacomel J. Dermoscopy of Non-Pigmented Skin Tumors. Boca Raton, FL: CRC Press; 2016

6.2 NEVOGÉNESIS

Aimilios Lallas, Zoe Apalla, Elvira Moscarella, Caterina Longo, Teresa Deinlein, Iris Zalaudek

The formation and evolution of nevi is, to a large extend, genetically determined, being though influenced also by environmental factors.[1]

Since the middle of the previous century it has been clarified that melanocytes do not derive from keratinocytes, but are of neural crest origin.[2] For decades, nevi have been thought to originate from proliferating epidermal melanocytes, which later in life extend into the dermis, where eventually they follow a regressive process.[3] This traditional model of downward migration has been challenged by the modern stem cell theory and by novel insights into the morphology of nevi, provided by dermoscopy and newer imaging techniques like reflectance confocal microscopy (RCM).[4]

Two Pathways of Nevogénesis

Combining all the aforementioned novel information, a dual concept of nevogénesis has been recently introduced.[5] According to it, nevi might be either of dermal origin, formed via the "constitutional" pathway, or of epidermal origin, formed via the "acquired" pathway. This dual concept is mainly based on the knowledge that precursor (stem) cells first differentiate into melanocytes within the dermis and, then, epidermal chemotactic factors guide their migration in the epidermis (Fig. 6.32).[2] During this procedure, a disturbance or delay of the "upward" migration of melanocytes in the epidermis might lead to the formation of a nevus from dermal melanocytes ("constitutional" pathway; Fig. 6.33). This pathway is minimally, or not at all, affected by environmental factors. Instead, melanocytes that have normally migrated into the epidermis might later proliferate in response to exogenous factors [like ultraviolet (UV) radiation], giving rise to nevi of epidermal origin ("acquired" pathway; Fig. 6.34). In simple words, nevi might develop early, within the dermis and independent of the environment, or later, in the epidermis and in response to environmental factors (Table 6.1).[5]

Several morphologic, genetic, and epidemiological data support this dual concept. Dermoscopy brought to light novel information on the morphology of nevi and dermoscopic criteria have been shown to perfectly correlate to histopathologic alterations.[4] Dermoscopically, the majority of nevi are known to display either a globular or a reticular pattern, with the globules corresponding to dermal nests of melanocytes and the pigment network corresponding to a lentiginous junctional proliferation (Figs. 6.35 and 6.36).[6] Recent evidence suggests that the globular and reticular dermoscopic patterns do not only represent two morphologic variants, but characterize two subgroups of nevi with clearly distinct epidemiological characteristics and different biology. For example, globular nevi are known to remain relatively stable during

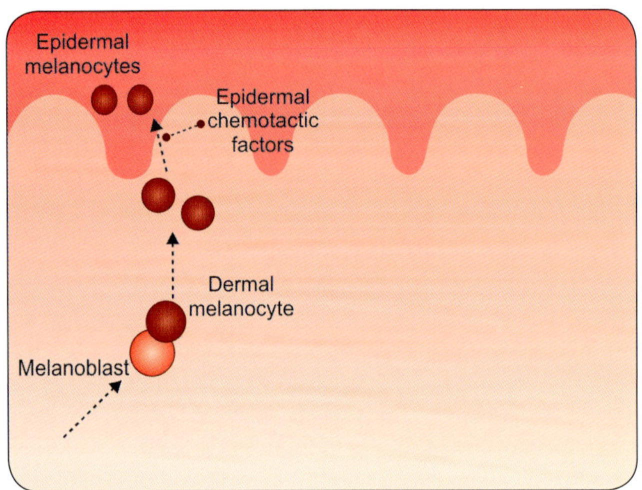

Fig. 6.32: Route of melanocyte migration in the skin.

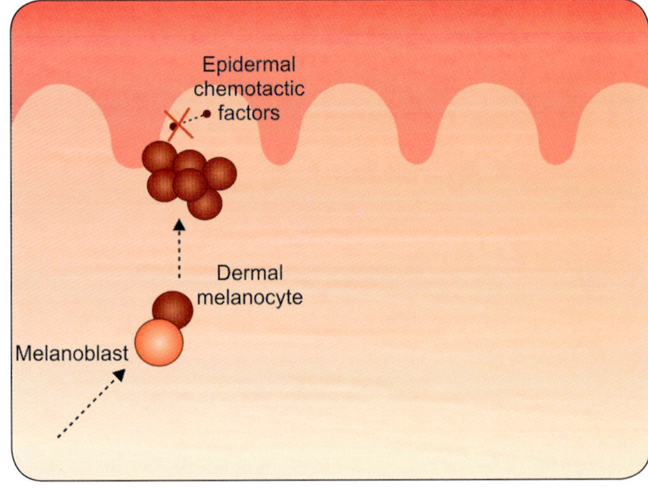

Fig. 6.33: Constitutional pathway of nevogénesis. A disturbance or delay of the "upward" migration of melanocytes in the epidermis leads to the formation of a nevus from dermal melanocytes.

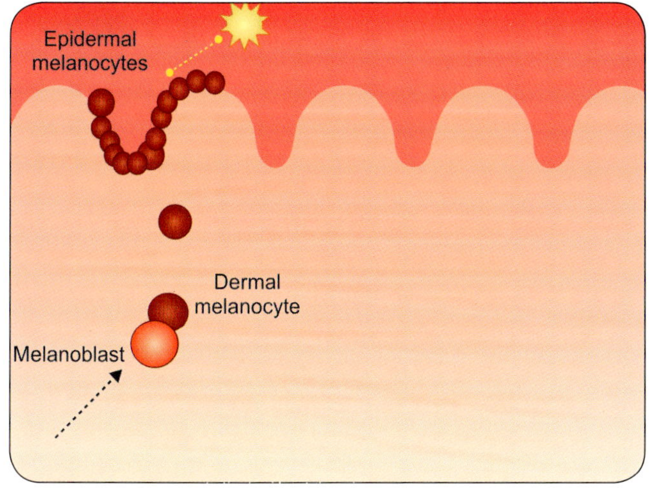

Fig. 6.34: Constitutional pathway of nevogénesis. Melanocytes that have normally migrated into the epidermis proliferate in response to exogenous factors (like ultraviolet radiation), giving rise to nevi of epidermal origin.

Table 6.1: Dual concept of nevogénesis.

	Constitutional pathway	*Acquired pathway*
Dermoscopic pattern	Globular	Reticular
Age	Embryonic life and early childhood	Late childhood and adulthood
Anatomic sites	Head/neck and upper trunk	Extremities
Environmental factors	No	Yes
Duration	Long (ofter a lifetime)	From 20s/30s to 60s

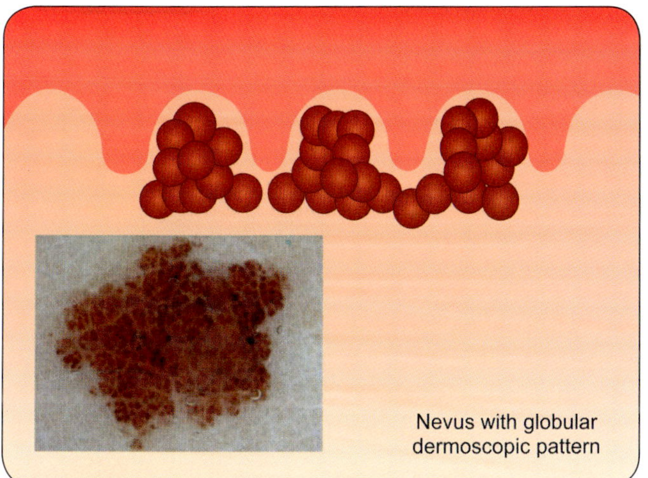

Fig. 6.35: Dermoscopic globules histopathologically correspond to dermal nests of melanocytes.

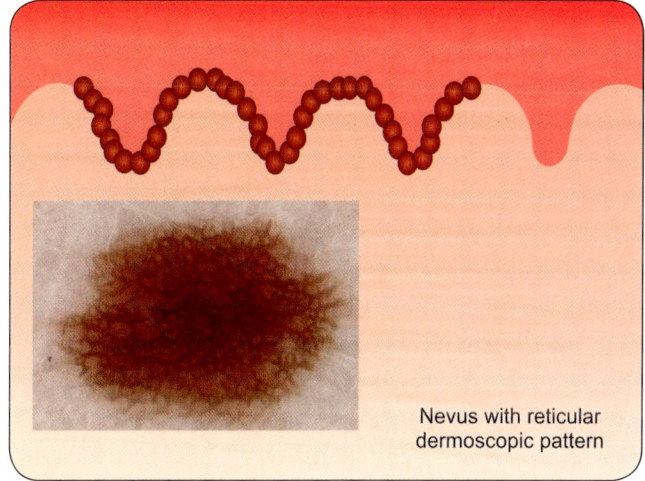

Fig. 6.36: Dermoscopic pigment network histopathologically corresponds to lentiginous melanocytic proliferation at the level of the dermoepidermal junction.

lifetime, while reticular nevi appear later and involute earlier, being exceptionally uncommon in elderly patients (Figs. 6.37 and 6.38).[7,8] Furthermore, there is a significant difference between globular and reticular nevi regarding their distribution on the body sites.[8] All these observations originated mainly from dermoscopic studies seem to be adequately explained by the dual concept of nevogénesis described above.

It has been shown that the dermoscopic pattern of nevi is significantly influenced by age, with the globular pattern predominating in children and the reticular pattern in adults (Fig. 6.39).[7] In more detail, virtually all congenital nevi display a globular pattern (the "cobblestone" is a variation of the globular pattern), as do also the nevi developing in early childhood, which is in line with the hypothesis that nevi appearing within the first years of life are in fact congenital nevi that become evident a few months or years later. This strong correlation between the globular dermoscopic pattern and young age is absolutely consistent with the "constitutional" pathway of nevogénesis, which

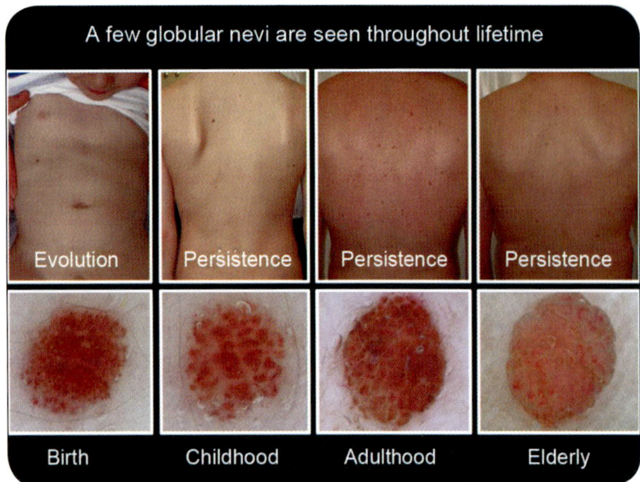

Fig. 6.37: Evolution of globular nevi throughout lifetime.

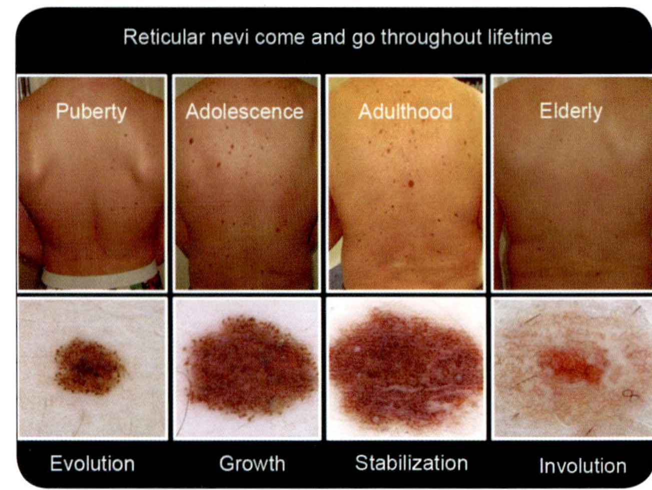

Fig. 6.38: Evolution of reticular nevi throughout lifetime.

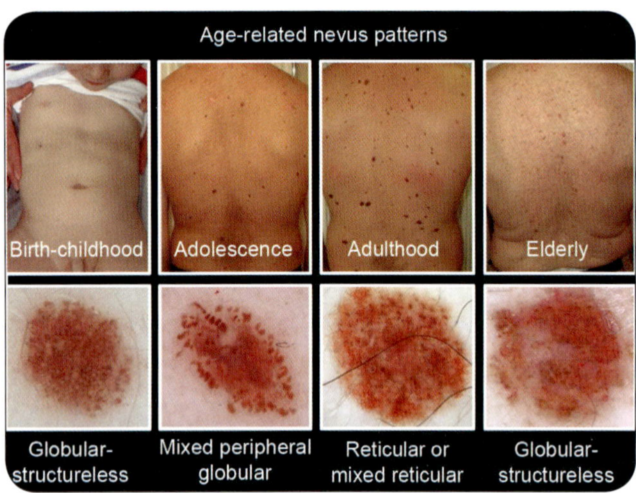

Fig. 6.39: Age-related nevus patterns.

suggests that an early perturbation or delay of the upward migration of melanocytes results in their retention within the dermis, giving rise to dermal nevi.[5] Moreover, dermoscopic studies suggest that globular nevi mainly develop on the head/neck area and on the upper trunk, while reticular nevi prevail on the extremities.[8] At the same time, the melanoblast migration is known to follow a cephalocaudal and proximal-to-distal sequence.[1] In simple words, the precursor cells of melanocytes arrive earlier on the head/neck and finally on the extremities. The two latter observations are perfectly combined in the proposed "constitutional" pathway of nevogénesis, since globular nevi (which are proposed to result from an early disturbance) tend to develop exactly on the body sites where melanoblasts arrive early in embryonic life.

In contrast, reticular nevi are suggested to originate at a later stage, from melanocytes, which have normally migrated from the dermis to the epidermis or reached at least the dermoepidermal junction. These nevi may develop in response to both endogenous and exogenous factors, such as growth hormones during puberty and UV radiation. Indeed, it has been shown that the total nevus count correlates with sun exposure.[9] Reticular nevi are dynamic tumors, typically developing from early childhood until midlife and afterward, the majority of them, involuting, so that they are rarely seen in elderly individuals.[4,9]

While the dual concept of nevogénesis seems to perfectly correlate with the dermoscopic morphology of globular and reticular nevi, it is inadequate to explain the existence of nevi with a mixed dermoscopic pattern, namely globular in the center and reticular at the periphery or centrally reticular with peripheral globules. These nevi have been hypothesized to originate from melanocytes at or immediately beneath the dermoepidermal junction, which are likely capable of migrating and proliferating in and between the dermis and the epidermis.[1]

In addition to improving our knowledge on the natural evolution of nevi, these novel insights into nevogénesis generated speculations on the possibility of a similar concept of a dermal origin of nodular melanoma (NM) and an epidermal origin of superficial spreading melanoma (SSM).[4,10,11] This hypothesis has been based on significant morphologic and epidemiologic similarities between dermal nevi and NM and between junctional nevi and SSM. Specifically, both dermal nevi and NM dermoscopically display a predominantly globular pattern, while junctional nevi and SSM typically exhibit a pigment network. The vast majority of nevi in children are globular and melanoma in childhood, although extremely rare, is usually nodular.[12] In adulthood, the majority of nevi are reticular and SSM is, by far, the most frequent subtype in this age group.[13] Persisting nevi in elderly individuals are usually dermal nevi with a globular pattern and NM patients are significantly older, compared to SSM patients.[14] Finally, junctional (reticular) nevi and SSM are known to be associated with intermittent sun exposure, while globular nevi and NM lack such an association.[13] However, these speculations definitely need to be further elucidated.

In conclusion, recent evidence on the morphology and biology of melanocytic lesions strongly challenged the traditional knowledge and turned nevogénesis into a highly emerging topic of research. Accumulating data from new studies aiming to correlate morphology with the genetic background of nevi and melanoma are expected to further shed light in the field and deepen our understanding of the biology of melanocytic lesions.

REFERENCES

1. Zalaudek I, Catricalà C, Moscarella E, et al. What dermoscopy tells us about nevogenesis. J Dermatol. 2011;38:16-24.
2. Cramer SF. Speckled lentiginous nevus (nevus spilus): the “roots” of the “melanocytic garden”. Arch Dermatol. 2001;137:1654-5.
3. Cramer SF. The origin of epidermal melanocytes. Implications for the histogenesis of nevi and melanomas. Arch Pathol Lab Med. 1991;115:115-9.
4. Zalaudek I, Leinweber B, Hofmann-Wellenhof R, et al. The epidermal and dermal origin of melanocytic tumors: theoretical considerations based on epidemiologic, clinical, and histopathologic findings. Am J Dermatopathol. 2008;30:403-6.
5. Zalaudek I, Hofmann-Wellenhof R, Kittler H, et al. A dual concept of nevogenesis: theoretical considerations based on dermoscopic features of melanocytic nevi. J Dtsch Dermatol Ges. 2007;5:985-92.
6. Hofmann-Wellenhof R, Blum A, Wolf IH, et al. Dermoscopic classification of atypical melanocytic nevi (Clark nevi). Arch Dermatol. 2001;137:1575-80.
7. Zalaudek I, Grinschgl S, Argenziano G, et al. Age-related prevalence of dermoscopy patterns in acquired melanocytic naevi. Br J Dermatol. 2006;154:299-304.
8. Zalaudek I, Schmid K, Marghoob AA, et al. Frequency of dermoscopic nevus subtypes by age and body site: a cross-sectional study. Arch Dermatol. 2011;147:663-70.
9. Kincannon J, Boutzale C. The physiology of pigmented nevi. Pediatrics. 1999;104:1042-5.
10. Zalaudek I, Marghoob AA, Scope A, et al. Three roots of melanoma. Arch Dermatol. 2008;144:1375-9.
11. Zalaudek I, Moscarella E, Longo C, et al. No one should die of melanoma: a vision or impossible mission. Melanoma Management. 2014;1:41-6.
12. Ferrari A, Bono A, Baldi M, et al. Does melanoma behave differently in younger children than in adults? A retrospective study of 33 cases of childhood melanoma from a single institution. Pediatrics. 2005;115:649-54.
13. Bauer J, Garbe C. Acquired melanocytic nevi as risk factor for melanoma development. A comprehensive review of epidemiological data. Pigment Cell Res. 2003;16:297-306.
14. Liu W, Dowling JP, Murray WK, et al. Rate of growth in melanomas: characteristics and associations of rapidly growing melanomas. Arch Dermatol. 2006;142:1551-8.

6.3 CONGENITAL MELANOCYTIC NEVI

Horacio A Cabo

The term "melanocytic nevi" comprises a heterogeneous group of benign melanocytic proliferations with different epidemiologic, clinical, dermoscopic, and histopathologic characteristics. Within this ample spectrum, it is possible to distinguish two main characteristics: congenital melanocytic nevi (CMN) and acquired melanocytic nevi (AMN). The former include also blue nevus and spilus nevus, while the latter comprise junction nevus, compounded and intradermal, Clark's nevus (also known as dysplastic or atypical nevus), and Spitz nevus.

Congenital melanocytic nevi are benign nevocytic hamartomas arising from a congenital malformation in which there appears to be a precocious terminal differentiation of the melanocytic precursors and/or a blockage of the migration at the dermal or hypodermal levels. Their cells derive from the neural crest.

In general, CMN are present at birth, although they may become evident months or even years later. They affect 1-6% of the general population. According to their size, they are classified into: small (<1.5 cm), medium (1.5-20 cm), and large or giant (>20 cm).

In the giant forms, which are rare, there is a 5-20% possibility that a melanoma will develop.

Their clinical appearance is varied from a simple macula or raised pigmented tumor, either smooth or verrucous, with or without hair, and small in size, to the involvement of large anatomical areas. Color usually ranges from light brown to dark brown or black.

Congenital melanocytic nevi have their own histologic features that differentiate them from AMN:

- Nevus cell nests in reticular dermis and hypodermis
- Adnexal, vascular, and/or neural involvement
- Arrangement of nevocytes between fibers of dermal collagen

The nevoid cell nests are accompanied by other hamartomatous structures, such as hair follicles, sebaceous glands, and fatty tissue, among others.

In some CMN, the histology is similar to that of acquired melanocytic nevus, especially the small ones.

Small CMN

Both from a clinical and a dermoscopic point of view, small CMN are generally indistinguishable from Clark's nevi.

With the exception of Spitz nevus and blue nevus (see Spitz nevus and Blue nevus and Combined nevus), nevi in general, and congenital nevi in particular, present three basic dermoscopic patterns. At the same time, these three basic patterns may show variants.

The basic patterns are:

- Reticular pattern
- Globular pattern
- Mixed pattern
  - Central
  - Peripheral

Reticular pattern: The pigment network extends over the whole lesion with similar features as regards shape and color (Figs. 6.40A to E).

- *Variant: Patched reticular pattern*: Pigment network areas alternating with areas without pigment network, usually skin-colored (Figs. 6.41A to C).

Globular pattern: Globules distributed over the entire lesion with similar features regarding shape, size, and color (Figs. 6.42A to C).

- *Variant: Cobblestone pattern*: A globular pattern where the globules are large and angulated (Figs. 6.43A and B).

Mixed pattern: Presence of both reticular and globular patterns in the same lesion. Globule location defines whether it is central or peripheral.

- *Central mixed pattern:* Globules in the central area and pigment network in the periphery (Figs. 6.44A and B).
  - *Variant: Hyperpigmented*: The central globules are highly pigmented and a brown zone can be seen in the central area (Fig. 6.45).
  - *Hypopigmented:* The central globules show little pigment and there is a central whitish or skin-colored area (Figs. 6.46A to C).
- *Peripheral mixed pattern*: Globules in the peripheral area. This variant can be observed in young people and is related to the nevi growth. In general, there are one to three lines of globules. These should not appear in adults, since at maturity nevi have to remain stable (Figs. 6.47A to D).

Other Variants

Homogeneous pattern: Homogeneous brown lesions, due to an even pigmentation over the entire lesion, which prevents structure distinction (Figs. 6.48A to D).

Half and half pattern: Half globules and half pigment network (Figs. 6.49A to D).

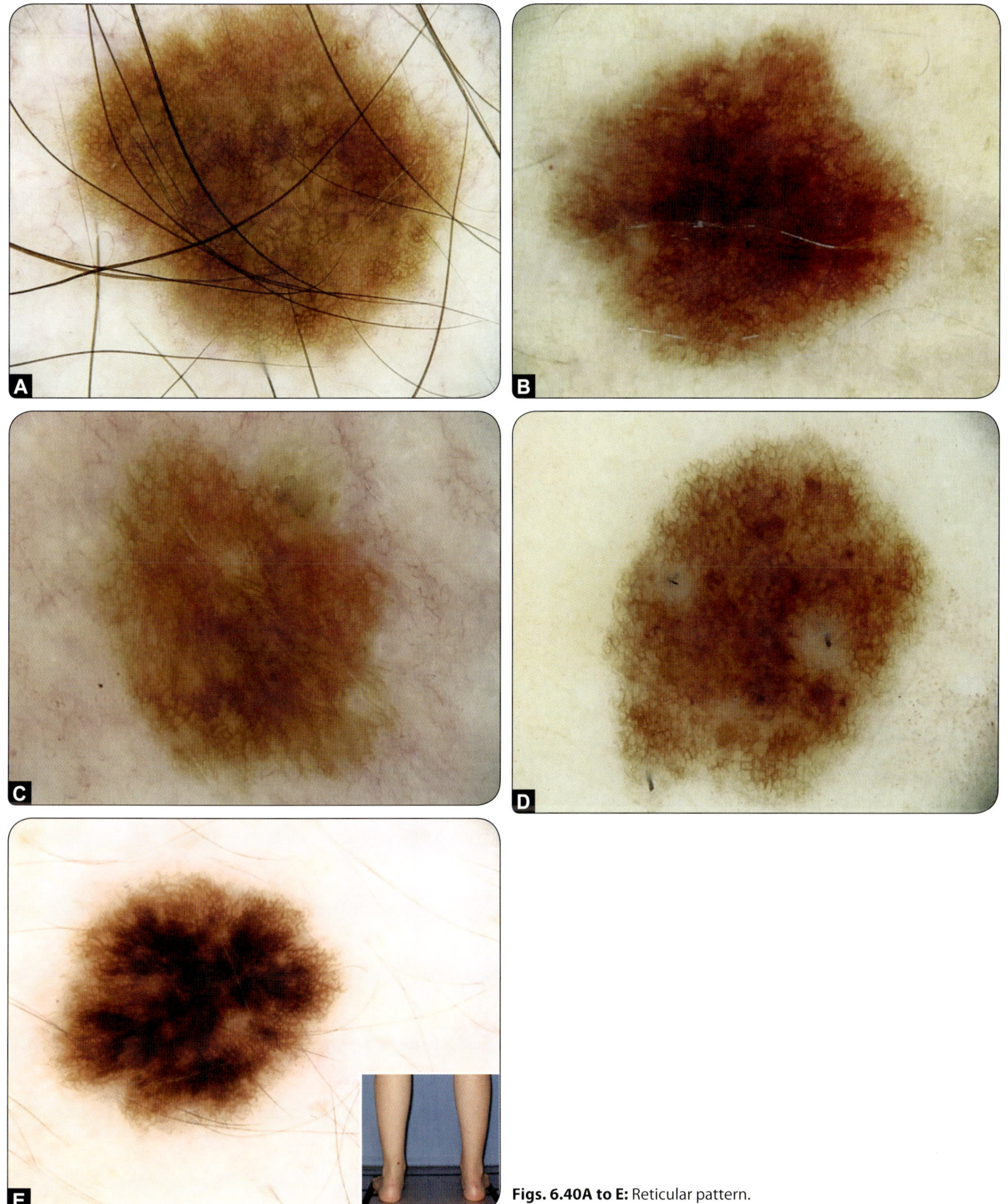

Figs. 6.40A to E: Reticular pattern.

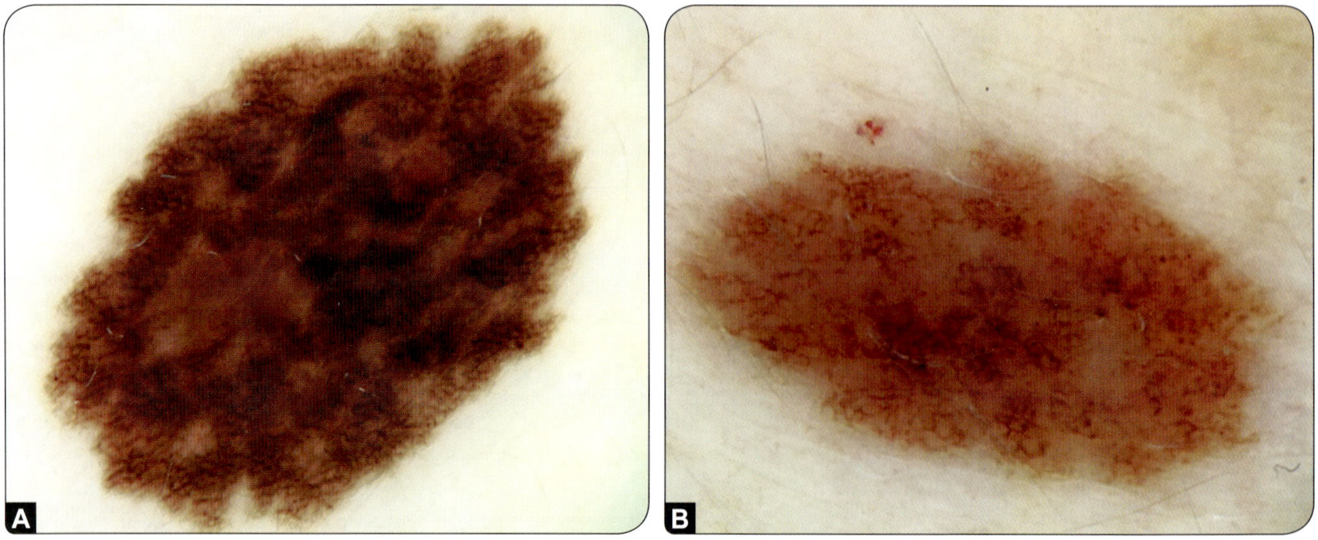

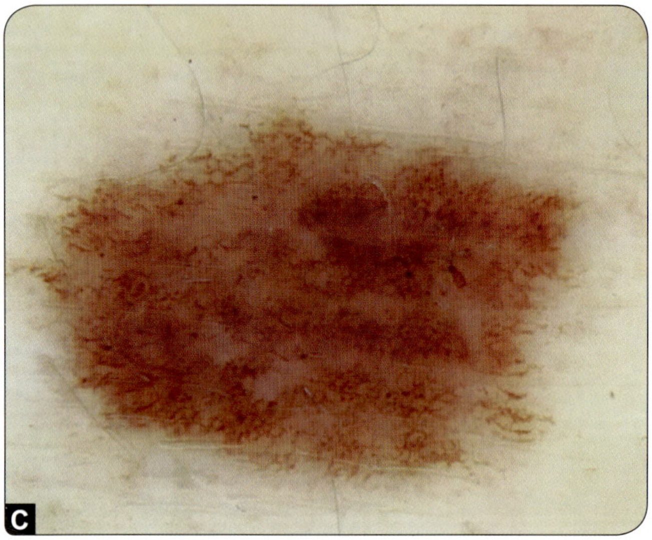

Figs. 6.41A to C: Patched reticular pattern.

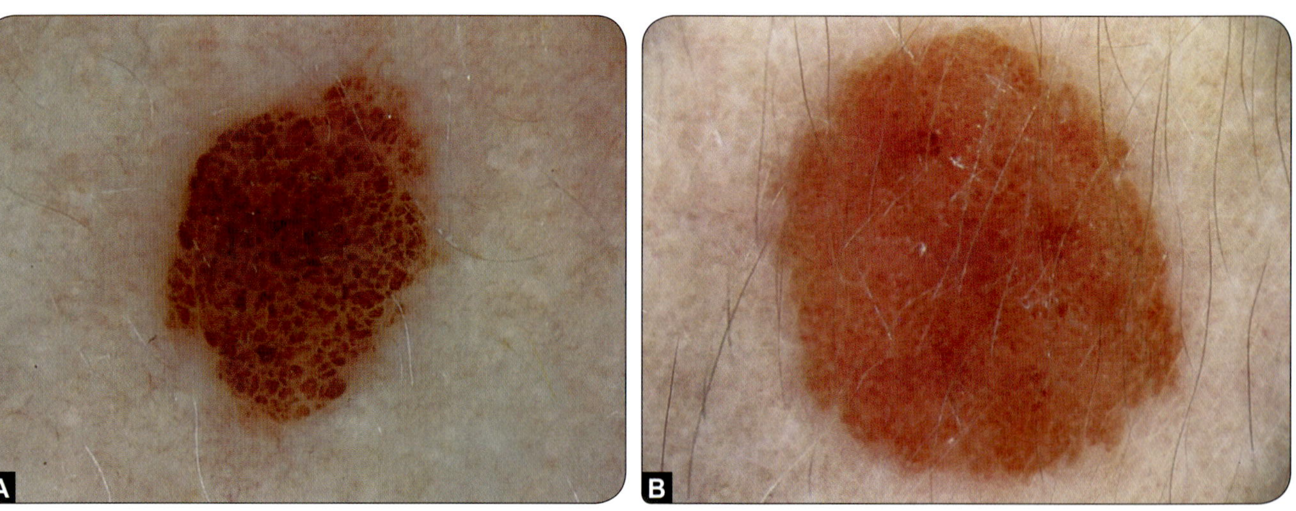

Figs. 6.42A and B

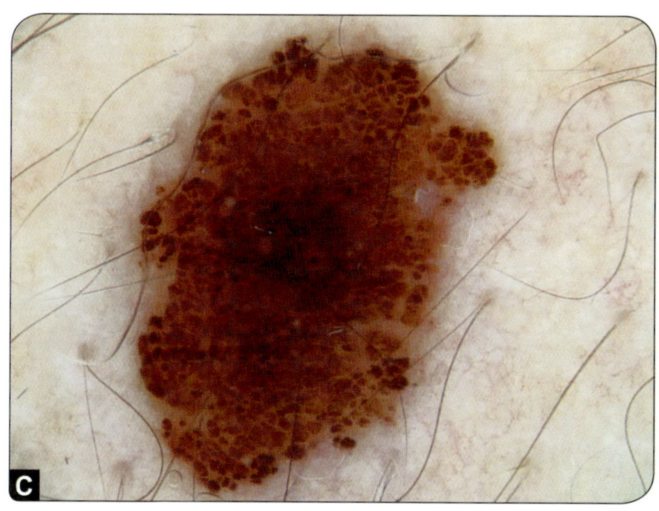

Figs. 6.42A to C: Globular pattern.

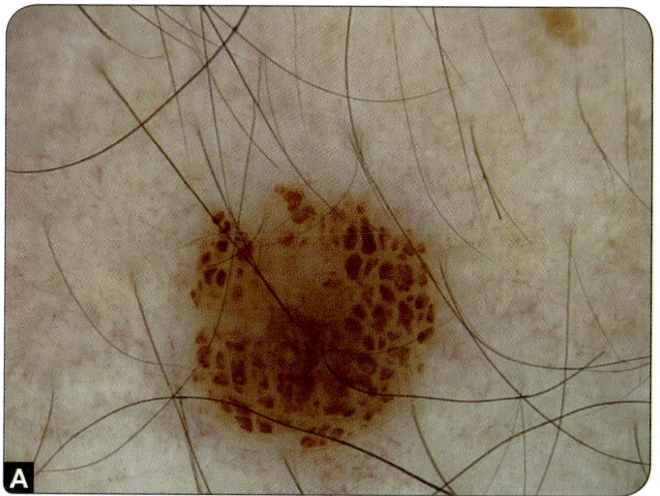

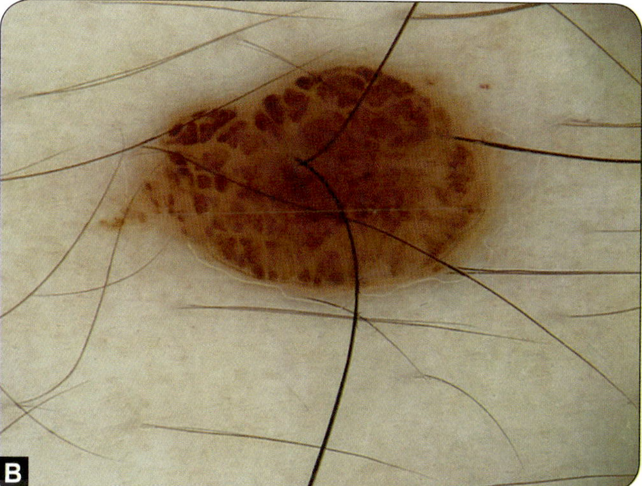

Figs. 6.43A and B: Cobblestone pattern.

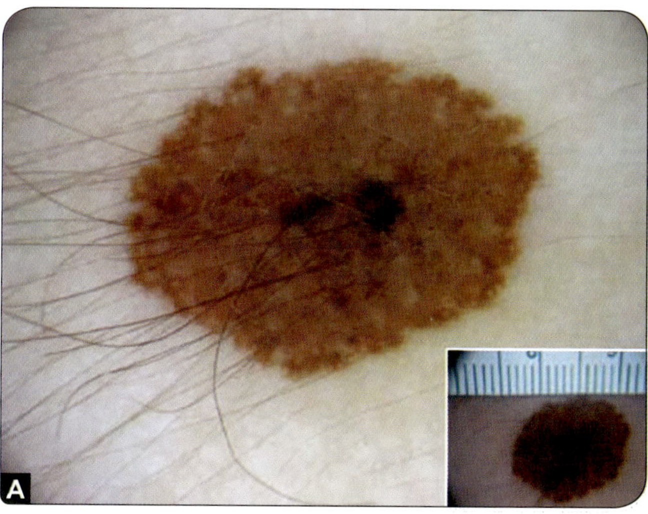

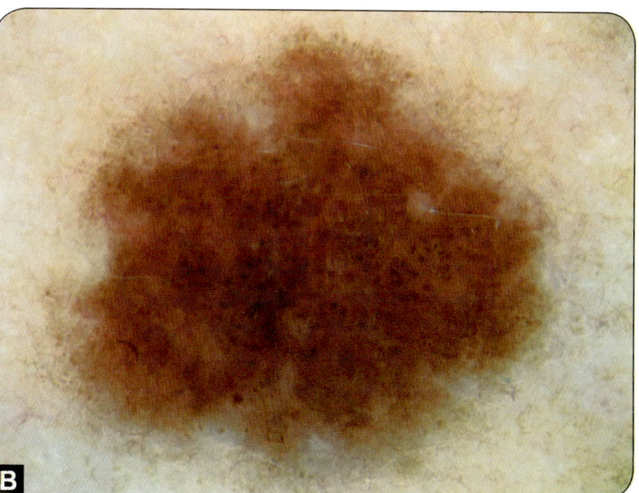

Figs. 6.44A and B: Central mixed pattern.

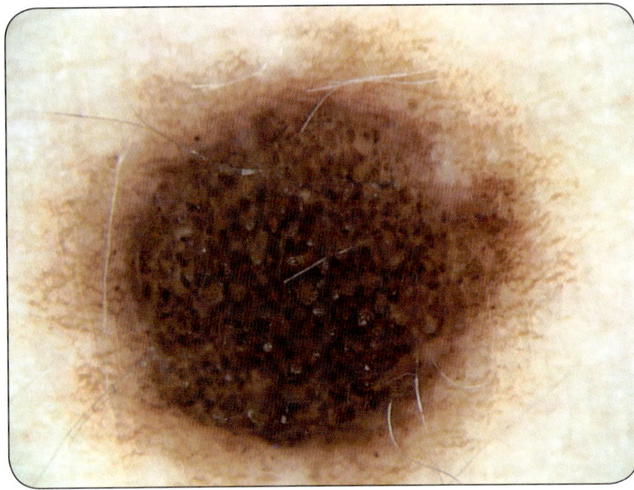

Fig. 6.45: Hyperpigmented central mixed pattern.

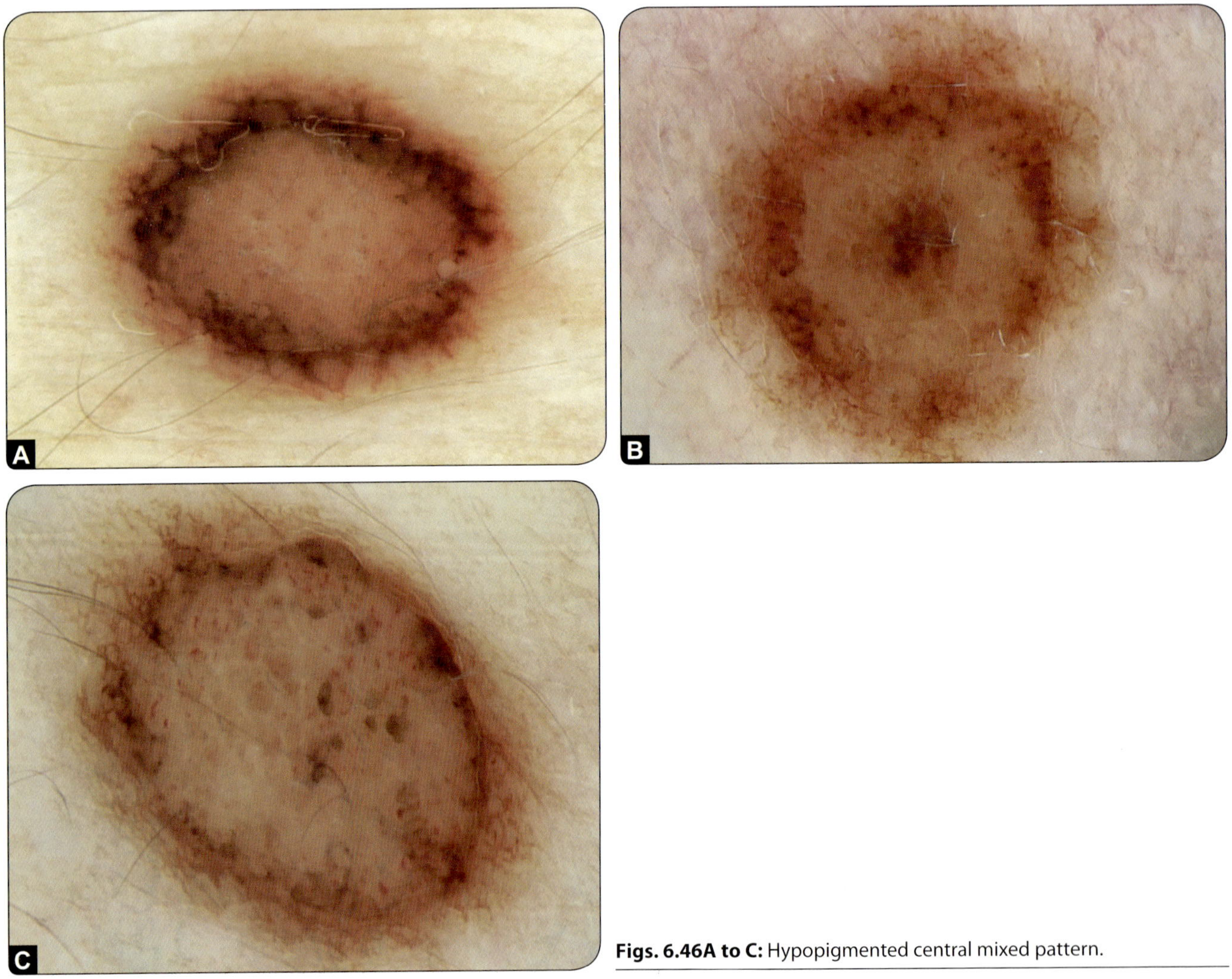

Figs. 6.46A to C: Hypopigmented central mixed pattern.

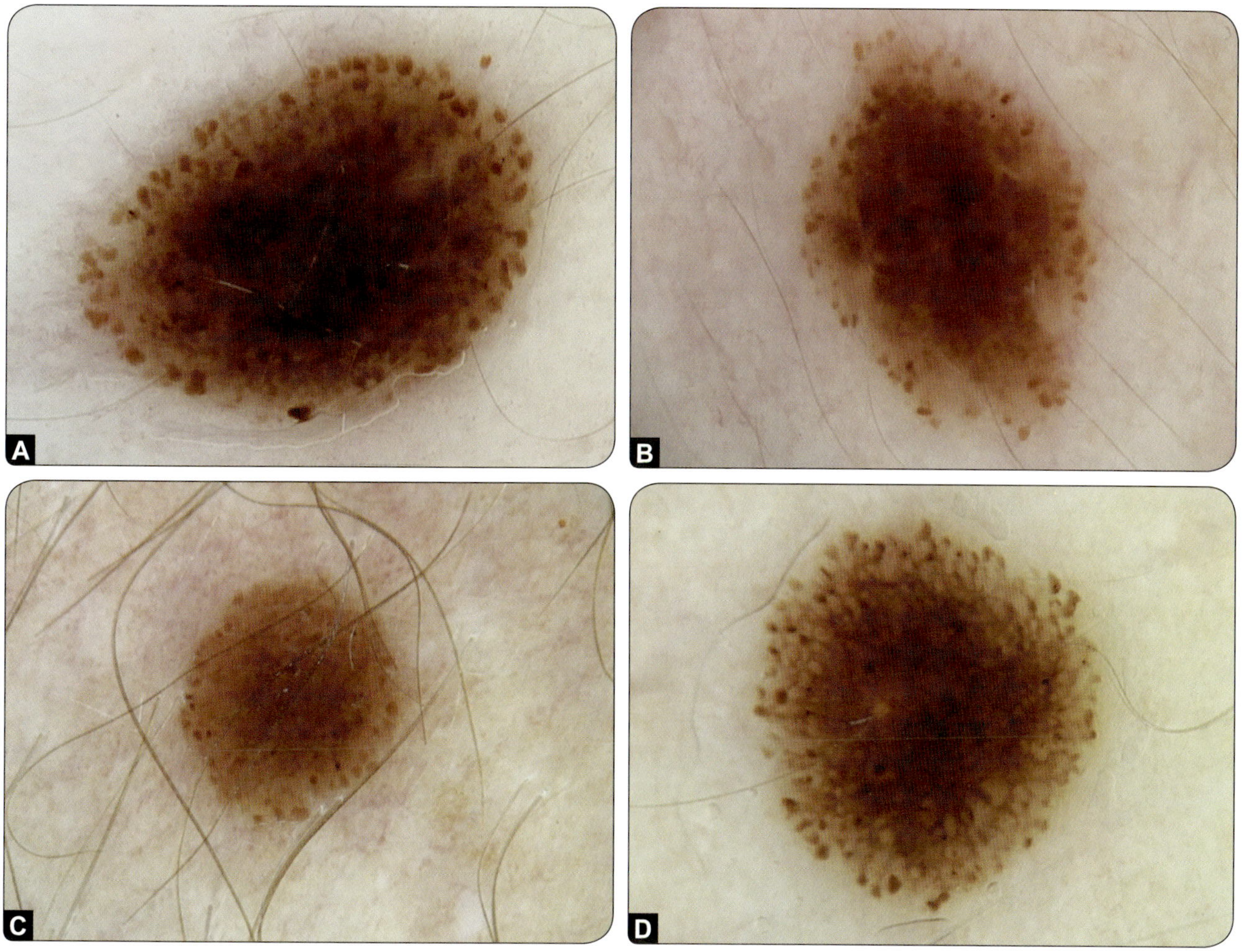

Figs. 6.47A to D: Peripheral mixed pattern.

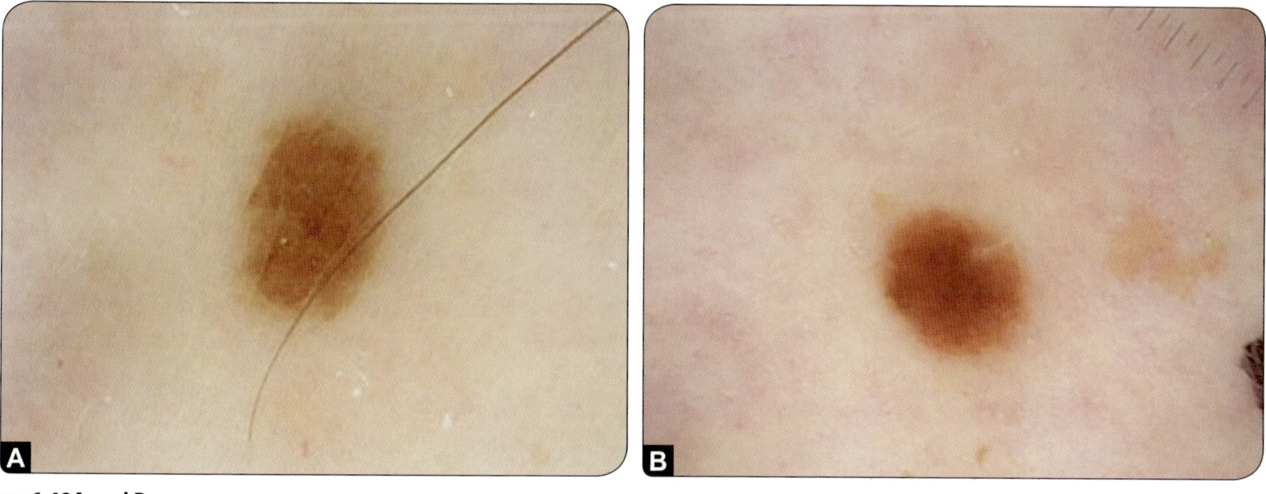

Figs. 6.48A and B

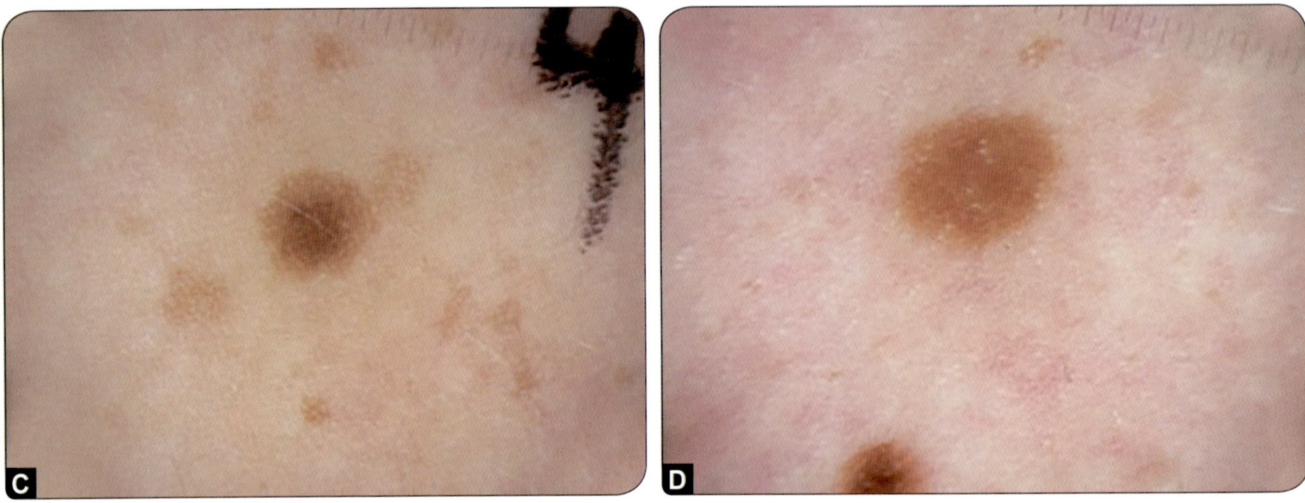

Figs. 6.48A to D: Homogeneous pattern.

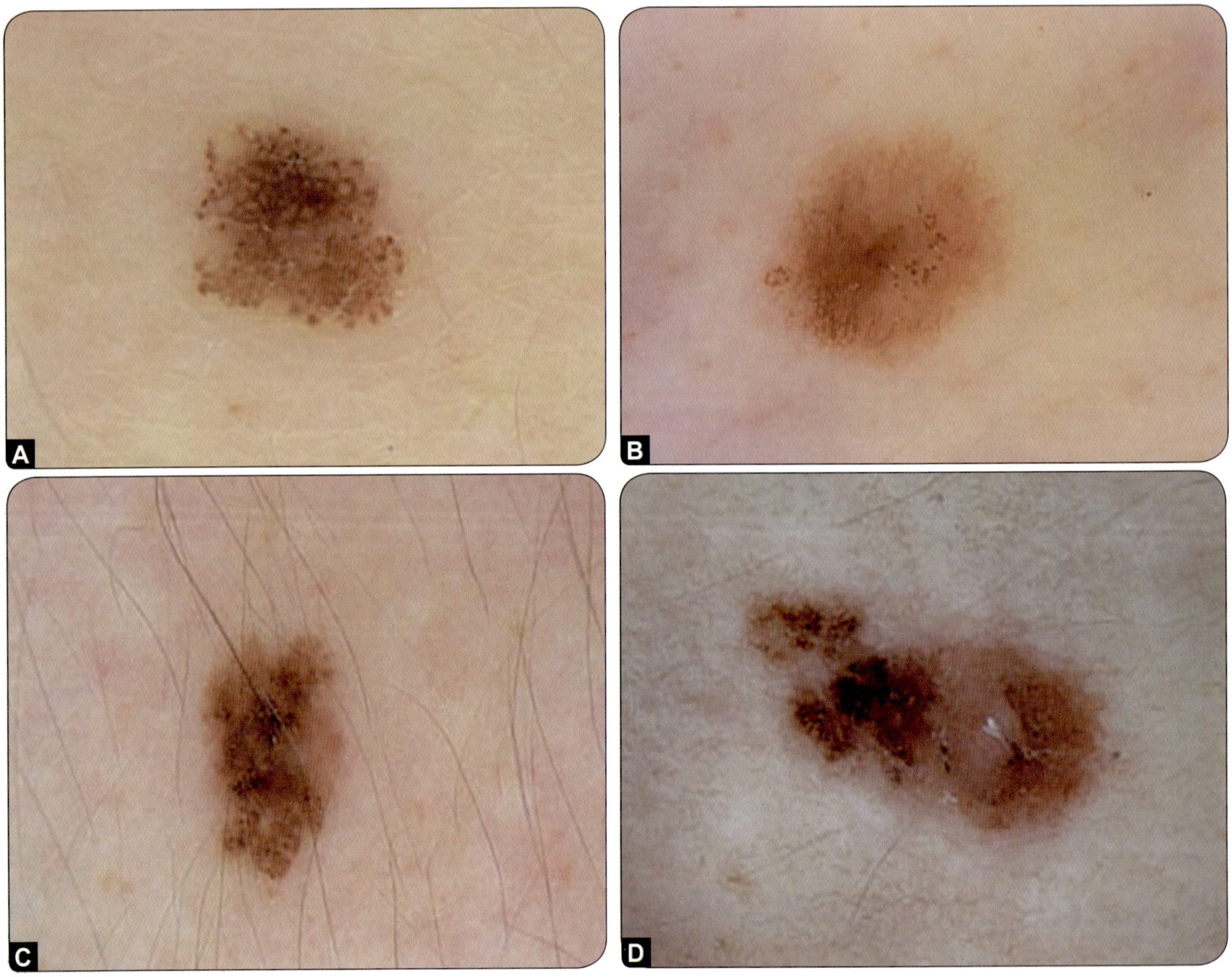

Figs. 6.49A to D: Half and half pattern.

Multicomponent pattern: Presence of three or more dermoscopic structures. It is associated with atypical nevi or melanoma (Figs. 6.50A to C).

It is very important to know the different dermoscopic patterns of the nevi and to be able to distinguish them from the dermoscopic patterns for melanoma.

On the basis that nevi are nevi and melanoma is melanoma, and that nevi do not become melanomas, follow-up of patients with multiple nevi is easier if we know the patient's nevi type, also known as nevi signature pattern.

Medium, Large, and Giant CMN (Figs. 6.51 to 6.58)

There are some dermoscopic structures mostly observed in CMN, which appear from infancy or at birth.

In relation with the reticular pattern:

- Lineal network fragments (fungal hypha-like) (Figs. 6.53 to 6.55)

In relation with the globular pattern:

- Cobblestone pattern (*see* Fig. 6.43)
- Target globules (globules within the network gaps) (Figs. 6.56 and 6.57)

Other features present in CMN include:

- *Milia-like cysts*: Round yellow-white small structures that correspond to intraepidermal keratin accumulation).
- *Hypertrichosis:* This means an increase in terminal hairs (Figs. 6.58A to C).
- *Perifollicular pigmentary changes*: Hyperpigmentation or hypopigmentation around the hair follicle.

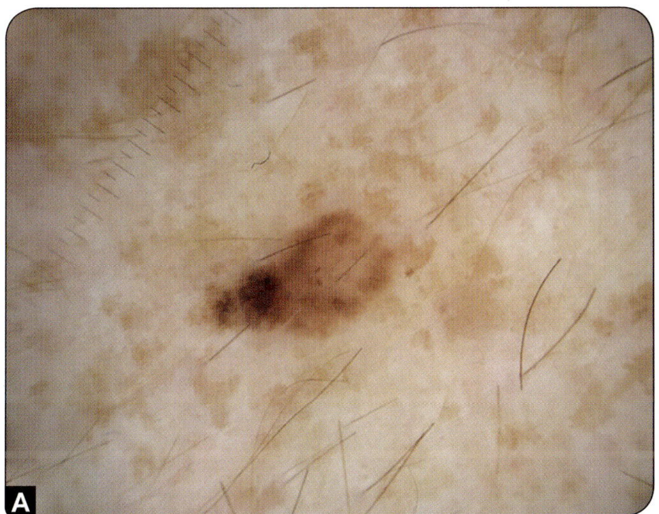

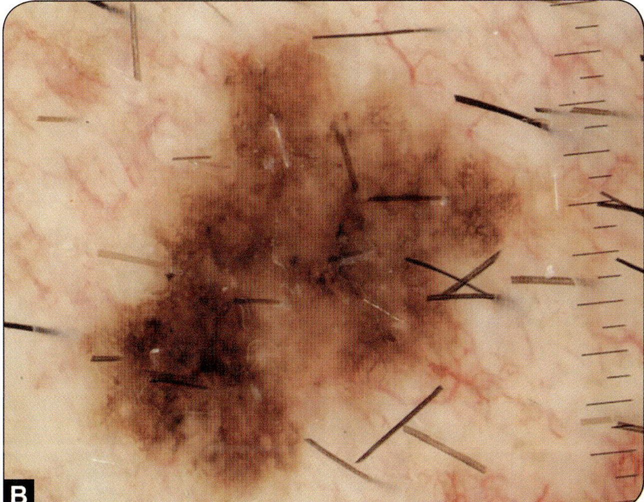

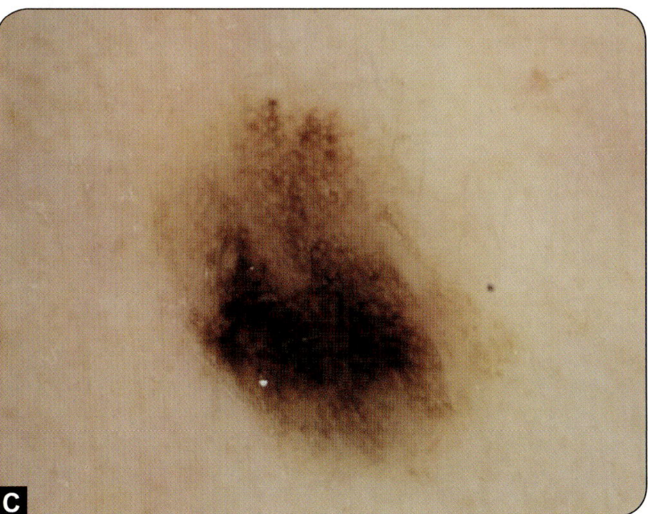

Figs. 6.50A to C: Multicomponent pattern.

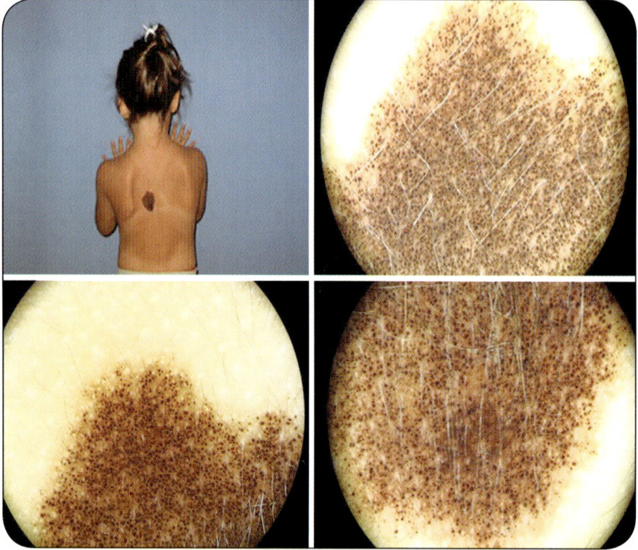

Fig. 6.51: Medium congenital melanocytic nevus.

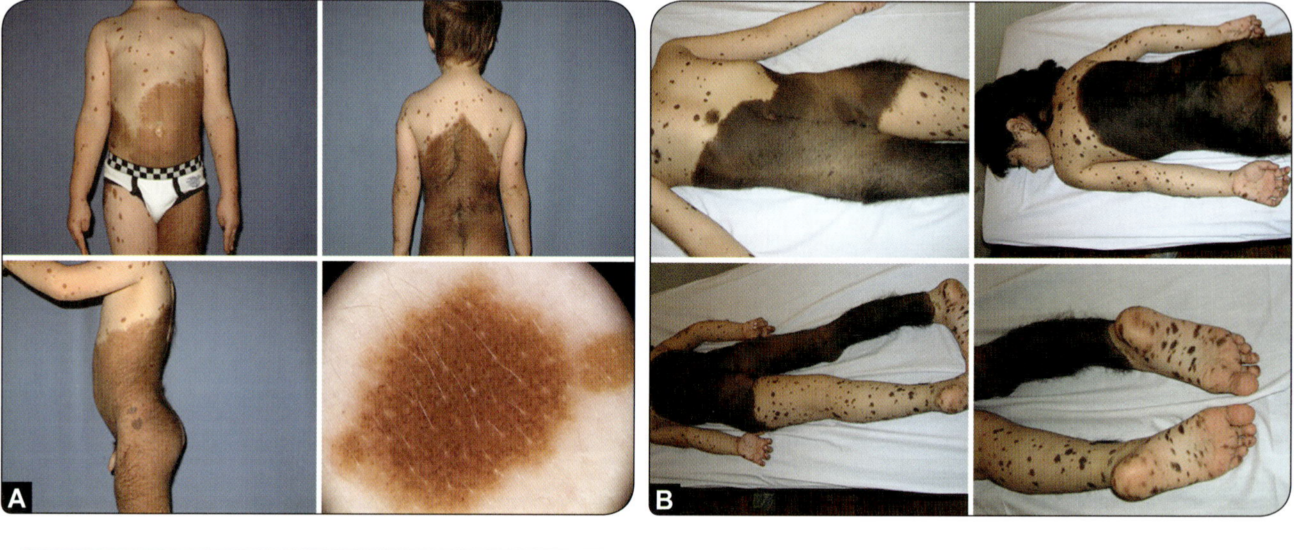

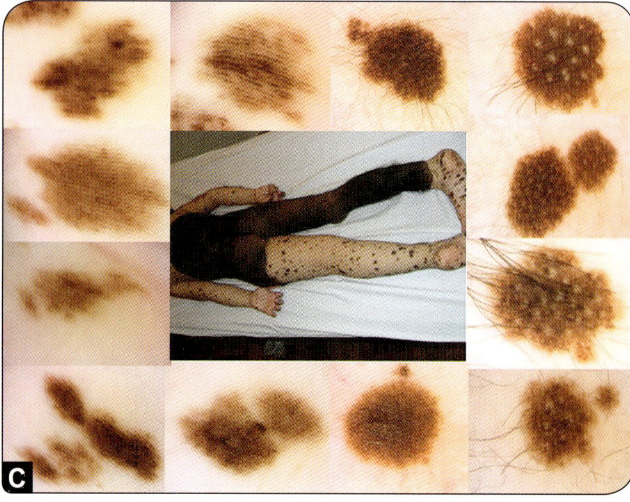

Figs. 6.52A to C: Giant congenital melanocytic nevus.

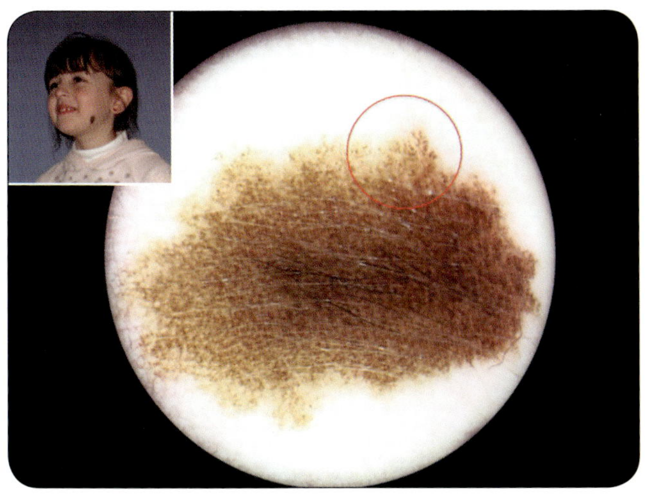

Fig. 6.53: Lineal network fragments (fungal hypha-like) (red circle).

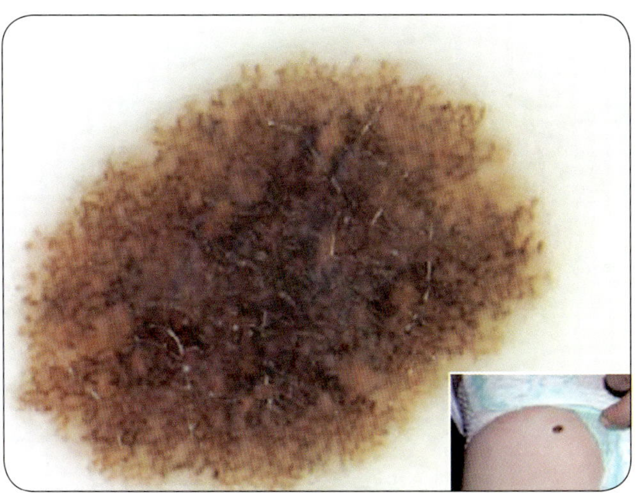

Fig. 6.54: Lineal network fragments (fungal hypha-like) at the periphery of the lesion.

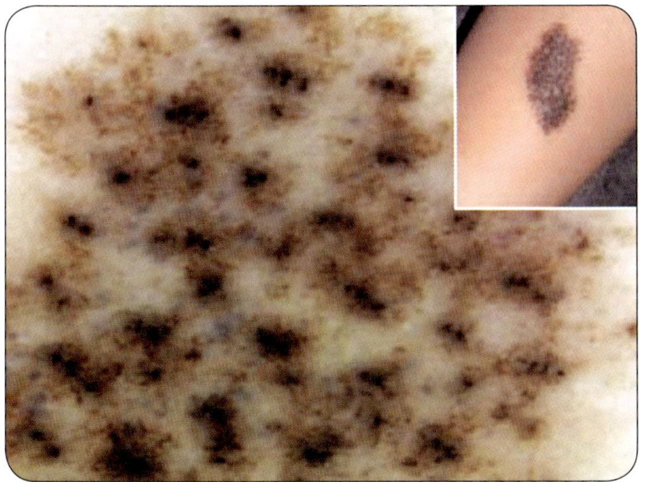

Fig. 6.55: Lineal network fragments (fungal hypha-like) throughout the lesion.

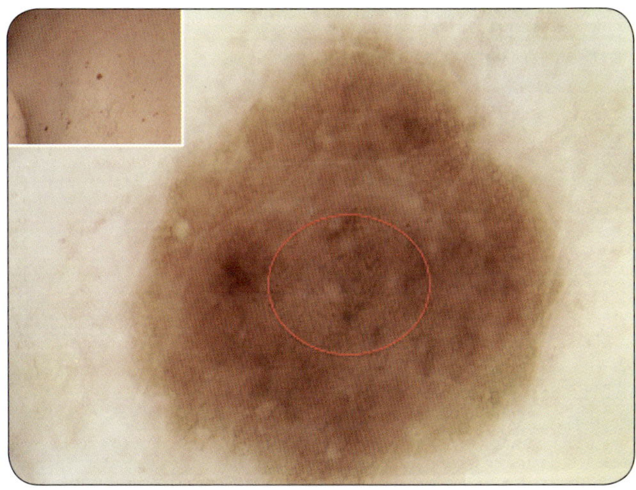

Fig. 6.56: Target globules (red circle).

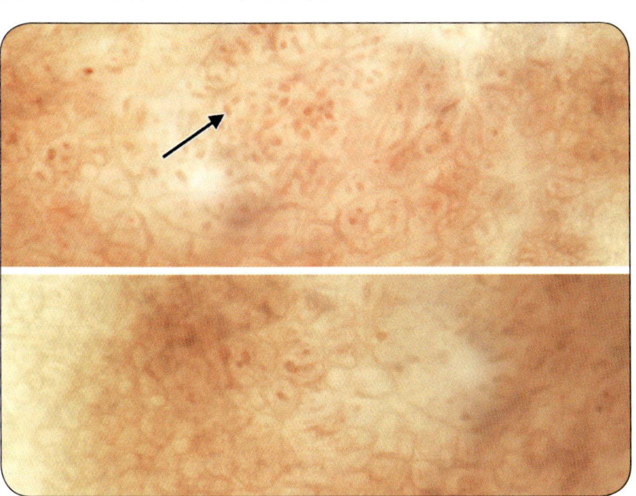

Fig. 6.57: Close-up target globules (arrow).

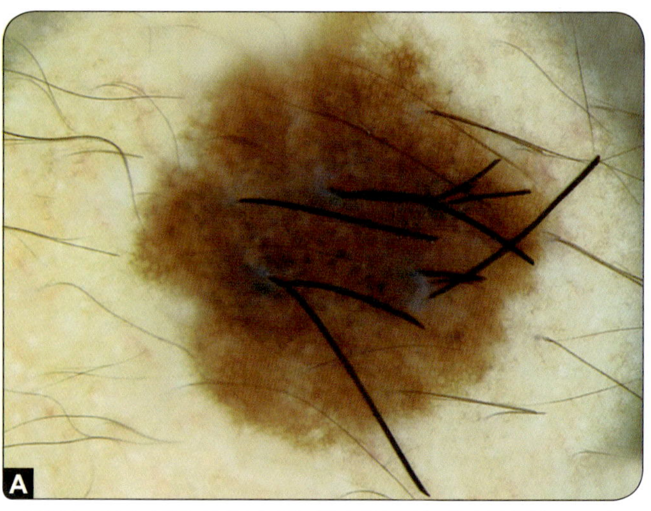
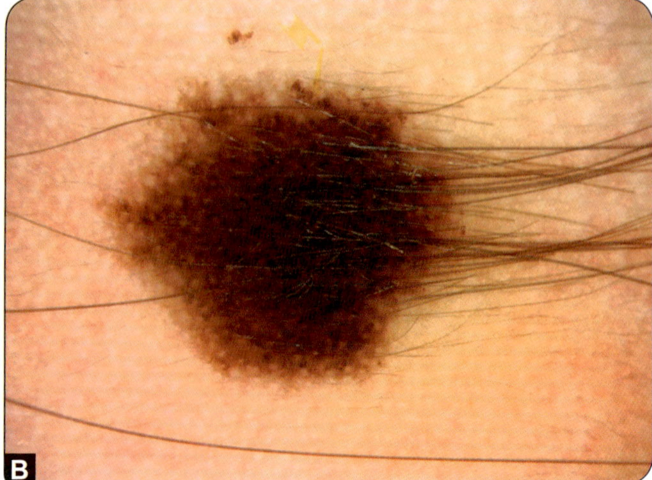
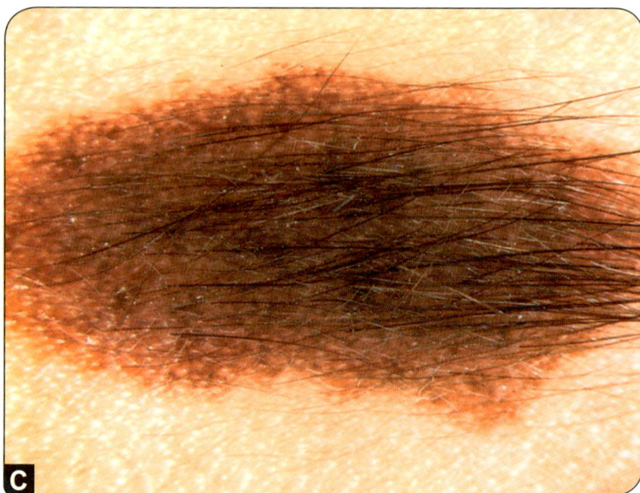

Figs. 6.58A to C: Congenital nevus with hypertrichosis.

SUGGESTED READING

Argenziano G, Soyer P, De Giorgio V, et al. Interactive Atlas of Dermoscopy. Milán: EDRA Medical Publishing & New Media; 2000.

Cabo H. Dermatoscopia. Buenos Aires, Argentina: Weber Ferro; 2000.

Cabo H. Dermatoscopia, 2nd edition. Buenos Aires, Argentina: Ediciones Journal; 2012.

Ingordo V, Iannazzone SS, Cusano F, et al. Dermoscopic features of congenital melanocytic nevus and Becker nevus in an adult male population: an analysis with a 10-fold magnification. Dermatology. 2006;212:354-60.

Johr R, Stolz W. Dermoscopy: An Illustrated Self-Assessment Guide, 2nd edition. New York: McGraw-Hill Education; 2015.

Jorh R, Soyer P, Argenziano G, et al. Dermoscopy. The Essentials (MOABT). New York: Elsevier Ltd; 2004.

Kittler H. Dermatoscopy. An Algorithmic Method Based on Pattern Analysis. Austria: Facultas.wuv; 2011.

Kopf AW, Bart RS, Hennessey P, et al. Congenital nevocytic nevi and malignant melanomas. J Am Acad Dermatol. 1979;1:123.

Lallas A. Dermoscopy in General Dermatology. Dermatol Clin. 2013;3:679-94.

Malvhey J, Puig S. Principles of Dermoscopy. Barcelona: Creaciones Gráficas; 2009.

Marghoob A, Braun R, Kopf A. Atlas of Dermoscopy. London: Taylor & Francis; 2005.

Menzies S, Crotty K, Ingvar C, et al. An Atlas of Surface Microscopy of Pigmented Skin Lesions. Sydney: McGraw-Hill Book Company; 1996.

Rabinovitz H, Kopf A. Dermoscopy: A Practical Guide. Miami: American Academy of Dermatology; 1999.

Soyer P, Argenziano G, Chimenti S, et al. Dermoscopy of Pigmented Skin Lesions. An Atlas Based on the Consensus Net Meeting on Dermoscopy. Milán: EDRA Medical Publishing & New Media; 2001.

Stolz W, Braun-Falco O, Bilek P, et al. Color Atlas of Dermatoscopy. Germany: Blackwell Science; 1994.

Zalaudek I, Argenziano G, Giacomel J. Dermoscopy of nonpigmented skin tumors. Boca Raton, FL: CRC Press; 2016.

6.4 ACQUIRED MELANOCYTIC NEVI

Horacio A Cabo

As previously mentioned, the term melanocytic nevi comprises a heterogeneous group of benign melanocytic proliferations with different epidemiologic, clinical, dermoscopic, and histopathologic features. We can classify them into two main categories: congenital melanocytic nevi (CMN)—including blue nevi and spilus nevi—and acquired melanocytic nevi (AMN). The latter conform a group comprising junction, compound and intradermal nevi, Clark nevus (also known as dysplastic nevus or atypical nevus), and Spitz nevus.

Acquired melanocytic nevi are melanocytic proliferations that are not present at birth. These nevi show a dynamic vital cycle starting at puberty and reaching its maximum incidence in the fourth and fifth decades of life. However, in the sixth and seventh decades their number decreases. There is evidence to support the idea that these nevi develop as a result of exposure to UV rays, and in other cases owing to hereditary factors (atypical nevus syndrome). Acquired melanocytic nevi may vary significantly in number, color, size, and/or clinical characteristics. A great number of common nevi or Clark nevi points to a high risk of melanoma development.

Color is very important in dermoscopy, especially in melanocytic lesions. Clearly, most of these lesions will be in different shades of brown. Other colors will depend on the localization of the pigment and blood vessels. Some nevi in people with high phototypes will be darker while others, in phototypes I or II, will be lighter.

Dermoscopic Classification of AMN

Like CMN, AMN also present three basic dermoscopic patterns. At the same time, these three basic patterns may present variants.

The basic patterns are:

- Reticular pattern
- Globular pattern
- Mixed pattern
  - Central
  - Peripheral

Reticular pattern: The pigment network appears in the entire lesion, presenting similar features as regards form and color. This is generally in different shades of brown. Nevi appearing in youth and in response to sun exposure frequently present this pattern (Figs. 6.59A to C).

- *Variant: Patched reticular pattern*: Areas with pigment network alternating with areas without pigment network and usually skin-colored (Fig. 6.60).

Globular pattern: Globules distributed in the entire lesion with similar features regarding shape, size, and color (Fig. 6.61).

- Light or dark brown nevi depending on phototype.
- This pattern is more frequently observed in CMN.
- Variant: Pebbled pattern: This is a globular pattern where the globules are bigger and angulated. It is mostly found in CMN (Fig. 6.62).

Mixed pattern: It is characterized by the presence of both reticular and globular patterns in the same lesion. The location of the globules determines whether it is central or peripheral.

- *Central mixed*: Globules in the central part and pigment network in the periphery (Fig. 6.63).
  - *Hyperpigmented variant*: The central globules are highly pigmented and only a brown area can be observed at the center of the lesion (Fig. 6.64).
  - *Hypopigmented variant*: The central globules show little pigmentation and a whitish or skin-colored area is observable at the center of the lesion (Fig. 6.65).
- *Peripheral mixed*: Globules in the peripheral area. This pattern is seen in young people and is related to the growth of the nevi. In general, there are between one and three lines of globules. It should not be found in adults, since at this time of life nevi are supposed to remain stable (Figs. 6.66A and B).

Other Variants

Homogeneous pattern: Homogeneous brown lesions, due to a uniform pigmentation over the entire lesion, which impedes the observation of structures (Fig. 6.67).

Half and half pattern: Half globules and half pigment network (Fig. 6.68).

Multicomponent pattern: Three or more desmoscopic structures present. It is associated with atypical nevi or melanoma (Fig. 6.69).

It is very important to know the different dermoscopic patterns of the nevi and distinguish them from those of melanoma (*see* Management of Patients with Multiple Nevi).

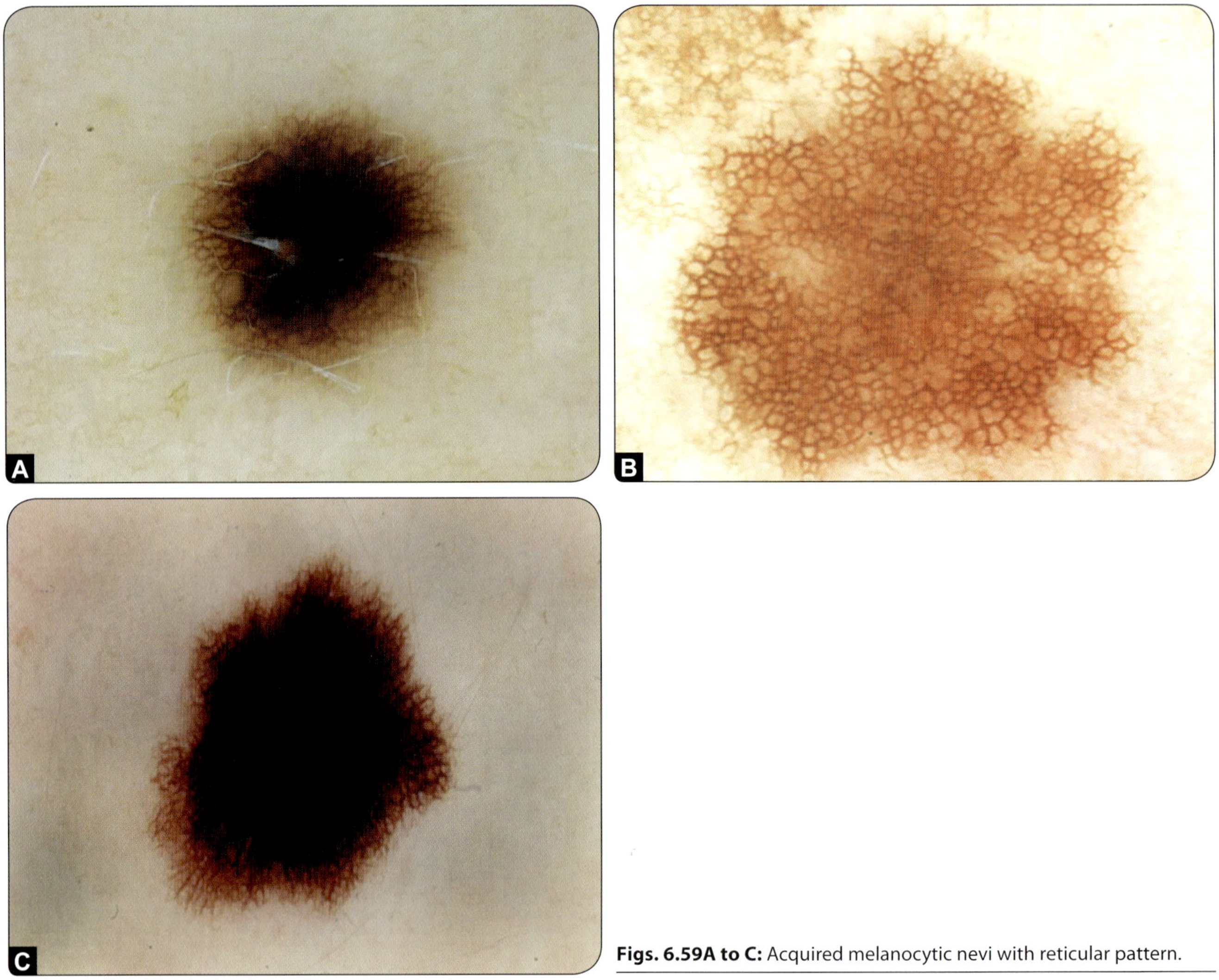

Figs. 6.59A to C: Acquired melanocytic nevi with reticular pattern.

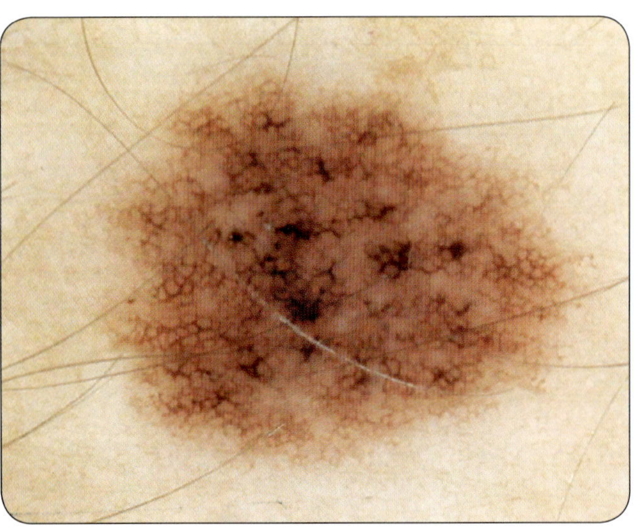

Fig. 6.60: Acquired melanocytic nevi with patched reticular pattern.

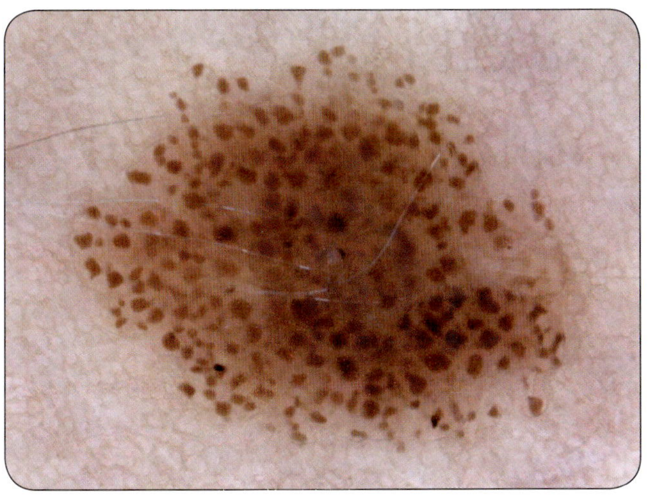

Fig. 6.61: Acquired melanocytic nevi with globular pattern.

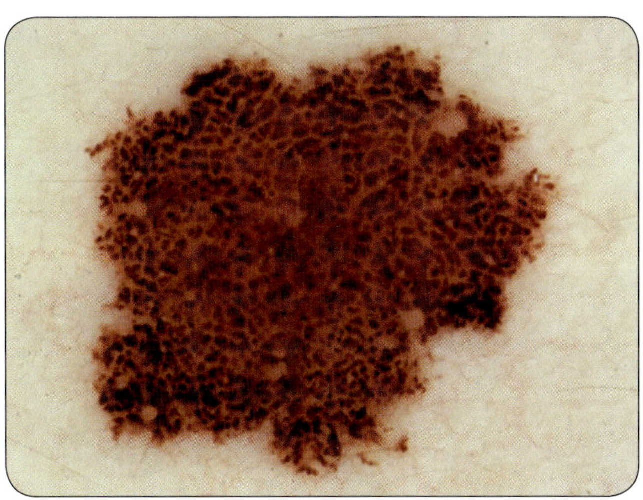

Fig. 6.62: Acquired melanocytic nevi with globular (pebbled) pattern.

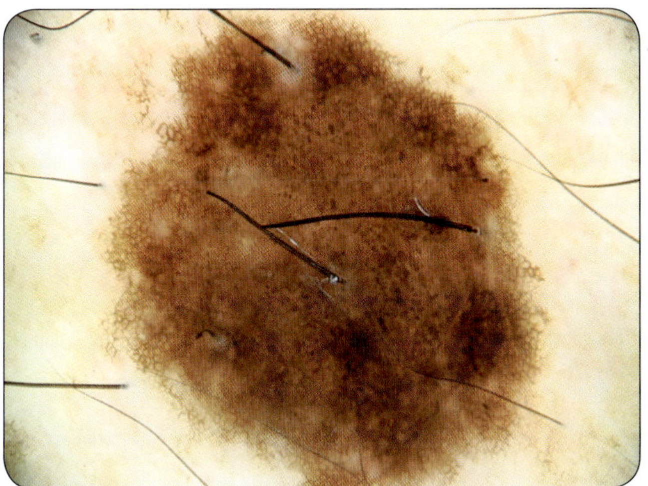

Fig. 6.63: Acquired melanocytic nevi with mixed central pattern.

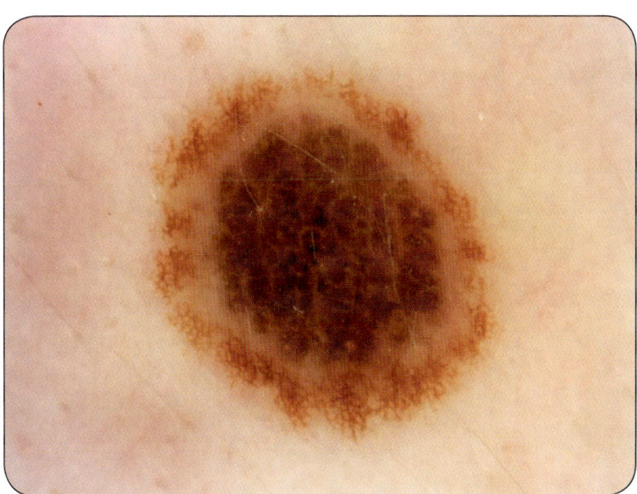

Fig. 6.64: Acquired melanocytic nevi with mixed central hyperpigmented pattern.

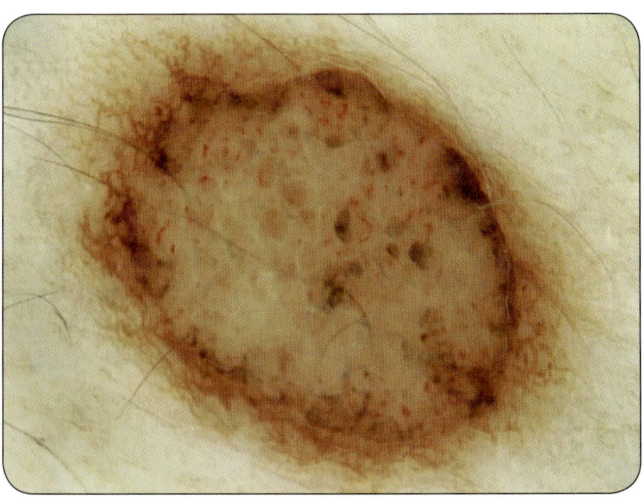

Fig. 6.65: Acquired melanocytic nevi with mixed central hypopigmented central pattern.

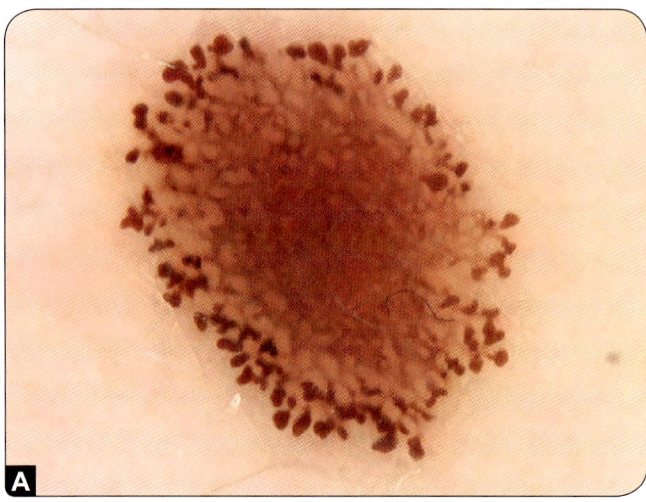

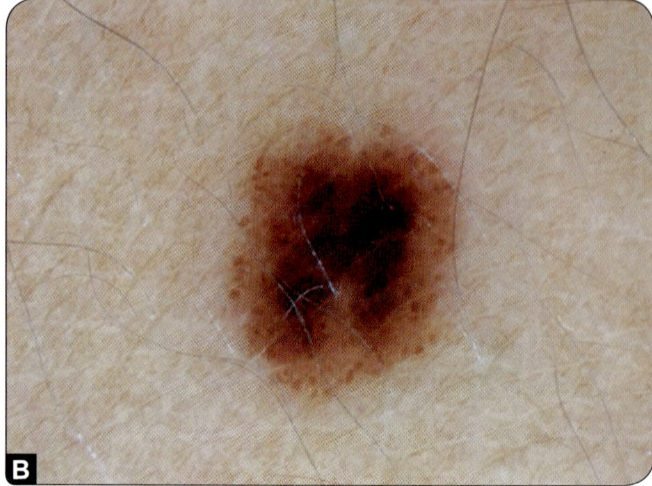

Figs. 6.66A and B: Acquired melanocytic nevi with peripheral mixed pattern.

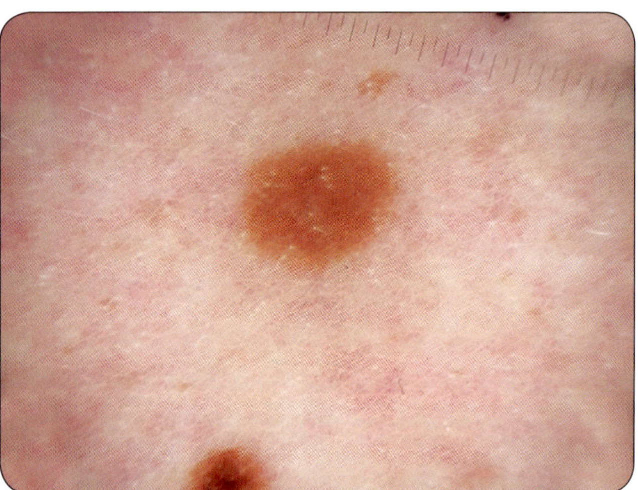

Fig. 6.67: Acquired melanocytic nevi with homogeneous pattern.

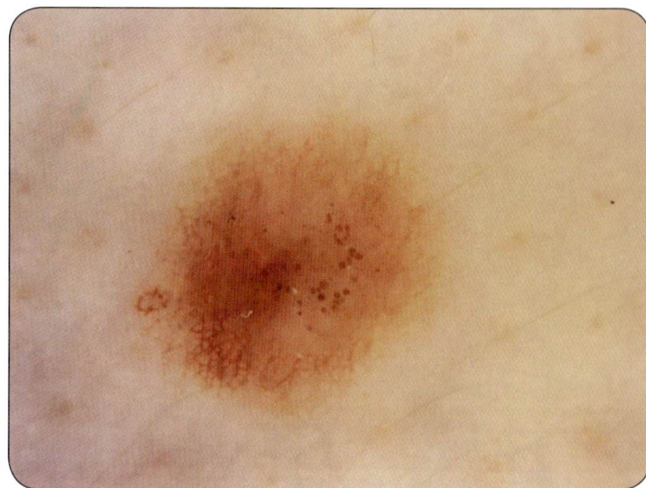

Fig. 6.68: Acquired melanocytic nevi with half and half pattern.

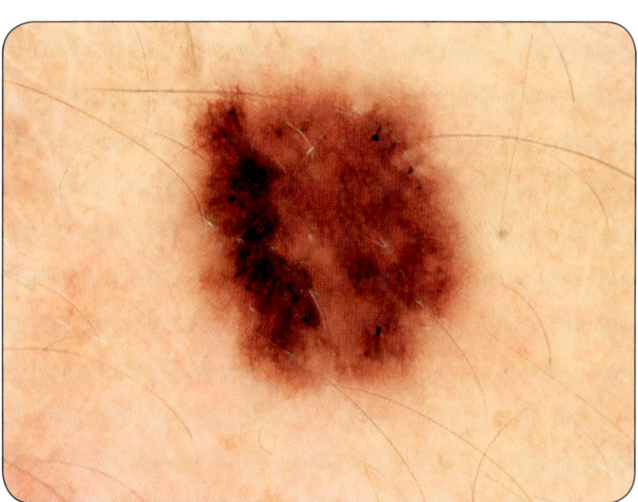

Fig. 6.69: Acquired melanocytic nevi with multicomponent pattern.

SUGGESTED READING

Argenziano G, Soyer P, De Giorgio V, et al. Interactive Atlas of Dermoscopy. Milán: EDRA Medical Publishing & New Media; 2000.

Cabo H. Dermatoscopia. Buenos Aires, Argentina: Weber Ferro; 2000.

Cabo H. Dermatoscopia, 2nd edition. Buenos Aires, Argentina: Ediciones Journal; 2012.

Johr R, Stolz W. Dermoscopy: An Illustrated Self-Assessment Guide, 2nd edition. New York: McGraw-Hill Education; 2015.

Jorh R, Soyer P, Argenziano G, et al. Dermoscopy. The Essentials (MOABT). New York: Elsevier Ltd; 2004.

Kittler H. Dermatoscopy. An Algorithmic Method Based on Pattern Analysis. Austria: Facultas.wuv; 2011.

Lallas A. Dermoscopy in general dermatology. Dermatol Clin. 2013;3:679-94.

Malvhey J, Puig S. Principles of Dermoscopy. Barcelona: Creaciones Gráficas; 2009.

Marghoob A, Braun R, Kopf A. Atlas of Dermoscopy. London: Taylor & Francis; 2005.

Menzies S, Crotty K, Ingvar C, et al. An Atlas of Surface Microscopy of Pigmented Skin Lesions. Sydney: McGraw-Hill Book Company; 1996.

Rabinovitz H, Kopf A. Dermoscopy: A Practical Guide. Miami: American Academy of Dermatology; 1999.

Soyer P, Argenziano G, Chimenti S, et al. Dermoscopy of Pigmented Skin Lesions. An Atlas Based on the Consensus Net Meeting on Dermoscopy. Milán: EDRA Medical Publishing & New Media, 2001.

Stolz W, Braun-Falco O, Bilek P, et al. Color Atlas of Dermatoscopy. Germany: Blackwell Science; 1994.

Zalaudek I, Argenziano G, Giacomel J. Dermoscopy of Non-Pigmented Skin Tumors. Boca Raton, FL: CRC Press; 2016.

6.5 ATYPICAL NEVUS (DYSPLASTIC)

Horacio A Cabo

Atypical nevi (AN) are those sharing all or some of the characteristics of melanoma of the clinical ABCD rule (Asymmetric lesion, irregular Borders, multiple Colors, and a Diameter >0.7 mm).

The term AN is a clinical term. Some of these AN under clinical examination, may present, histologic features different from those of common nevi and are called dysplastic.

It is then clear that clinical atypia may or may not be correlated to histologic dysplasia.

Therefore, dysplastic nevi (DN) must be regarded as histologic variants of common nevi.

That is to say, atypical-DN do not become nor are they precursors of melanoma.

Nevi are nevi and melanoma is melanoma. Primary melanoma appears in the skin in two ways: de novo (around 70%) or growing on a nevus (around 30%) and in these latter cases about 60% are common or not AN.

The presence of multiple nevi and DN is a genetic risk marker for cutaneous melanoma.

Histologic dysplasia may be mild, moderate, or severe.

In patients with AN and severe dysplasia, the excision margin must be extended, not because they may be melanoma precursors, but because it is occasionally difficult to distinguish them from melanoma, both clinically and dermoscopically, and even histologically.

Obviously, prophylactic excision of clinically AN does not reduce the risk of melanoma.

There are no doubts that the clinical acronym ABCD has failed when it comes to differentiating melanoma from DN, especially because by definition, both lesions share the same characteristics. However, dermoscopy offers a means to distinguish malignant from benign lesions in clinically indeterminate cases. The presence or absence of specific dermoscopic structures and patterns may help the dermatologist to decide which lesions may be controlled by means of short- or long-term monitoring and which ones require a biopsy.

Dermoscopy improves clinical diagnosis because it enables us to see structures that are not visible with the naked eye.

Thus, with the dermoscope we can recognize dermoscopic characteristics of the different types of nevi and distinguish them from melanoma. In contrast, it is difficult to distinguish the different types of nevi clinically, and besides some nevi are clinically atypical but are not so under dermoscopic examination. Therefore, under clinical and dermoscopic examination we face different scenarios.

Clinical Definition of AN

Atypical nevi sharing some or all ABCD characteristics of melanoma (Fig. 6.70).

Dermoscopic Definition of AN

- Clinically AN with benign dermoscopic patterns (*see* Congenital Melanocytic Nevi and Acquired Melanocytic Nevi). These patterns include:
  - Reticular pattern
  - Globular pattern
  - Mixed pattern
    - Central
    - Peripheral
- Clinically AN with indefinite dermoscopic patterns
  - These nevi present a dermoscopic pattern known as multicomponent, where it is possible to observe three or more dermoscopic criteria.
  - It is possible to see a wide range of alterations
  - *Mild alterations*: Suitable for short-term digital dermoscopy follow-up with sequential images (Figs. 6.71 to 6.75).

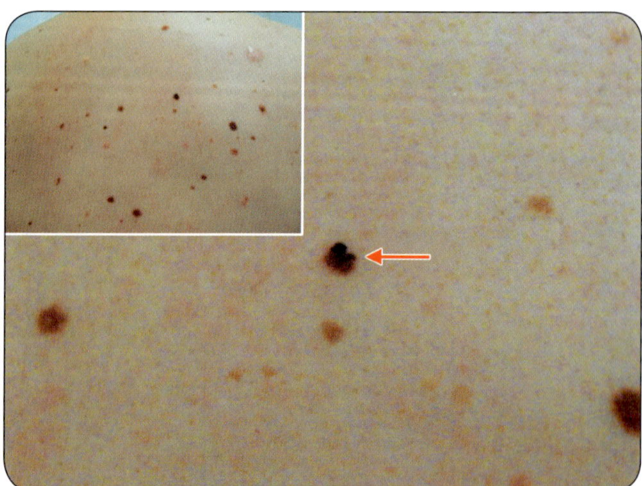

Fig. 6.70: Atypical nevus—clinical view (arrow). The clinical ABCD rule is positive (asymmetry, irregular borders, multiple colors, and 0.9 mm of diameter).

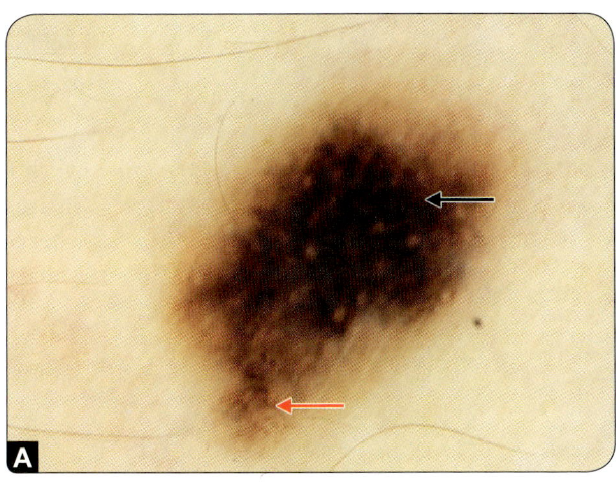

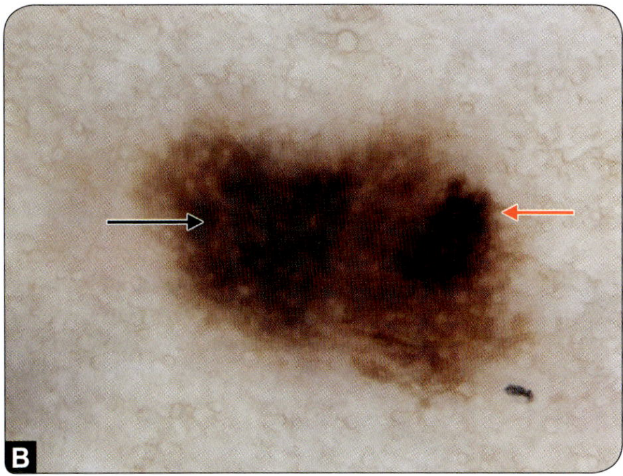

Figs. 6.71A and B: Atypical nevus (mild dysplasia) with different colors (black, gray, dark brown, and light brown) atypical pigment network (red arrow) and eccentric pigmentation (black arrow).

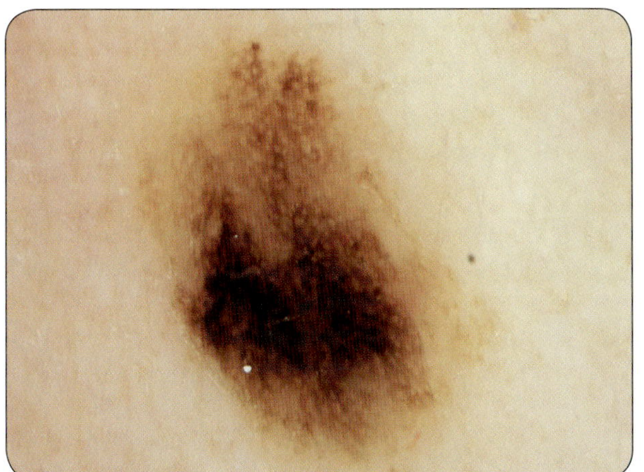

Fig. 6.72: Atypical nevus (mild dysplasia) with atypical pigment network.

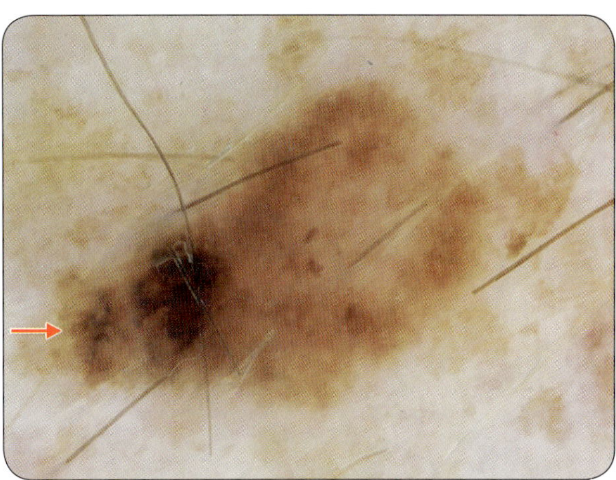

Fig. 6.73: Atypical nevus (mild dysplasia): asymmetric lesion with eccentric areas of regression (arrow).

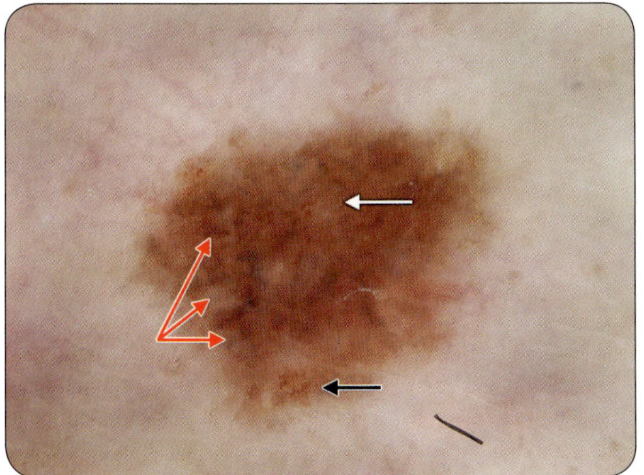

Fig. 6.74: Atypical nevus (mild dysplasia): areas of regression (red arrows); atypical pigment network (black arrow); and negative pigment network (white arrow).

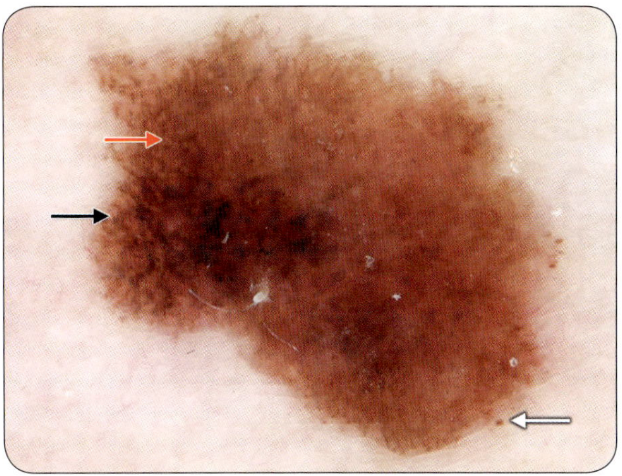

Fig. 6.75: Atypical nevus (mild dysplasia): atypical pigment network (red arrow); irregular streaks (black arrow); and irregular brown globules (white arrow).

- *Severe alterations*: Very difficult to differentiate from melanoma and requiring biopsy. These dermoscopy features include (Figs. 6.76 to 6.82):
  - Atypical pigment network
  - Negative pigment network
  - Irregular projections/streaks
  - Blue whitish-veil
  - Irregular dots and globules
  - Regression
  - Multiple colors

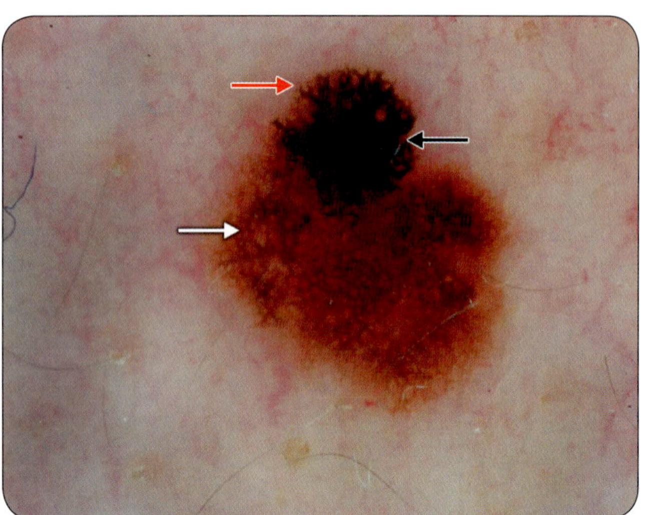

Fig. 6.76: Atypical nevus (severe dysplasia): irregular streaks (red arrow); atypical pigment network (white arrow); and asymmetric pigmentation (black arrow).

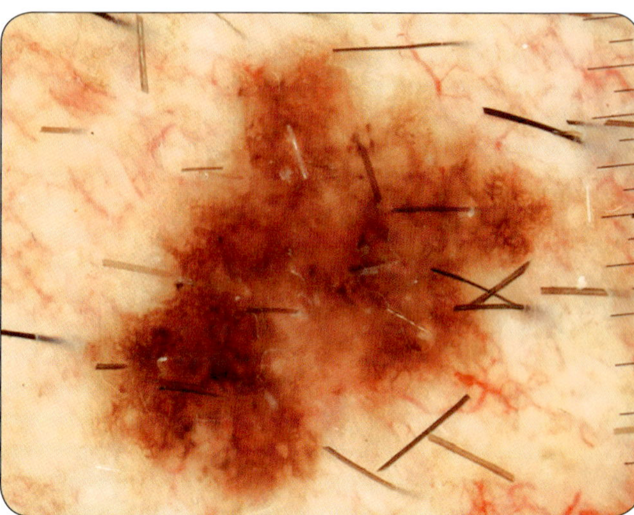

Fig. 6.77: Atypical nevus (severe dysplasia) with atypical pigment network.

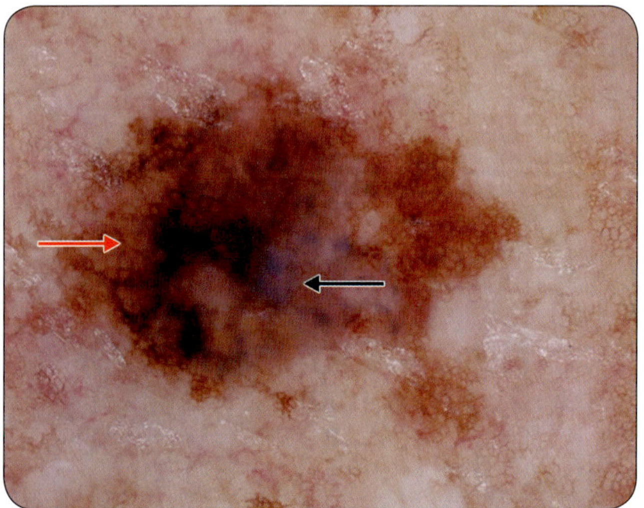

Fig. 6.78: Atypical nevus (severe dysplasia): atypical pigment network (red arrow); regression (black arrow).

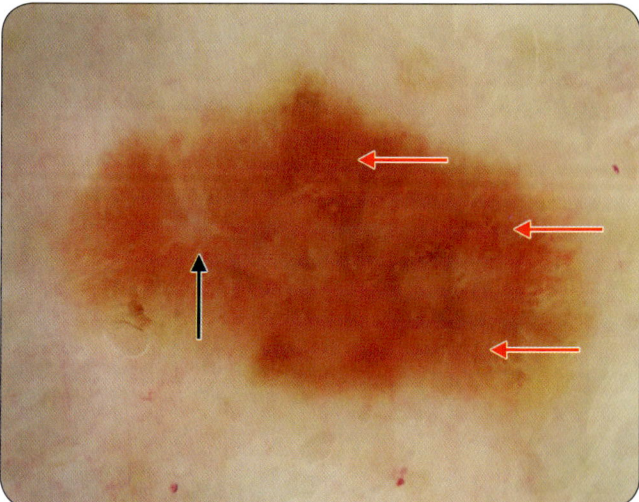

Fig. 6.79: Atypical nevus (severe dysplasia): atypical negative network (red arrows); regression (black arrow).

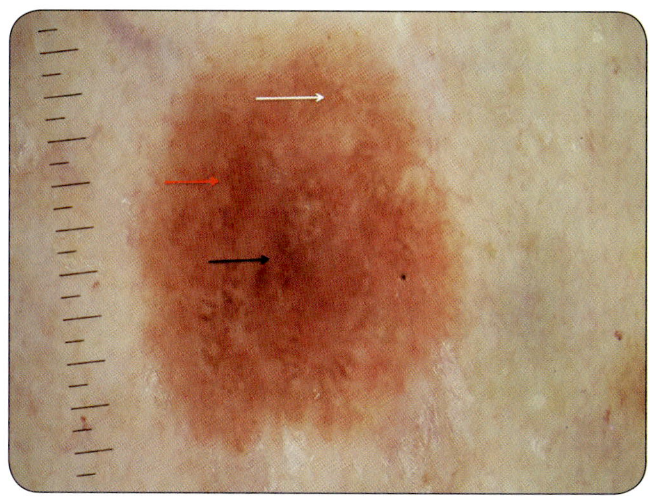

Fig. 6.80: Atypical nevus (severe dysplasia): red dots with irregular distribution (red arrow); atypical negative network (white arrow); and lineal irregular vessels (black arrow).

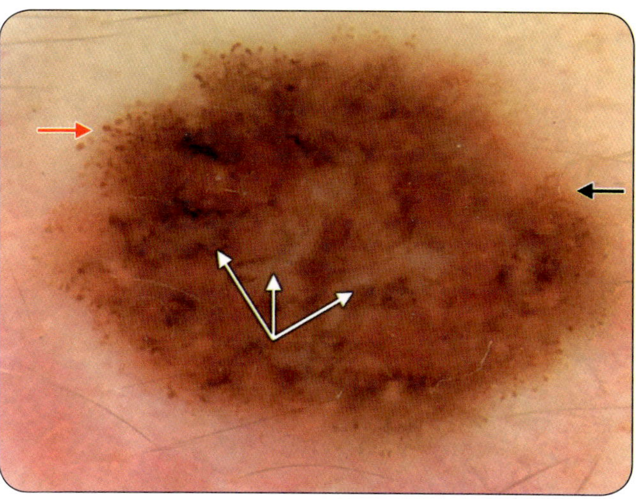

Fig. 6.81: Atypical nevus (severe dysplasia): multiple brown globules with irregular distribution (red arrow); irregular streaks (black arrow); and regression (white arrows).

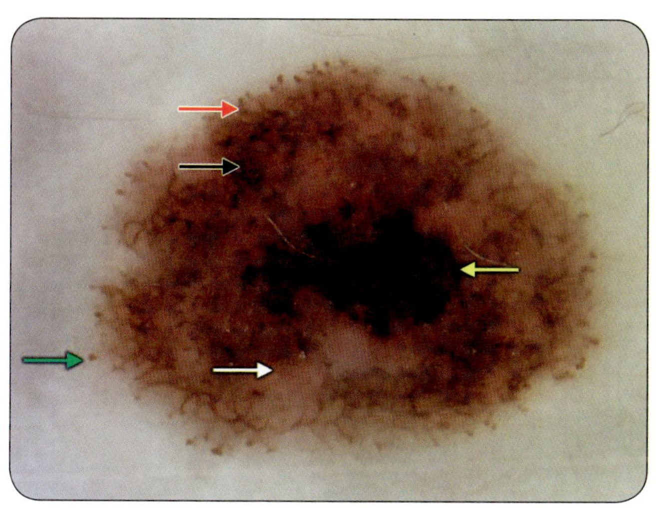

Fig. 6.82: Atypical nevus (severe dysplasia): irregular streaks (red arrow); atypical pigment network (black arrow); regression (white arrow); ulceration (yellow arrow); and brown globules with irregular distribution (green arrow).

SUGGESTED READING

Argenziano G, Soyer P, De Giorgio V, et al. Interactive Atlas of Dermoscopy. Milán: EDRA Medical Publishing & New Media; 2000.

Cabo H. Dermatoscopia. Buenos Aires, Argentina: Weber Ferro; 2000.

Cabo H. Dermatoscopia, 2nd edition. Buenos Aires, Argentina: Ediciones Journal; 2012.

Duffy K, Grossman D. The dysplastic nevus: from historical perspective to management in the modern era. Part 1 Historical, histologic and clinical aspects. J Am Acad Dermatol. 2012;67(1):1.e1-18.

Duffy K, Grossman D. The dysplastic nevus: from historical perspective to management in the modern era. Part 2 Molecular aspects and clinical management. J Am Acad Dermatol. 2012;67(1):19.e1-32.

Hoffmann-Wellenhof R, Blum A, Wolf IH, et al. Dermoscopic classification of atypical nevi (Clark Nevi). Arch Dermatol. 2001;137:1575-80.

Johr R, Stolz W. Dermoscopy: An Illustrated Self-Assessment Guide, 2nd edition. New York: McGraw-Hill Education; 2015.

Jorh R, Soyer P, Argenziano G, et al. Dermoscopy. The Essentials (MOABT). New York: Elsevier Ltd, 2004.

Kittler H, Tschandl P. Dysplastic nevus: why this term should be abandoned in dermatoscopy. Dermatol Clin. 2013;31: 579-88.

Kittler H. Dermatoscopy. An Algorithmic Method Based on Pattern Analysis. Austria: Facultas.wuv; 2011.

Lallas A. Dermoscopy in General Dermatology. Dermatol Clin. 2013;3:679-94.

Malvhey J, Puig S. Principles of Dermoscopy. Barcelona: Creaciones Gráficas; 2009.

Marghoob A, Braun R, Kopf A. Atlas of Dermoscopy. London: Taylor & Francis; 2005.

Menzies S, Crotty K, Ingvar C, et al. An Atlas of Surface Microscopy of Pigmented Skin Lesions. Sydney: McGraw-Hill Book Company; 1996.

Rabinovitz H, Kopf A. Dermoscopy: A Practical Guide. Miami: American Academy of Dermatology; 1999.

Rosendahl C, Grant-Kels JM, Que SK. Dysplastic nevus: facts and fiction. J Am Acad Dermatol. 2015;73:507-12.

Soyer P, Argenziano G, Chimenti S, et al. Dermoscopy of Pigmented Skin Lesions. An Atlas Based on the Consensus Net Meeting on Dermoscopy. Milán: EDRA Medical Publishing & New Media; 2001.

Stolz W, Braun-Falco O, Bilek P, et al. Color atlas of Dermatoscopy. Germany: Blackwell Science; 1994.

Strazzula L, Vedak P, Hoang MP, et al. The utility of re-excising mildly and moderately dysplastic nevi: a retrospective analysis. J Am Acad Dermatol. 2014;71:1071-6.

Zalaudek I, Argenziano G, Giacomel J. Dermoscopy of Non-Pigmented Skin Tumors. Boca Raton, FL: CRC Press; 2016.

6.6 SPITZ NEVUS

Stefano Caccavale, Alessio Gambardella, Amalia Lupoli, Gabriella Brancaccio, Giuseppe Argenziano

Clinical Features

Spitz nevi can occur in any body site. The most frequent location is on the limbs, particularly the lower limbs (30–41% of cases). Spitz nevi can present as macules, papules, nodules, or plaques and their size is usually <6 mm, rarely exceeding 10 mm.

The hypopigmented variant is defined as the "classic" type and is characterized by a pink-reddish appearance because of its abundant vascularity. This variety usually arises as a fast growing nodule or papule and is often located in the head-neck district (especially among infants and younger patients). The majority of Spitz nevi are pigmented. The pigmented type shows a brown-to-black appearance and is more common in adults.

Currently, pigmented Spitz nevi are excised more frequently than classical pink Spitz nevi. This may be due to the improved ability to recognize pigmented Spitz nevi using dermoscopy. The "pink" nodular Spitz nevi have the highest chances of manifesting atypical histopathological features. Although infrequent, these pink Spitz nevi are also the ones that most frequently contribute to the group of "atypical Spitz nevi/tumors". Spitzoid neoplasms are usually asymptomatic and have a sudden onset, with a relatively fast growth and visible changes in size (Figs. 6.83A and B).

Dermoscopic Criteria

In the last 20 years, dermoscopy has become the practical link between clinical dermatology and histopathology, allowing the clinicians to visualize structures not discernable by the naked eye. In order to confirm the diagnosis of a Spitz nevus, dermoscopy represents a useful tool, although histopathology is often mandatory. Dermoscopy has contributed significantly to improving the clinical diagnosis of pigmented and nonpigmented Spitz nevi and, more recently, digital dermoscopic follow-up has allowed a better understanding of the evolution of this peculiar group of nevi. The diagnostic accuracy of Spitz nevi has been shown to increase from 56 to 93% with the use of dermoscopy compared to the naked eye alone. Moreover, the better clinical recognition due to dermoscopy has contributed significantly to find out that Spitz nevi are pigmented in about 70–90% of histopathologically examined cases.

The dermoscopic patterns of spitzoid lesions were first described by Pehamberger et al. in 1987 and later reviewed by several authors. The main dermoscopic patterns ascribed to Spitz nevi are six, namely the reticular, globular, starburst, homogenous and atypical patterns, for pigmented lesions, and the vascular pattern (homogenous pink pattern, dotted vessels, and inverse network) in hypopigmented or amelanotic lesions. Dermoscopically, the globular and the starburst are the two predominant patterns; the former is more frequently associated with classical Spitz nevi, while the latter characterizes Reed nevi. Less common dermoscopic patterns are the homogeneous black pattern, the homogeneous pink pattern (with dotted or irregular vessels), and the inverse network pattern (with interconnected hypopigmented serpiginous lines, which form a network that circumscribes irregular pigmented globular-like structures or dotted vessels and which can be associated with crystalline or chrysalis structures). However, 20% of Spitz nevi dermoscopically exhibit an atypical or multicomponent pattern, characterized by an asymmetric or disorganized distribution of structures and colors and by pigmented structures suggestive of melanoma.

Most of these different dermoscopic patterns probably represent different phases of the natural evolution of Spitz nevi. In the growing phase, pigmented Spitz nevi can evolve from a globular to a starburst pattern: they reveal regular streaks, pseudopods, finger-like or globule-like pigmented projections regularly distributed on the periphery. The presence of streaks is not pathognomonic in Spitz nevi because they can also be found in melanoma, representing the tendency of both tumors to grow horizontally. After a variable number of months, the peripheral projections disappear and the lesion becomes stable, manifesting a homogenous pattern, typified by structureless brown-to-black pigmentation. After a variable number of years, when the lesion enters an apparent state of senescence, it manifests loss of pigment and undergoes spontaneous involution. Spontaneous involution seems, therefore, a plausible explanation for the epidemiologic data reporting the frequency of Spitz nevi as being inversely correlated to patient age. Not only pigmented but also nonpigmented Spitz nevi might go through spontaneous involution over time.

The dermoscopic recognition of amelanotic Spitz nevi is much more difficult. Dotted vessels, tan globules, and reticular depigmentation are common findings but the diagnosis should always be based on a combination of clinical and dermoscopic features. After a growing phase of several months, the lesion starts to become smaller until it finally disappears. Spitzoid melanoma can also display some of these features (peripheral streaks, dotted vessels, or inverse network), but it usually lacks the characteristic symmetric shape of Spitz nevi.

Reticular Pattern

This pattern is characterized by a homogeneous and regular pigment network covering most part of the lesion (Figs. 6.84A and B). The network in Spitz nevi is typified by a grid of black line segments (honeycomb-like) over a tan to gray-blue background. This black network is due to pigmented parakeratosis, which is thus partially removable by tape stripping. This is different from the classic network found in Clark nevi, which is due to pigmented keratinocytes in the basal layer. In this case, the network holes correspond to the tips of dermal papillae and the network itself to the projection of the pigmented ridges to the skin surface.

Globular Pattern

Pigmented Spitz nevi often present gray-brown, relatively large globules, distributed throughout the lesion or at the periphery (Figs. 6.85A and B). A globular pattern is found in about 22% of Spitz nevi but it can be found also in common, congenital or acquired (Clark), melanocytic nevi. While globules in common nevi are relatively small and brown, globules in Spitz nevi are larger and more irregular in terms of color and size. Histopathologically, globules correlate to nests of pigmented melanocytes located at the dermoepidermal junction and/or the superficial dermis, thus they can be found in melanoma as well.

Starburst Pattern

This is the most frequent pattern, being found in about 53% of pigmented Spitz nevi (Figs. 6.86A and B). It may represent one of the morphologic stages in the evolution of Spitz nevi and corresponds to the radial growth phase of this lesion. In most cases, peripheral black to gray globules are fused with the central body of the lesion (forming the so-called streaks, pseudopods, or radial streaming) and are responsible for the starburst appearance, similar to an exploding star. When present, the starburst pattern allows a diagnostic sensitivity of >90%.

Homogenous Pattern

This pattern is characterized by a diffuse, uniform, structureless, pink, dark brown or black-bluish color, which fills most of the lesion and lacks evidence of clear-cut streaks at the periphery (Figs. 6.87A and B). It may correspond to the stable phase of a Spitz nevus.

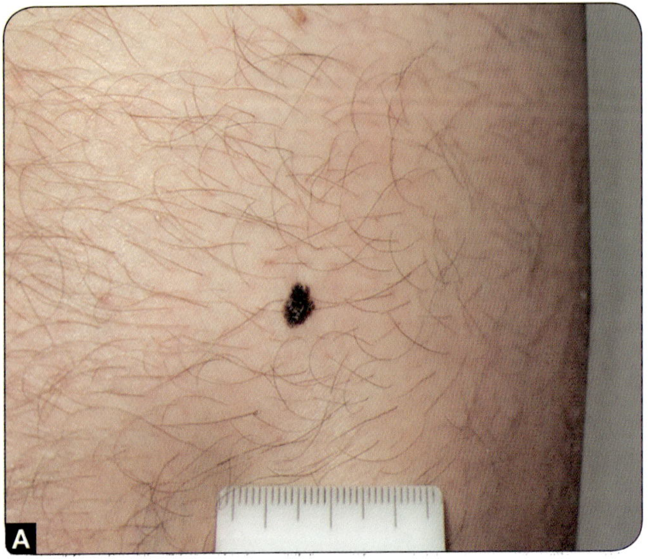

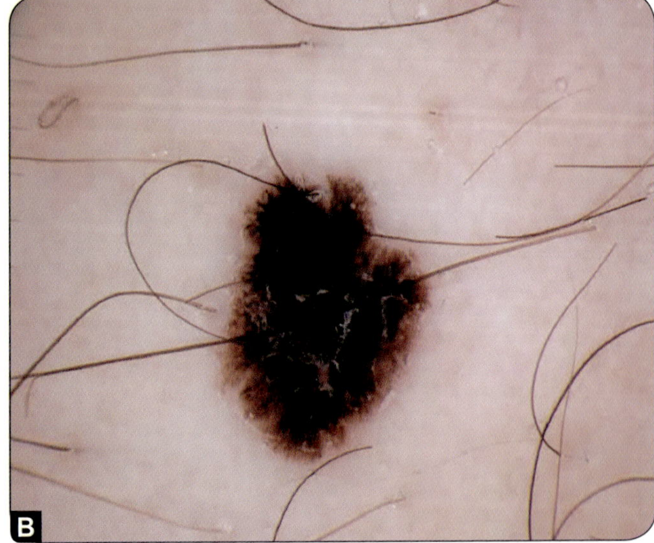

Figs. 6.83A and B: (A) Clinical image of a spitzoid melanoma. (B) Dermoscopy reveals a flat, hyperpigmented lesion with an atypical starburst pattern.

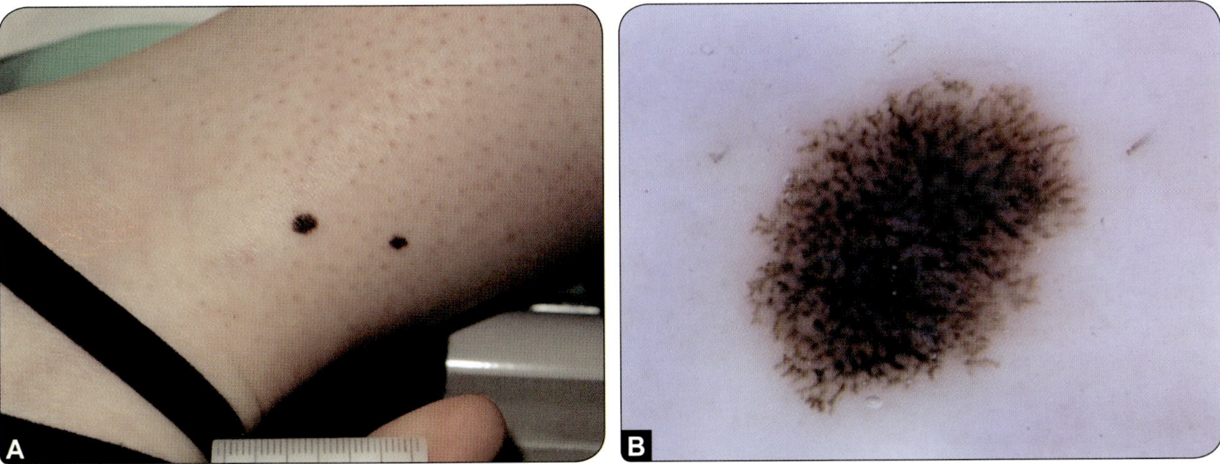

Figs. 6.84A and B: (A) Clinical image of a pigmented Spitz nevus. (B) Dermoscopy of a small, flat, hyperpigmented Spitz nevus with superficial black network.

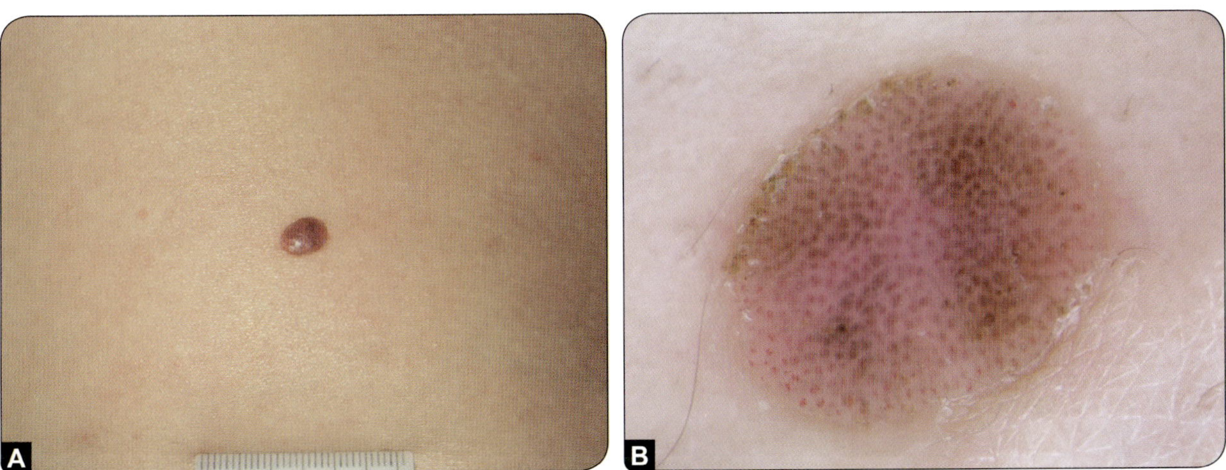

Figs. 6.85A and B: (A) Clinical image of a Spitz nevus. (B) Dermoscopy reveals a pigmented Spitz nevus, with large brown globules and dotted vessels.

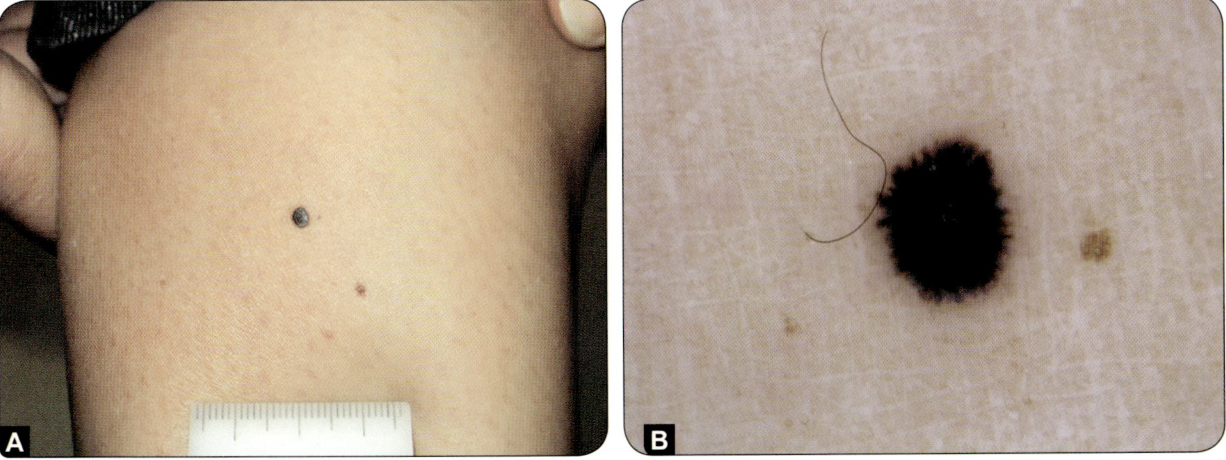

Figs. 6.86A and B: (A) Clinical image of a pigmented Spitz nevus. (B) A small Spitz nevus with stereotypical starburst pattern. The starburst pattern in this lesion consists of streaks (pseudopods) around the entire perimeter of the lesion.

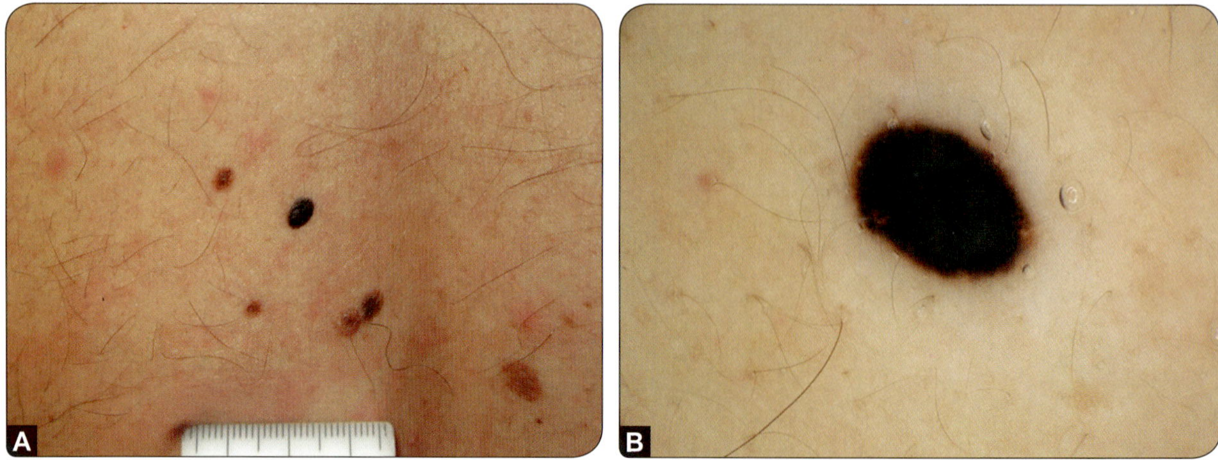

Figs. 6.87A and B: (A) Clinical image of a pigmented Spitz nevus. (B) Pigmented Spitz nevus with a diffuse, uniform, structureless, dark brown color.

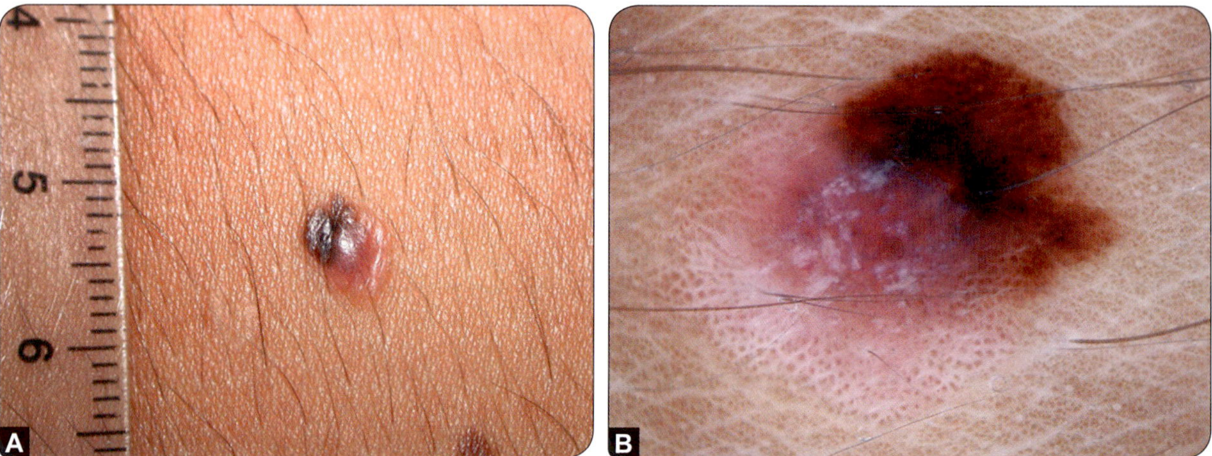

Figs. 6.88A and B: (A) Clinical image of a Spitz nevus. (B) Pigmented Spitz nevus with melanoma-like pattern, typified by irregular reticular pattern, blue-white veil, and irregular globules.

Atypical Pattern

Features suggestive of melanoma are present in about 20% of Spitz nevi (Figs. 6.88A and B). The irregularity in the distribution of colors and structures, and the presence of blue-white veil, black blotches, irregular streaks, and irregular globules make it difficult to differentiate a Spitz nevus from melanoma.

Vascular Pattern

This pattern is more frequent in hypopigmented or amelanotic Spitz nevi. It consists of dotted vessels and inverse network (Figs. 6.89A and B). Dotted vessels, in most cases, tend to be regularly distributed throughout the lesion but, in some cases, vessels acquire a nondotted morphology in atypical lesions. In this case, it is important to exclude the diagnosis of amelanotic melanoma. The inverse network is composed by interconnected hypopigmented lines, which form a network circumscribing dotted vessels. Chrysalis or crystalline structures may also frequently be seen under polarized dermoscopy. They consist of shiny white lines orientated orthogonally to each other and correspond to altered papillary dermal collagen.

Unusual Variants of Spitz Nevi

Some variants of Spitz nevi described mainly in their histopathological aspects have been reported rarely for their clinical and dermoscopic presentation. These are the desmoplastic, angiomatoid, and verrucous variants.

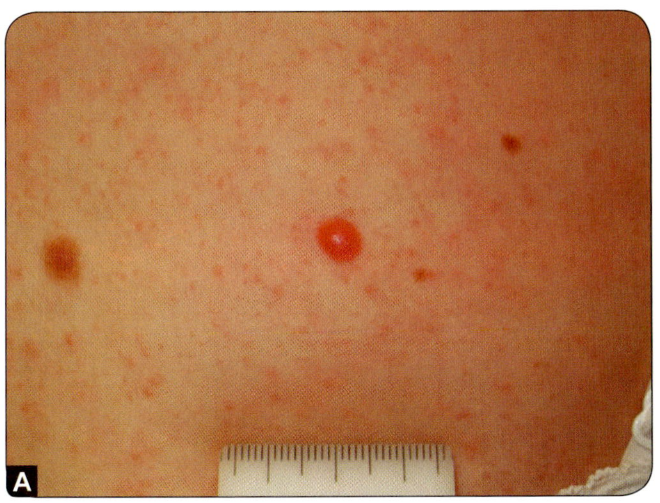

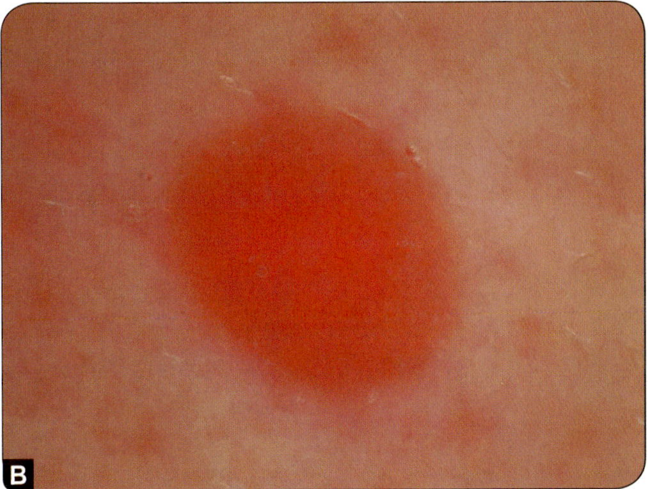

Figs. 6.89A and B: (A) Clinical image of a Spitz nevus. (B) A small pink nevus with irregular vessels.

Desmoplastic Spitz nevi mainly are symmetrical and well circumscribed. They are difficult to differentiate from dermatofibroma clinically, and from melanoma dermoscopically.

Angiomatoid Spitz nevi typically present as solitary papules on the extremities of young women and are characterized by a distinctive dermal vascular proliferation. They can commonly be mistaken for either vascular tumors or regressing melanoma. On dermoscopy, almost all cases show a prominent vascular pattern, mainly constituted of dotted and linear vessels.

Clinical and dermoscopic features of few verrucous Spitz nevi have been described recently. In these cases, the lesions showed clinical and dermoscopic features of a verruca vulgaris, a dermal nevus, or a melanoma. Under dermoscopy, comma vessels and brown background pigmentation, commonly seen in dermal nevi, were not detected. Despite their unusual clinical features, they show reassuring morphological clues histologically, which allow the differential diagnosis from an atypical spitzoid tumor.

Atypical Spitz Tumors

Atypical Spitz tumors (AST) are defined as melanocytic proliferations with intermediate histopathologic features between Spitz nevi and spitzoid melanoma, carrying uncertain malignant potential. The exact clinicopathologic definition of AST is a matter of ongoing debate among dermatopathologists. Some opinion leaders assert that only two diagnostic categories can be ascribed to spitzoid lesions, namely, Spitz nevi and spitzoid melanoma. Others suggest that spitzoid lesions are on a morphobiologic spectrum ranging from benign to clear-cut malignant lesions, with AST placed in the middle of this spectrum. Since the first description, by Smith and coworkers in 1989, several studies have investigated the histopathologic features of AST, but only few have described the clinical and dermoscopic features of AST.

Different clinical parameters have been used to differentiate classic Spitz nevi from AST. First of all, younger age (<10 years) is associated with more probably benign Spitz nevus; conversely, AST usually affect older ages (10–20 years). Location is another important parameter, with extremities being more likely related to Spitz nevi, while the back is the main location of AST. Smaller size (<5–6 mm) is usually common in classic Spitz nevus, while lesions >1 cm are likely to be atypical. Other benign features are the plaque silhouette, the symmetry in shape, and the well-defined borders. Conversely, AST often present as an asymmetric, not uniformly colored, ulcerated, and raised tumor (Figs. 6.90A and B). Under dermoscopy, AST potentially show all the dermoscopic elements typical of melanoma. A blue-white veil, resulting from deep dermal pigmentation with overlying epidermal hyperplasia, can often be seen. About half of AST are hypo- or nonpigmented and in these cases a typical spitzoid pattern can be seen, typified by dotted vessels and reticular depigmentation. Consequently, our attitude is to excise nodular spitzoid-looking lesions, independently of the patient's age.

Management and Prognosis

A classic pink or pigmented Spitz nevus appearing before the age of 12 years can be managed conservatively and

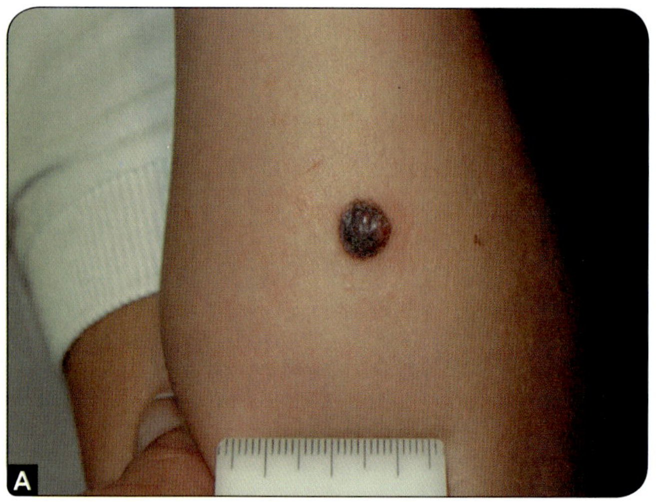

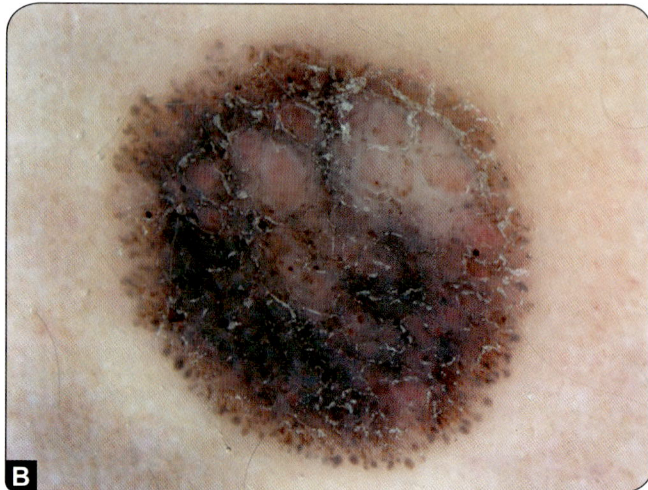

Figs. 6.90A and B: (A) Clinical image of an atypical Spitz tumor. (B) Dermoscopy reveals a melanoma-like pattern, typified by blue-white veil and an irregular tiered globular pattern.

monitored if it is relatively small (up to 1 cm) and shows no atypical clinical and dermoscopic features. The expected evolution of Spitz/Reed nevi includes a stabilization phase followed by a slow involution until disappearance. In the absence of irregular changes in color, shape, or size, a follow-up can be continued until the lesion enters senescence and/or manifests a homogenous pattern. In contrast, Spitz nevi developing in individuals >12 years, or spitzoid-looking lesions that are >1 cm, nodular, ulcerated, or otherwise atypical, even if seen during childhood, should warrant excision.

The management of AST is a matter of ongoing discussion. Parameters associated with a bad prognosis in ASTs seem to be ulceration, large size, asymmetry, and presence of mitosis. In 2000, Kelley and Cockerell suggested that sentinel lymph node (SLN) biopsy should be performed along with wide excision for patients with AST. However, there are no data proving the benefit of performing SLN biopsy and a conservative management strategy should be applied in the vast majority of AST.

SUGGESTED READING

Argenziano G, Agozzino M, Bonifazi E, et al. Natural evolution of Spitz nevi. Dermatology. 2011;222:256-60.

Argenziano G, Soyer HP, Chimenti S, et al. Dermoscopy of pigmented skin lesions: results of a consensus meeting via the Internet. J Am Acad Dermatol. 2003;48:679-93.

Barnhill RL, Barnhill MA, Berwick M, et al. The histologic spectrum of pigmented spindle cell nevus: a review of 120 cases with emphasis on atypical variants. Hum Pathol. 1991; 22:52-8.

Broganelli P, Titli S, Lallas A, et al. Spitz/Reed nevi: proposal of management recommendations by the Dermoscopy Study Group of the Italian Society of Dermatology (SIDeMaST). G Ital Dermatol Venereol. 2014;149:601-6.

Brunetti B, Nino M, Sammarco E, et al. Spitz naevus: a proposal for management. J Eur Acad Dermatol Venereol. 2005;19:391-3.

Ferrara G, Argenziano G, Soyer HP, et al. The spectrum of Spitz nevi: a clinicopathologic study of 83 cases. Arch Dermatol. 2005;141:1381-7.

Kelley SW, Cockerell CJ. Sentinel lymph node biopsy as an adjunct to management of histologically difficult to diagnose melanocytic lesions: a proposal. J Am Acad Dermatol. 2000;42:527-30.

Lallas A, Kyrgidis A, Ferrara G, et al. Atypical Spitz tumours and sentinel lymph node biopsy: a systematic review. Lancet Oncol. 2014;15:e178-e183.

Marghoob A, Malvehy J, Braun R. Taylor & Francis Group. 2013; CRC press, 2nd edition.

Moscarella E, Al Jalbout S, Piana S, et al. The stars within the melanocytic garden: unusual variants of Spitz nevi. Br J Dermatol. 2015;172:1045-51.

Moscarella E, Lallas A, Kyrgidis A, et al. Clinical and dermoscopic features of atypical Spitz tumors: a multicenter, retrospective, case-control study. J Am Acad Dermatol. 2015;73(5):777-84.

Neri I, Dika E, Ravaioli GM, et al. Spitz nevi: defining features and management in children. G Ital Dermatol Venereol. 2014;149:675-82.

Paniago-Pereira C, Maize JC, Ackerman AB. Nevus of large spindle and/or epithelioid cells (Spitz's nevus). Arch Dermatol. 1978;114:1811-23.

Pehamberger H, Steiner A, Wolff K. In vivo epiluminescence microscopy of pigmented skin lesions. I. Pattern analysis of pigmented skin lesions. J Am Acad Dermatol. 1987;17:571-83.

Peris K, Ferrari A, Argenziano G, et al. Dermoscopic classification of Spitz/Reed nevi. Clin Dermatol. 2002;20:259-62.

Piccolo V, Moscarella E, Zalaudek I, et al. Analysis of clinical and dermoscopic features in melanocytic lesions with special emphasis on problematic lesions in children. Expert Rev Dermatol. 2013;8:155-70.

Reed RJ, Ichinose H, Clark WH Jr, et al. Common and uncommon melanocytic nevi and borderline melanomas. Semin Oncol. 1975;2:119-47.

Requena C, Requena L, Kutzner H, et al. Spitz nevus: a clinicopathological study of 349 cases. Am J Dermatopathol. 2009;31:107-16.

Smith KJ, Barrett TL, Skelton HG 3rd, et al. Spindle cell and epithelioid cell nevi with atypia and metastasis (malignant Spitz nevus). Am J Surg Pathol. 1989;13:931-9.

Spitz S. Melanomas of childhood. Am J Pathol. 1948;24:591-609.

Weedon D, Little JH. Spindle and epithelioid cell nevi in children and adults. A review of 211 cases of the Spitz nevus. Cancer. 1977;40:217-25.

6.7 BLUE NEVUS AND COMBINED NEVUS

Horacio A Cabo

The blue nevus (BN) is a melanocytic nevus that may be classified as common and cellular. Common BN is a nodular lesion (<0.5 cm), bluish-gray or bluish-black. It usually appears as a single lesion, and it may manifest in any tegument area, although it is more frequent in the back of hands and feet, the scalp, and mucosae. It habitually appears in infancy, yet it can also manifest in adulthood.

Cellular BN is a larger nodule (>0.5–3 cm), blue or black in color, which preferably locates in the sacrocoxal area or in the buttocks (Fig. 6.91). Appears in infancy and manifests less frequently than the common BN.

Some blue nevi are asymmetrical, in different shades of blue, and may simulate a melanoma (Fig. 6.92).

For a correct diagnosis, it is very important to know the duration of the nevi if possible, since it generally appears in youth, as has already been pointed out.

Melanoma metastasis, tattoos, and radiotherapy marks may be mistaken with common new nevi, among others (Figs. 6.93 to 6.96).

The combined nevus (CN) is a melanocytic nevus characterized by the association of a BN with a nevocellular nevus (dermal, compound or juncture) in the same lesion. On occasion, it is possible to observe a BN associated to a Spitz nevus.

In the clinical aspect, the features of the BN prevail in the lesion. It may be similar to a BN or present a targetoid form (combined targetoid nevus), which presents a blue central area and a light or dark brown coloration in the peripheral area of the lesion.

Due to the overlapping of lesions with different histology, on occasion CN is considered a melanoma simulator. Histology depends on the type of nevi associated in the lesion.

The most frequent scenario is a common or cellular BN combined with a melanocytic nevus.

Dermoscopic Criteria

Blue Nevus

It shows a homogeneous blue coloration with generally uniform pigmentation (Figs. 6.97 to 6.99).

This blue pigmentation looks different under polarized and nonpolarized light dermoscopes (Figs. 6.100A and B).

Sclerotic BN is a variant that presents a central hypopigmented area (Fig. 6.101).

Combined Nevus (Figs. 6.102 to 6.104)

They may present a homogeneous blue coloration that makes them indistinguishable from blue nevi.

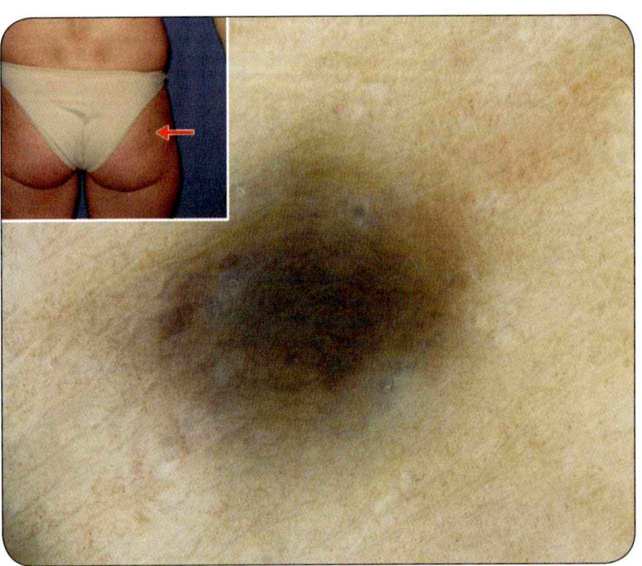

Fig. 6.91: Blue cellular nevus (clinical view: arrow).

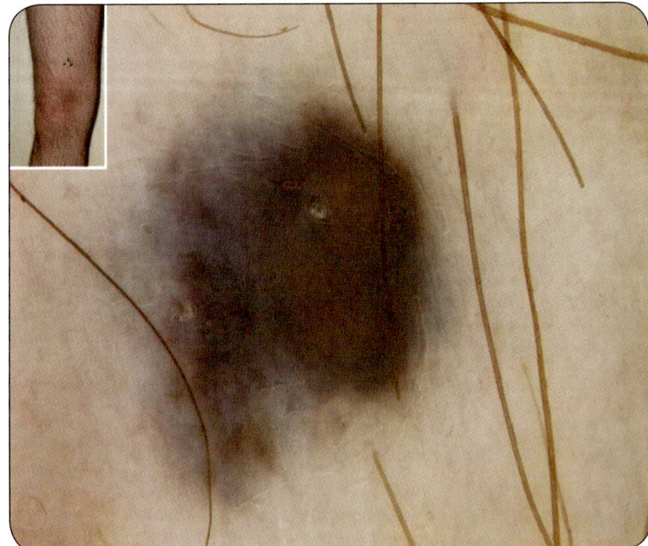

Fig. 6.92: Asymmetric blue nevus.

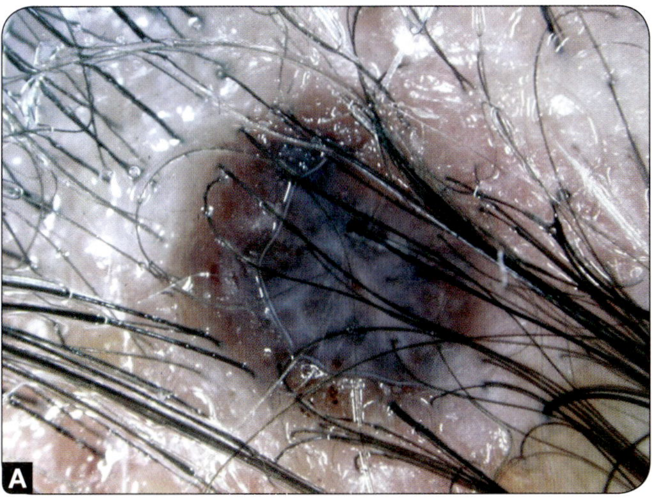

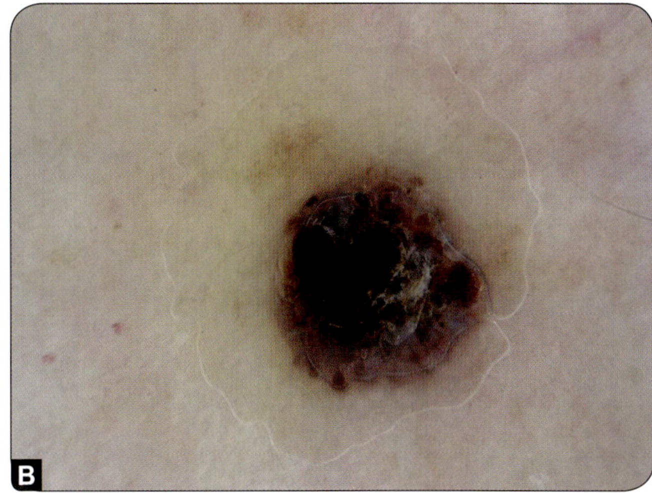

Figs. 6.93A and B: Melanoma metastasis.

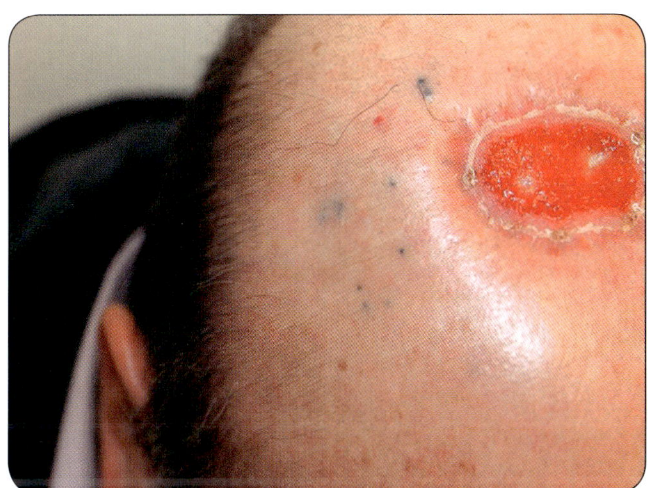

Fig. 6.94: Melanoma metastasis—clinical view.

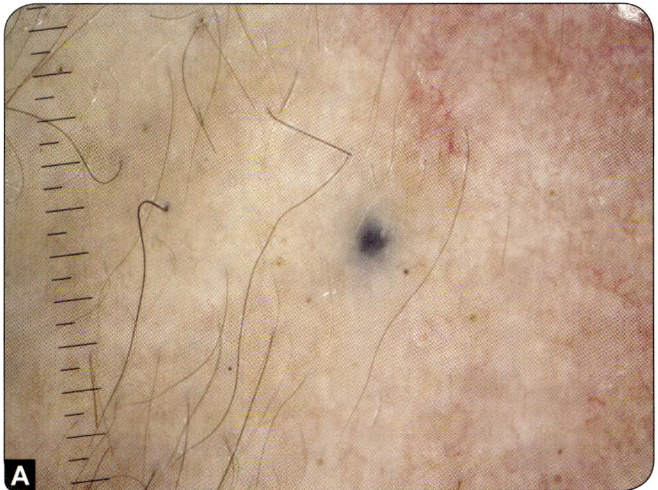

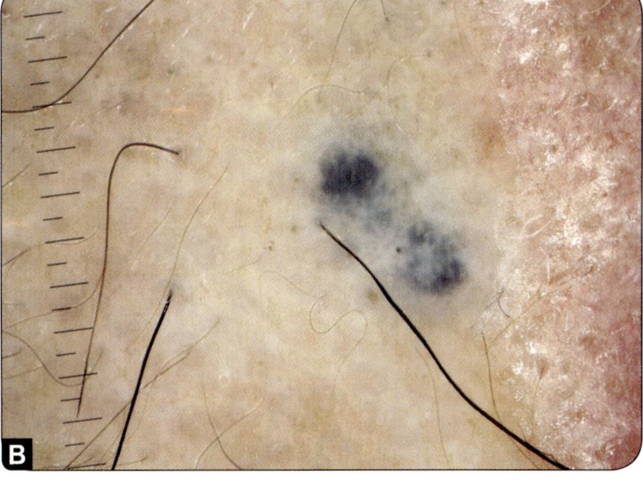

Figs. 6.95A and B: Melanoma metastasis (blue nevus-like).

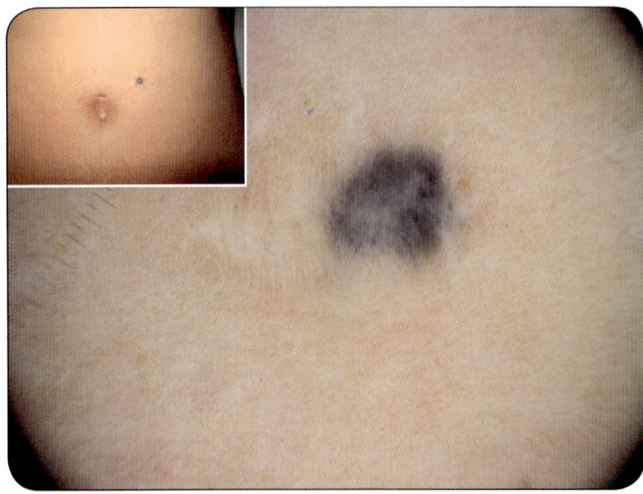

Fig. 6.96: Tattoo in the scar.

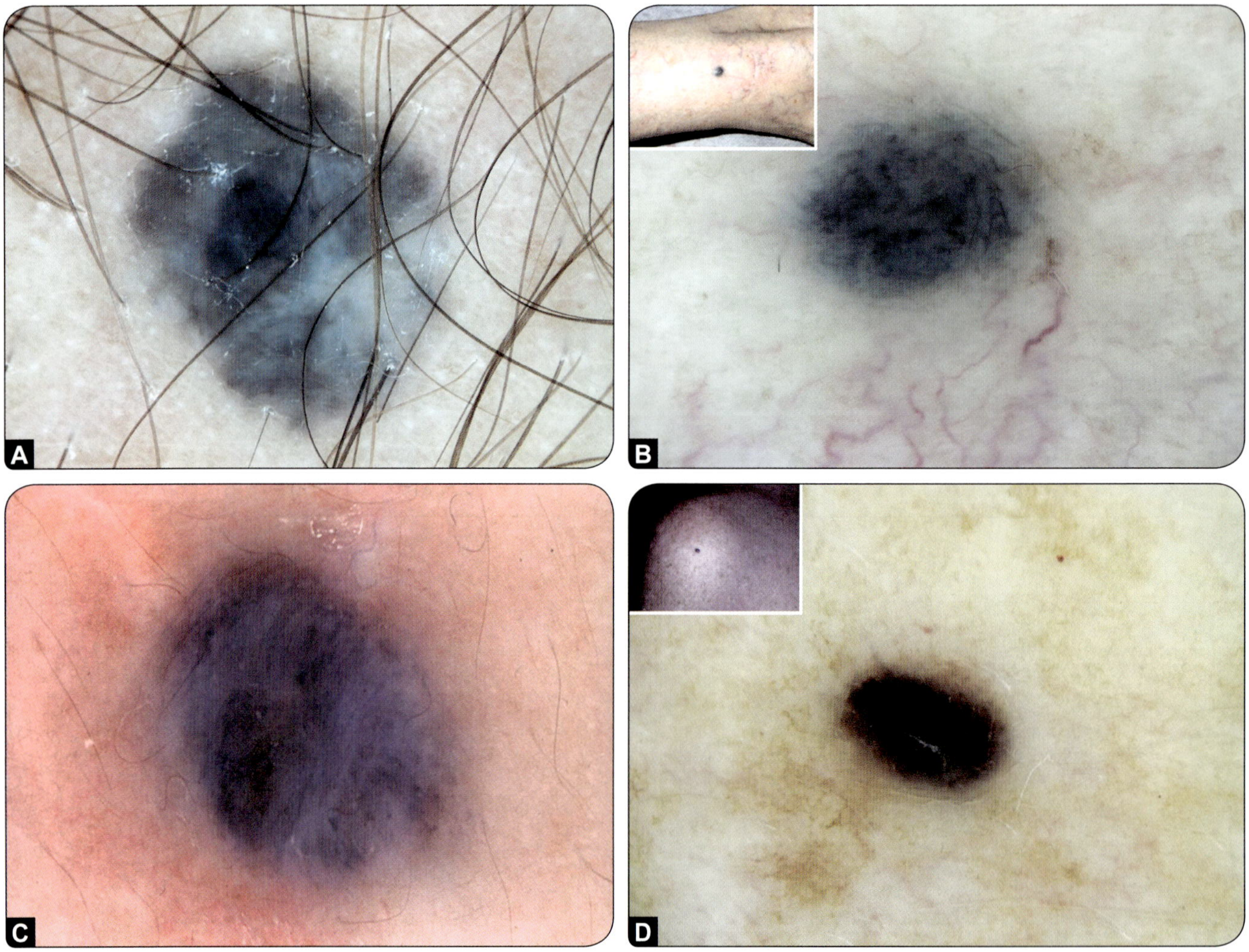

A B C D

Figs. 6.97A to D

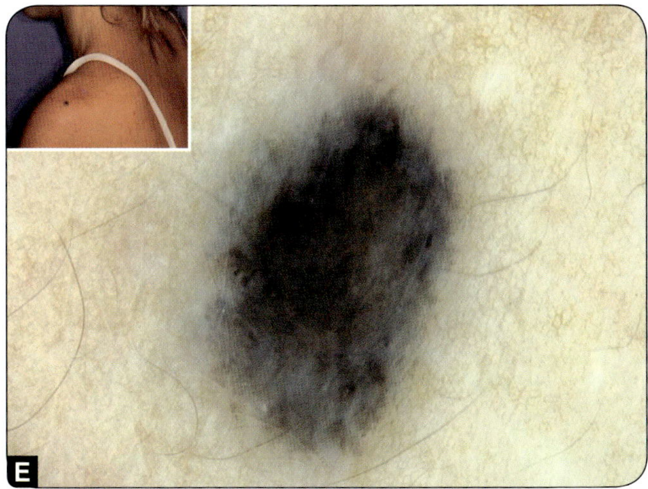

Figs. 6.97A to E : Blue nevus.

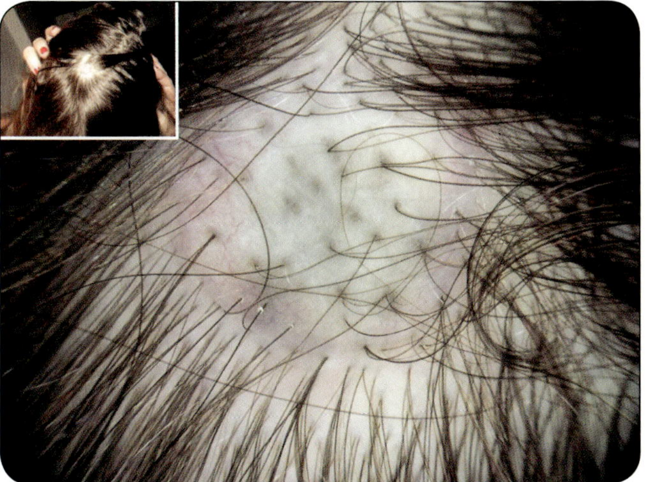

Fig. 6.98: Blue nevus in the scalp.

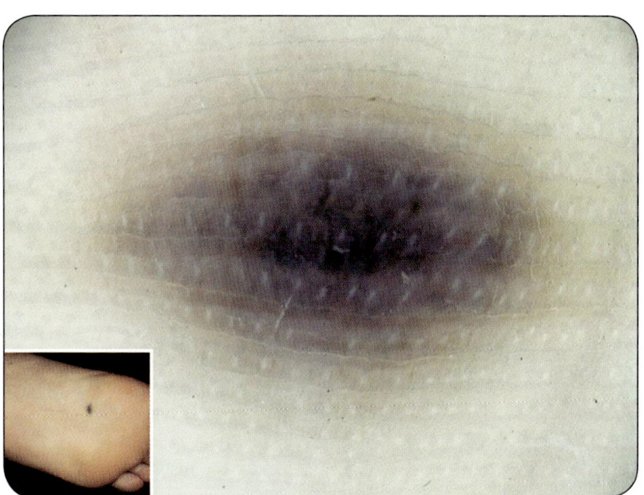

Fig. 6.99: Blue nevus in the sole.

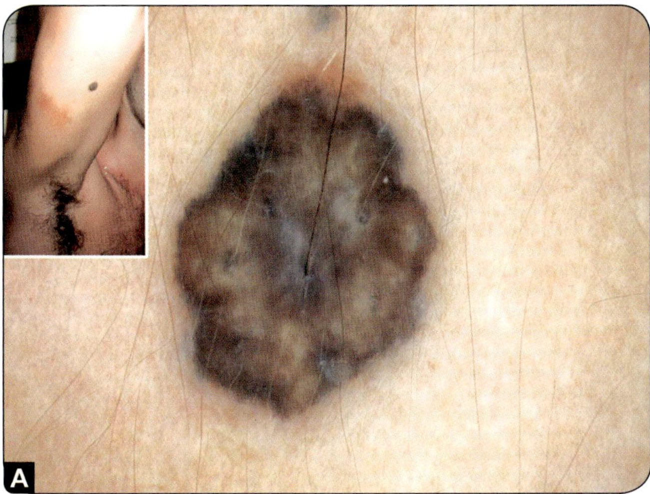

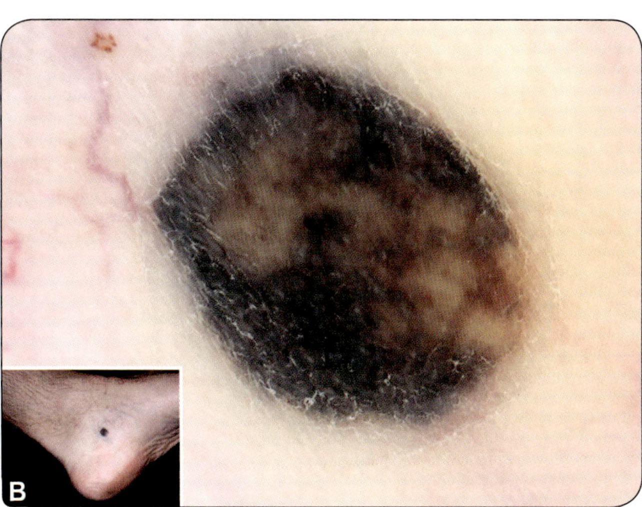

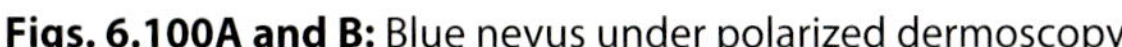

Figs. 6.100A and B: Blue nevus under polarized dermoscopy.

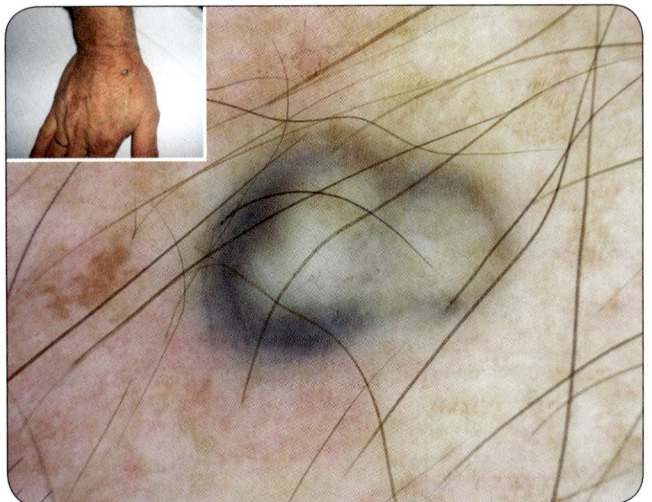

Fig. 6.101: Sclerotic blue nevus.

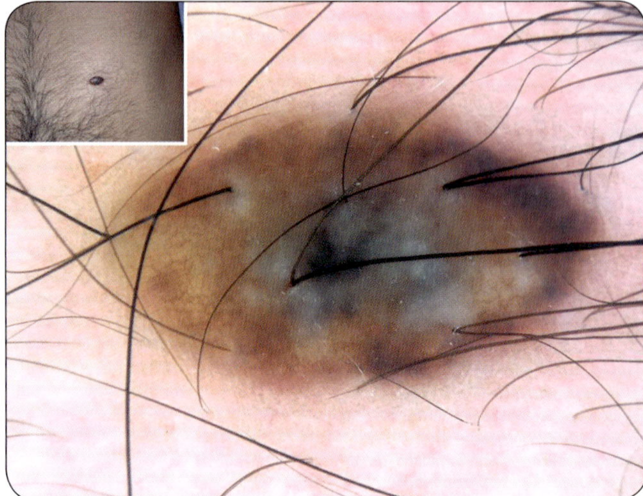

Fig. 6.102: Combined nevus (intradermal nevus + blue nevus).

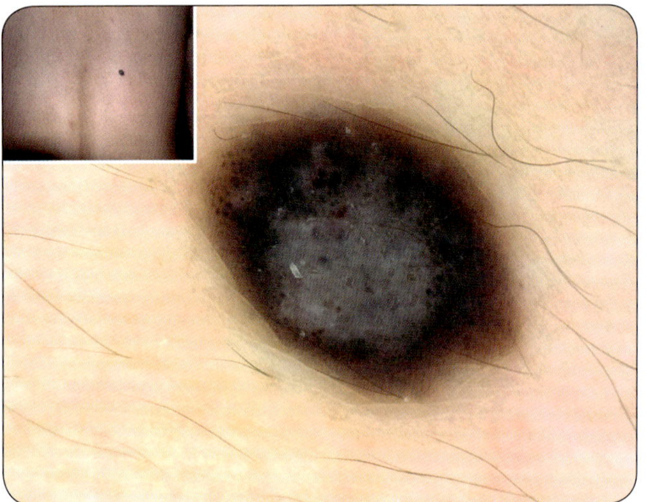

Fig. 6.103: Combined nevus (junction nevus + blue nevus).

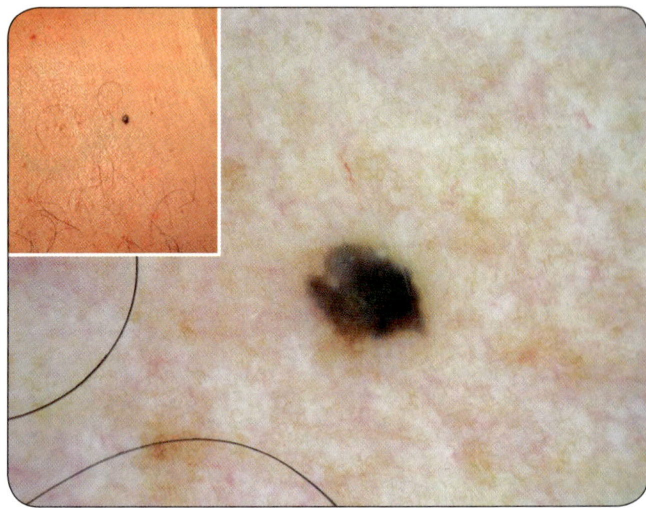

Fig. 6.104: Combined nevus.

There may also be combined nevi with two colors, a homogeneous blue, dark blue, or black central zone and a peripheral zone in different shades of brown with structureless areas, globules, or pigment network. All these structures corresponding to the superficial component (generally a nevocellular nevus) are invisible in the central zone owing to a black or blue color that stems from the deep component of the lesion (BN). If the superficial component were highly pigmented, the lesion would appear totally dark.

SUGGESTED READING

Argenziano G, Soyer P, De Giorgio V, et al. Interactive Atlas of Dermoscopy. Milán: EDRA Medical Publishing & New Media; 2000.

Cabo H. Dermatoscopia. Buenos Aires, Argentina: Weber Ferro; 2000.

Cabo H. Dermatoscopia, 2nd edition. Buenos Aires, Argentina: Ediciones Journal; 2012.

Johr R, Stolz W. Dermoscopy: An Illustrated Self-Assessment Guide, 2nd edition. New York: McGraw-Hill Education; 2015.

Jorh R, Soyer P, Argenziano G, et al. Dermoscopy. The Essentials (MOABT). New York: Elsevier Ltd; 2004.

Kittler H. Dermatoscopy. An Algorithmic Method Based on Pattern Analysis. Austria: Facultas.wuv; 2011.

Lallas A. Dermoscopy in general dermatology. Dermatol Clin. 2013;3:679-94.

Malvhey J, Puig S. Principles of Dermoscopy. Barcelona: Creaciones Gráficas; 2009.

Marghoob A, Braun R, Kopf A. Atlas of Dermoscopy. London: Taylor & Francis; 2005.

Menzies S, Crotty K, Ingvar C, et al. An Atlas of Surface Microscopy of Pigmented Skin Lesions. Sydney: McGraw-Hill Book Company; 1996.

Rabinovitz H, Kopf A. Dermoscopy: A Practical Guide. Miami: American Academy of Dermatology; 1999.

Soyer P, Argenziano G, Chimenti S, et al. Dermoscopy of Pigmented Skin Lesions. An Atlas Based on the Consensus Net Meeting on Dermoscopy. Milán: EDRA Medical Publishing & New Media; 2001.

Stolz W, Braun-Falco O, Bilek P, et al. Color Atlas of Dermatoscopy. Germany: Blackwell Science; 1994.

Zalaudek I, Argenziano G, Giacomel J. Dermoscopy of non-pigmented skin tumors. Boca Raton, FL: CRC Press; 2016.

6.8 RECURRENT NEVUS

Horacio A Cabo

The recurrent or persistent nevus (RN) constitutes the recurrence of pigmentation that manifests after the incomplete excision of a nevus, generally compound or intradermal.

Although most RN are secondary to an incomplete excision (shave excision), they can also appear after laser surgery, radiotherapy, or nevus traumatism. The most frequent site of appearance is the trunk.

Due to its clinical and dermoscopic features, it is included among melanoma simulators. In relation to a differential diagnosis, it is fundamental to bear in mind the following parameters:

- History of previous excision
- Histopathologic study, if it possible
- Time span between appearance and recurrence
  - Recurrent nevus: 4–10 months after excision
  - *Melanoma:* More than a year
- Pigment location
  - *RN:* Scar pigmented
  - *Melanoma:* Pigmented lesions spread beyond the scar

The term RN comprises two scenarios: one is reactive pigmentation of the scar; the other is nevus recurrence.

Reactive Pigmentation

It is most frequently seen after excisions followed by suture. The histologic scenario goes from hyperpigmentation of the basal layer at one end, through lentiginous epidermal hyperplasia, to melanocytic hyperplasia, without the presence of melanocytic nests.

- *Streaks or lines:* It is possible to observe brown lines that may be:
  - Thin and radiated from the center to the peripheral area of the scar (Figs. 6.105 and 6.106).

(On occasion we can see different variation of this: like thick homogeneous strip perpendicular to the scar central axis or thin and parallel to the lesion central axis).

True RN

Appear after trauma of a nevus or a shave, laser surgery or radiotherapy of a nevus. Histopathology shows melanocytic nests in the dermoepidermal and dermal junction.

Dermoscopy (Figs. 6.107 to 6.114)

- Globules with different sizes and distribution
- Heterogeneous pigmentation
- Pigment network and lines: infrequent.

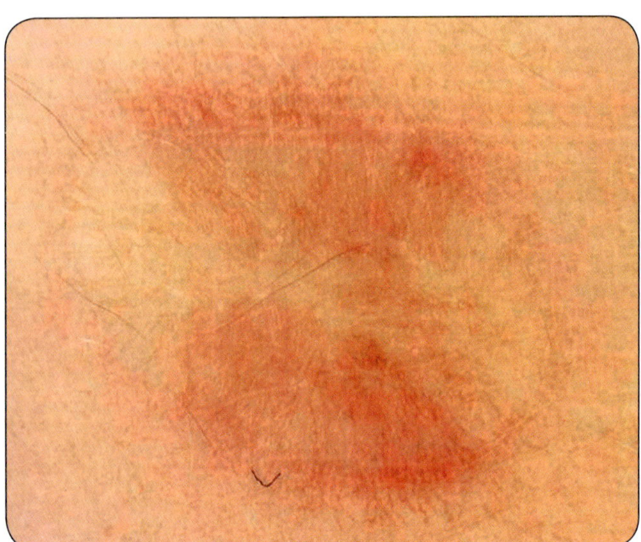

Fig. 6.105: Reactive pigmentation: streaks or lines thin and radiated from the center to the peripheral area of the scar.

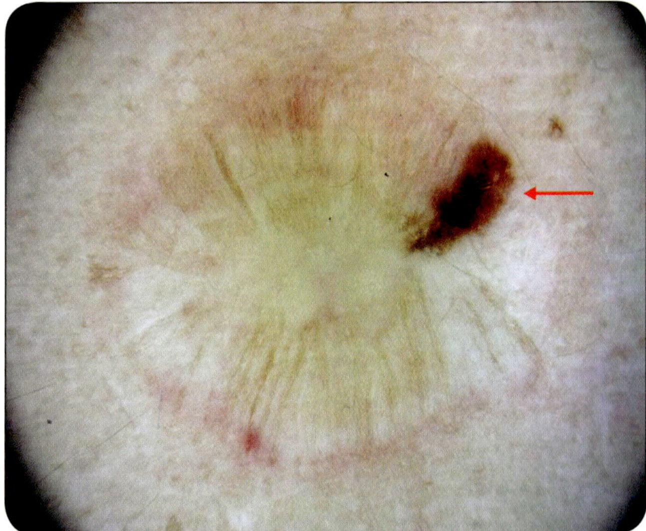

Fig. 6.106: Reactive pigmentation: streaks or lines thin and radiated from the center to the peripheral area of the scar and the presence of a recurrent nevus (arrow).

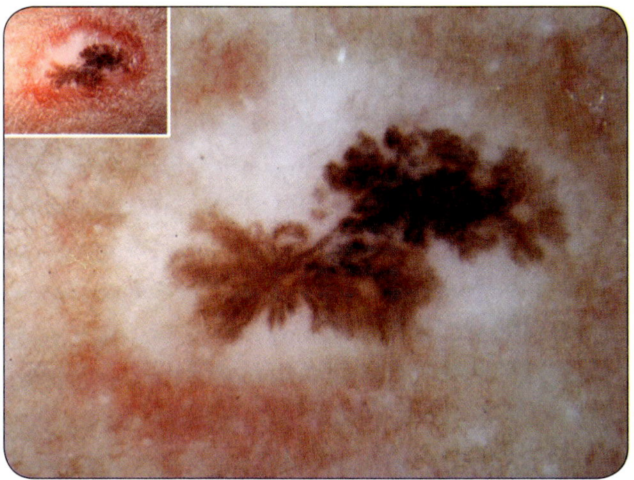

Fig. 6.107: Recurrent nevus: the pigmentation does not spread beyond the scar; heterogeneous pigmentation.

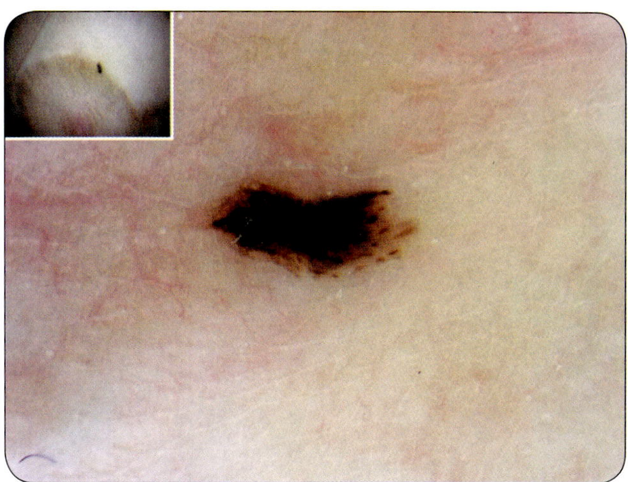

Fig. 6.108: Recurrent nevus: the pigmentation does not spread beyond the scar; different colors and parallel lines.

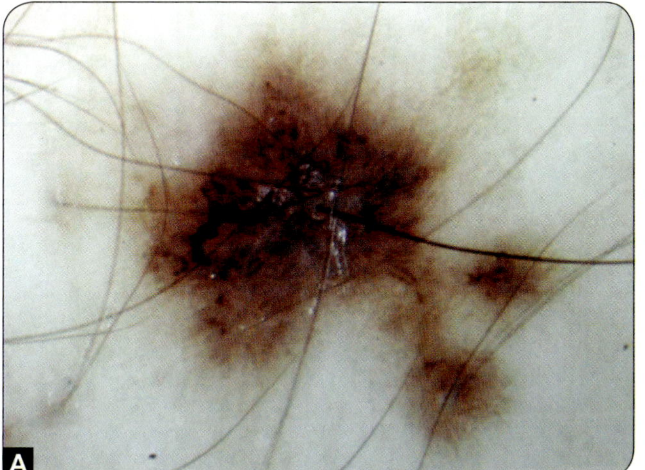

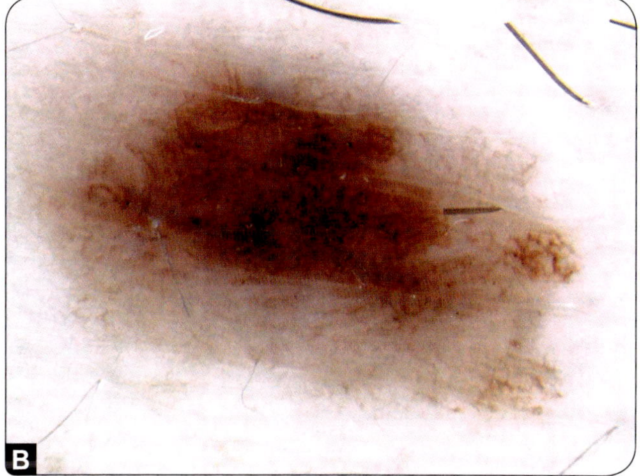

Figs. 6.109A and B: Recurrent nevus: the pigmentation does not spread beyond the scar with pigment network and lines.

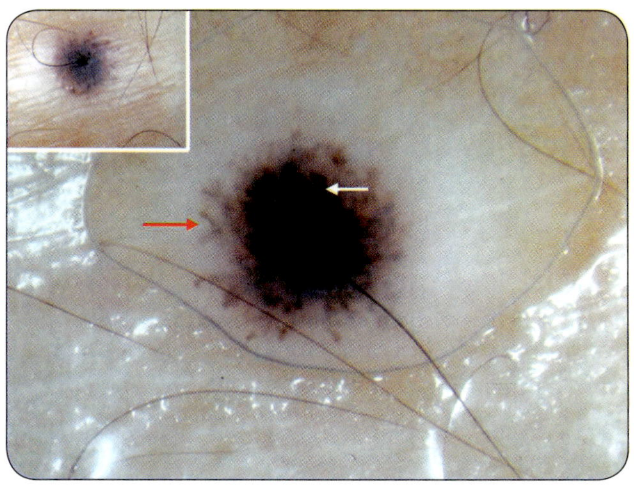

Fig. 6.110: Recurrent nevus: the pigmentation does not spread beyond the scar with globules (white arrow) and streaks (red arrow).

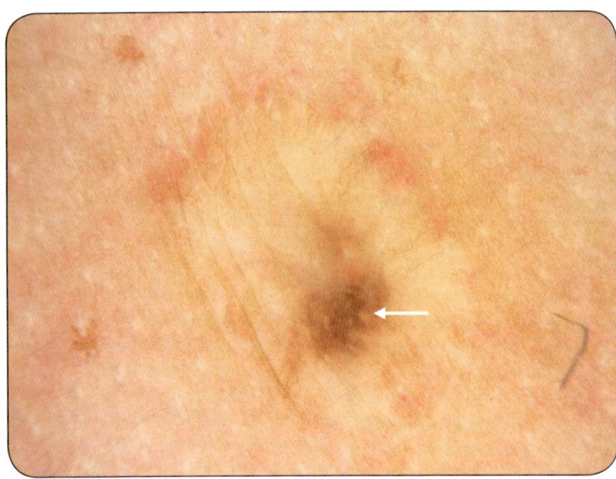

Fig. 6.111: Recurrent nevus: the pigmentation does not spread beyond the scar with globules (arrow).

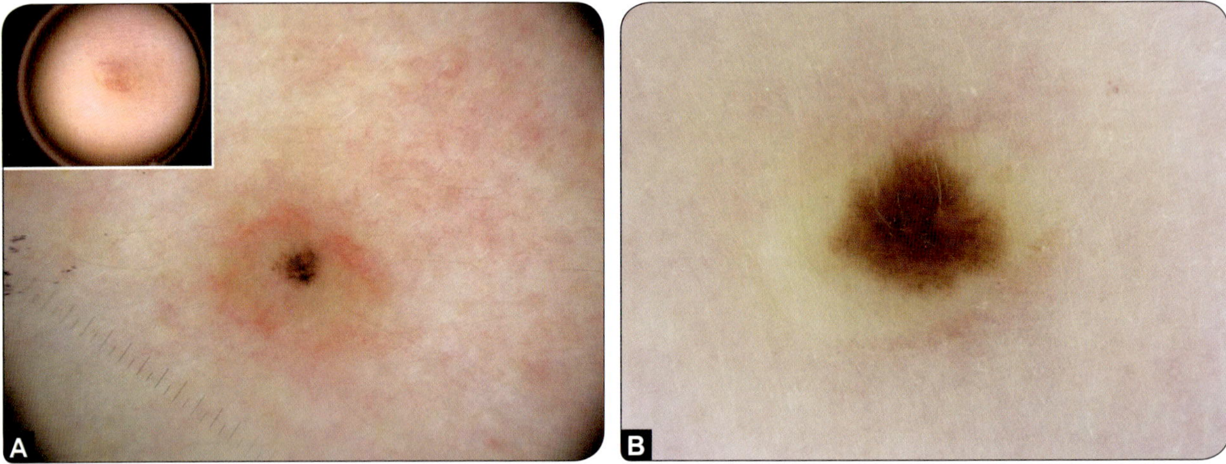

Figs. 6.112A and B: Recurrent nevus: the pigmentation does not spread beyond the scar with pigment network and lines in the center of the lesion.

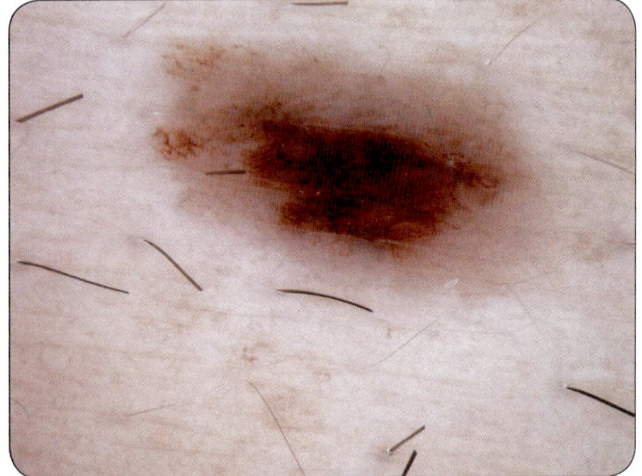

Fig. 6.113: Recurrent nevus: the pigmentation does not spread beyond the scar with pigment network and lines.

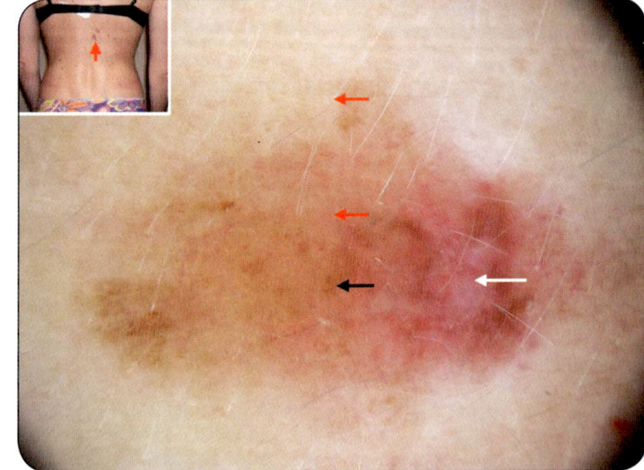

Fig. 6.114: Recurrent nevus: the pigmentation does not spread beyond the scar. Atypical vascular pattern with red areas (white arrow); linear irregular vessels (red arrows); and brown globules (black arrow).

SUGGESTED READING

Argenziano G, Soyer P, De Giorgio V, et al. Interactive Atlas of Dermoscopy. Milán: EDRA Medical Publishing & New Media; 2000.

Blum A, Hofmann-Wellenhof R, Marghoob AA, et al. Recurrent melanocytic nevi and melanomas in dermoscopy: results of a multicenter study of the International Dermoscopy Society. JAMA Dermatol. 2014;150(2):138-45.

Cabo H. Dermatoscopia. Buenos Aires, Argentina: Weber Ferro; 2000.

Cabo H. Dermatoscopia, 2nd edition. Buenos Aires, Argentina: Ediciones Journal; 2012.

Johr R, Stolz W. Dermoscopy: An Illustrated Self-Assessment Guide, 2nd edition. McGraw-Hill Education; 2015.

Jorh R, Soyer P, Argenziano G, et al. Dermoscopy. The Essentials (MOABT). New York: Elsevier Ltd; 2004.

Kittler H. Dermatoscopy. An Algorithmic Method Based on Pattern Analysis. Austria: Facultas.wuv; 2011.

Lallas A. Dermoscopy in general dermatology. Dermatol Clin. 2013;3:679-94.

Malvhey J, Puig S. Principles of Dermoscopy. Barcelona: Creaciones Gráficas; 2009.

Marghoob A, Braun R, Kopf A. Atlas of Dermoscopy. London: Taylor & Francis; 2005.

Menzies S, Crotty K, Ingvar C, et al. An Atlas of Surface Microscopy of Pigmented Skin Lesions. Sydney: McGraw-Hill Book Company; 1996.

Rabinovitz H, Kopf A. Dermoscopy: A Practical Guide. Miami: American Academy of Dermatology; 1999.

Soyer P, Argenziano G, Chimenti S, et al. Dermoscopy of Pigmented Skin Lesions. An atlas based on the consensus net meeting on Dermoscopy. Milán: EDRA Medical Publishing & New Media; 2001.

Stolz W, Braun-Falco O, Bilek P, et al. Color Atlas of Dermatoscopy. Germany: Blackwell Science; 1994.

Zalaudek I, Argenziano G, Giacomel J. Dermoscopy of Non-Pigmented Skin Tumors. Boca Raton, FL: CRC Press; 2016.

6.9 MELANOMA

6.9.1 Superficial Spreading Melanoma

Horacio A Cabo

Superficial spreading melanoma (SSM) is the most common type of melanoma. Its incidence is slightly higher in men than in women. It lies in areas with intermittent solar exposure and preferably in the lower limbs of females and the back of males.

In recent years, the frequency of its appearance has increased. It has a phase of radial growth that may be of variable but prolonged duration, until finally entering the vertical invasive growth phase with the possibility of metastasis and of causing the death of the patient.

As it is widely known, the best treatment for melanoma is the early diagnosis since in the case of in situ forms, excision with adequate margins ensures a cure rate close to 100%. Having said that, it is necessary to perform an early diagnosis in initial lesions to ensure a good therapeutic result.

Clinical examination is very good, but not highly effective in small lesions, where dermoscopy has increased diagnostic accuracy by 30% and proved to have very high specificity (80%) and sensitivity (90%).

In pattern analysis, which is the method most widely used by experts, the procedure is to evaluate general patterns and local patterns.

General Patterns for SSM

- *Multicomponent pattern*: Stems from the combination of three or more dermoscopic patterns in the same lesion. It is the pattern most frequently associated with the existence of melanoma, although it can also be observed in other lesions such as Clark nevus, Spitz-Reed nevus, and congenital nevus.
- *Atypical reticular pattern*: The lesion is fundamentally composed of a pigment reticule or atypical pigment network.
- *Atypical globular pattern*: Composed of dots and globules with irregular shape, size, and distribution.
- *Peripheral streaks pattern (starburst pattern)*: It is characterized by the presence of projections or lines adopting a regular radial distribution along the periphery of the pigmented lesion, which is characteristic of Spitz-Reed nevus. However, some melanomas may present this pattern, especially in adults.
- *Unspecific pattern*: This is present in those lesions that cannot be classified within any of the previous patterns. In the presence of this pattern, it is essential to rule out the existence of a possible melanoma in all cases.

Local SSM Patterns

Almost all these methods evaluate the presence of the following local dermoscopic features:

- Atypical pigment network
- Negative pigment network
- Irregular streaks
- Irregular dots and globules
- Blue-white veil
- Regression structures with white or blue areas
- Irregular pigmentation
- Irregular vascular pattern
- Shiny white structures

When analyzing the different lesions we must consider that:

- The presence of a criterion is more important than its absence, as none of these criteria is 100% specific for melanoma.
- Only one criterion is not enough to proceed to a melanoma diagnosis.
- Some criteria are more important than others.
- The absence of definite criteria leading to a dermoscopic diagnosis must suggest the possibility that the lesion should correspond to a melanoma.

Atypical Pigment Network (Figs. 6.115 to 6.118)

A black, gray, or brown network with irregular mesh and wide lines.

Negative Pigment Network (Figs. 6.119 to 6.124)

It is a structure composed of a network of slightly pigmented lines and dark openings, and provides a "negative" image of the pigment reticule. At a histologic level, the pigmented openings are large nests of melanocytic cells located in the dermal papillae, and the network lines are elongated interpapillary processes. This structure appears in melanoma and Spitz nevi.

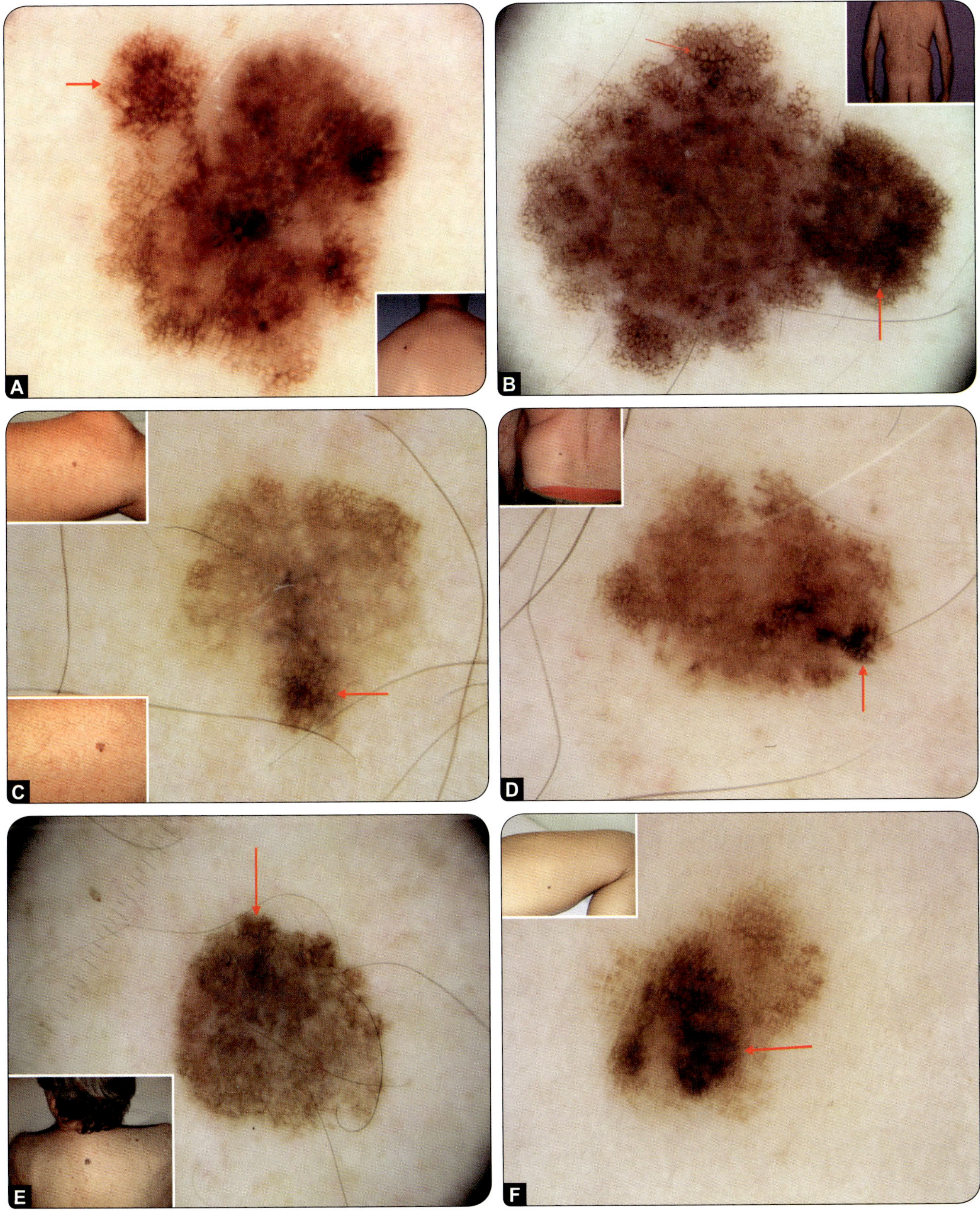

Figs. 6.115A to F

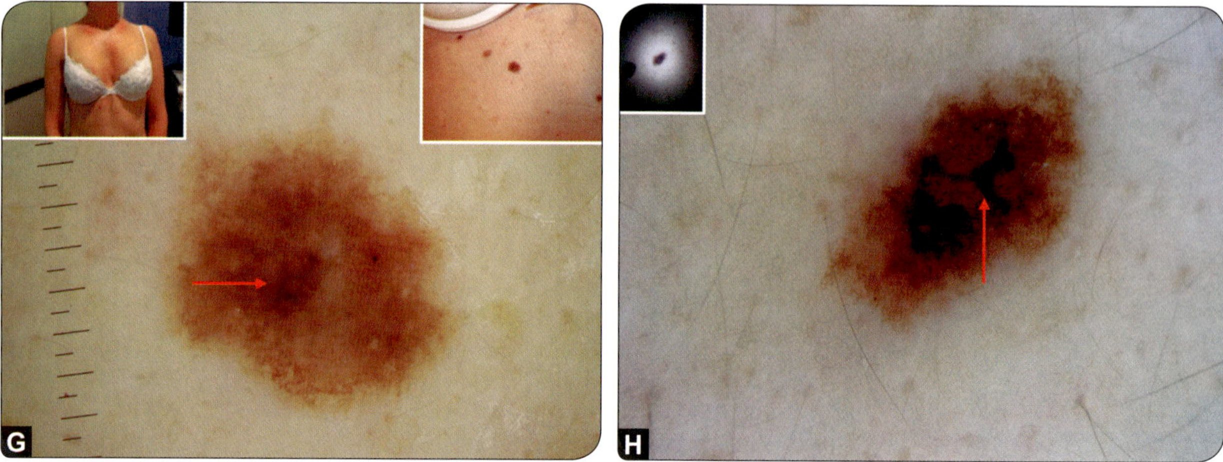

Figs. 6.115A to H: Melanoma in situ: atypical pigment network (arrow).

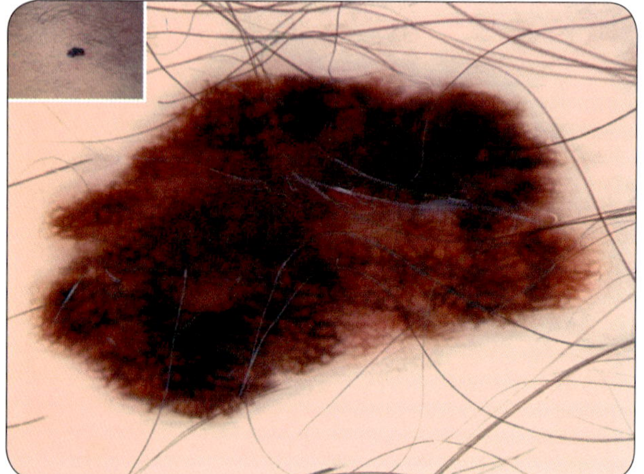

Fig. 6.116: Melanoma in situ: atypical reticular pattern with atypical pigment network.

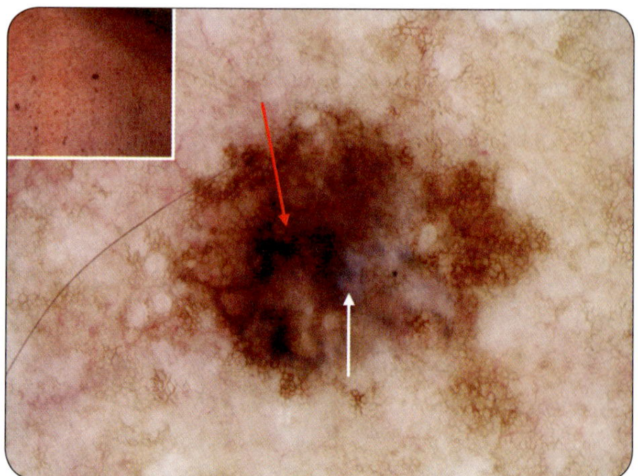

Fig. 6.117: Melanoma in situ: atypical pigment network (red arrow); regression structures with blue areas (white arrow).

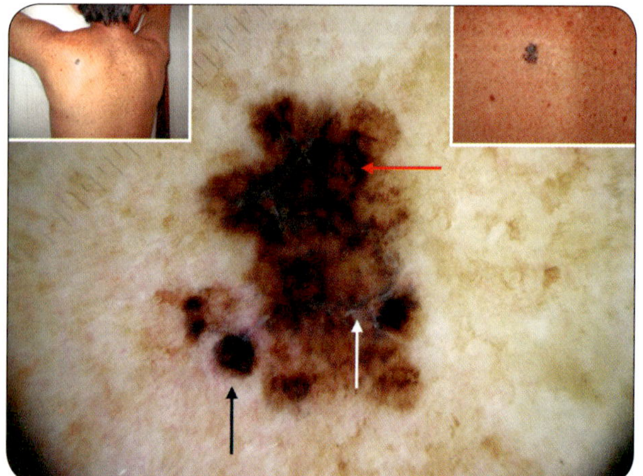

Fig. 6.118: Melanoma in situ: atypical pigment network (red arrow); regression structures with blue areas (white arrow) and white areas (black arrow).

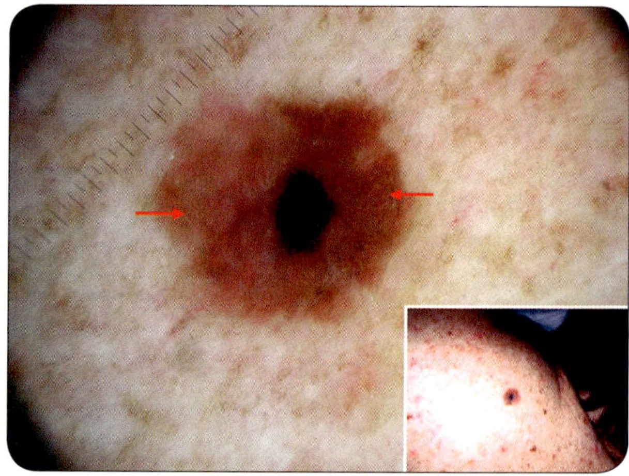

Fig. 6.119: Superficial spreading melanoma B 0.3: atypical negative pigment network (red arrows).

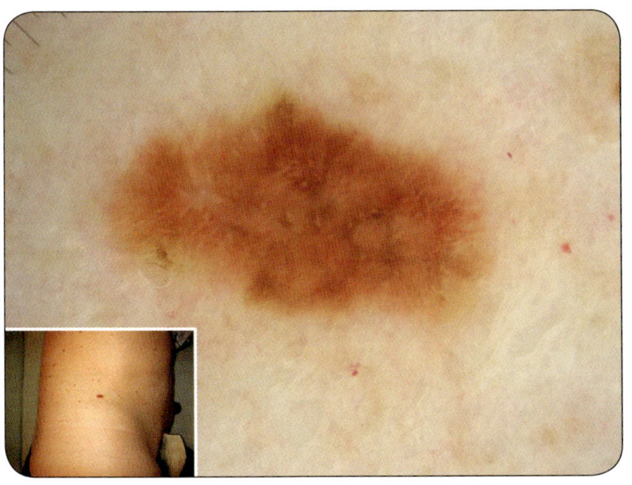

Fig. 6.120: Superficial spreading melanoma B 0.3: atypical negative pigment network in different areas of the lesion.

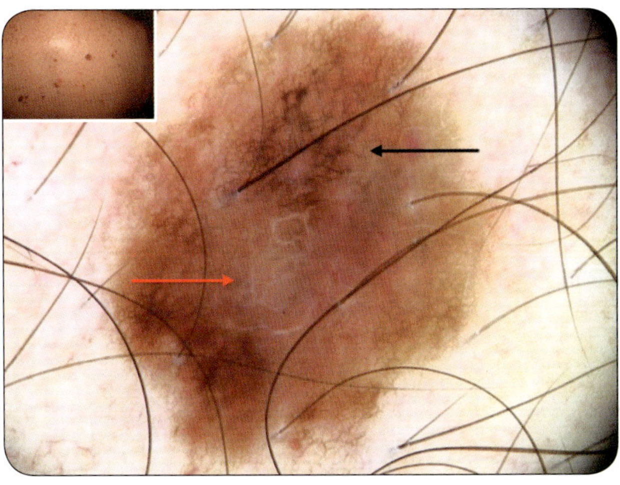

Fig. 6.121: Superficial spreading melanoma: negative pigment network (red arrow); atypical pigment network (black arrow).

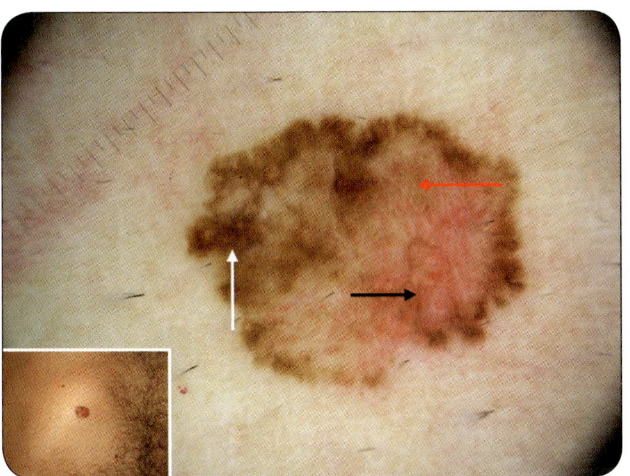

Fig. 6.122: Superficial spreading melanoma: atypical negative pigment network (red arrow); irregular vascular pattern (black arrow); and regression structures with blue areas (white arrow).

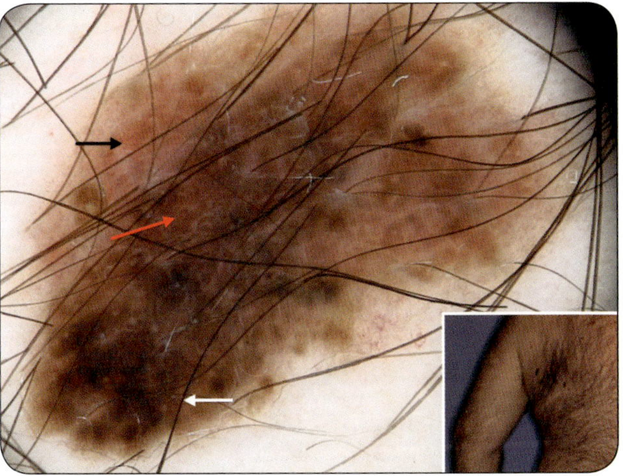

Fig. 6.123: Superficial spreading melanoma: atypical negative pigment network (red arrow); irregular vascular pattern (black arrow); and irregular pigmentation (white arrow).

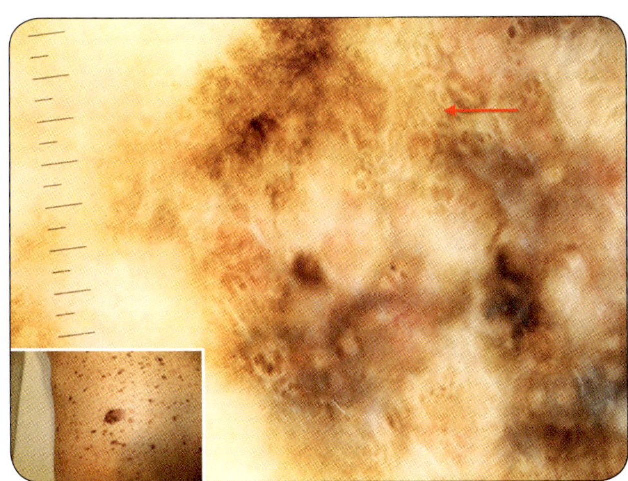

Fig. 6.124: Superficial spreading melanoma (B 0.86): atypical negative pigment network (arrow).

Irregular Streaks (Irregular Projections) (Figs. 6.125 to 6.129, 6.134 and 6.135)

There are two types of lines or streaks: pseudopods and radial or radiated projections. The former have a bulbous digit-formed appearance, while the latter are fine radiated lines.

Branching and pseudopods are considered as only one criterion. Both correlate histologically to nests of melanocytes convergent in the dermoepidermal junction.

Irregular Dots and Globules (Figs. 6.130 to 6.135)

The presence of dots and globules of different size and color distributed irregularly over the melanocytic lesion may suggest malignancy.

Blue-white Veil (Figs. 6.136 to 6.140)

This is the blue-grey or blue-white (blue-whitish) confluent diffuse pigmentation, with absence of structures within.

It is an important parameter; it is one of the most specific melanoma parameters; however, it may also be found in fusocelular nevi or combined lesions.

From a clinical point of view, it may correspond to a raised area of the lesion. Histologically, it corresponds to the presence of large confluent nests of highly pigmented tumorous cells, in the superficial dermis, which appear veiled due to the overlapping of compact orthokeratosis with more or less acanthosis and hypergranulosis.

Regression Structures with White or Blue Areas (Figs. 6.141 to 6.144)

Blue and white areas are considered together, reflecting the two main morphological aspects of regression: fibrosis and melanosis (melanofagia).

Clinically, they correspond to the flat part of the lesion. In the case of large regression areas, it is necessary to rule out a melanoma.

Irregular Pigmentation (Figs. 6.145 to 6.147)

These areas correspond, inside a melanocytic lesion, to areas within which it is impossible to distinguish structures. They may be either hyperpigmented brown, gray, or black areas, or areas of hypopigmentation. The distribution of these structures is very important, since when localized irregularly and focally, they are more characteristic of a malignant lesion. Asymmetric hyperpigmented eccentric areas are more frequently associated to melanoma than hypopigmented ones.

Irregular Vascular Pattern (Figs. 6.148A to D)

In the hypopigmented areas of a melanoma or in hypomelanotic melanomas, it is possible to observe vessels with the following features:

- Dotted vessels with irregular distribution
- Lineal vessels with irregular shape and distribution
- Pink-whitish areas
- Vessels within regression areas.

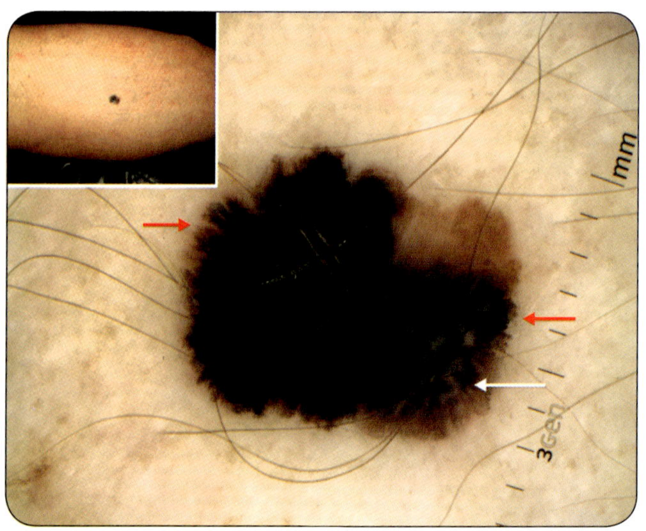

Fig. 6.125: Superficial spreading melanoma: irregular streaks (red arrows); shiny white structures (white arrow).

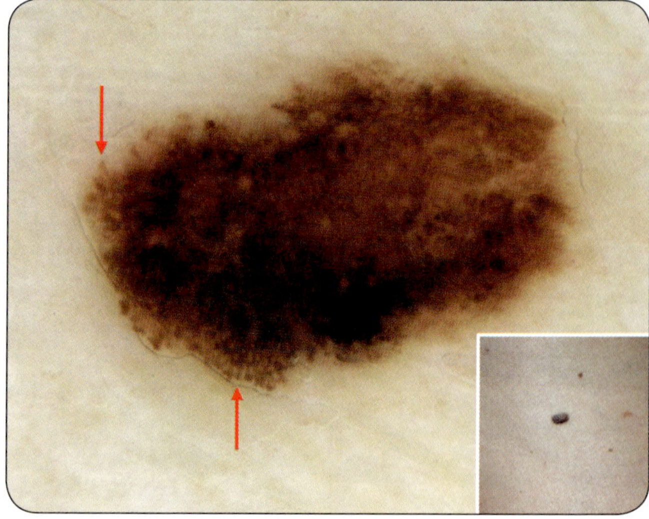

Fig. 6.126: Superficial spreading melanoma: irregular streaks (arrows).

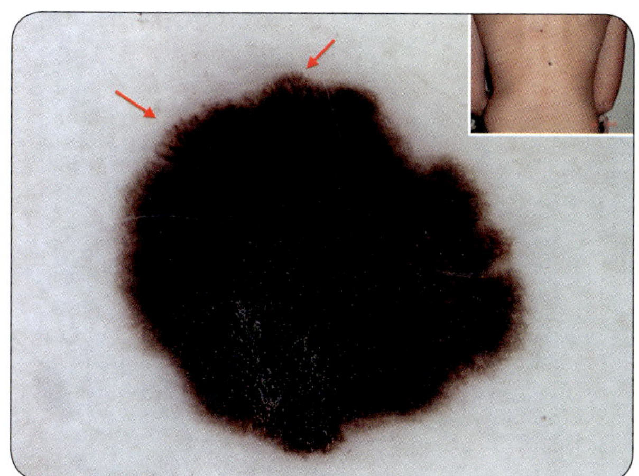

Fig. 6.127: Superficial spreading melanoma (B 0.3): irregular streaks (arrows).

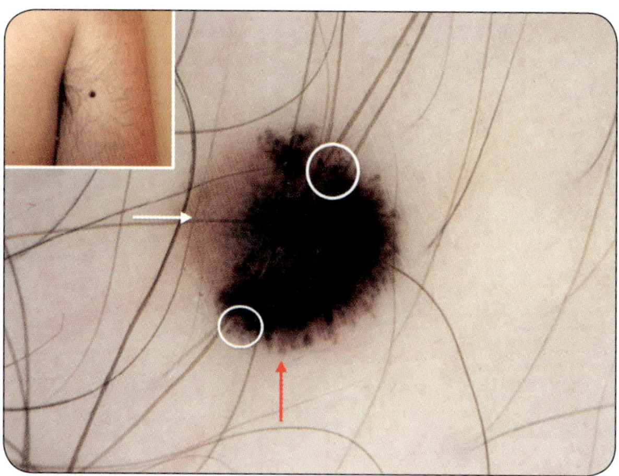

Fig. 6.128: Superficial spreading melanoma (B 0.5): irregular streaks (red arrow); negative pigment network (white arrow); and irregular dots and globules (white circles).

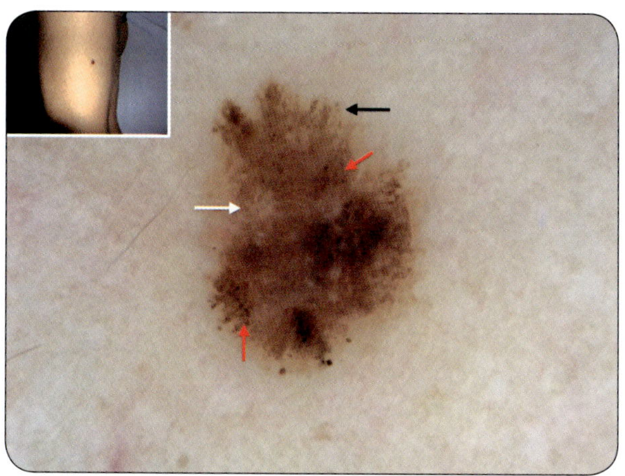

Fig. 6.129: Superficial spreading melanoma: irregular dots and globules (red arrows); irregular streaks (black arrow); and negative pigment network (white arrow).

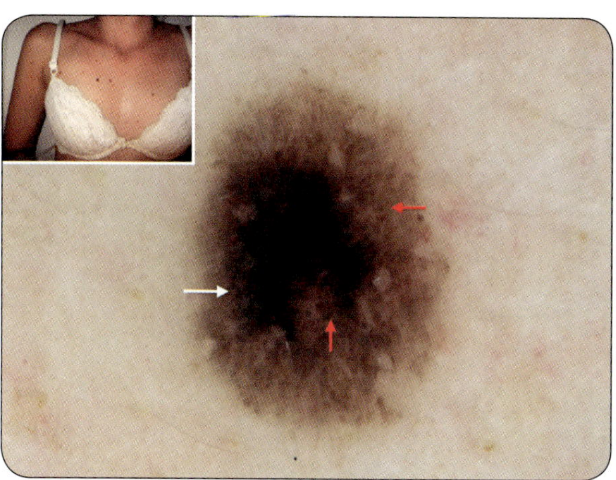

Fig. 6.130: Superficial spreading melanoma: irregular dots and globules (red arrows); regression structures with blue areas (white arrow).

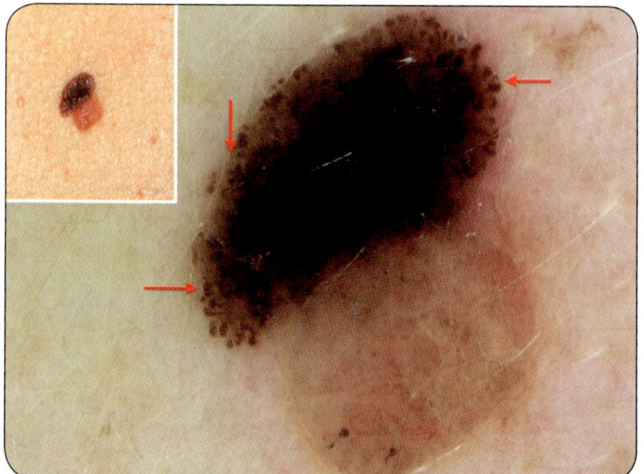

Fig. 6.131: Superficial spreading melanoma: irregular dots and globules (arrows).

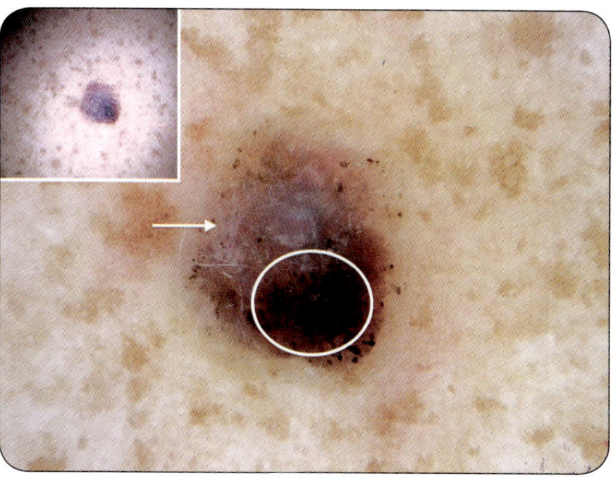

Fig. 6.132: Superficial spreading melanoma: irregular dots and globules (white circle); shiny white structures (white arrow).

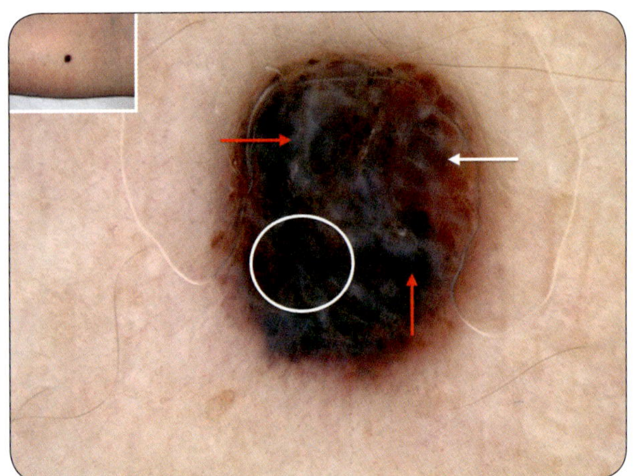

Fig. 6.133: Superficial spreading melanoma: irregular dots and globules (white circle); blue-white veil (red arrows); and negative pigment network (white arrow).

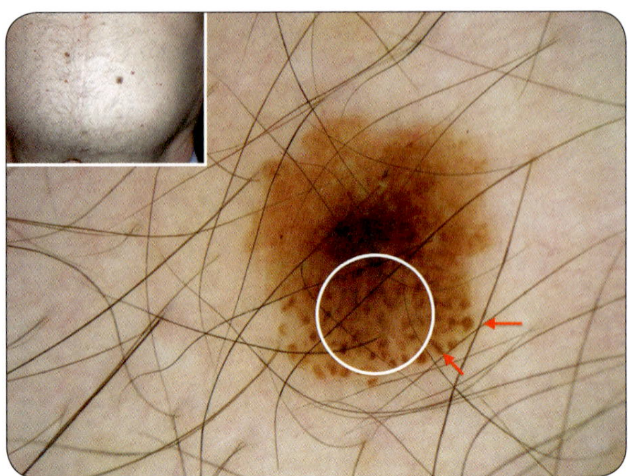

Fig. 6.134: Superficial spreading melanoma: irregular dots and globules (white circle); irregular streaks (red arrows).

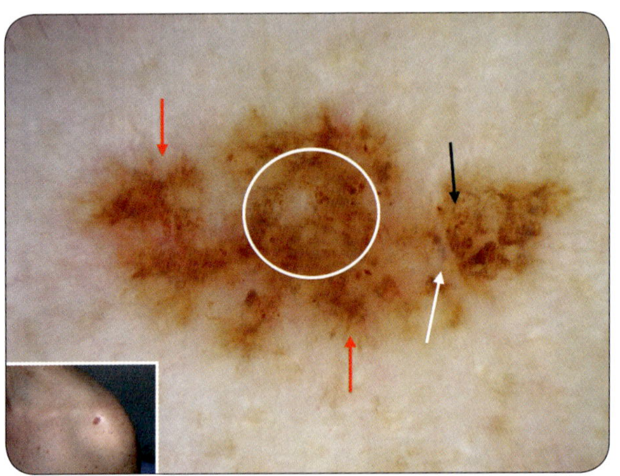

Fig. 6.135: Superficial spreading melanoma (B 0.4): irregular dots and globules (white circle); irregular streaks (red arrows); negative pigment network (black arrow); and regression (white arrow).

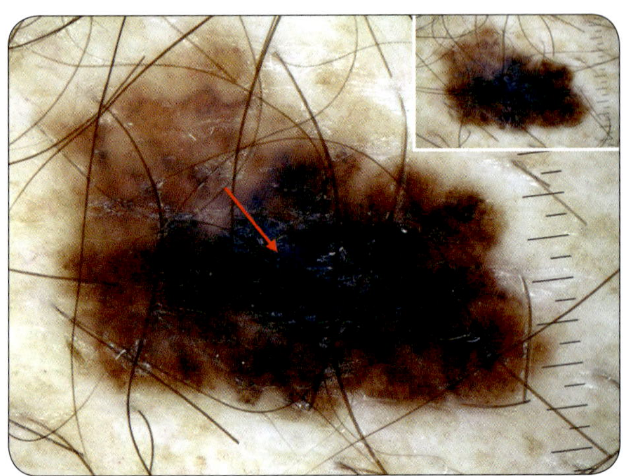

Fig. 6.136: Súperficial spreading melanoma B 0.7: blue-white veil (arrow).

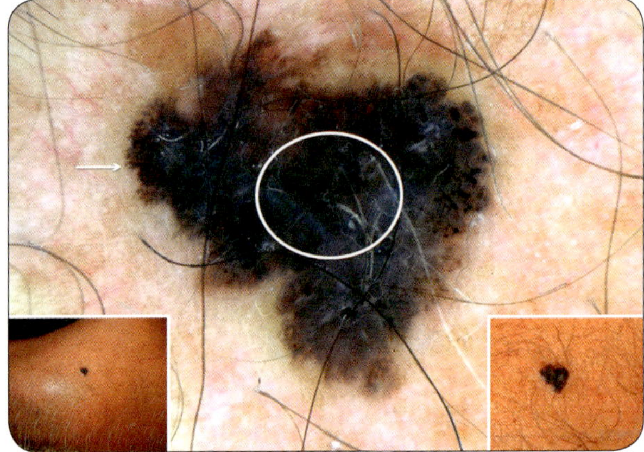

Fig. 6.137: Superficial spreading melanoma B 0.91: blue-white veil (white circle); irregular streaks (white arrow).

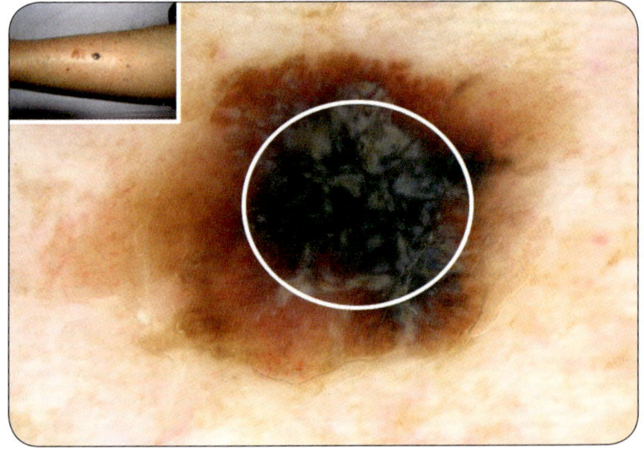

Fig. 6.138: Superficial spreading melanoma B 0.6: blue-white veil and shiny white structures (white circle).

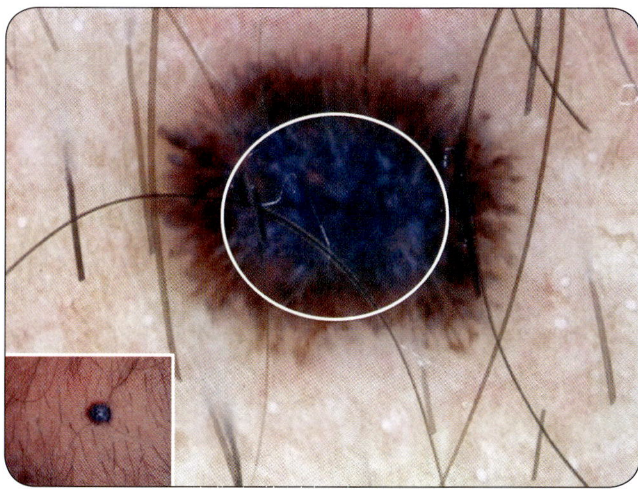

Fig. 6.139: Blue-white veil (white circle).

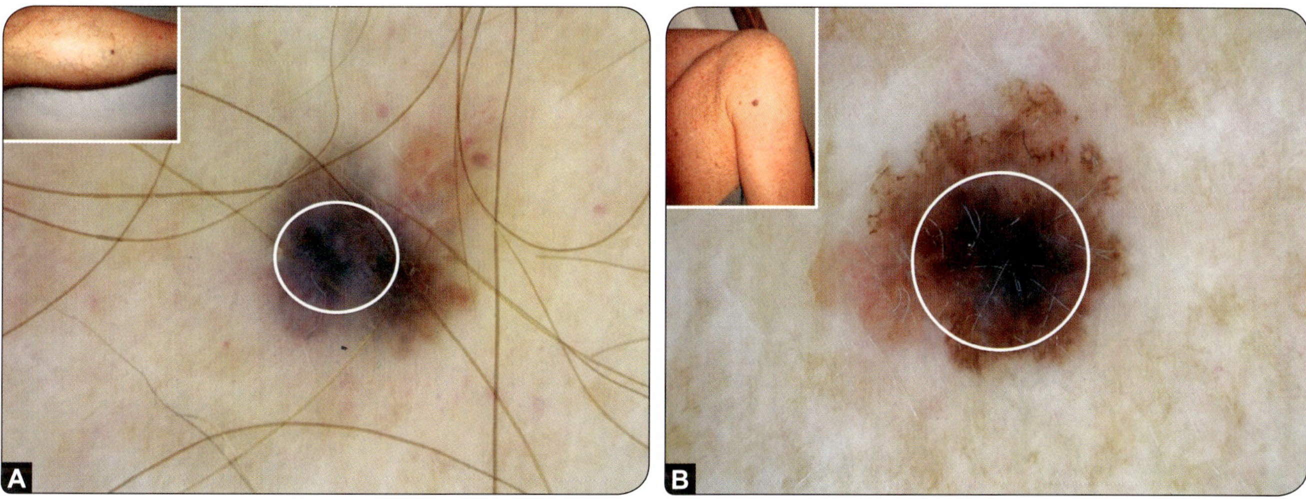

Figs. 6.140A and B: Superficial spreading melanoma B 0.9: blue-white veil (white circles).

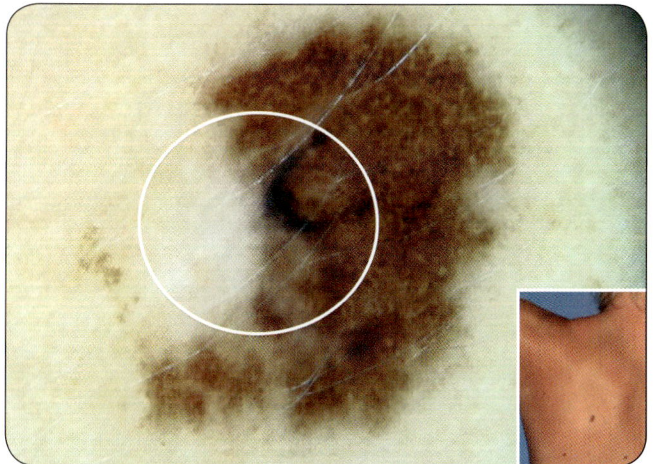

Fig. 6.141: Superficial spreading melanoma: regression structures with white and blue areas (white circle).

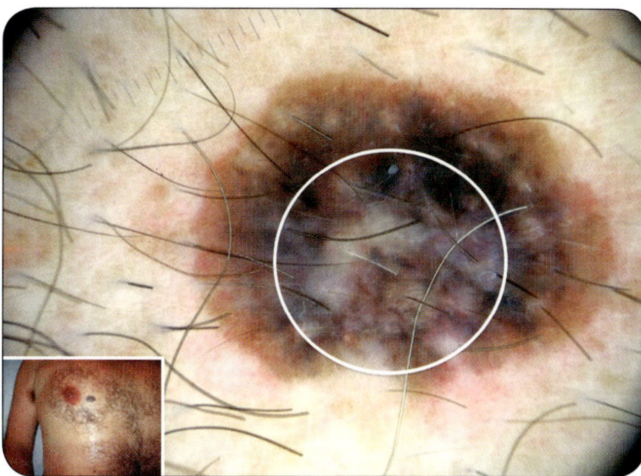

Fig. 6.142: Superficial spreading melanoma: regression structures with white and blue areas (white circle).

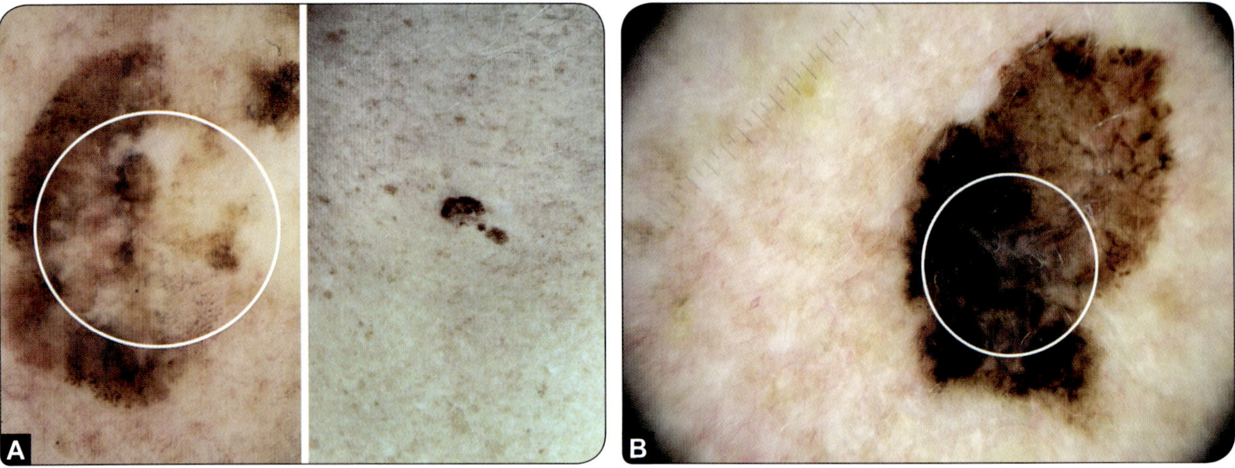

Figs. 6.143A and B: Melanoma in situ: regression structures with white and blue areas (white circle).

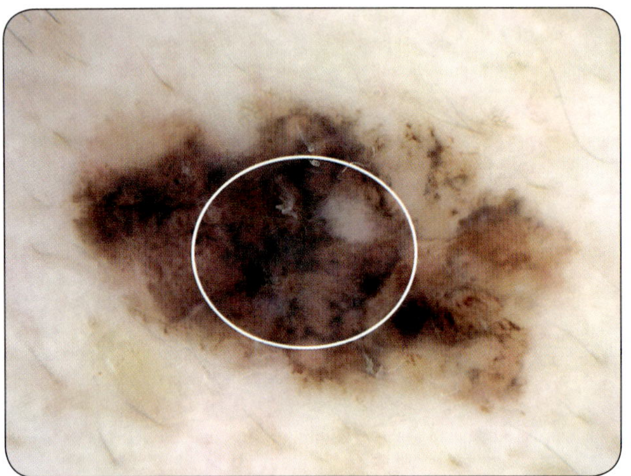

Fig. 6.144: Superficial spreading melanoma B 0.3: regression structures with white and blue areas (white circle).

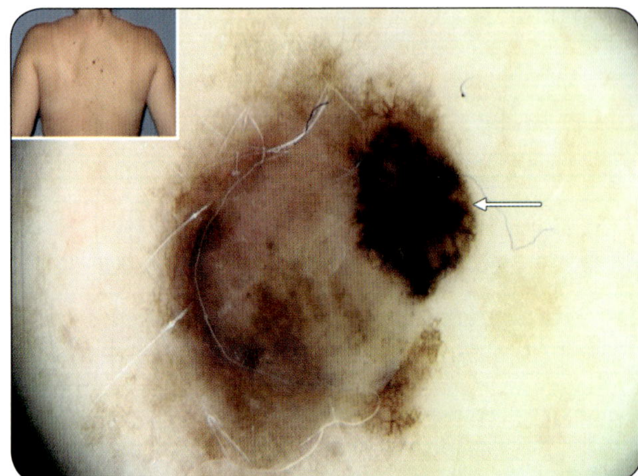

Fig. 6.145: Superficial spreading melanoma B 0.8: irregular pigmentation (white arrow).

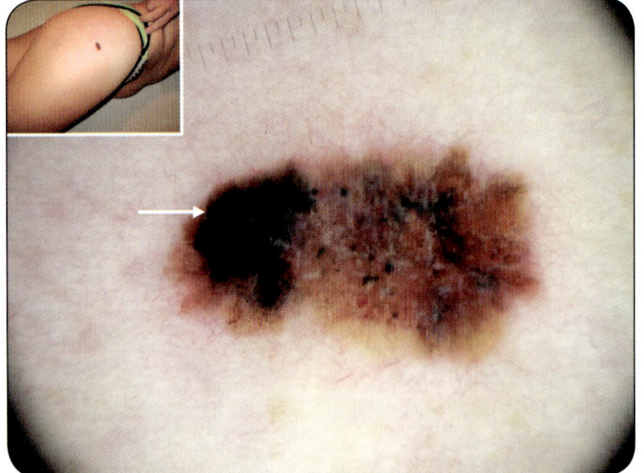

Fig. 6.146: Superficial spreading melanoma B 1.5: irregular pigmentation (arrow).

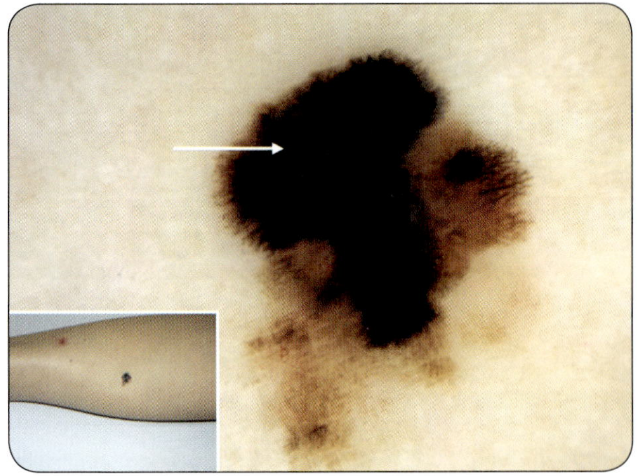

Fig. 6.147: Superficial spreading melanoma: irregular pigmentation (arrow).

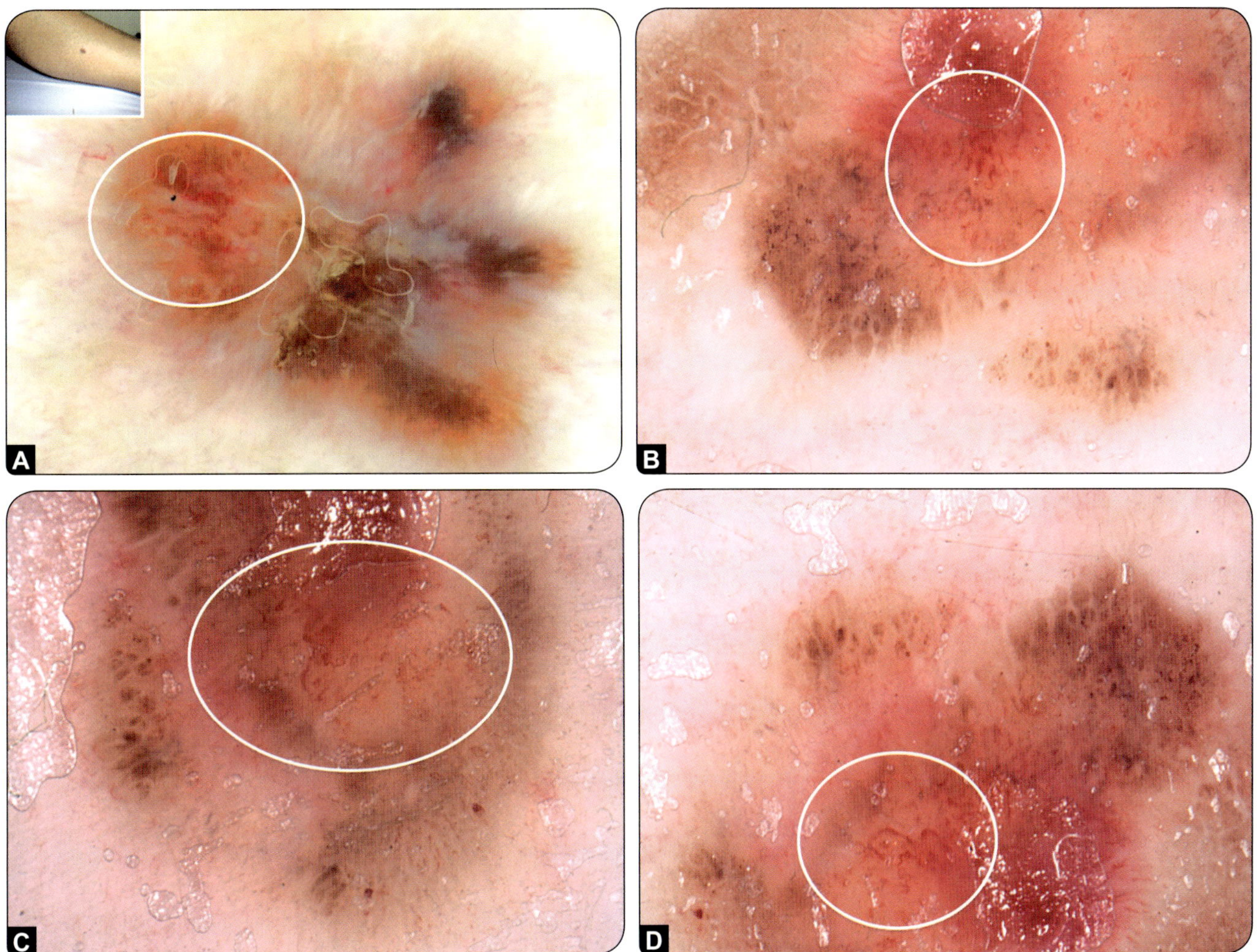

Figs. 6.148A to D: Irregular vascular pattern (white circles).

Shiny White Areas (Figs. 6.149 to 6.151)

Shiny white streaks are not visible with the naked eye or with the nonpolarized dermoscope. They can be seen in lesions with heightened collagen (melanoma, dermatofibroma, scars, and basal cell carcinoma). Collagen streaks are birefringent and this causes a fast randomization of the polarized light.

It is a dynamic polarized dermoscopy since by rotating the dermoscope while keeping it in contact with the cutaneous surface, the orientation of the crystalline structures changes owing to the angular dependence of the polarized light, reflecting the nonrandomized distribution of the collagen fibers in the dermis.

Conclusion

The knowledge of these structures allows the dermoscopic diagnosis of SSM with a diagnostic accuracy index higher than under clinical examination.

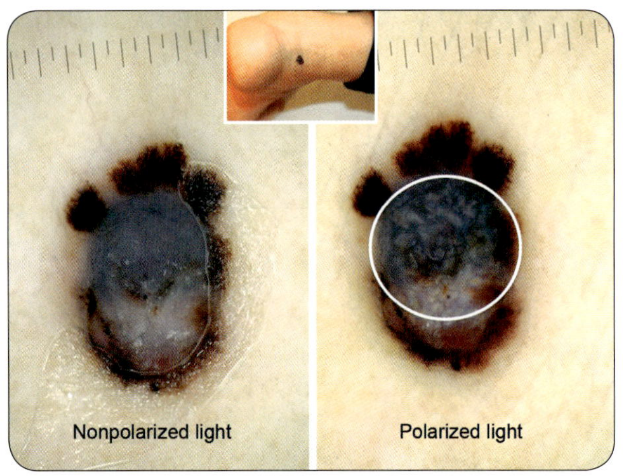

Fig. 6.149: Superficial spreading melanoma B 1.2: shiny white structures (white circle).

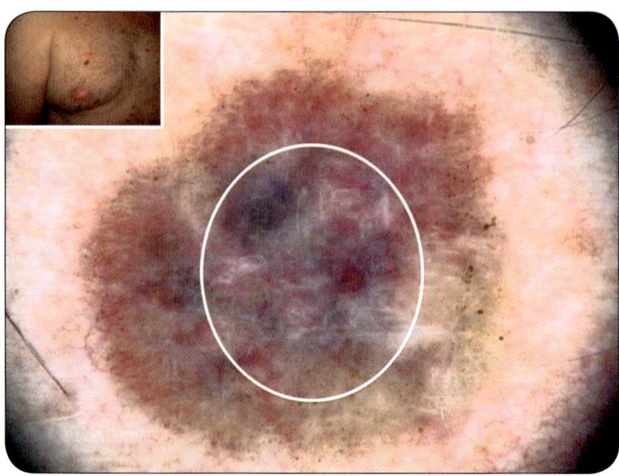

Fig. 6.150: Superficial spreading melanoma: shiny white structures (white circle).

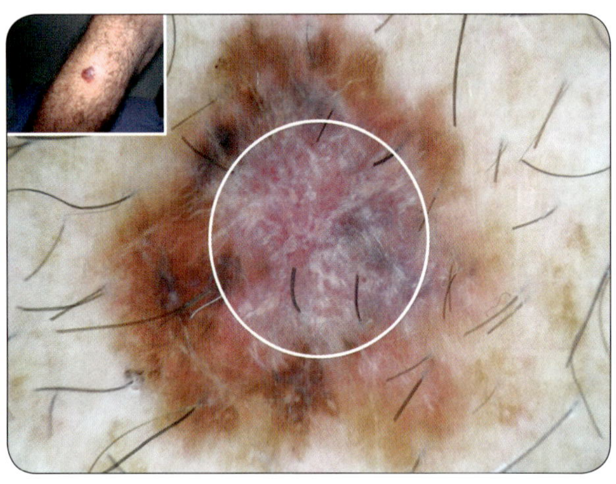

Fig. 6.151: Superficial spreading melanoma B 1.1: shiny white structures (white circle).

SUGGESTED READING

Argenziano G, Soyer P, De Giorgio V, et al. Interactive Atlas of Dermoscopy. Milán: EDRA Medical Publishing & New Media; 2000.

Cabo H. Dermatoscopia. Buenos Aires, Argentina: Weber Ferro; 2000.

Cabo H. Dermatoscopia, 2nd edition. Buenos Aires, Argentina: Ediciones Journal; 2012.

Johr R, Stolz W. Dermoscopy: An Illustrated Self-Assessment Guide, 2nd edition. New York: McGraw-Hill Education; 2015.

Jorh R, Soyer P, Argenziano G, et al. Dermoscopy. The Essentials (MOABT). New York: Elsevier Ltd; 2004.

Kittler H. Dermatoscopy. An Algorithmic Method Based on Pattern Analysis. Austria: Facultas.wuv; 2011.

Lallas A. Dermoscopy in general dermatology. Dermatol Clin. 2013;3:679-94.

Malvhey J, Puig S. Principles of Dermoscopy. Barcelona: Creaciones Gráficas; 2009.

Marghoob A, Braun R, Kopf A. Atlas of Dermoscopy. London: Taylor & Francis; 2005.

Menzies S, Crotty K, Ingvar C, et al. An atlas of surface microscopy of pigmented skin lesions. Sydney: McGraw-Hill Book Company; 1996.

Pizzichetta M, Talamini R, Marghoob AA, et al. Negative pigment network: an additional dermoscopic feature for the diagnosis of melanoma. J Am Acad Dermatol. 2013;68:552-9.

Rabinovitz H, Kopf A. Dermoscopy: A Practical Guide. Miami: American Academy of Dermatology; 1999.

Soyer P, Argenziano G, Chimenti S, et al. Dermoscopy of Pigmented Skin Lesions. An Atlas Based on the Consensus Net Meeting on Dermoscopy. Milán: EDRA Medical Publishing & New Media; 2001.

Stolz W, Braun-Falco O, Bilek P, et al. Color Atlas of Dermatoscopy. Germany: Blackwell Science; 1994.

Zalaudek I, Argenziano G, Giacomel J. Dermoscopy of non-pigmented skin tumors. Boca Raton, FL: CRC Press; 2016.

Zalaudek I, Kittler H, Hofmann-Wellenhof R, et al. "White" network in Spitz nevi and early melanomas lacking significant pigmentation. J Am Acad Dermatol. 2013;69:56-60.

6.9.2 Nodular Melanoma

Horacio A Cabo

The name nodular melanoma (NM) is given to an invasive melanoma of vertical growth without a radial growth phase. Nodular melanoma must be distinguished from the nodular component that may develop in a superficial spreading melanoma (Fig. 6.152). Nodular melanoma represents 14% of invasive melanoma and 56% of thick melanoma (>3 mm).

Nodular melanoma has the highest death rate of all melanoma, despite being less frequent than spreading superficial melanoma (SSM), which causes the most deaths of all melanoma due to its high frequency.

It is therefore very important to bear in mind that for any raised lesion we should never proceed to a short- or long-term follow-up when suspecting an atypical lesion, since if it were a case of NM the prognosis might be much worse. If in doubt it is better to perform a biopsy.

Nodular melanomas have clinical and dermoscopic features different from those of the other types of melanoma.

Clinical Characteristics

It usually appears as a fast growing nodule, occasionally ulcerated, with asymmetric pigmentation pattern, yet less pronounced than in the case of more superficial forms.

The characteristic brown or black color may contain red, white, and/or blue foci. On occasion, the pigment is scarce or even lacking, and it is possible to see skin-color lesions (amelanotic melanoma), which may hinder the diagnosis.

In order to achieve a diagnosis, it is necessary to trace additional signs in the patient's record, such as changes in size, color, and shape of the lesion, or any ulceration sign or spontaneous bleeding.

Nodular melanomas are fast growing melanomas and their onset is hidden from the eye because they start under the skin.

They generally appear in patients with few nevi and it is thought that solar exposure does not play a major role in their development.

- *Clinical features*:
  - Fast growing nodule
  - Sometimes ulcerated
  - With symmetric or asymmetrical pigment pattern
  - The characteristic brown or black color may show red, white, and/or blue foci
  - On occasion it is amelanotic or hypomelanotic
- *Dermoscopic characteristics* (Figs. 6.153 to 6.156): These lesions do not usually show criteria related to radial growth and the pagetoid spreading of the tumor (lines or streaks, black dots/globules, and multiple gray dots), neither those observed in fine melanomas (pigment network) and in early regression stages [white areas (fibrosis) and blue areas (melanosis)], and multiple blue gray dots.

Dermoscopy characteristics of Nodular Melanoma

- Absence of radial growth and pagetoid spreading criteria
  - Lines and streaks
  - Irregular dots and globules
- Absence of criteria for fine melanoma
  - Atypical pigment network
- Absence of regression criteria
  - White or blue areas with multiple blue-gray dots

Neither can we find dermoscopic criteria for special locations (such as face, palms, and soles) owing to the destruction of specific anatomical structures during the growth of thick melanoma.

Dermoscopy characteristics of Nodular Melanoma

- Absence of dermoscopic criteria for special locations (such as face, palms and soles) owing to the destruction of anatomical structures specific during the growth of thick melanoma.

Dermoscopic examination of NM usually shows ordinary thick melanoma criteria, such as the presence of multiple colors (black, light brown, dark brown, blue, gray, red, and white), blue-white veil (blue-white or white-grayish diffuse confluent pigmentation), and atypical vascular pattern

Dermoscopy characteristics of Nodular Melanoma

Thick melanoma criteria

- Blue-white veil
- Multiple colors (5–6)
- Atypical vascular pattern
  - Irregularly distributed dots
  - Irregular lineal vessels
  - Milky-red globules
- Blue-black rule: The presence of blue and black color in the same lesion.

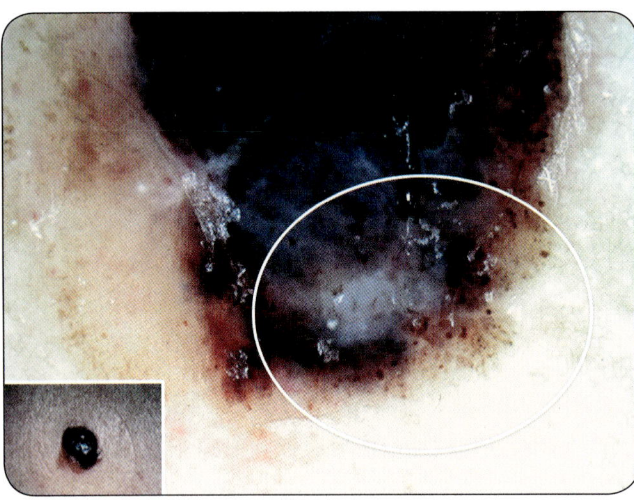

Fig. 6.152: Thick spreading superficial melanoma B 1.8 with irregular streaks, blue-white veil, and irregular dots and globules (white oval).

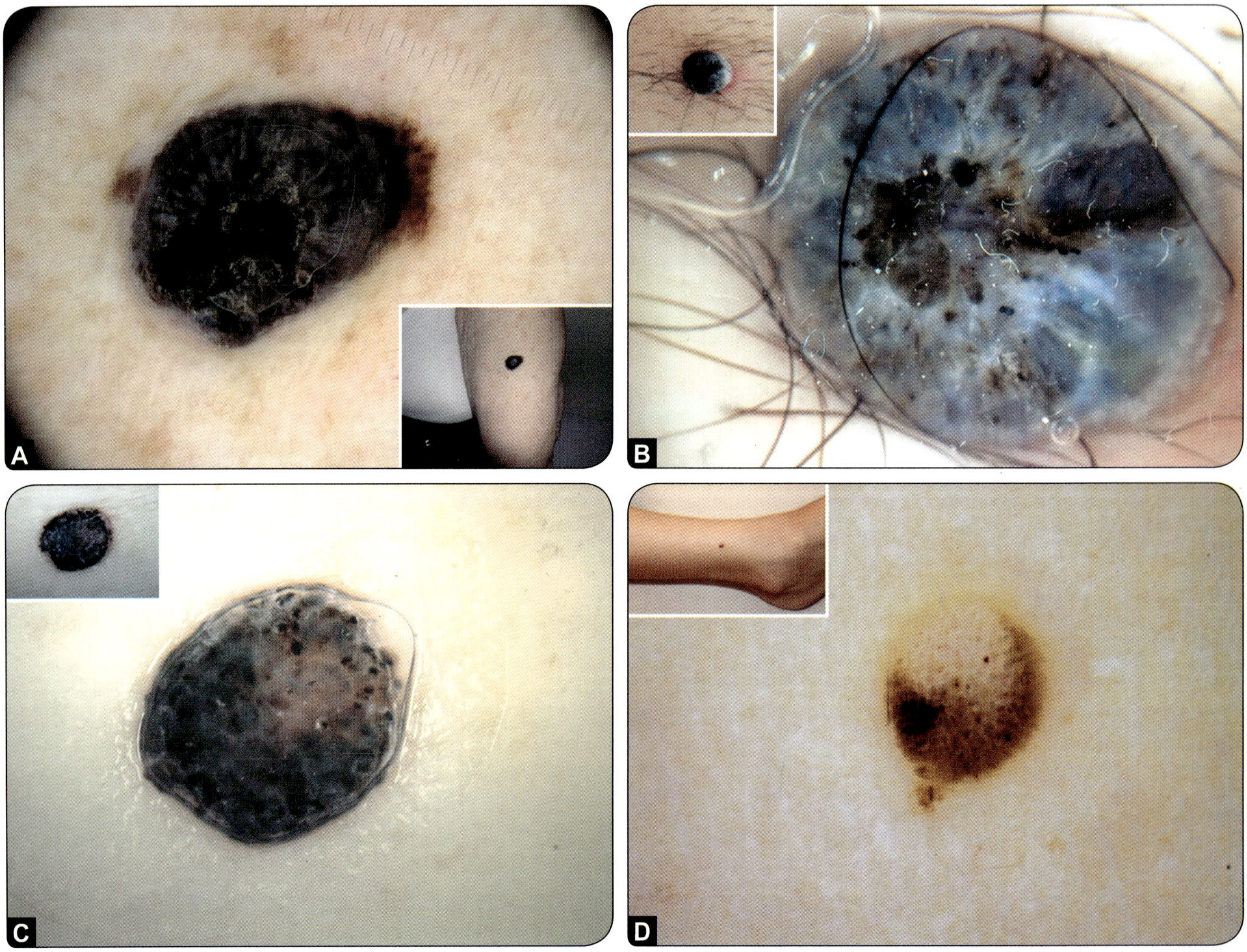

A B C D

Figs. 6.153A to D: Nodular melanoma: blue-white veil and multiple colors.

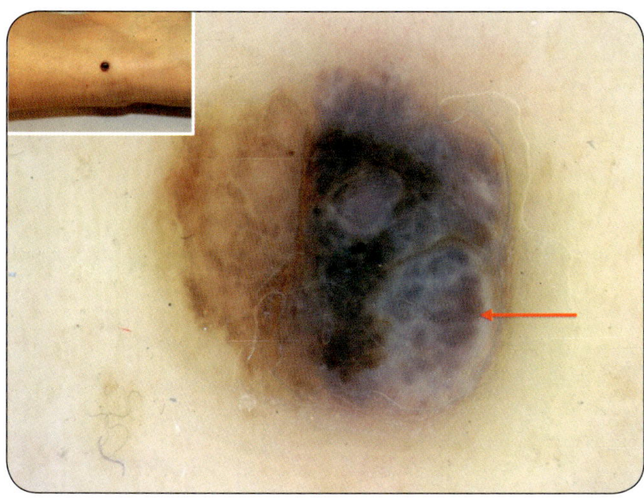

Fig. 6.154: Nodular melanoma: blue-white veil and multiple colors and atypical vascular pattern with irregularly distributed globules (arrow).

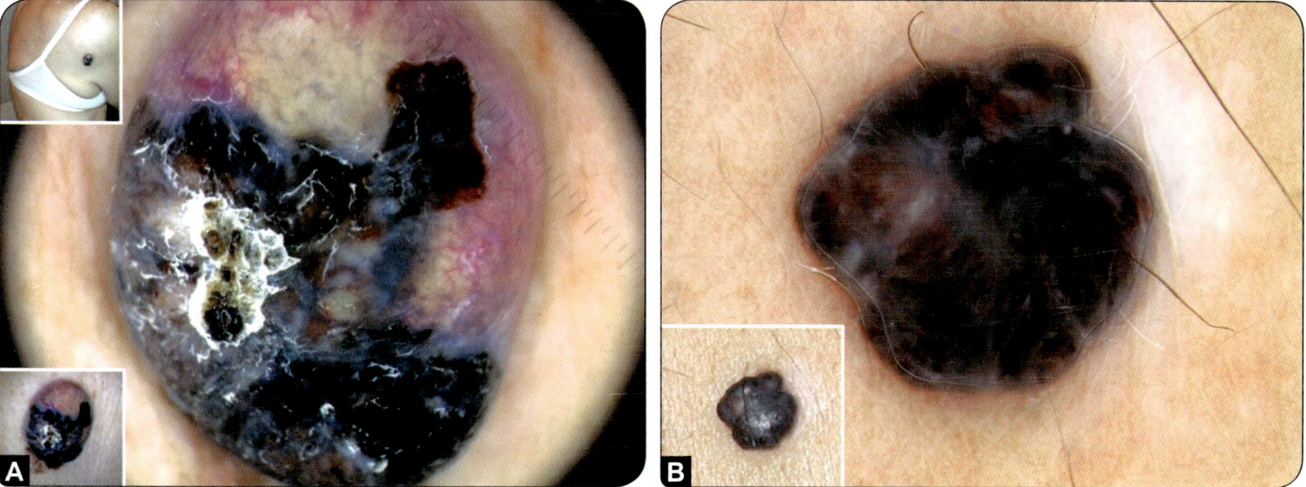

Figs. 6.155A and B: Nodular melanoma: blue-white veil and multiple colors and atypical vascular pattern with irregularly lineal vessels.

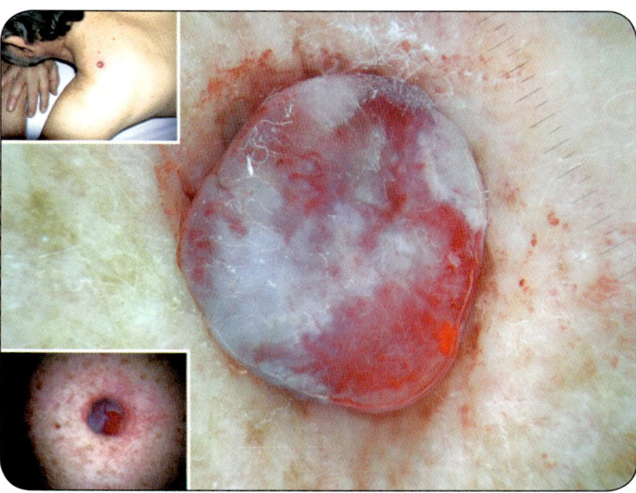

Fig. 6.156: Nodular melanoma: blue-white veil and atypical vascular pattern with irregularly lineal vessels and milky-red areas.

SUGGESTED READING

Argenziano, Longo C, Cameron A, et al. Blue-black rule: a simple dermoscopic clue to recognize pigmented nodular melanoma. BJD. 2011;165:1251-5.

Argenziano G, Soyer P, De Giorgio V, et al. Interactive Atlas of Dermoscopy. Milán: EDRA Medical Publishing & New Media; 2000.

Cabo H. Dermatoscopia. Buenos Aires, Argentina: Weber Ferro; 2000.

Cabo H. Dermatoscopia, 2nd edition. Buenos Aires, Argentina: Ediciones Journal; 2012.

Jorh R, Soyer P, Argenziano G, et al. Dermoscopy. The Essentials (MOABT). New York: Elsevier Ltd; 2004.

Johr R, Stolz W. Dermoscopy: An Illustrated Self-Assessment Guide, 2nd edition. New York: McGraw-Hill Education; 2015.

Kittler H. Dermatoscopy. An Algorithmic Method Based on Pattern Analysis. Austria: Facultas.wuv; 2011.

Lallas A. Dermoscopy in general dermatology. Dermatol Clin. 2013;3:679-94.

Malvhey J, Puig S. Principles of Dermoscopy. Barcelona: Creaciones Gráficas; 2009.

Mar V, Roberts H, Wolfe R, et al. Nodular melanoma: a distinct clinical entity and the largest contributor to melanoma deaths in Victoria, Australia. J Am Acad Dermatol. 2013;68:568-75.

Marghoob A, Braun R, Kopf A. Atlas of Dermoscopy. London: Taylor & Francis; 2005.

Menzies S, Crotty K, Ingvar C, et al. An Atlas of Surface Microscopy of Pigmented Skin Lesions. Sydney: McGraw-Hill Book Company; 1996.

Menzies SW, Moloney FJ, Byth K, et al Dermoscopic evaluation of nodular melanoma. JAMA Dermatol. 2013; 149(6): 699-709.

Rabinovitz H, Kopf A. Dermoscopy: A Practical Guide. Miami: American Academy of Dermatology; 1999.

Soyer P, Argenziano G, Chimenti S, et al. Dermoscopy of Pigmented Skin Lesions. An Atlas Based on the Consensus Net Meeting on Dermoscopy. Milán: EDRA Medical Publishing & New Media; 2001.

Stolz W, Braun-Falco O, Bilek P, et al. Color Atlas of Dermatoscopy. Germany: Blackwell Science; 1994.

Zalaudek I, Argenziano G, Giacomel J. Dermoscopy of Non-Pigmented Skin Tumors. Boca Raton, FL: CRC Press; 2016.

6.9.3 Lentigo Maligna Melanoma

Horacio A Cabo

Dermoscopy has decreased the number of cutaneous biopsies. However, in the case of the face it has increased them. This is due to the fact that with dermoscopy it is possible to distinguish the subtle changes and structures leading to an early diagnosis, of high importance in lentigo maligna melanoma (LMM). Lentigo maligna melanoma appears in skin that has been chronically exposed to light, usually on the face and in middle-aged and elderly people.

The face has a particular anatomic feature: in adult facial skin, the rete ridge is flattened or simply absent, which means that the pigment network is not observable (Fig. 6.157).

The hair follicles, as well as the sebaceous and sweat glands, have no pigment and it is possible to observe a pseudonetwork made up of a thick mesh resulting from the skin color and the white openings, which correspond to the follicular openings, since these areas lack melanin pigment. This pseudonetwork is present in melanocytic and nonmelanocytic lesions on the face. Therefore, in the case of the face it is not possible to differentiate between melanocytic and nonmelanocytic lesions by the pseudonetwork, which makes it necessary to use other criteria.

On the face, the most important differential diagnosis is between lentigo maligna (LM), solar lentigo (flat seborrheic keratosis), pigmented actinic keratosis, and liken planus-like keratosis.

Dermoscopy of pigmented lesions on the face

- General considerations
  - Classical pigmented network
    - Infrequent on the face
    - Flat rete ridge
  - Pigmented pseudonetwork
    - Frequent on the face
    - Hair follicle openings and sweat glands lack pigment
    - Present in melanocytic and nonmelanocytic lesions
    - Other criteria are necessary to differentiate these lesions from one another.

Lentigo maligna progression model: (Figs. 6.158A and B)

Annular-granular pattern

Annular pattern (initial criteria in the development of LM)

- Gray or black pigmentation of the follicular openings
- Asymmetric pigmentation of the follicular openings (also known as gray circles)
- Circle within a circle (gray dots within the follicular openings)

Granular pattern around the hair follicles

- Gray dots
- Gray globules
- Lines around the follicles

With greater progression:

- Rhomboidal structures (the lines become longer and cross each other)
- Blue-gray or black homogeneous areas with or without invasion of the follicular openings
- Whitish and pink structures

Dermoscopic Features (Figs. 6.159 to 6.174)

Classic Criteria

Blue-gray color: Sometimes this color is the only clue to suspect a malignant lentigo.

Blue, gray or black pigmented and asymmetrically pigmented follicular openings: are dark brown or black in color, which indicates the irregular proliferation of atypical melanocytes within the follicles. In LM (melanoma in situ) and in LMM (invasive melanoma), if the follicles are close together, it is possible to perceive a second pseudonetwork characterized by a thin mesh, as opposed to the pseudonetwork that depends on location and presents a thick mesh. These grid-like structures are pseudonetworks, since they do not arise from the pigmentation of the crests or ridges of the rete ridges but from the follicular openings in pigmented facial skin.

Two concentric circles (circle within a circle): This new criteria is highly useful and its significance, statistically

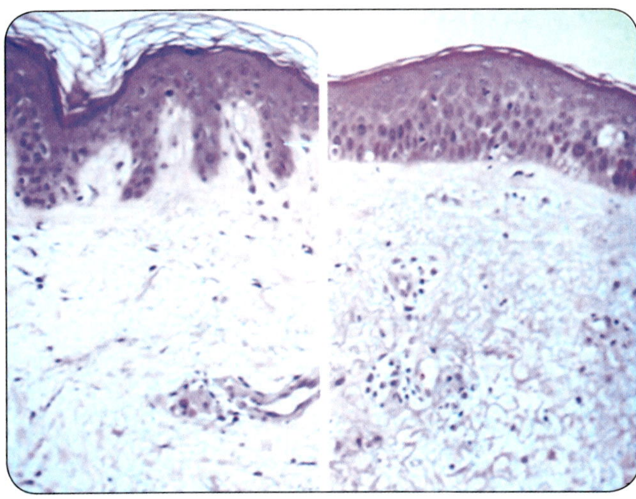

Fig. 6.157: The face has a particular anatomic feature: in adult facial skin, the rete ridge is flattened or simply absent, which means that the pigment network is not observable.

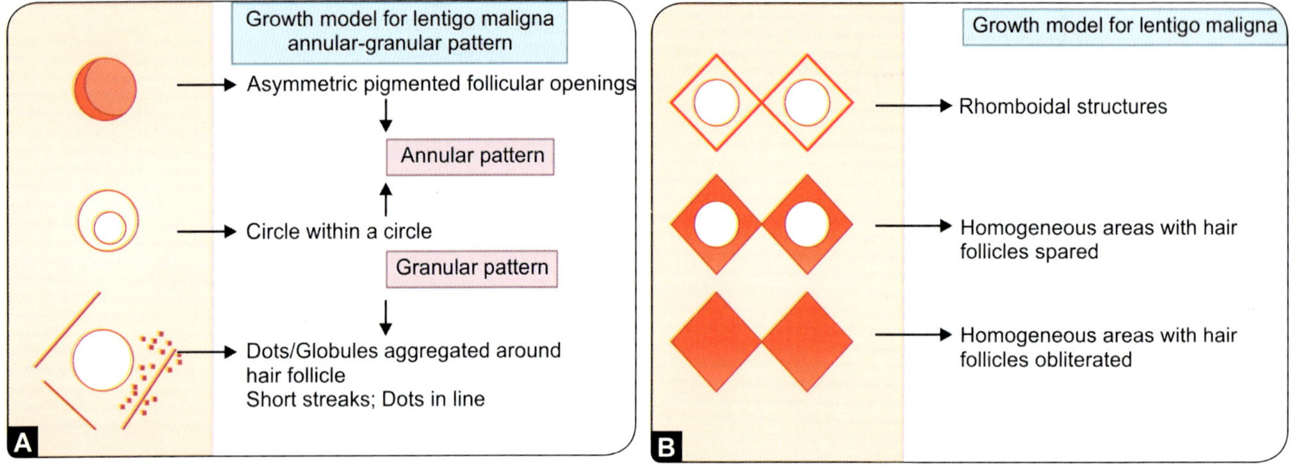

Figs. 6.158A and B: Lentigo maligna progression model.

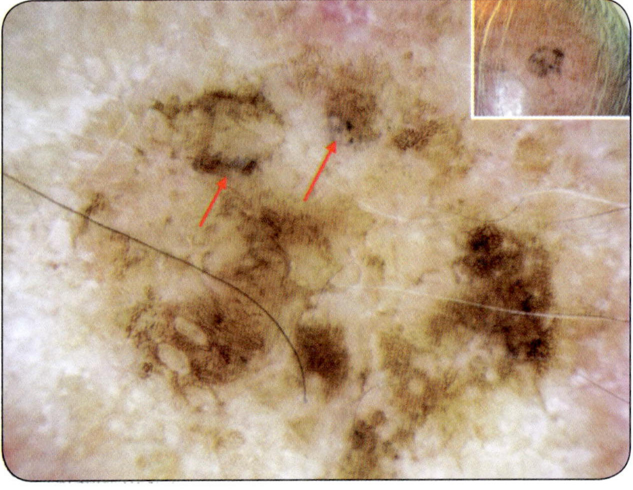

Fig. 6.159: Lentigo maligna: blue-gray color (arrows).

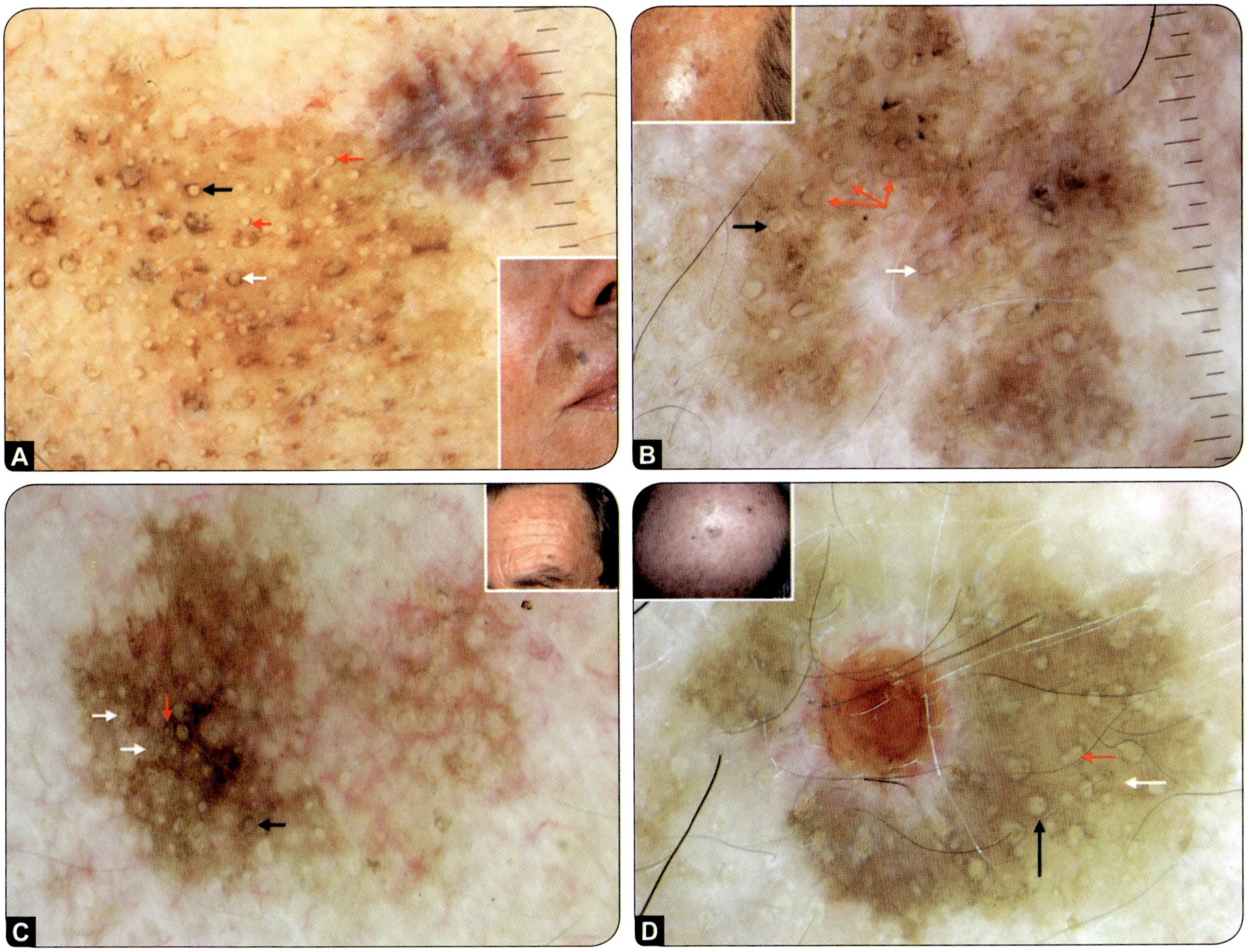

Figs. 6.160A to D: Lentigo maligna: blue-gray pigmented follicular openings (black arrows); asymmetric pigmentation of the follicular openings (red arrows); circle within a circle (white arrows).

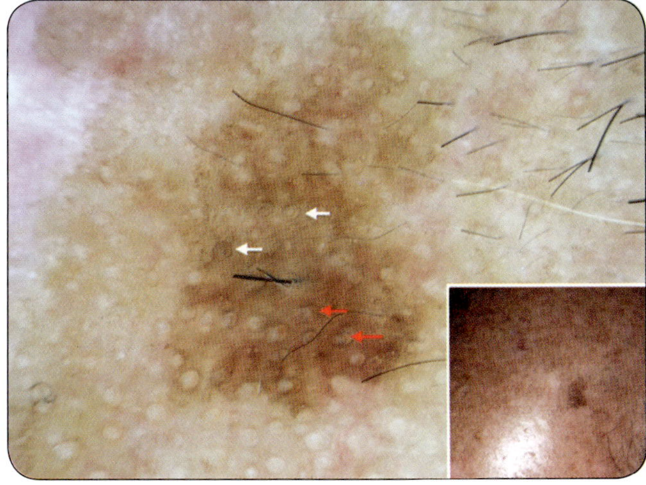

Fig. 6.161: Lentigo maligna: asymmetric pigmentation of the follicular openings (red arrows); circle within a circle (white arrows).

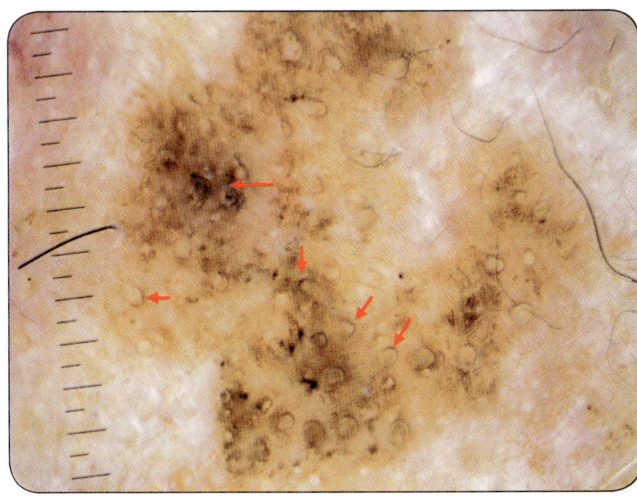

Fig. 6.162: Lentigo maligna: asymmetric pigmentation of the follicular openings (arrows).

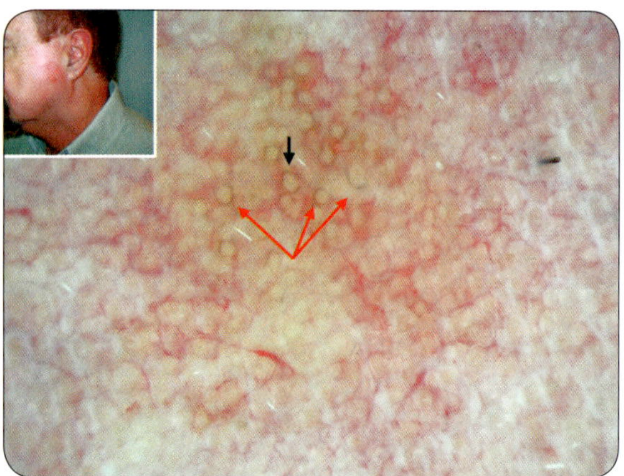

Fig. 6.163: Lentigo maligna: blue-gray pigmented follicular openings (black arrow); asymmetric pigmentation of the follicular openings (red arrows).

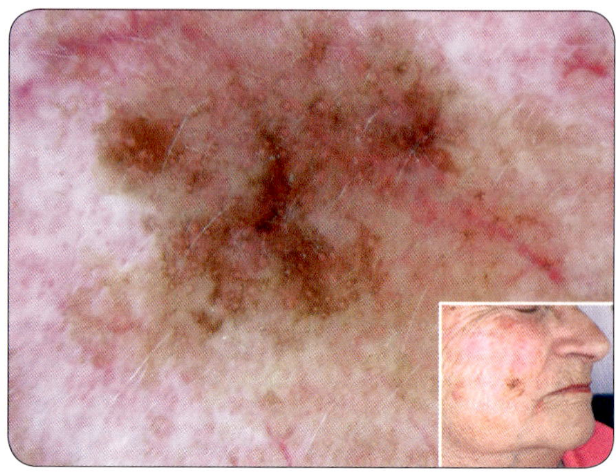

Fig. 6.164: Lentigo maligna: blue-gray pigmented and asymmetric pigmentation of the follicular openings.

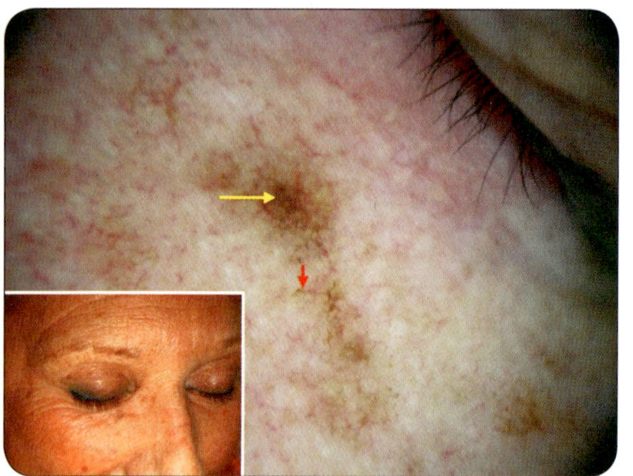

Fig. 6.165: Lentigo maligna: slate-gray dots around the follicular openings (yellow arrow); asymmetric pigmentation of the follicular openings (red arrow).

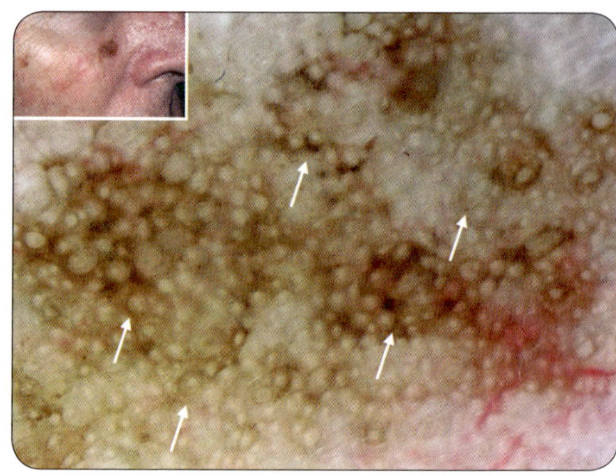

Fig. 6.166: Lentigo maligna: circle within a circle (arrows).

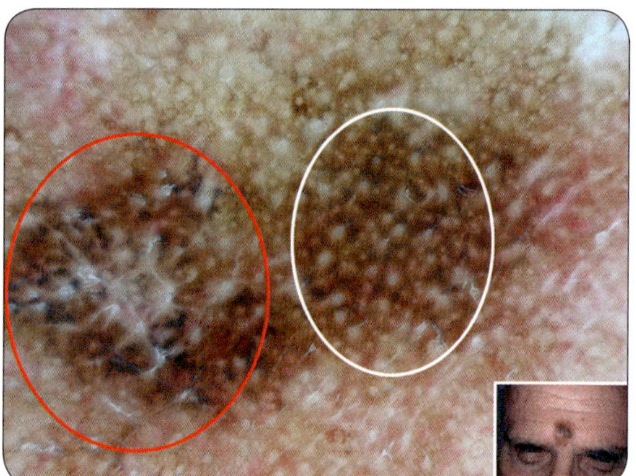

Fig. 6.167: Lentigo maligna: slate-grey dots around the follicular openings (red circle); rhomboidal structures (white circle).

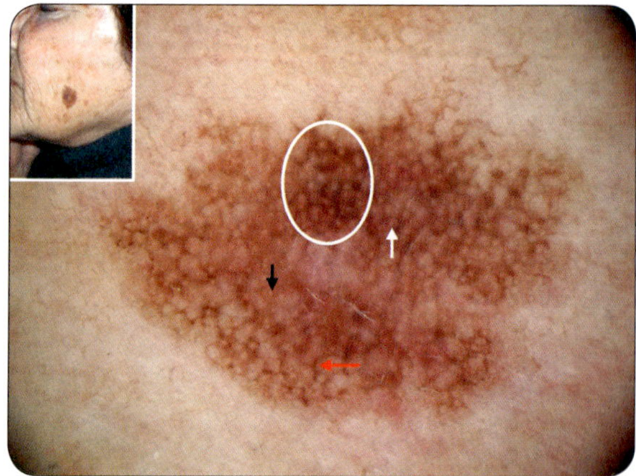

Fig. 6.168: Lentigo maligna: blue-gray pigmented follicular openings (black arrow); asymmetric pigmentation of the follicular openings (red arrow); circle within a circle (white arrow); rhomboidal structures (white circle).

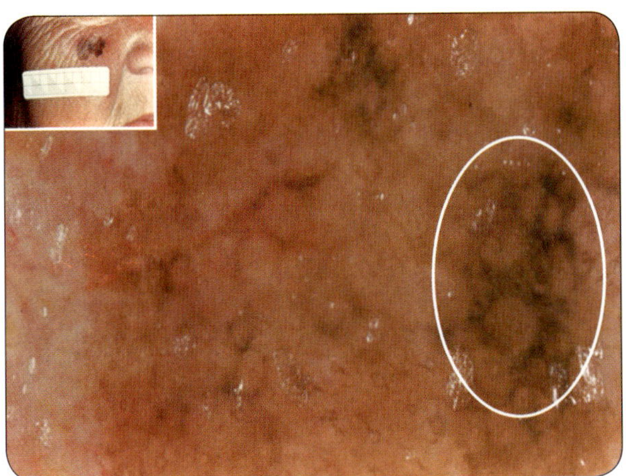

Fig. 6.169: Lentigo maligna: rhomboidal structures (white circle).

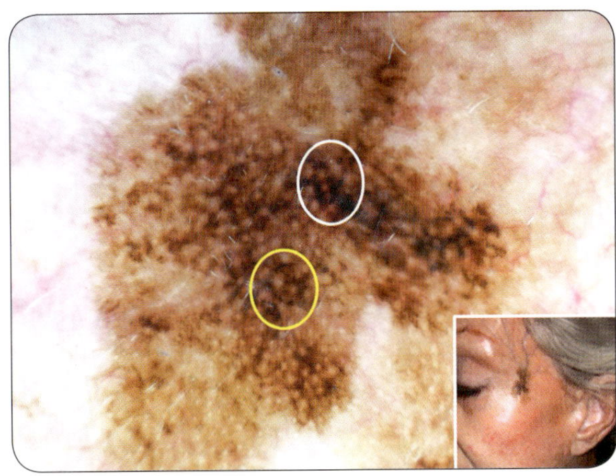

Fig. 6.170: Lentigo maligna: rhomboidal structures (white circle); slate-gray dots around the follicular openings (yellow circle).

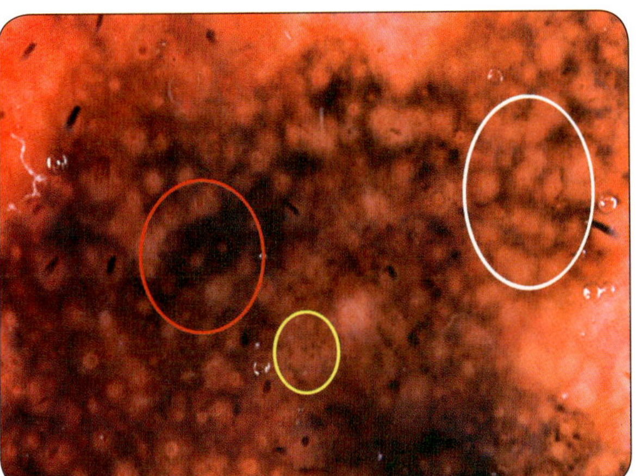

Fig. 6.171: Lentigo maligna melanoma: rhomboidal structures (white circle); slate-gray dots around the follicular openings (yellow circle); homogeneous blue-gray areas with the hair follicles spared (red circle).

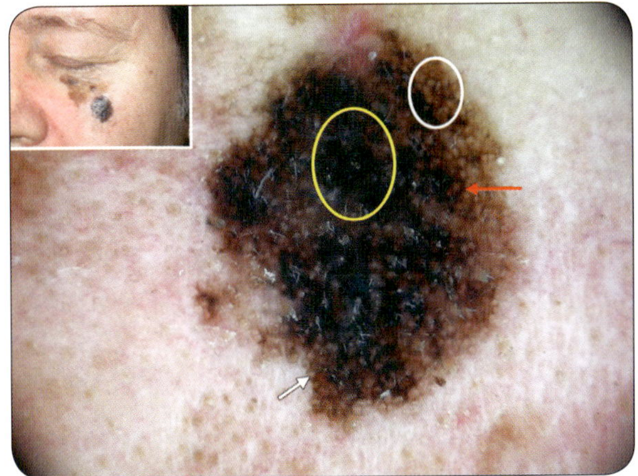

Fig. 6.172: Lentigo maligna melanoma: rhomboidal structures (white circle); homogeneous blue-gray areas with the hair follicles obliterated (yellow circle); asymmetric pigmentation of the follicular openings (red arrow); circle within a circle (white arrow).

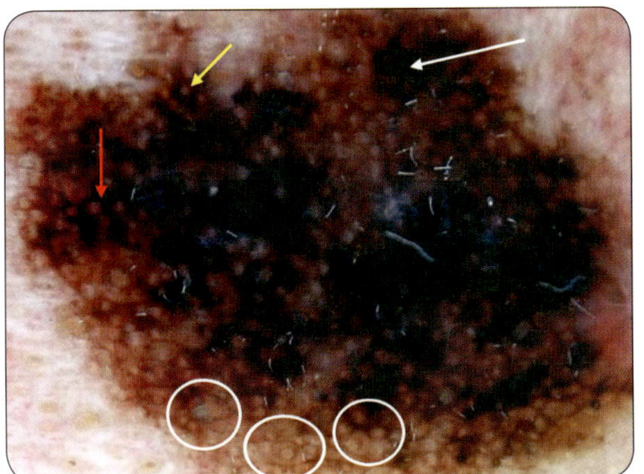

Fig. 6.173: Lentigo maligna melanoma: circle within a circle (white circles); homogeneous blue-gray areas with the hair follicles obliterated (white arrow) or spared (yellow arrow); rhomboidal structures (red arrow).

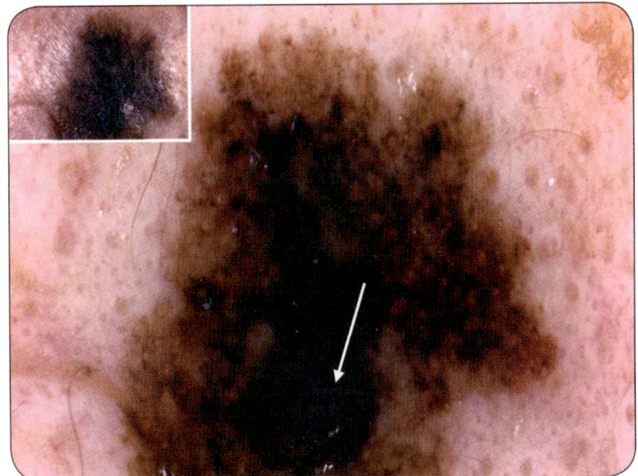

Fig. 6.174: Lentigo maligna melanoma: homogeneous blue-gray areas with the hair follicles obliterated (arrow).

undetermined yet, could be similar to that of the asymmetric pigmentation of the follicular openings.

Slate gray dots around the follicular openings: It is an early sign of LM and it is the beginning of granular-annular pattern.

Rhomboidal structures: At a later stage, it is possible to detect dark brown or black lines or short streaks, highly specific around the follicles.

Homogeneous blue-gray areas with the hair follicles spared or obliterated.

New Criteria (Figs. 6.175 to 6.178)

- Darkening at dermoscopic examination
- Target-like pattern
- Increased density of the vascular network
- Red rhomboidal structures

There are many lesions that may resemble the initial changes observed in malignant lentigo. In teenagers, melanocytic nevi may present slate-gray lines and dots. Liken planus-like keratosis and irritated form of seborrheic keratosis may also present gray lines and dots. In pigmented actinic keratosis, the main melanin location is the macrophages of the upper dermis, just as it happens in incipient malignant lentigo. Asymmetric follicular openings tend to be absent. There are some other indicators of pigmented actinic keratosis, including the habitual presence of multiple lesions and its rough surface. It is possible that the

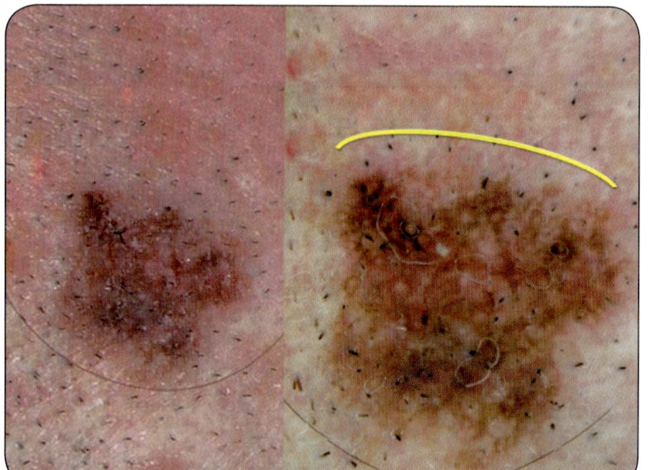

Fig. 6.175: Darkening at dermoscopic examination.

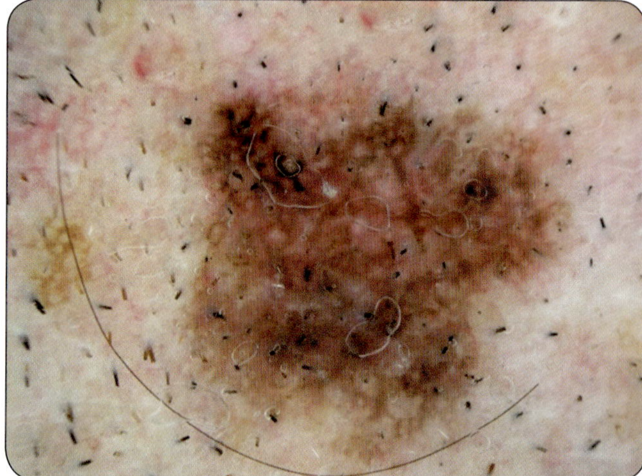

Fig. 6.176: Target-like pattern.

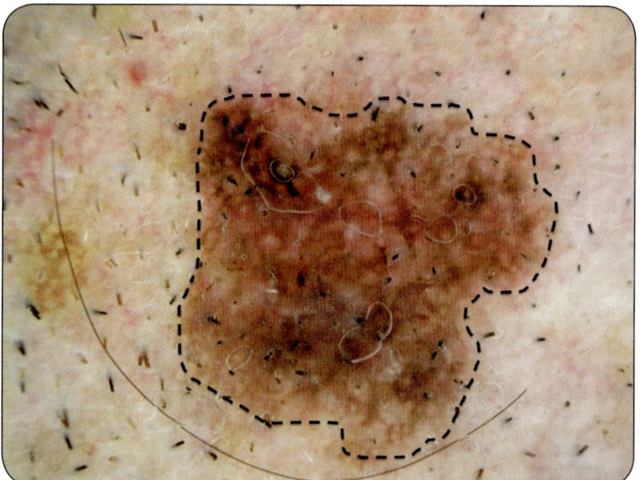

Fig. 6.177: Increased density of the vascular network.

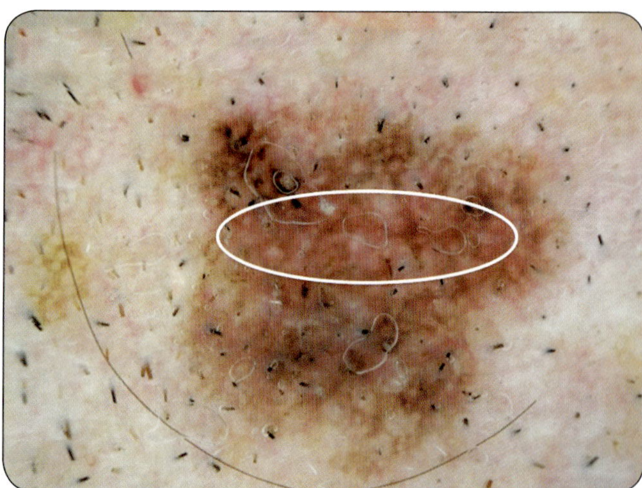

Fig. 6.178: Red rhomboidal structures (white oval).

differentiation may result microscopically difficult, since sun-damaged skin usually presents melanocytic atypia. If in doubt, a biopsy must be performed. All these simulators and malignant lentigo may present asymmetric follicular openings. This crucial fact is highly frequent in malignant lentigo and infrequent in the other lesions.

SUGGESTED READING

Argenziano G, Soyer P, De Giorgio V, et al. Interactive Atlas of Dermoscopy. Milán: EDRA Medical Publishing & New Media; 2000.

Cabo H. Dermatoscopia. Buenos Aires, Argentina: Weber Ferro; 2000.

Cabo H. Dermatoscopia, 2nd edition. Buenos Aires, Argentina: Ediciones Journal; 2012.

Johr R, Stolz W. Dermoscopy: An Illustrated Self-Assessment Guide, 2nd edition. New York: McGraw-Hill Education; 2015.

Jorh R, Soyer P, Argenziano G, et al. Dermoscopy. The Essentials (MOABT). New York: Elsevier Ltd; 2004.

Kittler H. Dermatoscopy. An Algorithmic Method Based on Pattern Analysis. Austria: Facultas.wuv; 2011.

Lallas A. Dermoscopy in general dermatology. Dermatol Clin. 2013;3:679-94.

Malvhey J, Puig S. Principles of Dermoscopy. Barcelona: Creaciones Gráficas; 2009.

Marghoob A, Braun R, Kopf A. Atlas of Dermoscopy. London: Taylor & Francis; 2005.

Menzies S, Crotty K, Ingvar C, et al. An Atlas of Surface Microscopy of Pigmented Skin Lesions. Sydney: McGraw-Hill Book Company; 1996.

Pralong P, Bathelier E, Dalle S, et al. Dermoscopy of lentigo maligna melanoma: report of 125 cases. BJD. 2012;167:280-7.

Rabinovitz H, Kopf A. Dermoscopy: A Practical Guide. Miami: American Academy of Dermatology; 1999.

Soyer P, Argenziano G, Chimenti S, et al. Dermoscopy of Pigmented Skin Lesions. An Atlas Based on the Consensus Net Meeting on Dermoscopy. Milán: EDRA Medical Publishing & New Media; 2001.

Stolz W, Braun-Falco O, Bilek P, et al. Color atlas of Dermatoscopy. Germany: Blackwell Science; 1994.

Tiodorovic-Zivkovic D, Argenziano G, Lallas A, et al. Age, gender, and topography influence the clinical and dermoscopic appearance of lentigo maligna. J Am Acad Dermatol. 2015;72:801-8.

Tschandl P, Rosendahl C, Kittler H. Dermoscopy of flat pigmented facial lesion. JEADV. 2015;29:120-7.

Zalaudek I, Argenziano G, Giacomel J. Dermoscopy of Non-Pigmented Skin Tumors. Boca Raton, FL: CRC Press; 2016.

6.9.4 Acral Melanoma

Horacio A Cabo

Acral melanoma represents 10% of all human melanomas and it is most frequently observed in Asian and black populations. In the past it was believed that melanocytic lesions in acral areas were more dangerous since friction might turn them malignant. For years, nevi were routinely excised under the misconception that they could become melanoma.

Besides, there were mistakes in the interpretation of these lesions, which delayed diagnosis with a worse prognosis and survival prospects, many times also due to inadequate treatment.

Dermoscopy is an extremely useful technique to confirm a suspected melanoma in locations and to distinguish benign lesions, which prevents many unnecessary biopsies.

This chapter specifically refers to localized melanoma in the acral zone, in the volar skin of this particular anatomical area.

Thus, it is necessary to interpret the cutaneous anatomical structure, which differs from that observed in the back of hands and feet. In these cases, the main surface characteristic consists in the presence of dermatoglyphics of furrows and ridges, which are particular to each individual by means of a genetic combination. The skin anatomy shows specific features due to the heightened depth of its corneal layer, the absence of hair follicles, the presence of eccrine glands, and a repetition of crista intermedia and crista limitans (Fig. 6.179).

Characteristically, eccrine glands are located in the crista intermedia; therefore, their eccrine ducts lead to the surface of the ridge (crista superficials).

In the case of benign melanocytic lesions, the nests of nevic cells tend to lie fundamentally in the sulci or furrows. This phenomenon, of unknown origin, gives rise to dermoscopic patterns described in another chapter of this book: parallel furrow-pattern, lattice-like pattern, fibrillar pattern. Benign acral lesions also present other characteristic patterns (globular, homogeneous, and reticular) and finally, an atypical pattern defining those lesions that cannot be classified in the same manner as the previous ones. In the case of localized lesions in the transition area between volar skin and back of hands and feet (Wallace line), a transition pattern can be observed combining benign parallel patterns and pigmented reticule.

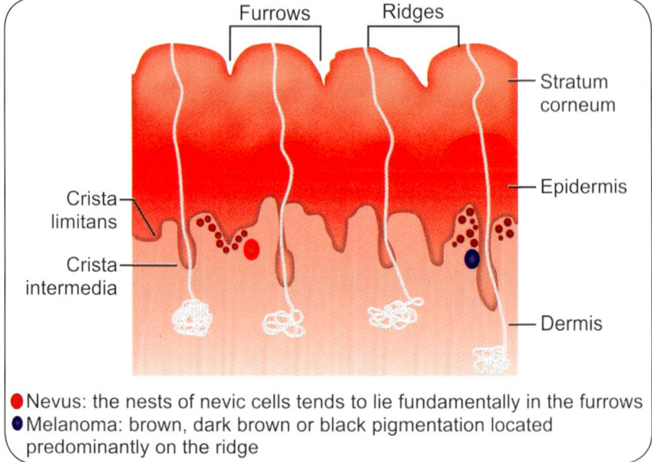

Fig. 6.179: Scheme of the skin anatomy in palms and soles.

Acral Melanoma Dermoscopic Patterns (Figs. 6.180 to 6.192)

- *Parallel ridge pattern*: It has 99% specificity and 86.4% sensitivity. It presents a brown, dark brown, or black pigmentation located predominantly on the ridge. It correlates to the in situ component of acral lentiginous melanoma and therefore may be observed in early lesions or peripheral areas of invasive melanoma.

  Exceptionally, this pigmentation has been described in some benign melanocytic lesion. (Ethnic pigmentation, in Peutz-Jeghers syndrome and subcorneal hemorrhages).
- Diffuse pigmentation with varying coloration
- Irregular and peripheral globules/dots
- Abrupt end of pigmentation at the periphery of the lesion.

In general, the behavior is:

- Typical benign patterns (*see* Chapter 9, part 2): no follow-up
- Parallel ridge pattern: biopsy in order to rule out melanoma
- Atypical pattern without the presence of parallel ridge pattern: follow-up or excision. In order to excise, the following points must be taken into account:
  - Size >7 mm, age, history, recent alterations, and any other data suspicious of melanoma.

Recently, it developed a new algorithm named BRAFF Checklist that significantly improves the diagnostic accuracy of dermoscopy for the diagnosis of acral melanoma.

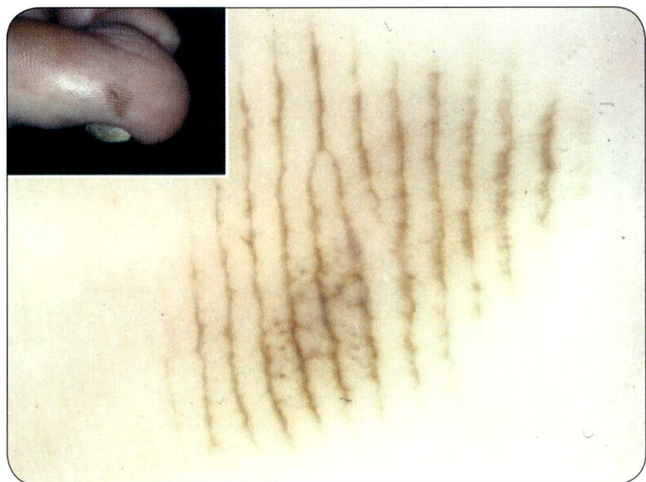

Fig. 6.180: Acral nevus: parallel furrow-pattern.

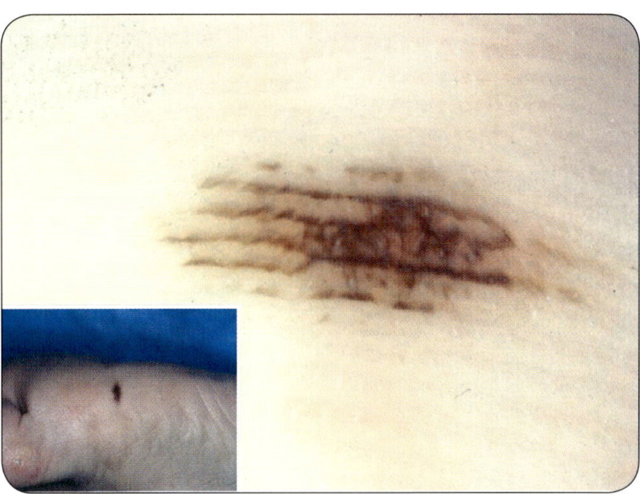

Fig. 6.181: Acral nevus: lattice-like pattern.

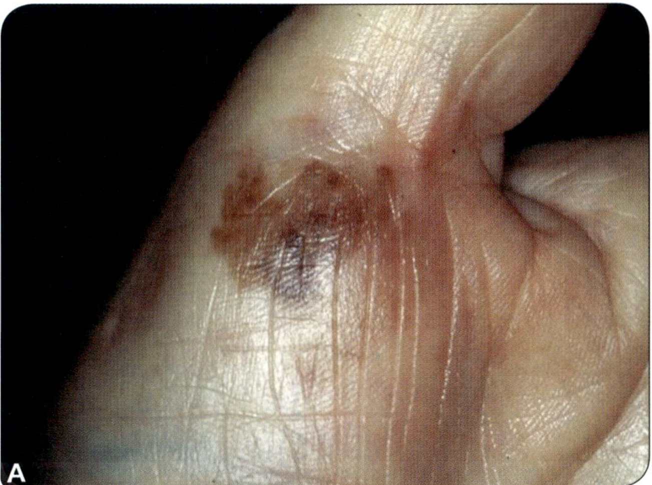

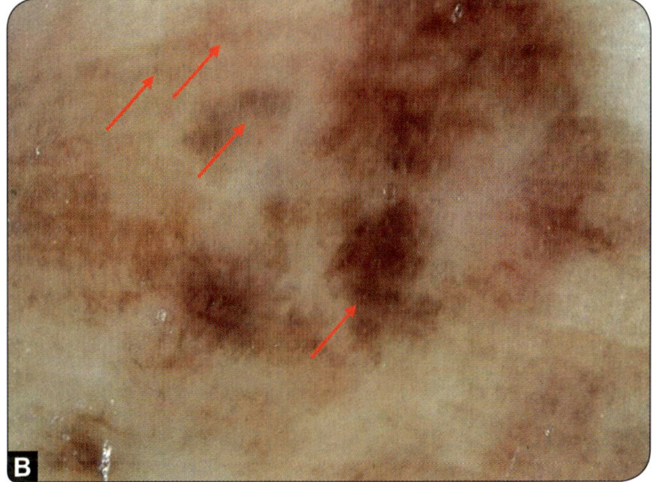

Figs. 6.182A and B: (A) Acral melanoma—clinical view. (B) Acral melanoma: parallel ridge pattern (arrows); diffuse pigmentation with varying coloration.

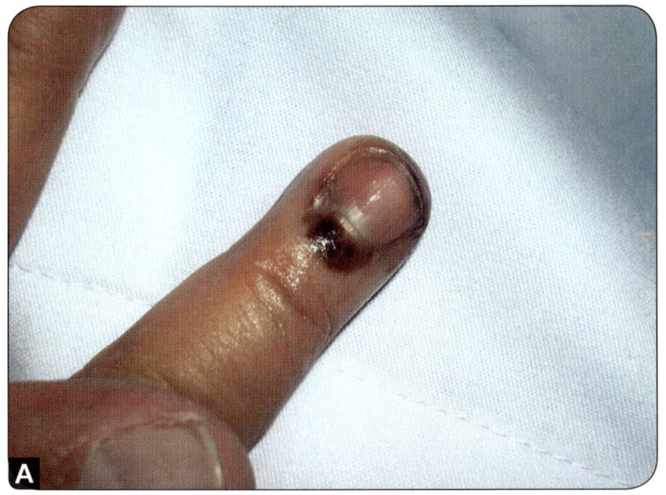

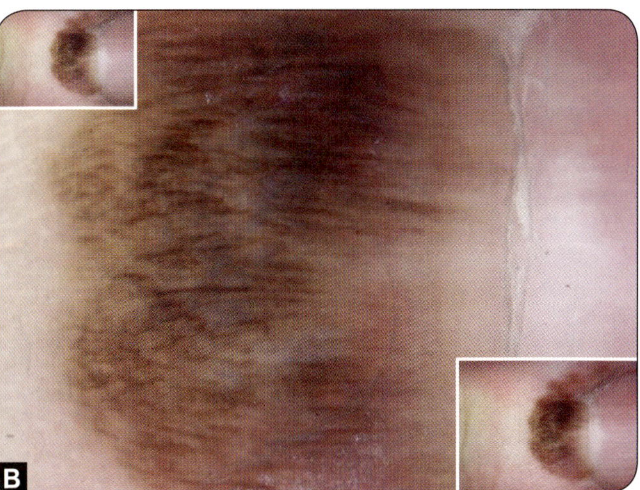

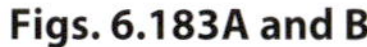

Figs. 6.183A and B

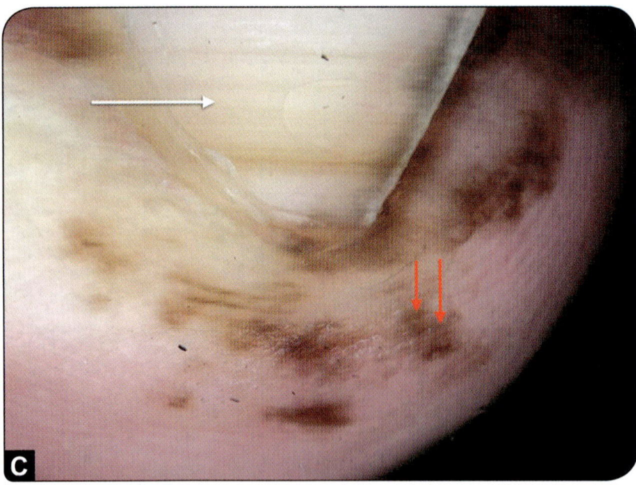

Figs. 6.183A to C: (A) Acral melanoma—clinical view. (B) Acral melanoma: diffuse pigmentation with varying coloration with irregular parallel arrangement. (C) Acral melanoma: irregular pattern of the overlying lines in their thickness, color, and spacing (white arrow); parallel ridge pattern (red arrows).

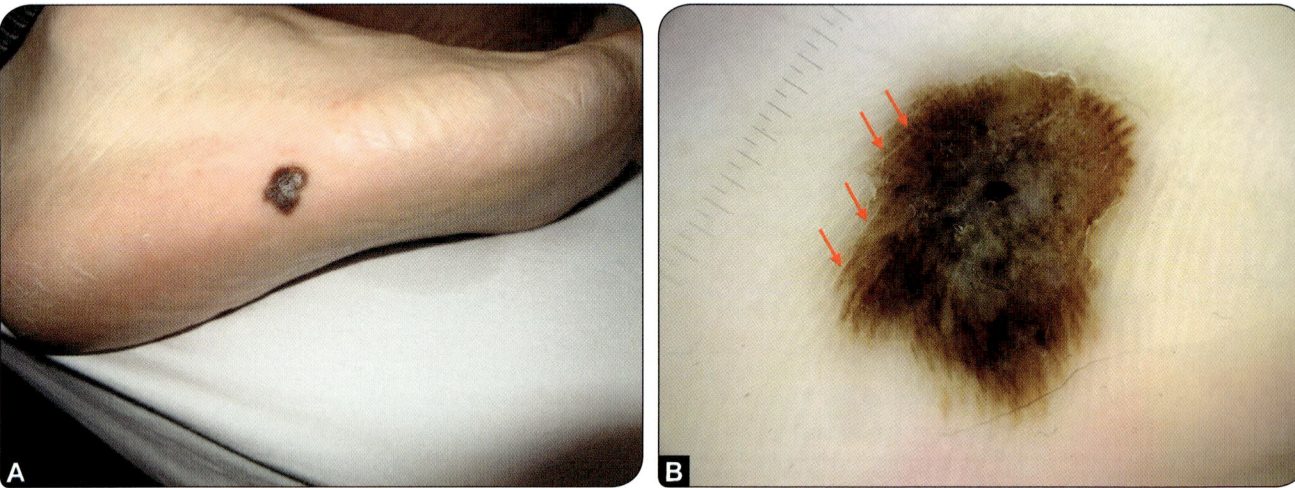

Figs. 6.184A and B: (A) Acral melanoma—clinical view. (B) Acral melanoma—parallel ridge pattern (arrows); diffuse pigmentation with varying coloration.

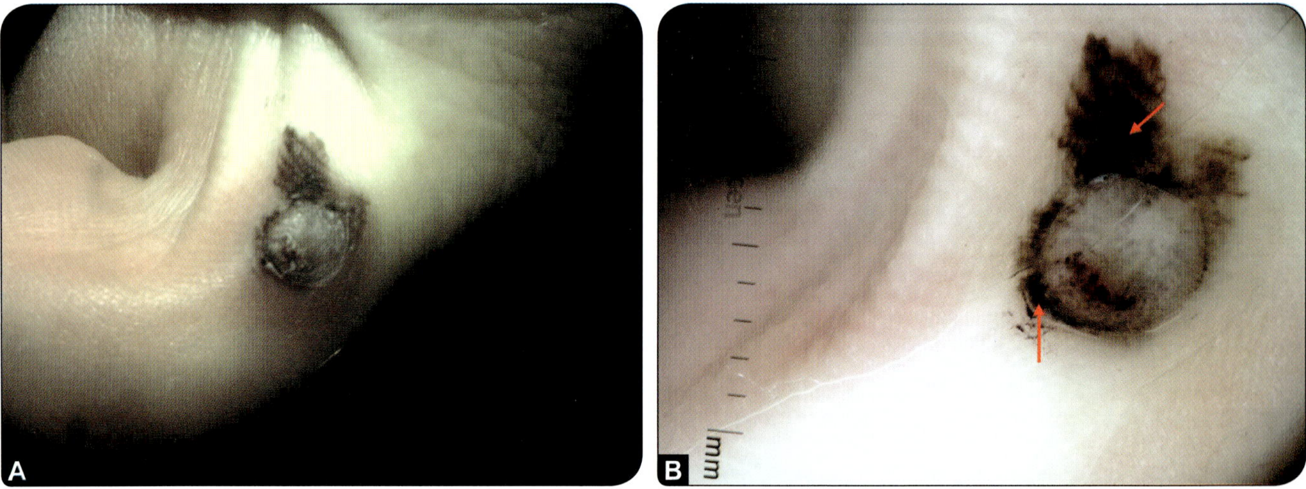

Figs. 6.185A and B: (A) Acral melanoma—clinical view. (B) Acral melanoma—parallel ridge pattern (arrows); diffuse pigmentation with varying coloration.

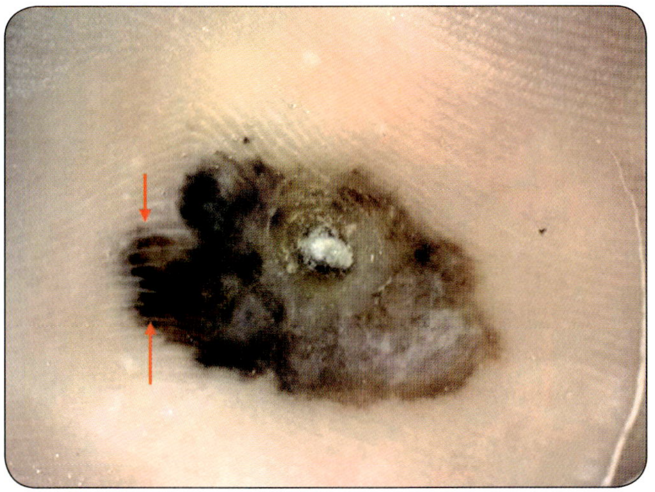

Fig. 6.186: Acral melanoma—parallel ridge pattern (arrows); diffuse pigmentation with varying coloration.

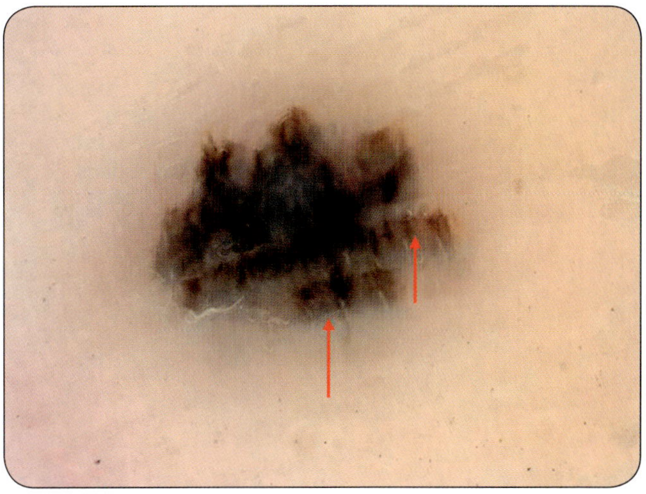

Fig. 6.187: Acral melanoma—parallel ridge pattern (arrows); diffuse pigmentation with varying coloration.

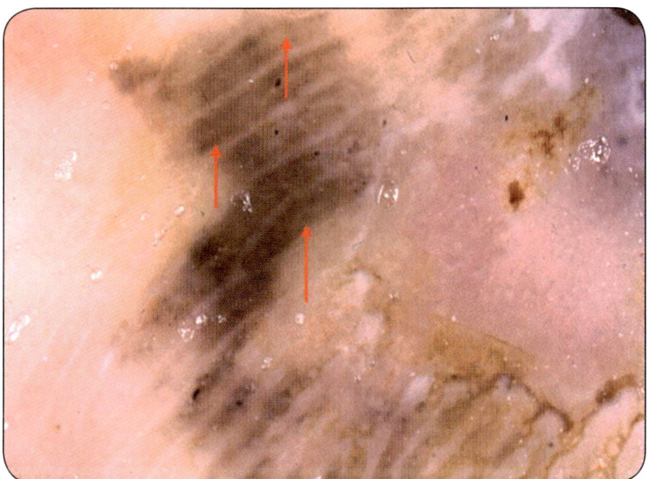

Fig. 6.188: Acral melanoma—parallel ridge pattern (arrows); diffuse pigmentation with varying coloration.

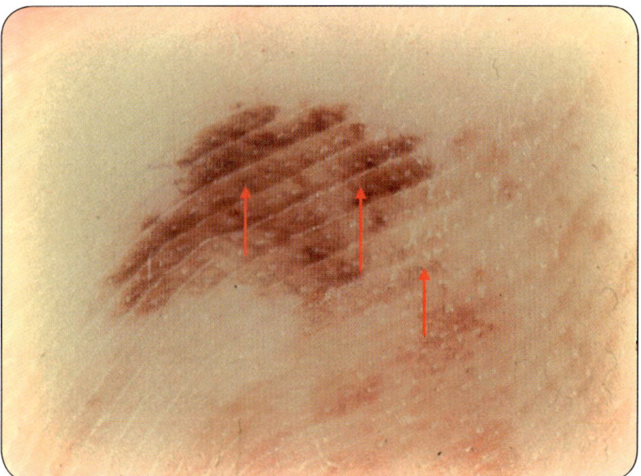

Fig. 6.189: Acral melanoma—parallel ridge pattern (arrows); diffuse pigmentation with varying coloration.

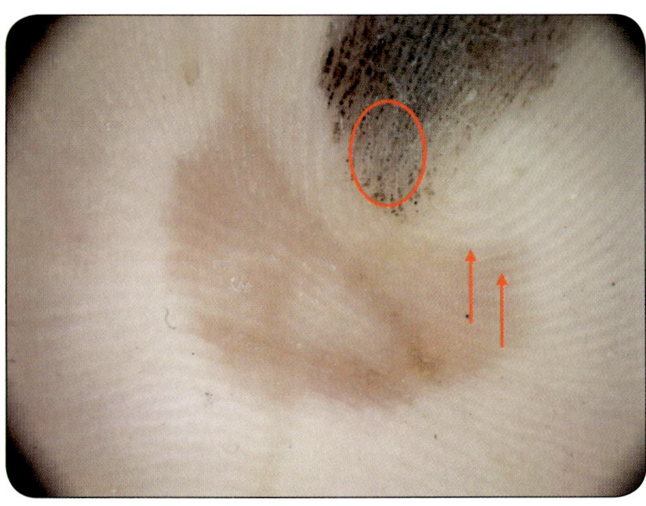

Fig. 6.190: Acral melanoma—parallel ridge pattern (arrows); diffuse pigmentation with varying coloration; irregular and peripheral globules/dots (circle).

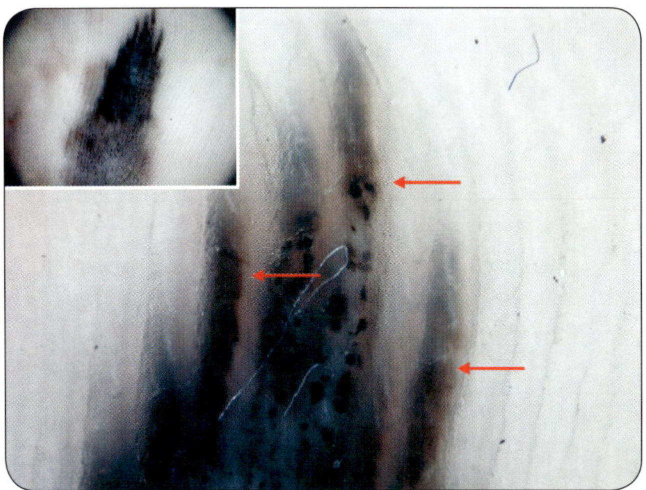

Fig. 6.191: Acral melanoma—parallel ridge pattern (arrows); diffuse pigmentation with varying coloration.

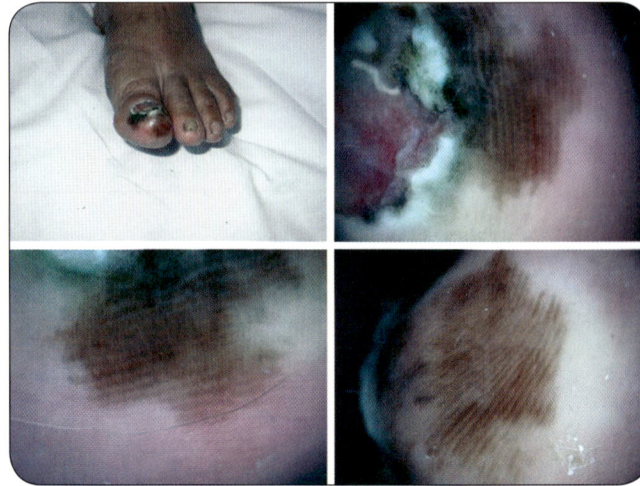

Fig. 6.192: Acral melanoma—parallel ridge pattern; diffuse pigmentation with varying coloration.

BRAAFF checklist includes six variables—four positive and two negative.

Positive predictors:

- Blotches (irregulars)
- Ridge pattern
- Asymmetry of structures
- Asymmetry of colors

Negative predictors:

- Furrow pattern
- Fibrillar pattern

SUGGESTED READING

Argenziano G, Soyer P, De Giorgio V, et al. Interactive Atlas of Dermoscopy. Milán: EDRA Medical Publishing & New Media; 2000.

Cabo H. Dermatoscopia. Buenos Aires, Argentina: Weber Ferro; 2000.

Cabo H. Dermatoscopia, 2nd edition. Buenos Aires, Argentina: Ediciones Journal; 2012.

Johr R, Stolz W. Dermoscopy: An Illustrated Self-Assessment Guide, 2nd edition. New York: McGraw-Hill Education; 2015.

Jorh R, Soyer P, Argenziano G, et al. Dermoscopy. The Essentials (MOABT). New York: Elsevier Ltd; 2004.

Kittler H. Dermatoscopy. An Algorithmic Method Based on Pattern Analysis. Austria: Facultas.wuv; 2011.

Lallas A, Kyrgidis A, Koga H, et al. The BRAAFF checklist: a new dermoscopic algorithm for diagnosing acral melanoma. Br J Dermatol. 2015;173:1041-9.

Lallas A. Dermoscopy in general dermatology. Dermatol Clin. 2013;3:679-94.

Malvhey J, Puig S. Principles of Dermoscopy. Barcelona: Creaciones Gráficas; 2009.

Marghoob A, Braun R, Kopf A. Atlas of Dermoscopy. London: Taylor & Francis; 2005.

Menzies S, Crotty K, Ingvar C, et al. An Atlas of Surface Microscopy of Pigmented Skin Lesions. Sydney: McGraw-Hill Book Company; 1996.

Rabinovitz H, Kopf A. Dermoscopy: A Practical Guide. Miami: American Academy of Dermatology; 1999.

Soyer P, Argenziano G, Chimenti S, et al. Dermoscopy of Pigmented Skin Lesions. An Atlas Based on the Consensus Net Meeting on Dermoscopy. Milán: EDRA Medical Publishing & New Media; 2001.

Stolz W, Braun-Falco O, Bilek P, et al. Color Atlas of Dermatoscopy. Germany: Blackwell Science; 1994.

Zalaudek I, Argenziano G, Giacomel J. Dermoscopy of Non-Pigmented Skin Tumors. Boca Raton, FL: CRC Press; 2016

6.9.5 Amelanotic Melanoma

Horacio A Cabo

A low percentage of cutaneous melanomas (>2%) show no pigmentation under clinical examination (amelanotic). These are frequently metastatic melanomas. Many amelanotic primary cutaneous melanomas are nodular. In these cases, we do not use the clinical ABCD rule, but the clinical EFG rule instead (elevated—firm—growing). This is generally a clinical issue rather than a histologic one, since histologically it is usual to find melanin evidence. Thus, the diagnosis difficulty lies on the clinical dermatologist, not the pathologist.

In cutaneous primary melanomas, clinical classification does not exactly correlate with dermoscopic observation, as this technique permits the observation of colors and structures not visible with the naked eye.

The dermoscopic classification of amelanotic melanomas is different since some of them present pigmentation traces and it is preferable to call them amelanotic/hypomelanotic.

Dermoscopic Classification of Amelanotic/Hypomelanotic Melanoma (Figs. 6.193 to 6.209)

- *Amelanotic melanoma*: No color derived from melanin pigment (light brown, dark brown, blue, gray, or black) is observed under the dermoscopic examination.
- ***Hypopigmented melanoma***:
  - *Lightly pigmented melanoma*: It presents light brown, pale blue, or pale gray pigmentation that may cover >25% of the total surface area, but no evidence of dark brown, deep blue, or black coloration.
  - *Partially pigmented melanoma*: Under dermoscopic examination, the melanin pigment is observable in <25% of the total tumor surface. In highly pigmented areas of the partially pigmented melanoma, it is possible to find other classical pigmented dermoscopic features of melanoma.
- *Melanoma with regression*: When the amelanosis in a melanoma is the result of regression, it is possible to visualize the classical dermoscopic features of scar-like depigmentation [white areas (fibrosis) and blue areas (melanosis)].

Dermoscopic Features of Amelanotic/Hypomelanotic

Under dermoscopic examination it is possible to observe:

- ***Pigment traces***
- ***Vascular structures within the amelanotic/hypomelanotic area:***
  - *Dotted vessels*: These are indicative of melanocytic tumors, with 90% positive predictive value (i.e. probability) that a lesion presenting such vessels should be melanocytic.
  - *Irregular lineal vessels*: They have 68% predictive value in melanoma diagnosis. They are a significant feature in thin melanomas (> 1 mm Breslow thickness) compared to benign melanocytic lesions, with 19% sensitivity and 199% specificity in melanoma diagnosis.
  - *Pink areas or globules (milky-red areas) (Figs. 6.199B and 6.200B)*: They present a blurred border as opposed to the highly demarcated and well-circumscribed borders of the hemangioma red lacunes. The milky-red globules and milky-red areas (larger in size) have a 78% prognostic predictive value in the melanoma diagnosis.
  - *Hairpin vessels (Figs. 6.194C and 6.201B)*: These are common in seborrheic keratosis but can also be found in amelanotic melanoma, particularly in the thick one.
  - ***Halo melanoma***: Asymmetrical white halo in a lesion with dermoscopic features of melanoma.

Recently, a diagnostic algorithms have been developed based on conclusions from the study of amelanotic and hypomelanotic melanoma to help detect this type of melanomas.

Diagnostic Algorithms of Amelanotic Melanoma

- Negative characteristic (must not be present)
  - More than three milia-like pseudocysts
- Positive characteristics (at least one must be present)
  - Brown dots and globules with irregular size and distribution
  - Multiple blue-gray dots
  - Blue-white veil
  - Irregular depigmentation
  - More than one shade of pink
  - Predominantly central vessels
  - Dotted vessels and irregular vessels.

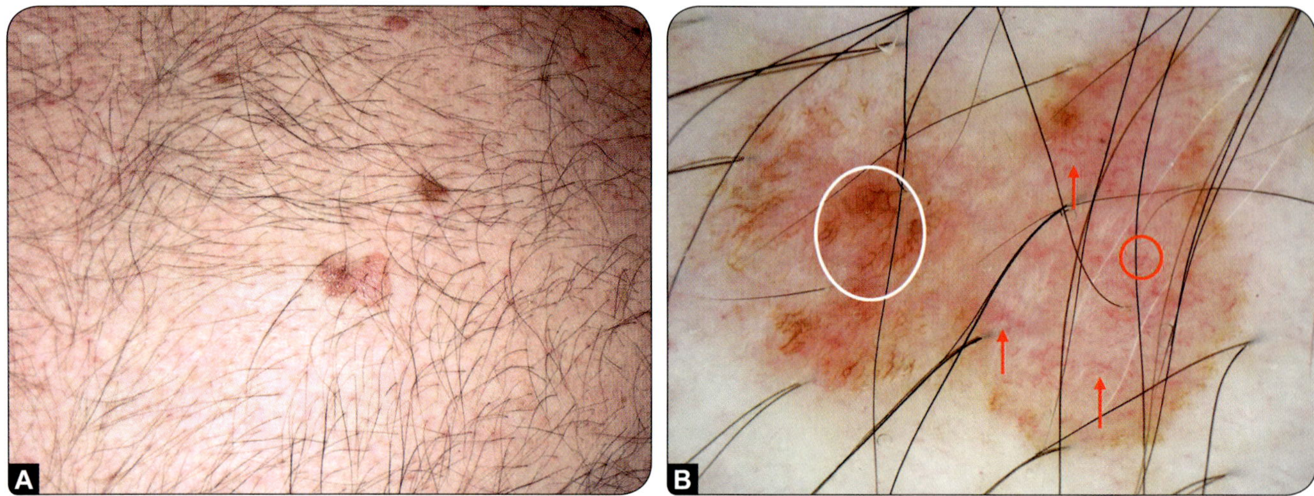

Figs. 6.193A and B: Hypomelanotic melanoma in situ (partially pigmented melanoma): (A) Clinical view. (B) Light brown reticular pigmentation (white circle); dotted vessels (red circle); irregular lineal vessels (red arrows).

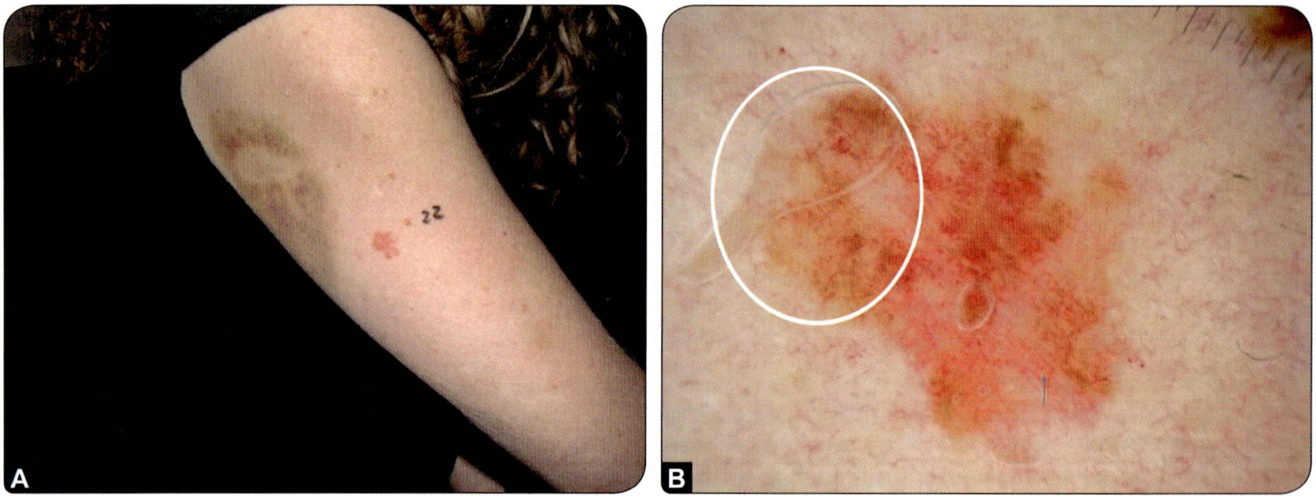

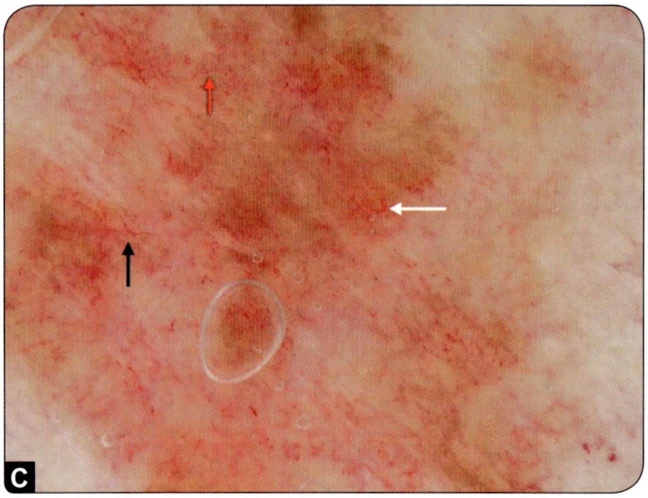

Figs. 6.194A to C: Hypomelanotic melanoma in situ (partially pigmented melanoma): (A) Clinical view. (B) Light brown pigmentation (white circle); dotted and irregular lineal vessels in the area without pigmentation. (C) Close-up Figure 6.194B—dotted vessels (red arrow); irregular lineal vessels (black arrow); hairpin vessels (white arrow).

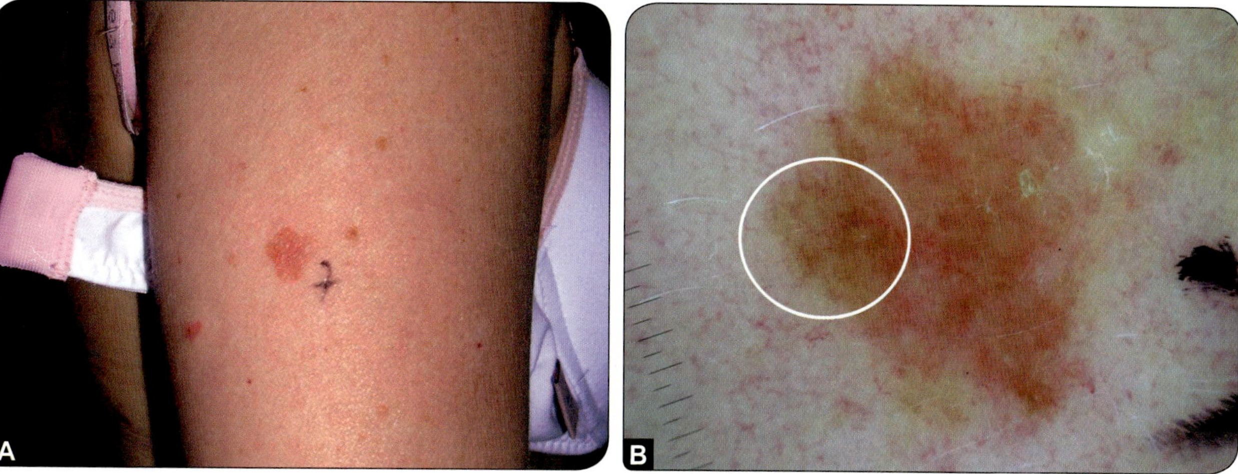

Figs. 6.195A and B: Hypomelanotic melanoma in situ (partially pigmented melanoma): (A) Clinical view. (B) Light brown pigmentation (white circle); dotted and irregular lineal vessels in the area without pigmentation.

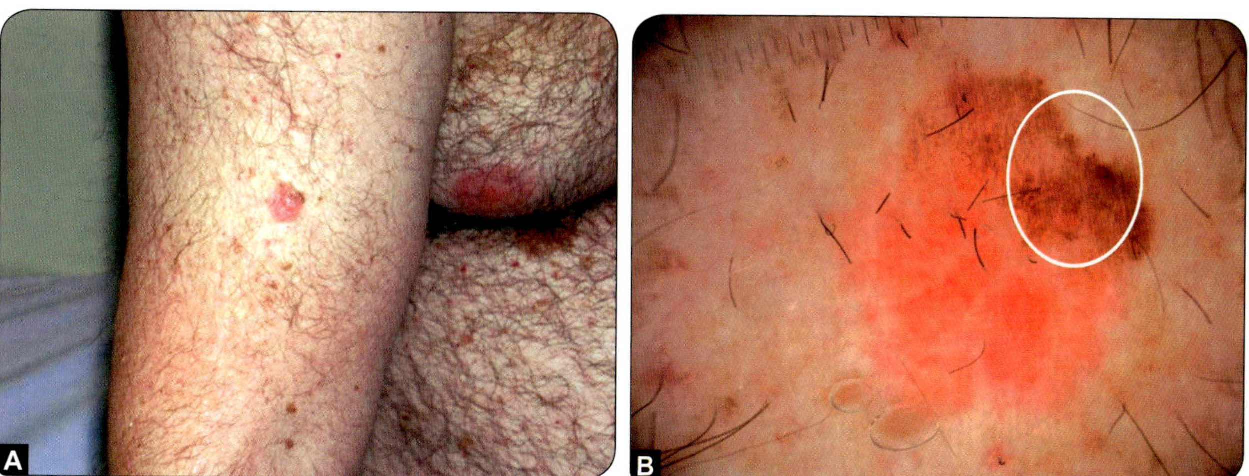

Figs. 6.196A and B: Hypomelanotic melanoma in situ (partially pigmented melanoma): (A) Clinical view. (B) Light brown reticular pigmentation (white circle); dotted and irregular lineal vessels in the area without pigmentation.

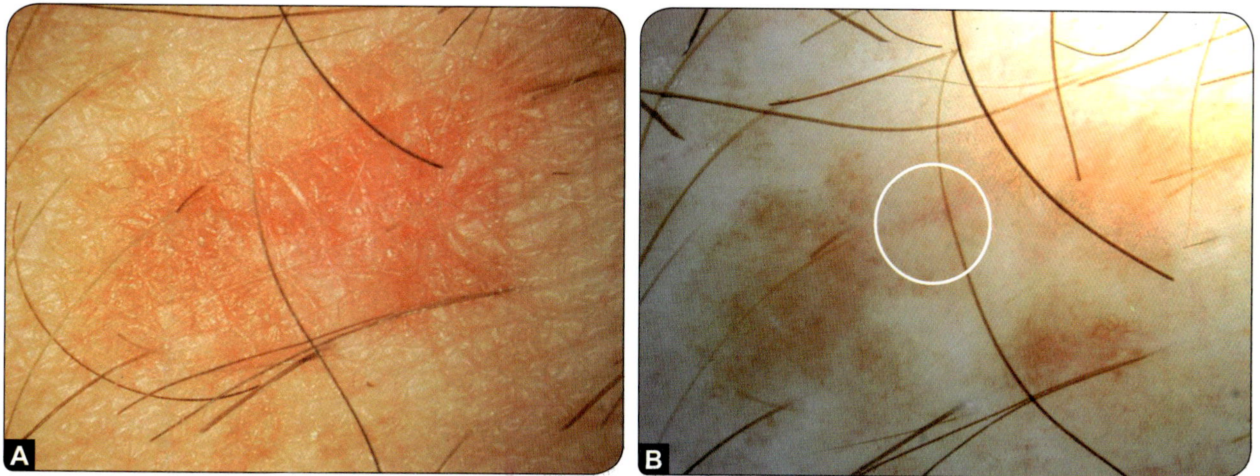

Figs. 6.197A and B: Hypomelanotic melanoma in situ (partially pigmented melanoma): (A) Clinical view. (B) Light brown pigmentation and irregular lineal vessels in the area without pigmentation (white circle). This image was taken with nonpolarized dermoscopy.

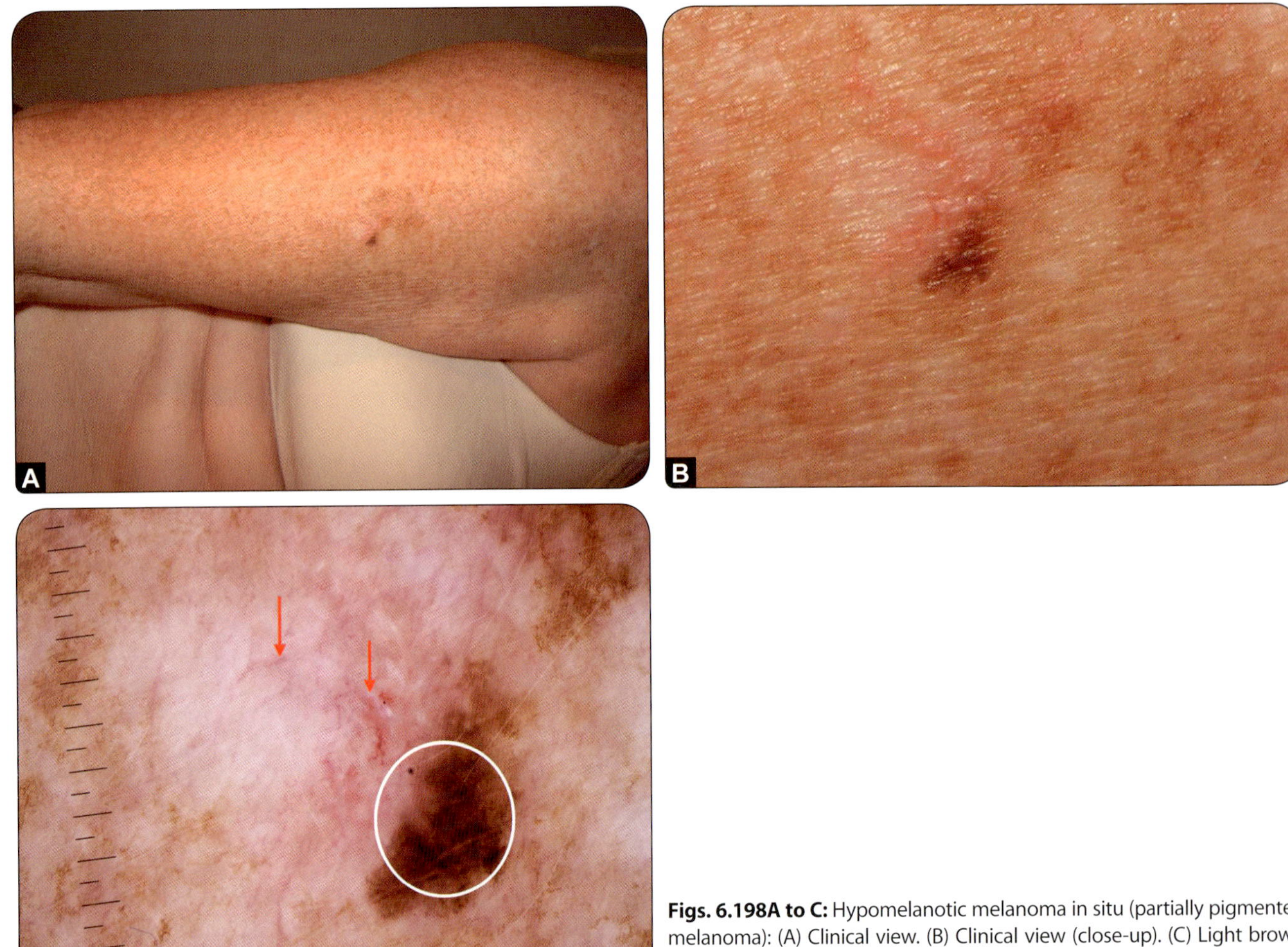

Figs. 6.198A to C: Hypomelanotic melanoma in situ (partially pigmented melanoma): (A) Clinical view. (B) Clinical view (close-up). (C) Light brown reticular pigmentation (white circle); irregular lineal vessels (red arrows).

Figs. 6.199A and B: Hypomelanotic melanoma in situ (partially pigmented melanoma): (A) Clinical view. (B) Light brown reticular pigmentation (white circle); irregular lineal vessels (red arrow); pink areas (milky-red areas) (black arrow).

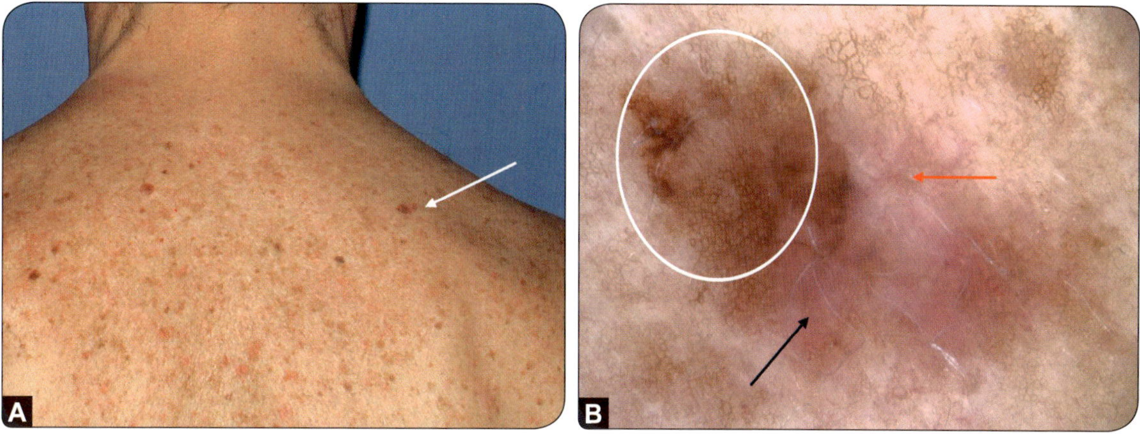

Figs. 6.200A and B: (A) Hypomelanotic melanoma in situ (lightly pigmented melanoma) clinical view (white arrow). (B) Hypomelanotic melanoma—superficial spreading melanoma B 0.3 mm (lightly pigmented melanoma) light brown reticular pigmentation (white circle); irregular lineal vessels (red arrow); pink areas (milky-red areas) (black arrow).

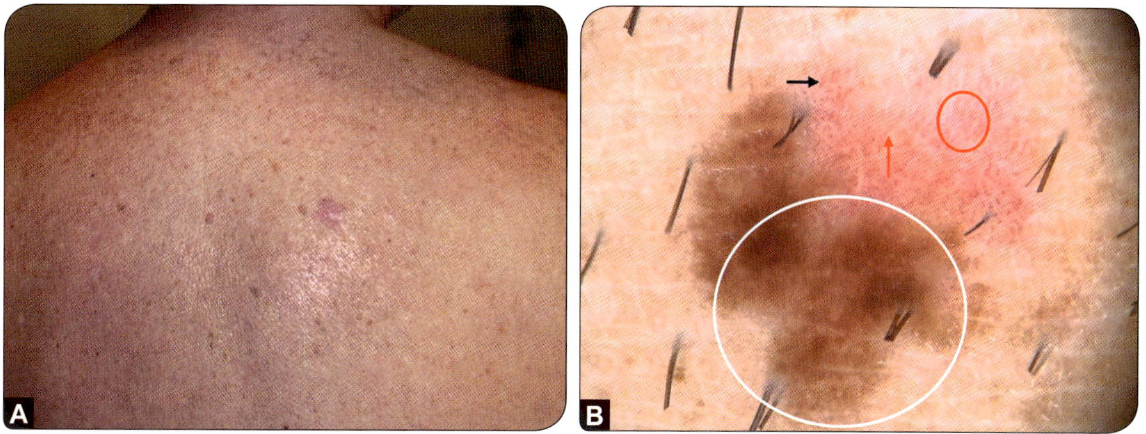

Figs. 6.201A and B: (A) Hypomelanotic melanoma in situ (lightly pigmented melanoma) clinical view. (B) Hypomelanotic melanoma—superficial spreading melanoma B 0.3 mm (lightly pigmented melanoma) light brown reticular pigmentation (white circle); irregular lineal vessels (red arrow); hairpin vessels (black arrow); dotted vessels (red circle).

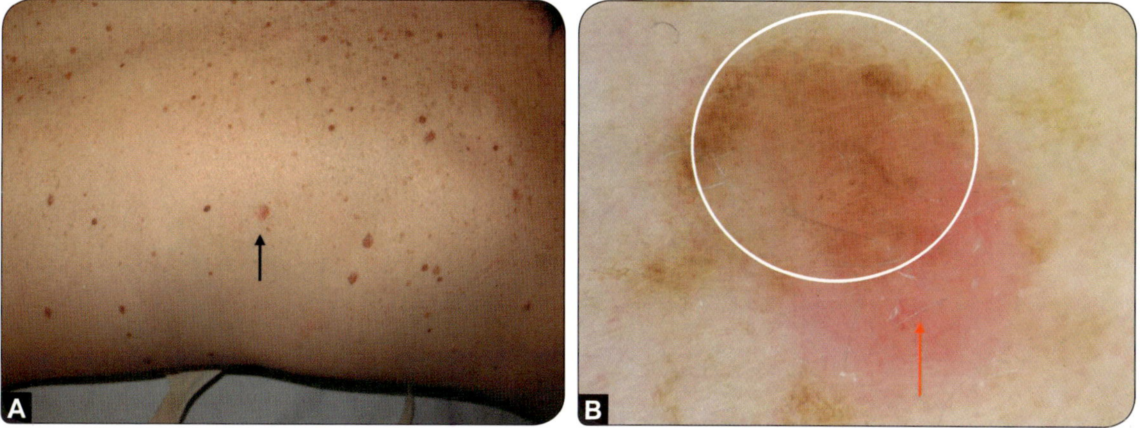

Figs. 6.202A and B: (A) Hypomelanotic melanoma in situ (lightly pigmented melanoma) clinical view (black arrow). (B) Hypomelanotic melanoma—superficial spreading melanoma B 0.3 mm (lightly pigmented melanoma) light brown reticular pigmentation (white circle); irregular lineal vessels (red arrow).

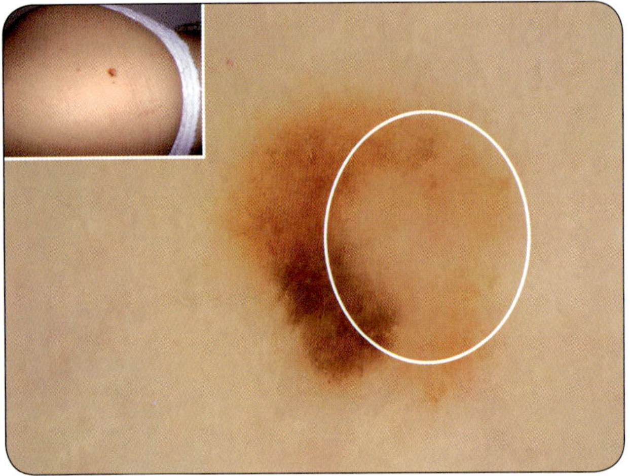

Fig. 6.203: Melanoma in situ with a large area of regression (white circle).

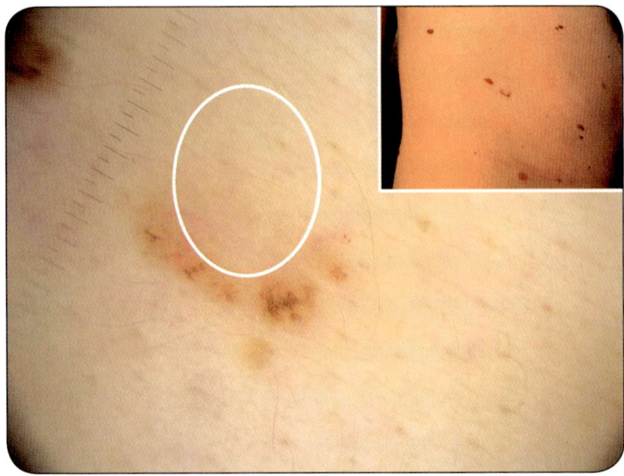

Fig. 6.204: Melanoma in situ with a large area of regression (white circle).

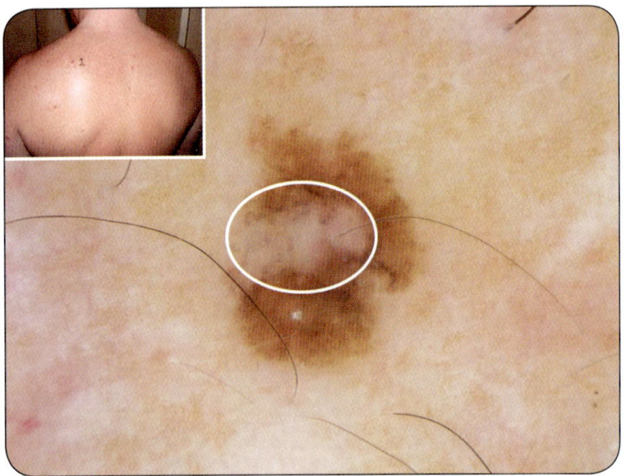

Fig. 6.205: Melanoma in situ with a large area of regression (white circle).

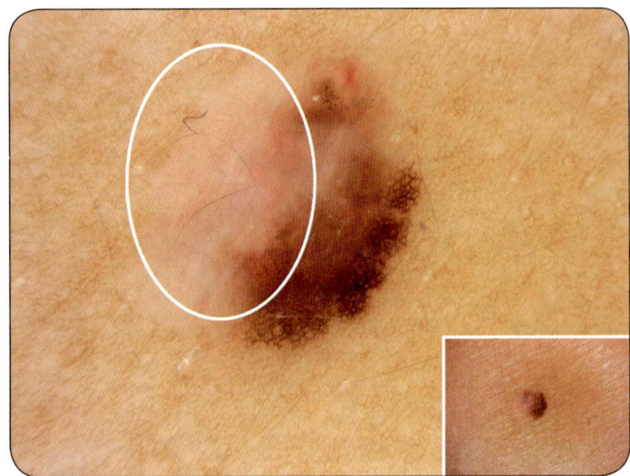

Fig. 6.206: Melanoma in situ with a large area of regression (white circle).

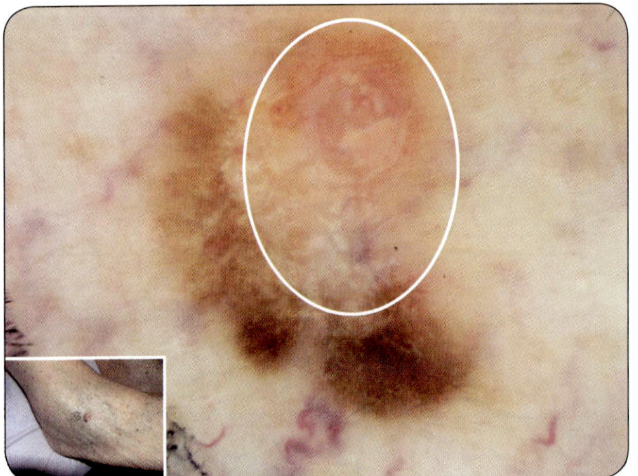

Fig. 6.207: Superficial spreading melanoma with a large area of regression (white circle).

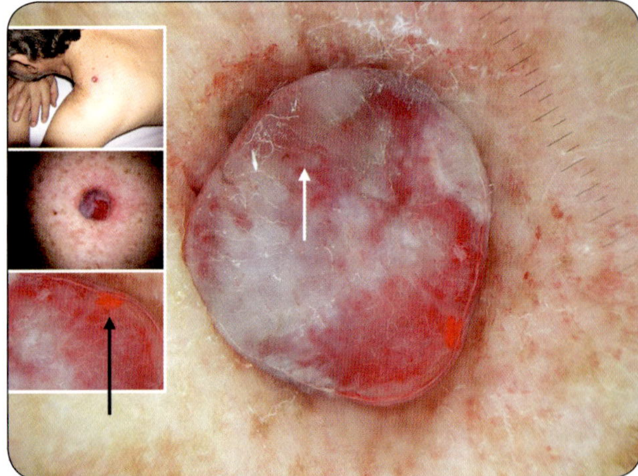

Fig. 6.208: Amelanotic nodular melanoma. Irregular lineal vessels (white arrow); pink areas (milky-red areas) (black arrow).

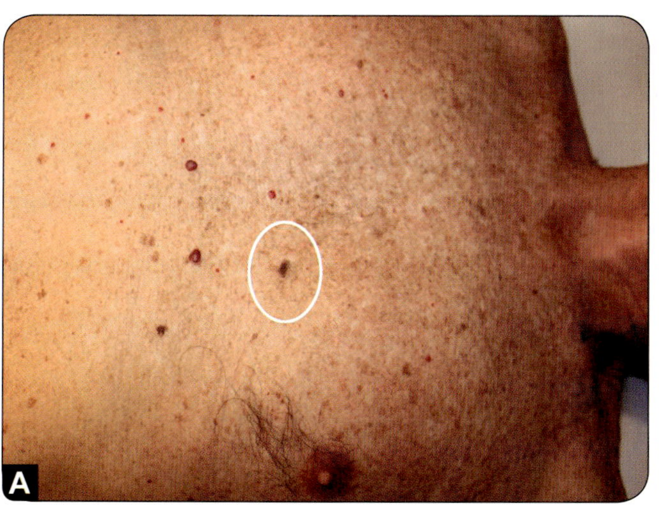

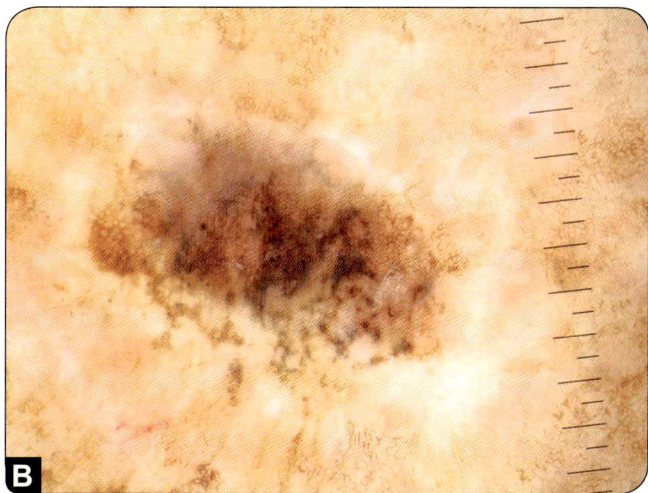

Figs. 6.209A and B: Superficial spreading melanoma B 0.6 with white halo: (A) Clinical view (white circle); (B) dermoscopy view.

SUGGESTED READING

Argenziano G, Soyer P, De Giorgio V, et al. Interactive Atlas of Dermoscopy. Milán: EDRA Medical Publishing & New Media; 2000.

Cabo H. Dermatoscopia, 2nd edition. Buenos Aires, Argentina: Ediciones Journal; 2012.

Johr R, Stolz W. Dermoscopy: An Illustrated Self-Assessment Guide, 2nd edition. New York: McGraw-Hill Education; 2015.

Johr R, Stolz W. Dermoscopy: An Illustrated Self-Assessment Guide, 2nd edition. McGraw-Hill Education; 2015

Kittler H. Dermatoscopy. An Algorithmic Method Based on Pattern Analysis. Austria: Facultas.wuv; 2011.

Lallas A. Dermoscopy in general dermatology. Dermatol Clin. 2013;3:679-94.

Malvhey J, Puig S. Principles of Dermoscopy. Barcelona: Creaciones Gráficas; 2009.

Marghoob A, Braun R, Kopf A. Atlas of Dermoscopy. London: Taylor & Francis; 2005.

Menzies S, Crotty K, Ingvar C, et al. An Atlas of Surface Microscopy of Pigmented Skin Lesions. Sydney: McGraw-Hill Book Company; 1996.

Menzies SW, Kreusch J, Byth K, et al. Dermoscopic evaluation of amelanotic and hypomelanotic melanoma. Arch Dermatol. 2008;144(9):1120-7.

Pizzichetta MA, Talamini R, Stanganelli I, et al. Amelanotic/hypomelanotic melanoma: clinical and dermoscopic features. Br J Dermatol. 2004;150:1117-24.

Rabinovitz H, Kopf A. Dermoscopy: A Practical Guide. Miami: American Academy of Dermatology; 1999.

Soyer P, Argenziano G, Chimenti S, et al. Dermoscopy of Pigmented Skin Lesions. An Atlas Based on the Consensus Net Meeting on Dermoscopy. Milán: EDRA Medical Publishing & New Media; 2001.

Stojkovic-Filipovic J, Kittler H. Dermatoscopy of amelanotic and hypomelanotic melanoma. JDDG. 2014;12(6):467-72.

Stolz W, Braun-Falco O, Bilek P, et al. Color atlas of Dermatoscopy. Germany: Blackwell Science; 1994.

Zalaudek I, Argenziano G, Kerl H, et al. Amelanotic/hypomelanotic melanoma: is dermatoscopy useful for diagnosis? J Deuts Dermatol Ges. 2003;1:369-73.

Zalaudek I, Argenziano G, Giacomel J. Dermoscopy of Nonpigmented Skin Tumors. Boca Raton, FL: CRC Press; 2016.

6.9.6 Dermoscopy Approach in Patients with Multiple Nevi

Horacio A Cabo

At present it is very common to receive patients who want to have their nevi (N) checked. On occasion we see patients who are deeply concerned about their N, but under examination are found to have almost none. They are low-risk patients and we generally check them less frequently. Since it may happen that a patient with few or without any N could present a melanoma (M) we check them anyway (Figs. 6.210 and 6.211).

But the case that most concerns dermatologists is that of patients with a high M risk. Among these risks, presenting multiple N is a very important factor (Figs. 6.212 and 6.213).

In relation to M detection in these patients, dermoscopy (Fig. 6.214):

- Has been proven to reduce the number of biopsies and unnecessary excisions by 40% depending on the experience of the observer.
- Decreases the benign/malignant ratio of excised lesions; this expresses how many benign lesions are necessary to excise in order to detect an M. In predermoscopic era this ratio was 18/1 and it has decreased to 4/1 in dermoscopic era.
- Has improved the sensitivity and, to a lesser extent, the specificity; sensibility refers to the capacity to detect M, while specificity refers to the capacity to detect non-M. In the formula of specificity are the false positives, which are mostly atypical N and may be confused with M, even under dermoscopic examination.
- This is the reason for the improved specificity, whereas the sensitivity shows a more moderate improvement (Figs. 6.215 to 6.218).

The fact is that the decrease in the number of biopsies, the fall in the benign/malignant relationship, and the improvement in sensitivity and specificity have been reached by studying individual lesions, but not in the context of patients with multiple N (Fig. 6.219).

What Can We Do? (Figs. 6.220 to 6.223)

It is also useless in the case of these patients to ***perform multiple excisions***, since the great majority of the excised lesions are N and not M. The ***clinical ABCD rule*** is not helpful in small lesions. And finally, ***just dermoscopy is not enough*** because many benign lesions in patients with multiple N present irregular dermoscopic patterns, which means that many unnecessary excisions are still performed.

So, What Can We Do? (Figs. 6.224 and 6.225)

It is therefore necessary to have a more reliable detection strategy than just the clinical and dermoscopic ones and the option is the ***comparative approach*** in which individual lesions are evaluated in the context of the patient's general N profile.

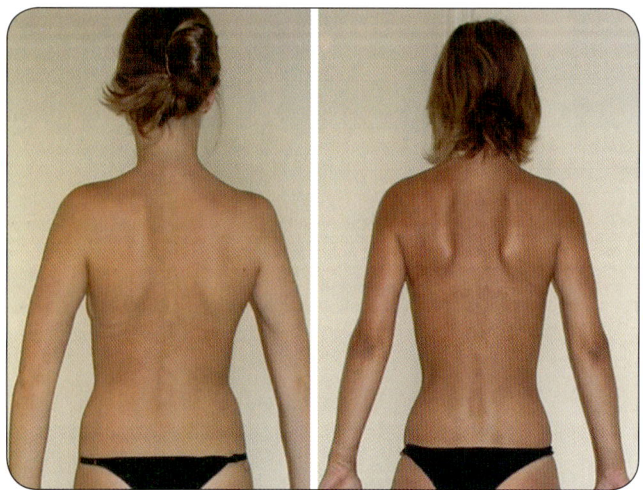

Fig. 6.210: Low-risk patients.

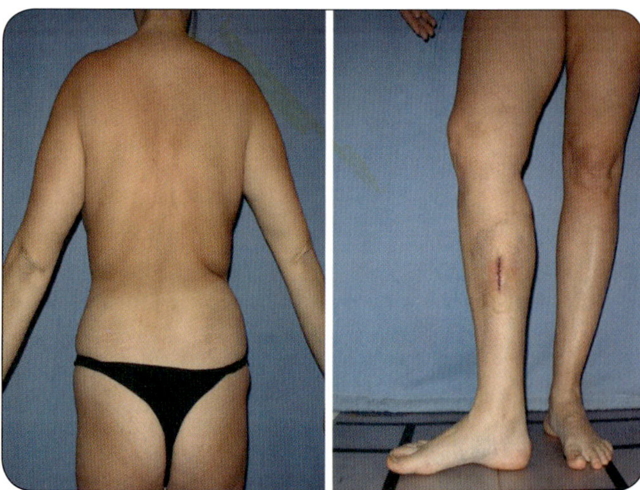

Fig. 6.211: Low-risk patients with very few nevi underwent a melanoma excision from the right leg.

High-risk patients

- Skin phototype I-II
- Blue or green eyes
- Freckles
- History of solar burns
- > 10 dysplastic nevi
- > 100 nevi (3-16)
- Family history of melanoma
- Previous melanoma
- Familial melanoma

Fig. 6.212: Clinical features of high-risk patients.

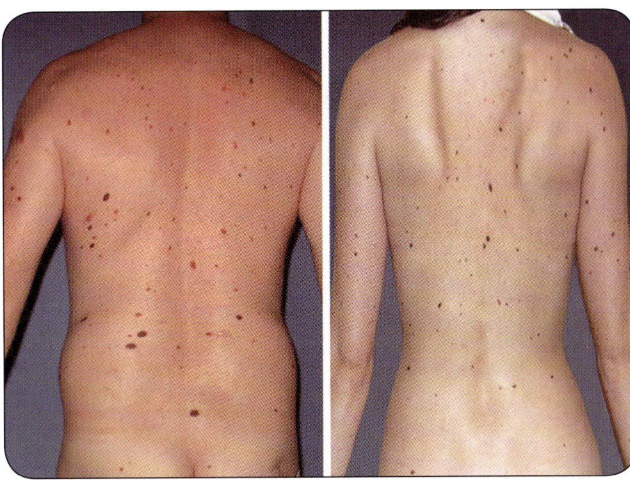

Fig. 6.213: High-risk patients with multiple nevi.

Dermoscopy approach in patients with multiple nevi

- **Dermoscopy**
  - Has been proved to reduce the number of skin biopsies and unnecessary excisions
  - Reduces the benign—malignant ratio for excised lesions
    - Pre-dermoscopy era 18:1
    - > Dermoscopy era 4:1
  - Improves the sensitivity and (to a lower extent) Specificity

Fig. 6.214: Usefulness of dermoscopy in melanoma detection.

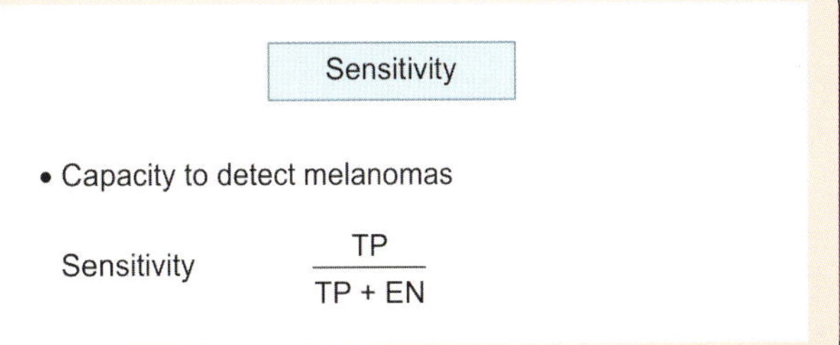

Fig. 6.215: Sensitivity refers to the capacity to detect melanoma.

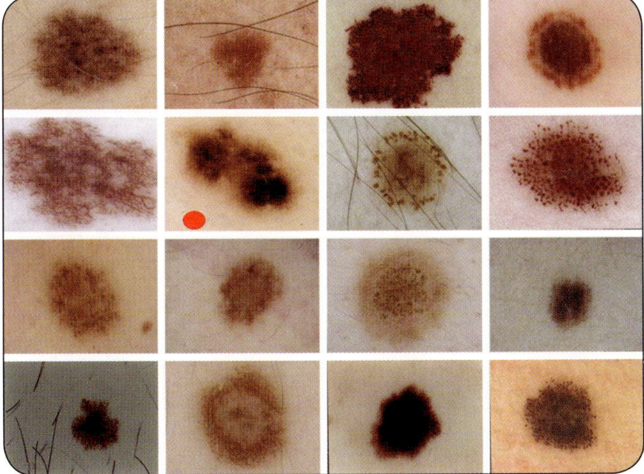

Fig. 6.216: Sensitivity refers to the capacity to detect melanoma. In these examples, the melanoma is quickly identified (red dot).

Specificity

- Capacity to detect nonmelanomas

Sensitivity $\frac{TP}{TP + EN}$

- False positive
  - Lesions clinically diagnosed as melanoma but found to be nevi under histopathological examination

Fig. 6.217: Specificity refers to the capacity to detect nonmelanomas.

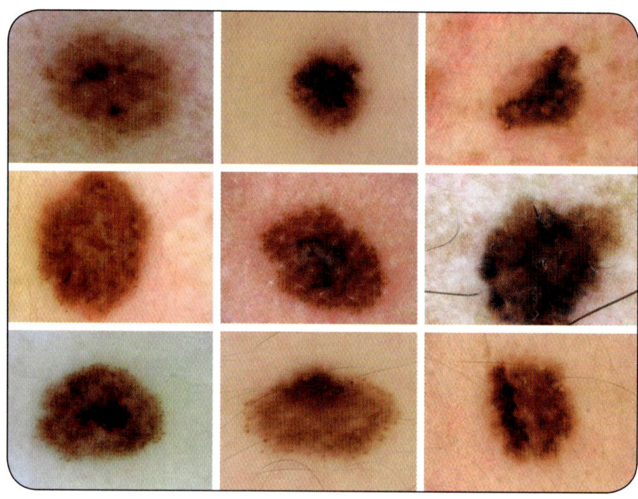

Fig. 6.218: Specificity refers to the capacity to detect nonmelanomas. In this example it is very difficult to distinguish which is the melanoma. In fact, any of them could be it since nevi with severe dysplasia are almost indistinguishable from melanoma in situ.

- Dermoscopy
  - Has been proved to reduce the number of skin biopsies and unnecessary excisions
  - Reduces the benign—malignant ratio for excised lesions
  - Improves the sensitivity and (to a lower extent) specificity
  - *These studies were performed evaluating individual lesions*

Fig. 6.219: The decrease in the number of biopsies, the fall in the benign/malignant relationship and the improvement in sensitivity and specificity has been reached by studying individual lesions.

Dermoscopy approach in patients with multiple nevi

What can we do?

- *Biopsies and excisions* of clinically suspicious lesions
- *Clinical ABCD rule*
- *Dermoscopy*

Fig. 6.220: Different strategies in patients with multiple nevi.

Dermoscopy approach in patients with multiple nevi

- *Biopsies and excisions* of clinically suspicious lesions—most are benign (false positives)
  - This is not useful because there are patients with multiple atypical lesions

A

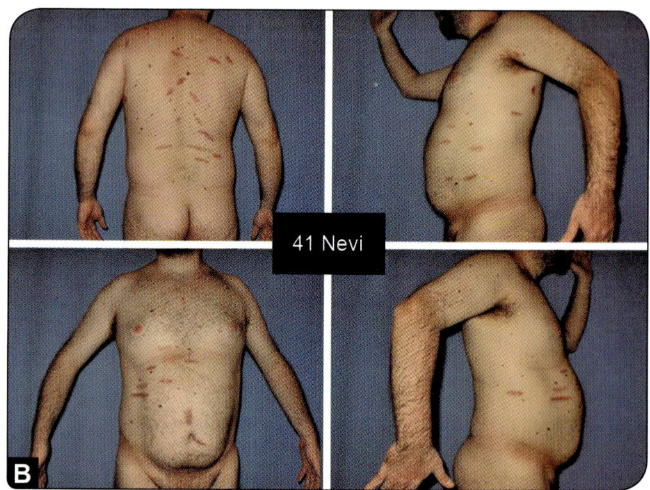

Figs. 6.221A and B

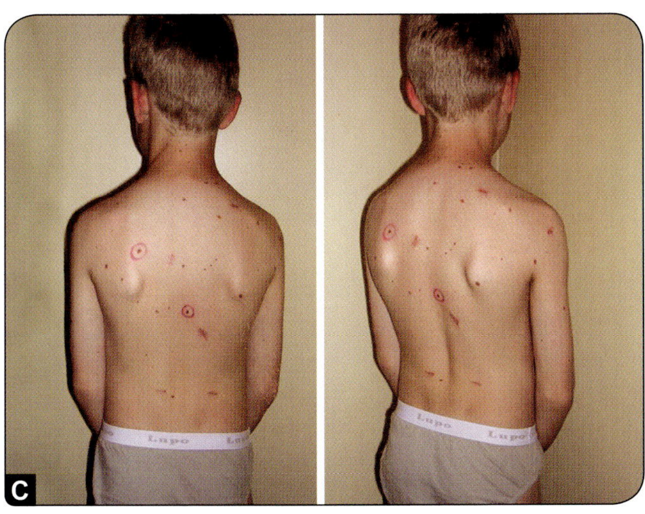

Figs. 6.221A to C: (A) Dermoscopy approach in patients with multiple nevi: biopsies and excisions. (B) Dermoscopy approach in patients (56-year-old) with multiple nevi: biopsies and excisions—this is an example of what not to do. (C) Dermoscopy approach in patients (11-year-old) with multiple nevi: biopsies and excisions—this is an example of what not to do.

Dermoscopy approach in patients with multiple nevi

- *Clinical ABCD rule*: *not useful* for these patients since many of the bening lesions are ABCD positive

?

ABCD rule

(a) (b)

Figs. 6.222A and B: (A) Dermoscopy approach in patients with multiple nevi: usefulness of clinical ABCD rule. (B) Dermoscopy approach in patients with multiple nevi: Nevus or melanoma? The clinical ABCD rule is not helpful in small lesions (b is melanoma).

Dermoscopy approach in patients with multiple nevi

Dermoscopy:

- Many *benign* lesions in patients with multiple nevi present *irregular dermoscopic* patterns
- So, there are still many unnecessary biopsies and excisions performed

Fig. 6.223: Dermoscopy approach in patients with multiple nevi: only dermoscopy is not enough because many benign lesions in patients with multiple nevi present irregular dermoscopic patterns, which means that many unnecessary excisions are still performed.

Dermoscopy approach in patients with multiple nevi

So, what can we do?

- We need more reliable detection strategies than just *clinical examination and dermoscopy*
- *Option*: ***Comparative approach*** in which individual lesions are assessed in the context of the patient's general nevi profile

Fig. 6.224: It is therefore necessary to have a more reliable detection strategy than just the clinical and dermoscopic ones and the option is the comparative approach.

Dermoscopy approach in patients with multiple nevi

- ***Two different (complementary) dermoscopic approaches***
  - *Morphological dermoscopic approach*
    - Assessment of one single lesion
  - *Comparative dermoscopic approach*
    - Multiple lesions assessment

Fig. 6.225: Two different (complementary) dermoscopic approaches.

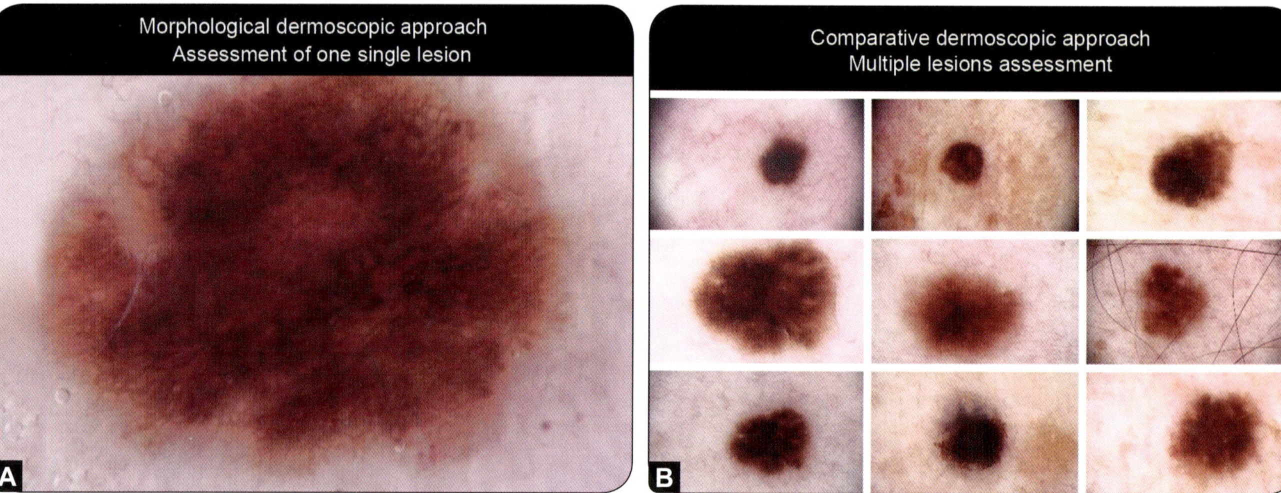

Figs. 6.226A and B: (A) The morphological dermoscopic approach: nevus with atypical dermoscopic features, we should remove this. (B) Comparative dermoscopic approach: the same patient as in Figure 6.226A, these nevi have atypical dermoscopic features but are all similar with one another. Now, with this comparative approach we do not need to remove.

In this manner we would have two different and complementary dermoscopic approaches (Figs. 6.226A and B):

- The morphological dermoscopic approach—assessment of only one lesion.
- Comparative dermoscopic approach (Fig. 6.227)
  - ***Assessment*** of multiple lesions with a view to recognizing the:
  - Predominant N pattern (signature N; Fig. 6.228)
  - The different lesion (Fig. 6.234)
    - Ugly duckling sign
    - Little red riding hood sign

Predominant N pattern (signature nevus): It is the predominant group of N sharing the same clinical or dermoscopic appearance; although they may present atypical dermoscopic features, they are all similar to one another (Figs. 6.229 to 6.233).

The different lesions are (Fig. 6.234):

- *Ugly duckling sign*: A lesion clinically or dermoscopically different from the predominant N pattern in a given patient. It may not present the specific dermoscopic criteria for M and yet be one (Figs. 6.235 to 6.237).
- *Little red riding hood sign*: Especially in patients with multiple atypical N. It is that lesion which is clinically similar to the others but under dermoscopy is highly suspicious of being an M (Figs. 6.238 to 6.241).

Conclusion: It has been proved that with the comparative approach about 30% fewer N are excised than with just the morphologic approach.

- ***Predominant nevus pattern***
  - *Signature nevus*
- ***The different lesion***
  - Clinically and dermoscopically
    - *Ugly duckling sign*
  - Dermoscopically
    - *Little red riding hood sign*

Fig. 6.227: Comparative dermoscopic approach.

- Prevailing group of nevi sharing the same clinical and dermoscopic appearance
  - They may present atypical dermoscopic features but are all similar to one another

Fig. 6.228: Signature nevus.

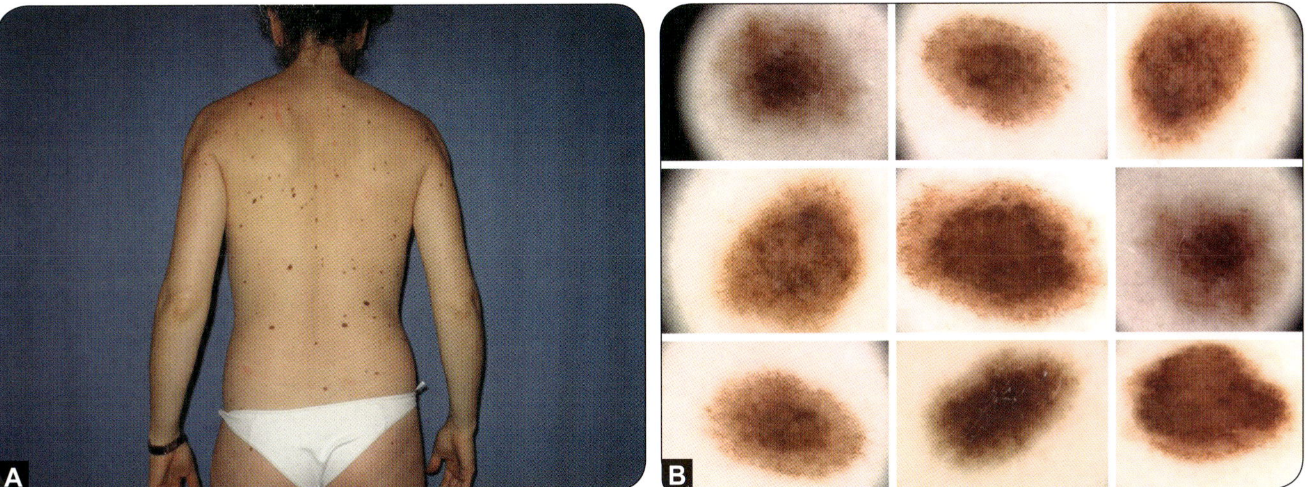

Figs. 6.229A and B: Signature nevi: (A) Patients with multiple clinical atypical nevi. (B) All of these nevi present the same typical dermoscopy pattern (mixed central pattern).

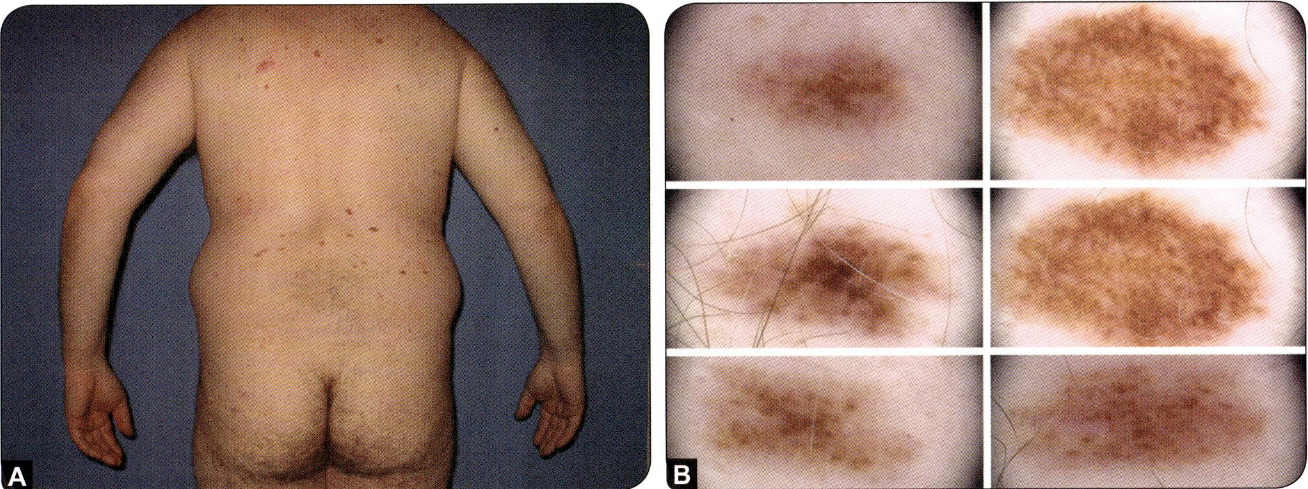

Figs. 6.230A and B: Signature nevi: (A) Patients with multiple clinical atypical nevi. (B) All of these nevi present the same typical dermoscopy pattern.

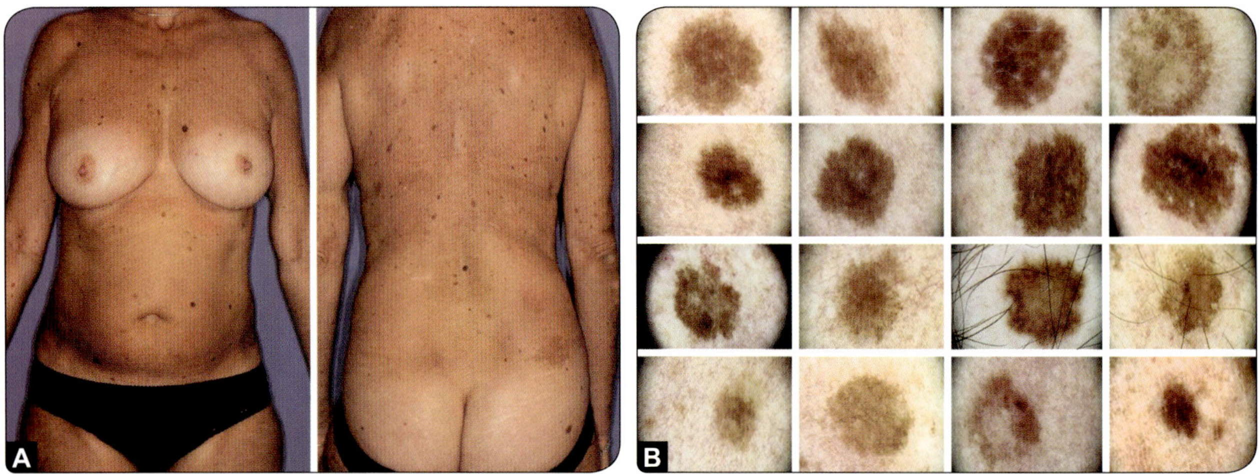

Figs. 6.231A and B: Signature nevi: (A) Patients with multiple clinical atypical nevi. (B) All of these nevi present the same typical dermoscopy pattern.

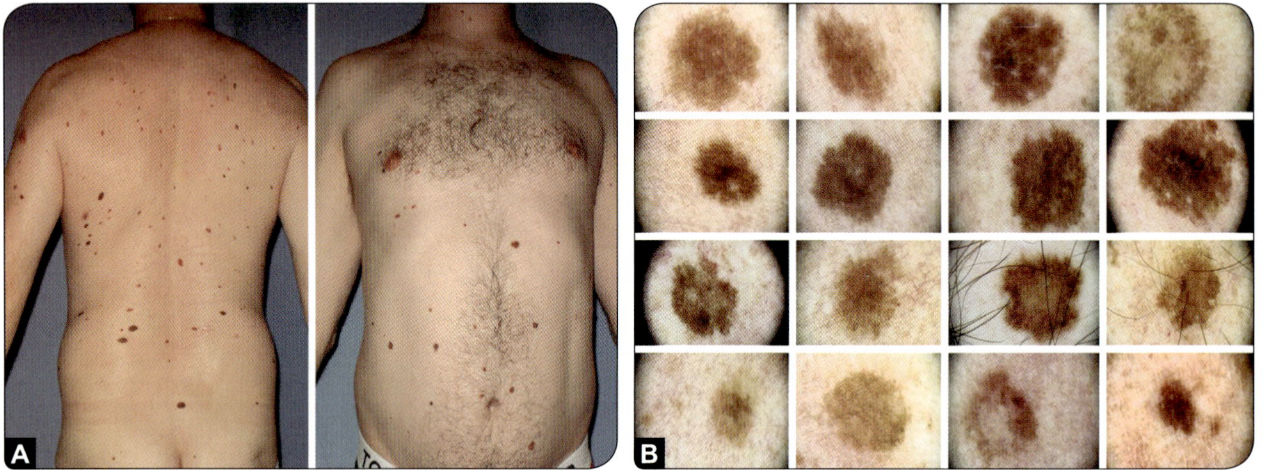

Figs. 6.232A and B: Signature nevi: (A) Patients with multiple clinical atypical nevi. (B) All of these nevi present an atypical dermoscopy pattern.

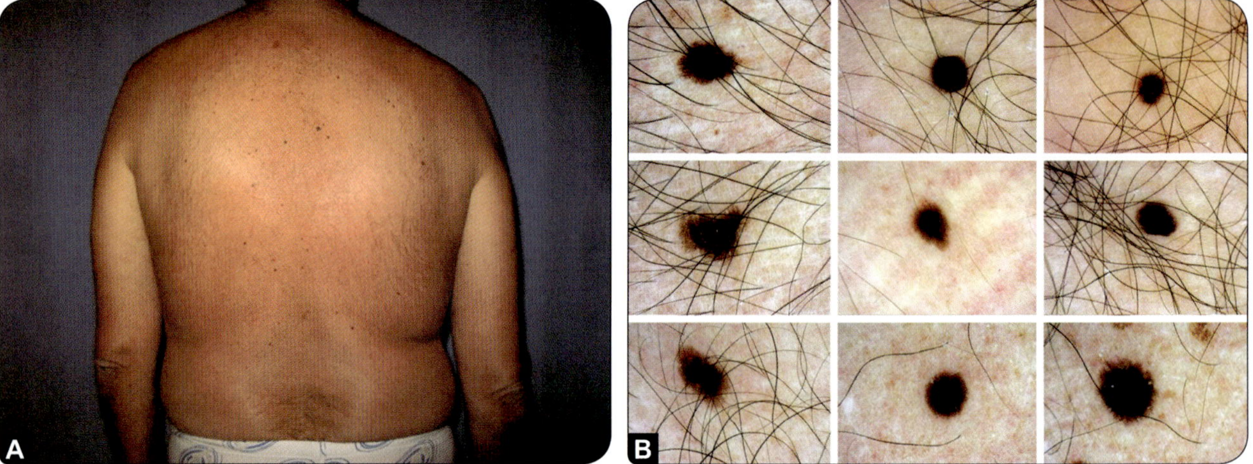

Figs. 6.233A and B: Signature nevi: (A) Patients with multiple clinical atypical nevi. (B) All of these nevi present the same typical dermoscopy pattern.

- *Clinically and dermoscopically*
  Ugly duckling sign
- *Dermoscopically*
  Little red riding hood sign

Fig. 6.234: The different lesion: ugly duckling sign and little red riding hood sign.

- Lesion different from the predominant nevus pattern in a given patient
  - May not present the specific dermoscopic criteria for melanoma

Fig. 6.235: Ugly duckling sign: a lesion clinically or dermoscopically different from the predominant nevi pattern in a given patient.

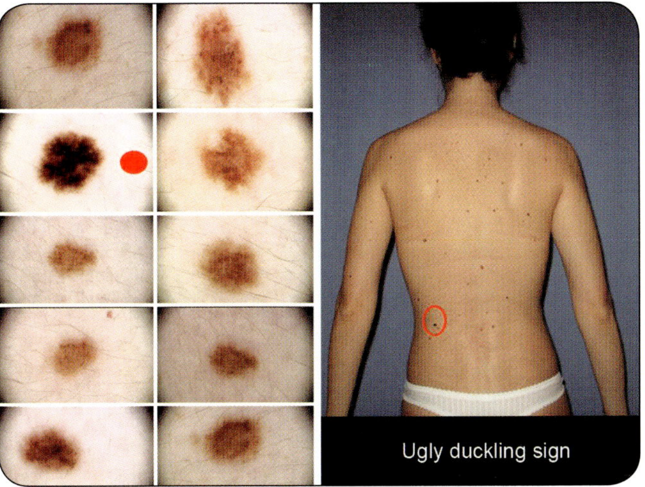

Fig. 6.236: Ugly duckling sign: this nevus is different under clinical (red dot) and dermoscopy (red dot) examination.

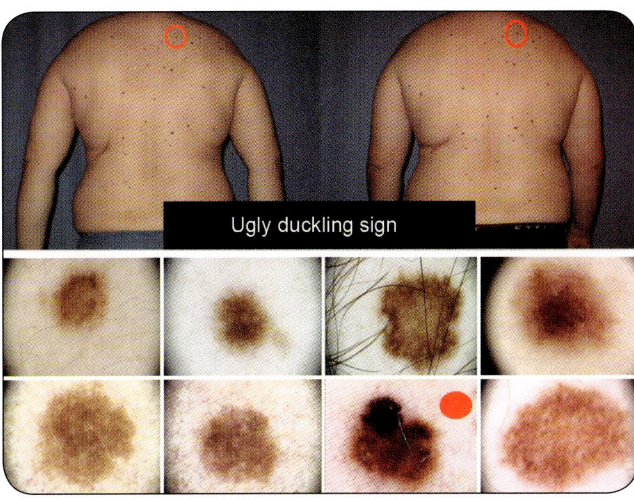

Fig. 6.237: Ugly duckling sign: this nevus is different under clinical (red dot) and dermoscopy examination.

- Especially in patients with multiple atypical nevi
- That lesion which *clinically resembles the others but has highly suspicious dermoscopy features*

Fig. 6.238: Little red riding hood sign: it is that lesion that is clinically similar to the others but under dermoscopy is highly suspicious of being a melanoma.

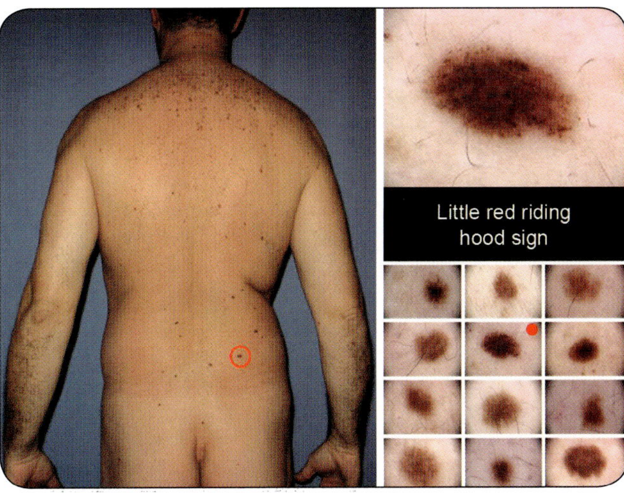

Fig. 6.239: Little red riding hood sign: the nevus in the red circle is clinically similar to the others but under dermoscopy (red dot) is highly suspicious of being a melanoma (superficial spreading melanoma B 0.30).

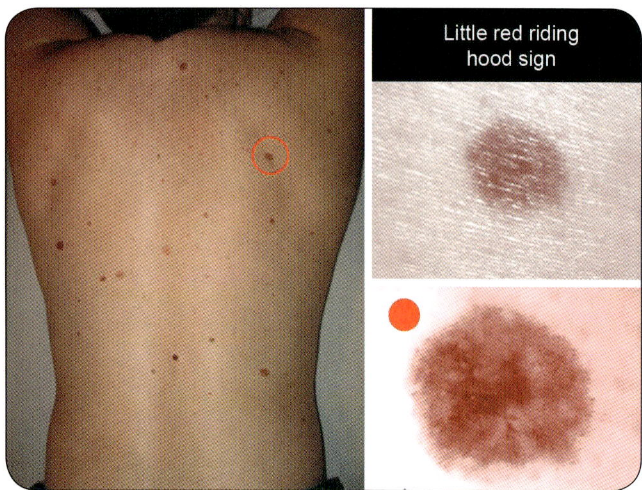

Fig. 6.240: Little red riding hood sign: the nevus in the red circle is clinically similar to the others but under dermoscopy (red dot) is highly suspicious of being a melanoma (superficial spreading melanoma in situ).

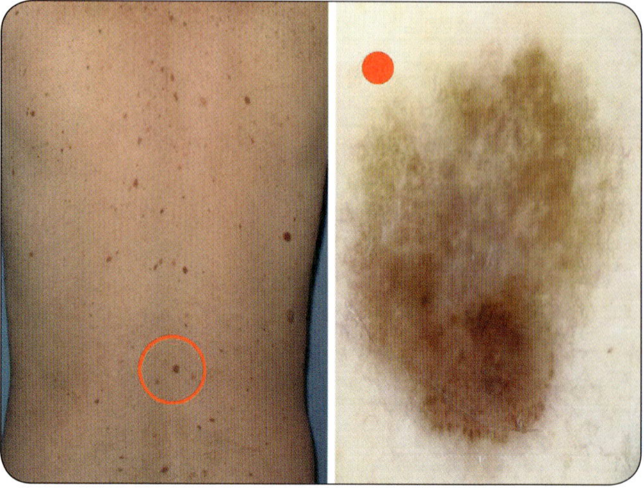

Fig. 6.241: Little red riding hood sign: the nevus in the red circle is clinically similar to the others but under dermoscopy (red dot) is highly suspicious of being a melanoma (superficial spreading melanoma B 0.40).

SUGGESTED READING

Argenziano G, Catricalà C, Ardigo M, et al. Dermoscopy of patients with multiple nevi. Improved management recommendations using a comparative diagnosis approach. Arch Dermatol. 2011;147(1):46-9.

Argenziano G, Cerroni L, Zalaudek I, et al. Accuracy in melanoma detection: a 10-year multicenter survey. J Am Acad Dermatol. 2012;67(1):54-9.

Argenziano G, Soyer P, De Giorgio V, et al. Interactive Atlas of Dermoscopy. Milán: EDRA Medical Publishing & New Media; 2000.

Argenziano G, Zalaudek I, Hofmann-Wellenhof R, et al. Total body skin examination for skin cancer screening in patients with focused symptoms. J Am Acad Dermatol. 2012;66(2):212-9.

Cabo H. Dermatoscopia. Buenos Aires, Argentina: Weber Ferro; 2000.

Cabo H. Dermatoscopia, 2nd edition. Buenos Aires, Argentina: Ediciones Journal; 2012.

Carli P, de Giorgi V, Chiarugi A, et al. Addition of dermoscopy to conventional naked-eye examination in melanoma screening: a randomized study. J Am Acad Dermatol. 2004;50:683-9.

Carli P, de Giorgi V, Crocetti E, et al. Improvement of malignant/benign ratio in excised melanocytic lesions in the "dermoscopy era": a retrospective study 1997-2001. Br J Dermatol. 2004;150(4):687-92.

Jaimes N, Dusza SW, Quigley EA, et al. Influence of time on dermoscopic diagnosis and management. Australas J Dermatol. 2013;54(2):96-104.

Johr R, Stolz W. Dermoscopy: An Illustrated Self-Assessment Guide, 2nd edition. New York: McGraw-Hill Education; 2015.

Jorh R, Soyer P, Argenziano G, et al. Dermoscopy. The Essentials (MOABT). New York: Elsevier Ltd; 2004.

Kittler H. Dermatoscopy. An Algorithmic Method Based on Pattern Analysis. Austria: Facultas.wuv; 2011.

Lallas A. Dermoscopy in general dermatology. Dermatol Clin. 2013;3:679-94.

Lin W, Luo S, Muzikansky A, et al. Outcome of patients with de novo versus nevus-associated melanoma. J Am Acad Dermatol. 2015;72:54-8.

Malvhey J, Puig S. Principles of Dermoscopy. Barcelona: Creaciones Gráficas; 2009.

Marghoob A, Braun R, Kopf A. Atlas of Dermoscopy. London: Taylor & Francis; 2005.

Menzies S, Crotty K, Ingvar C, et al. An Atlas of Surface Microscopy of Pigmented Skin Lesions. Sydney: McGraw-Hill Book Company; 1996.

Rabinovitz H, Kopf A. Dermoscopy: A Practical Guide. Miami: American Academy of Dermatology; 1999.

Soyer P, Argenziano G, Chimenti S, et al. Dermoscopy of Pigmented Skin Lesions. An Atlas Based on the Consensus Net Meeting on Dermoscopy. Milán: EDRA Medical Publishing & New Media; 2001.

Stolz W, Braun-Falco O, Bilek P, et al. Color Atlas of Dermatoscopy. Germany: Blackwell Science; 1994.

Terushkin V, Warycha M, Levy M, et al. Analysis of the benign to malignant ratio of lesions biopsied by a general dermatologist before and after the adoption of dermoscopy. Arch Dermatol. 2010;146(3):343-4.

Zalaudek I, Argenziano G, Giacomel J. Dermoscopy of Non-Pigmented Skin Tumors. Boca Raton, FL: CRC Press; 2016.

Zalaudek I, Argenziano G, Mordente I, et al. Nevus type in dermoscopy is related to skin type in white persons. Arch Dermatol. 2007;143(3):351-6.

MELANOMA SIMULATORS

7

Horacio A Cabo

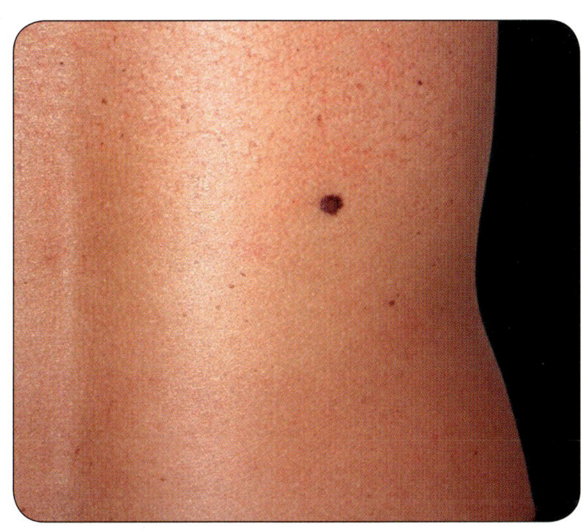

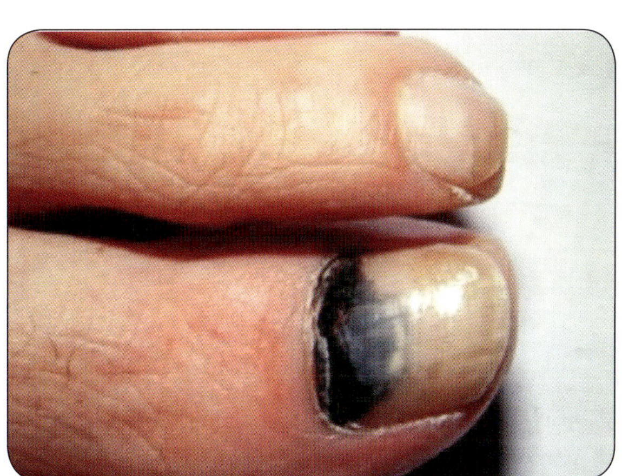

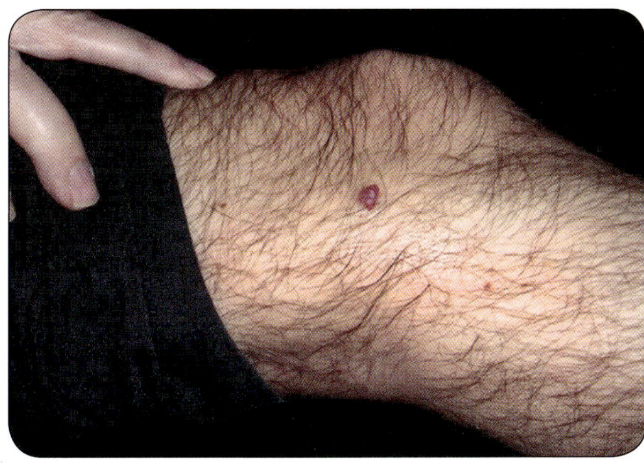

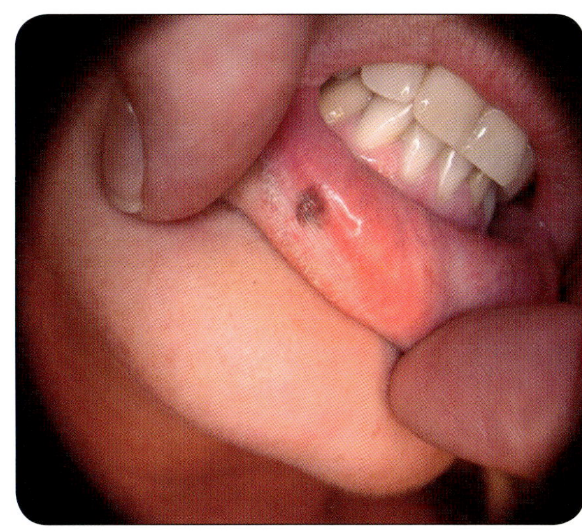

"In this chapter are included all those lesions that may simulate a melanoma, both clinically and dermoscopically.

They can be divided into two groups, nonmelanocytic melanoma simulators, such as basal cell carcinoma, squamous cell carcinoma and actinic keratosis, ink-spot lentigo, seborrheic keratosis, dermatofibroma, thrombosed hemangioma and hematomas, pyogenic granuloma, eccrine poroma and collision tumors; melanocytic melanoma simulators also will be treated, atypical nevus (Clark's nevus), recurrent nevus, combined nevus, blue nevus, Spitz-Reed nevus, melanocytic maculae and longitudinal melanonychia."

In this chapter all those lesions are included that may simulate a melanoma, both clinically and dermoscopically.

They can be divided into two groups.

NONMELANOCYTIC MELANOMA SIMULATORS (FIGS. 7.1 TO 7.12)

- Basal cell carcinoma
- Squamous cell carcinoma
- Actinic keratosis
- Ink-spot lentigo
- Seborrheic keratosis
- Dermatofibroma
- Thrombosed hemangioma
- Hematomas
- Pyogenic granuloma
- Eccrine poroma
- Collision tumors

MELANOCYTIC MELANOMA SIMULATORS (FIGS. 7.13 TO 7.20)

- Atypical nevus (Clark's nevus)
- Recurrent nevus
- Combined nevus
- Blue nevus
- Spitz-Reed nevus
- Melanocytic maculae
- Longitudinal melanonychia

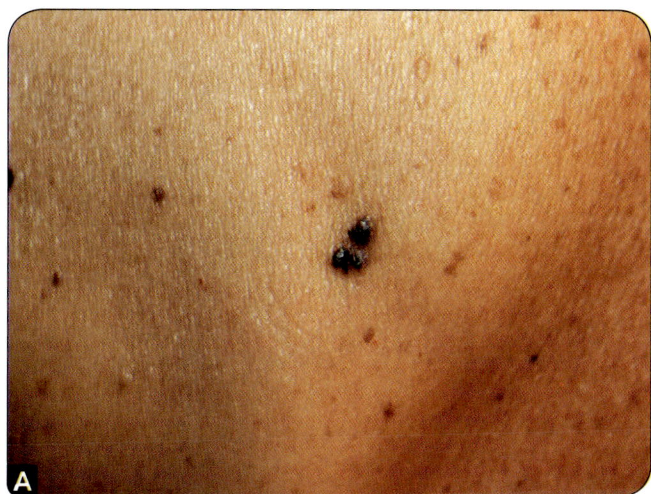

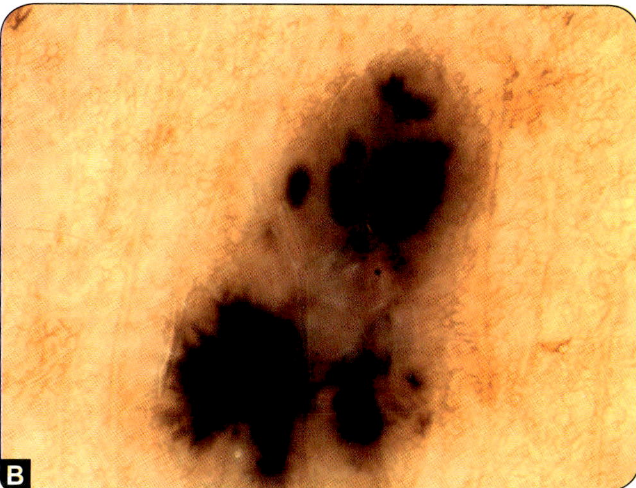

Figs. 7.1A and B: (A) Basal cell carcinoma (BCC); clinical view and (B) Pigmented BCC; dermoscopy view.

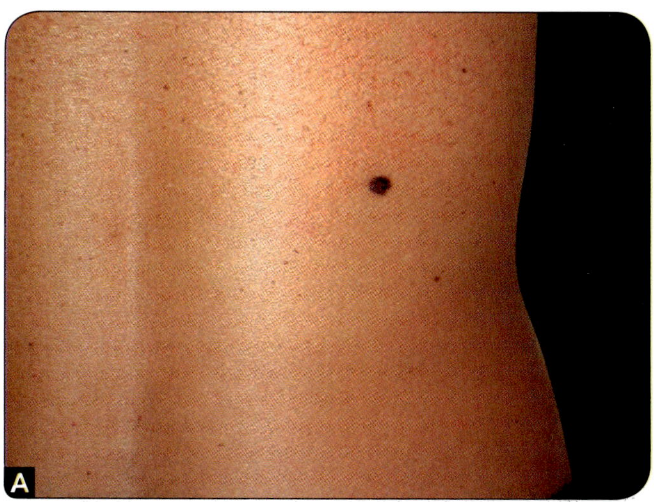

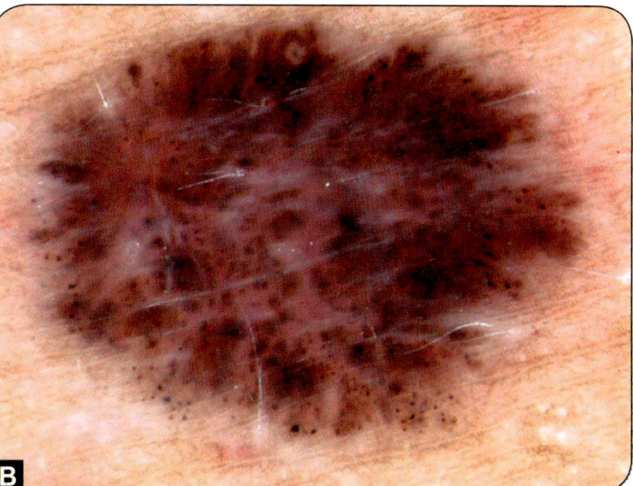

Figs. 7.2A and B: (A) Basal cell carcinoma (BCC); clinical view and (B) Pigmented BCC; dermoscopy view.

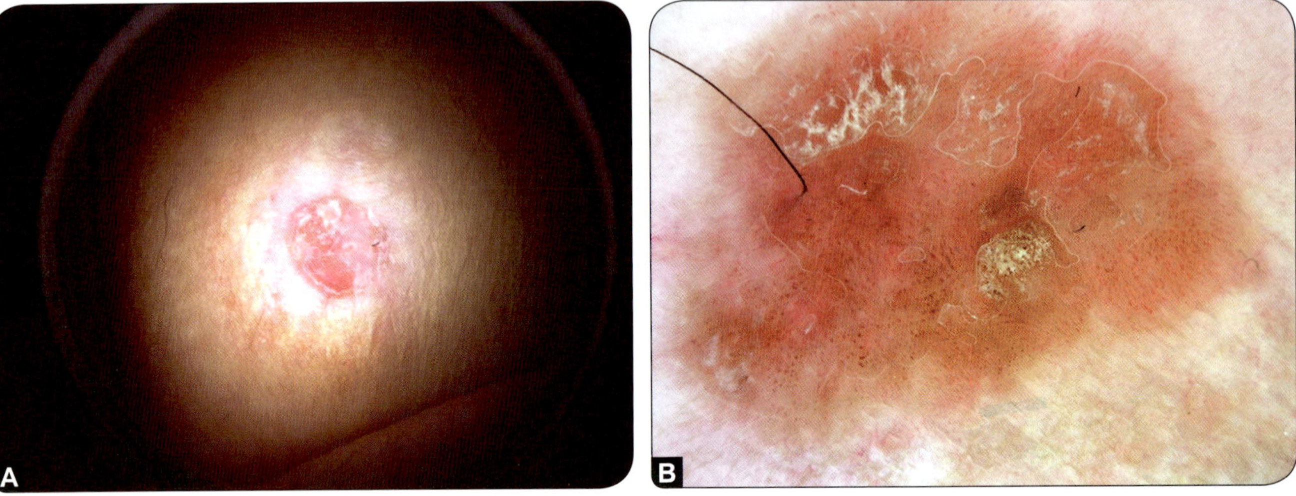

Figs. 7.3A and B: (A) Squamous cell carcinoma (SCC); clinical view and (B) Pigmented SCC; dermoscopy view.

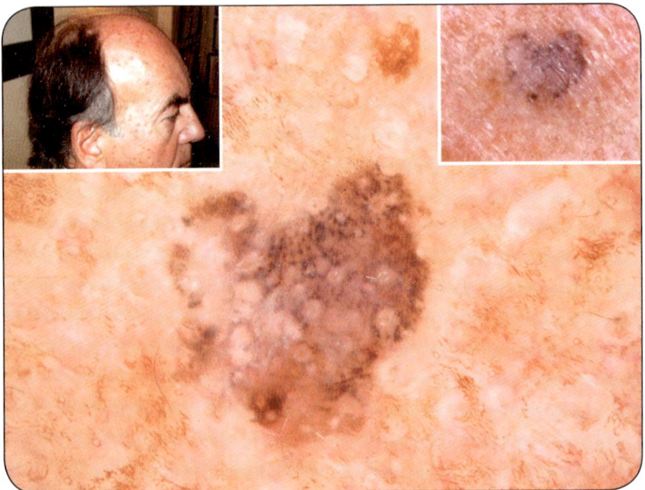

Fig. 7.4: Pigmented actinic keratosis.

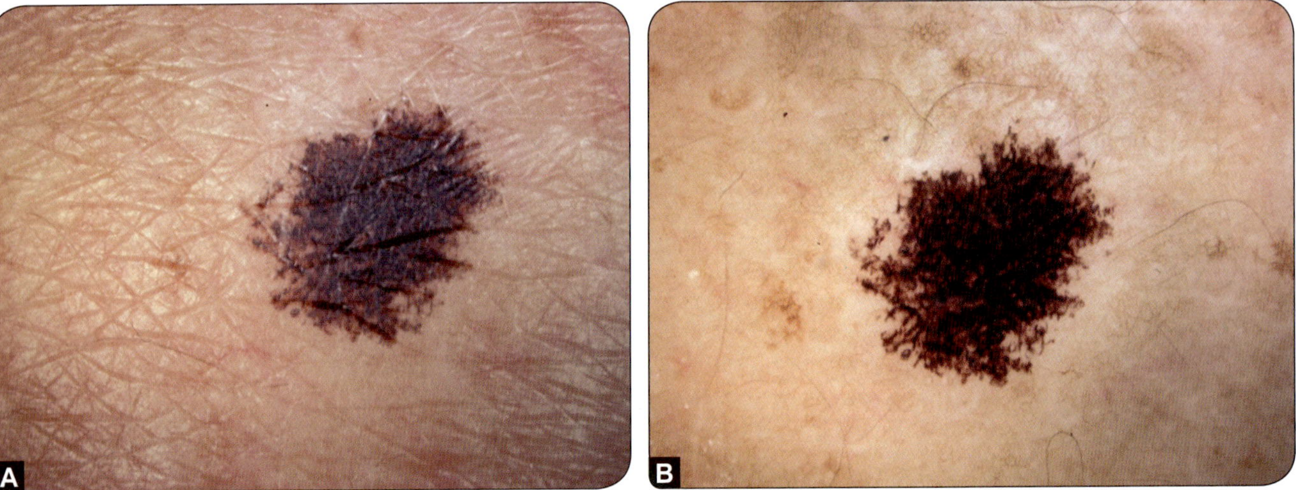

Figs. 7.5A and B: (A) Ink-spot lentigo; clinical view and (B) Ink-spot lentigo; dermoscopy view.

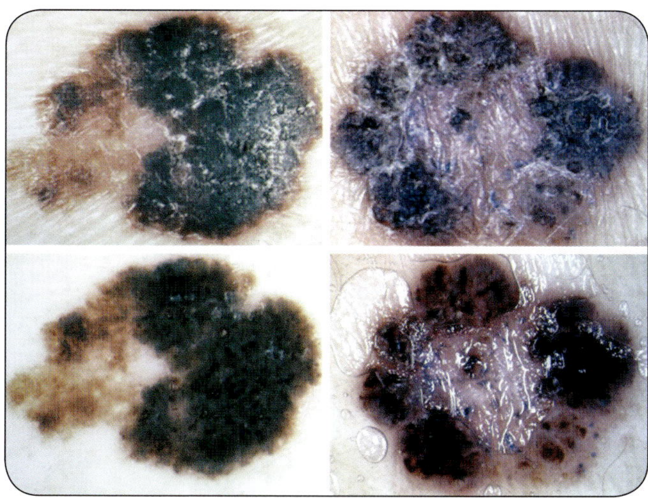

Fig. 7.6: Pigmented seborrheic keratosis; clinical and dermoscopy view.

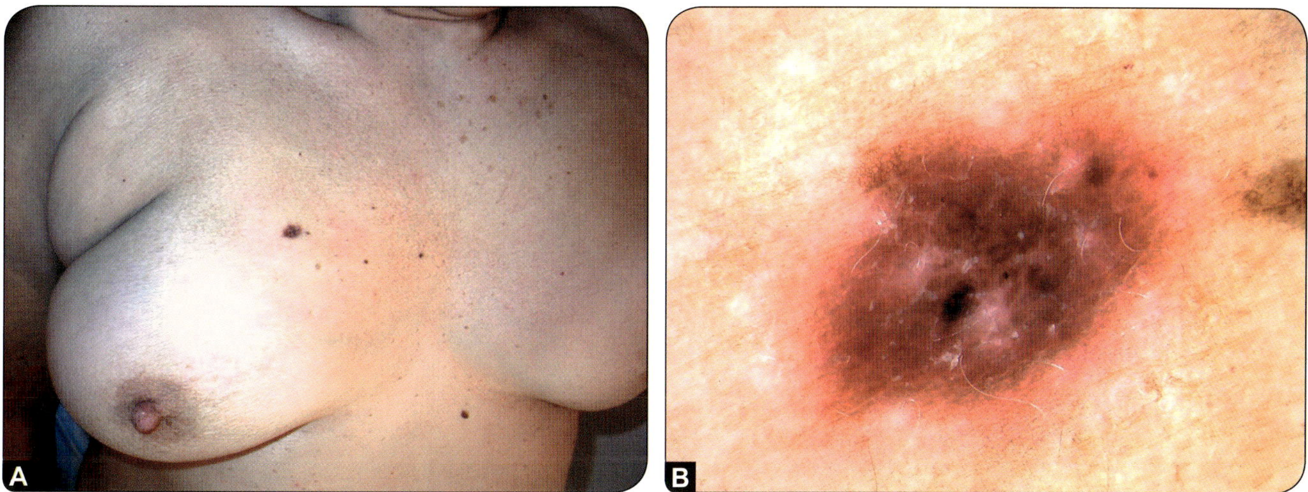

Figs. 7.7A and B: (A) Dermatofibroma; clinical view and (B) Dermatofibroma; dermoscopy view.

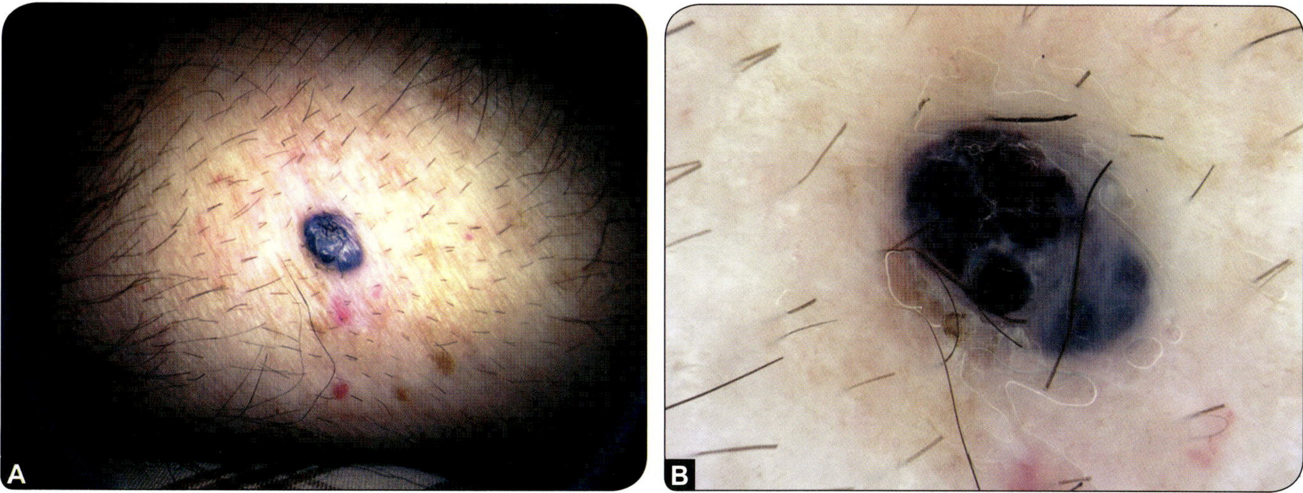

Figs. 7.8A and B: (A) Thrombosed hemangioma; clinical view and (B) Thrombosed hemangioma; dermoscopy view.

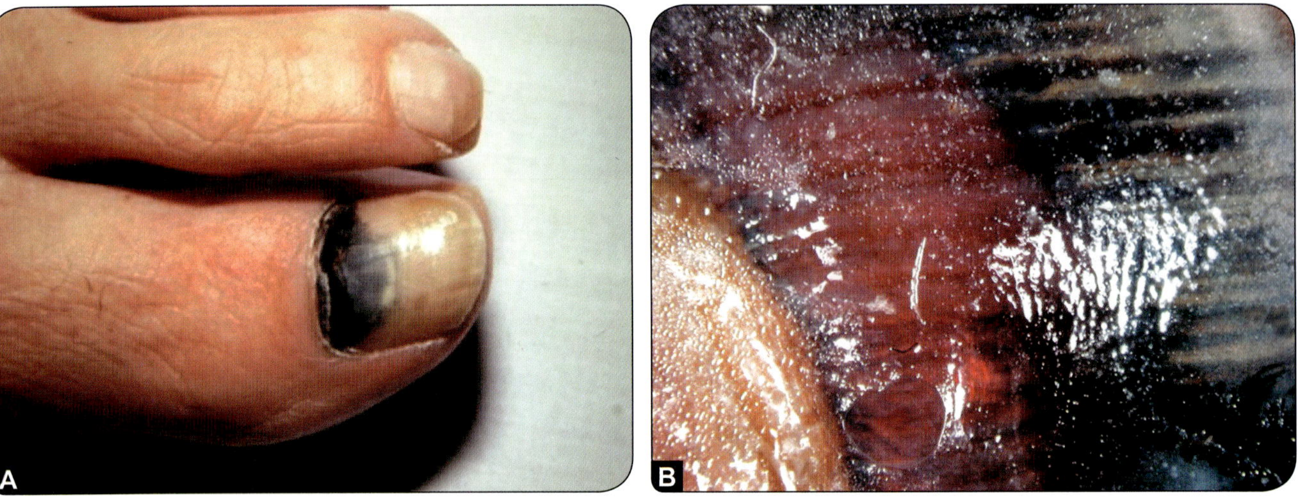

Figs. 7.9A and B: (A) Subungual hematomas; clinical image and (B) Subungual hematomas; dermoscopy view.

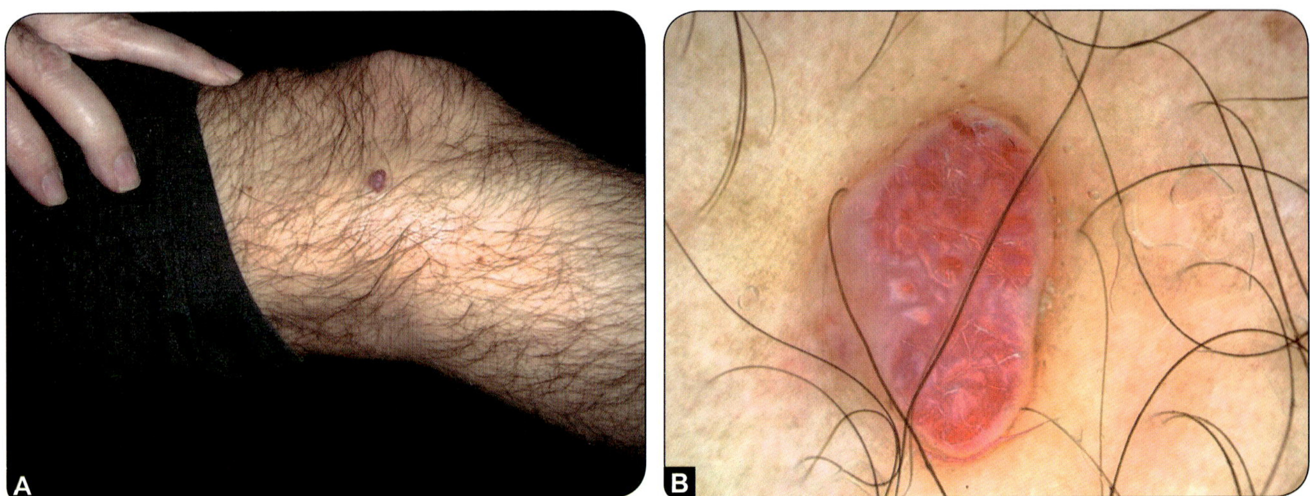

Figs. 7.10A and B: (A) Pyogenic granuloma; clinical image and (B) Pyogenic granuloma; dermoscopy image.

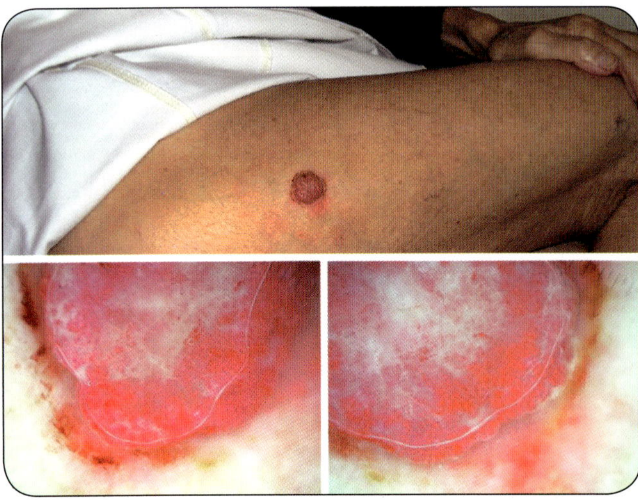

Fig. 7.11: Eccrine poroma; clinical and dermoscopy view.

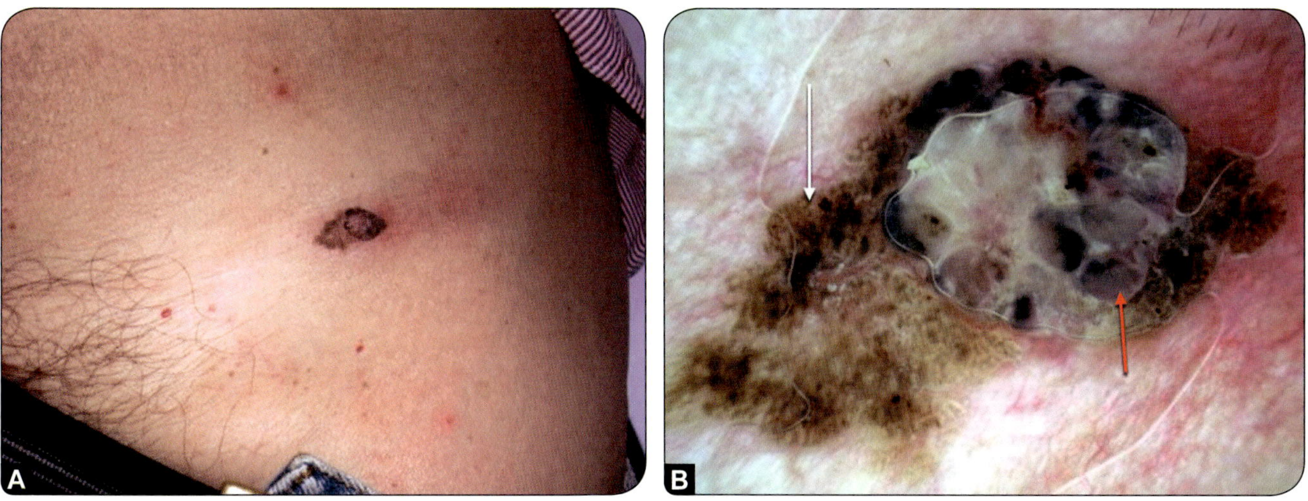

Figs. 7.12A and B: (A) Collision tumors clinical view and (B) Collision tumors dermoscopy view—basal cell carcinoma (red arrow) and seborrheic keratosis (white arrow).

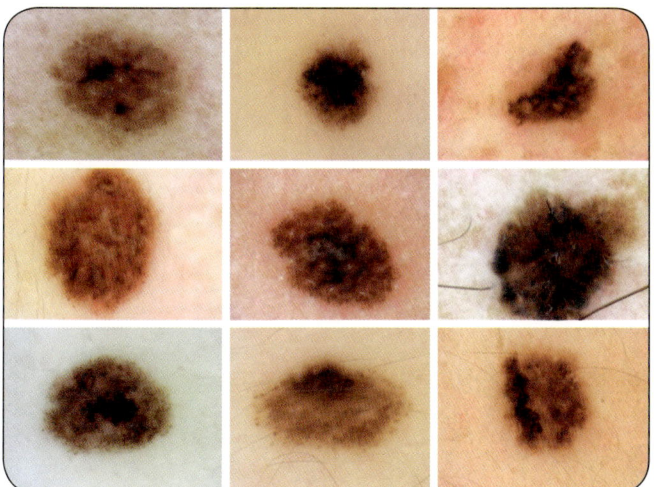

Fig. 7.13: Different dermoscopy images of atypical nevus (Clark's nevus).

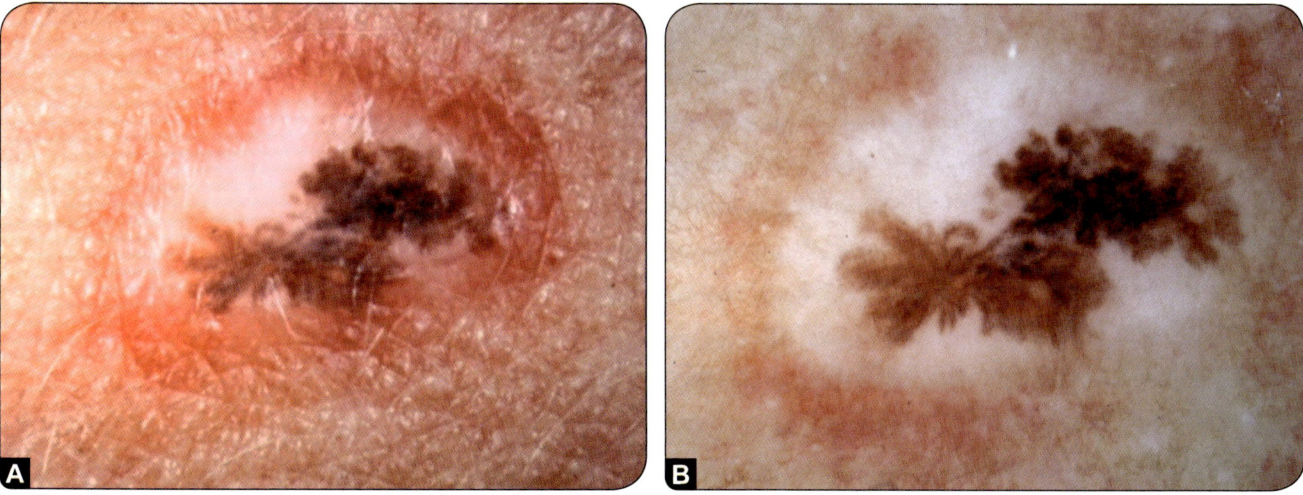

Figs. 7.14A and B: (A) Recurrent nevus; clinical view and (B) Recurrent nevus; dermoscopy image.

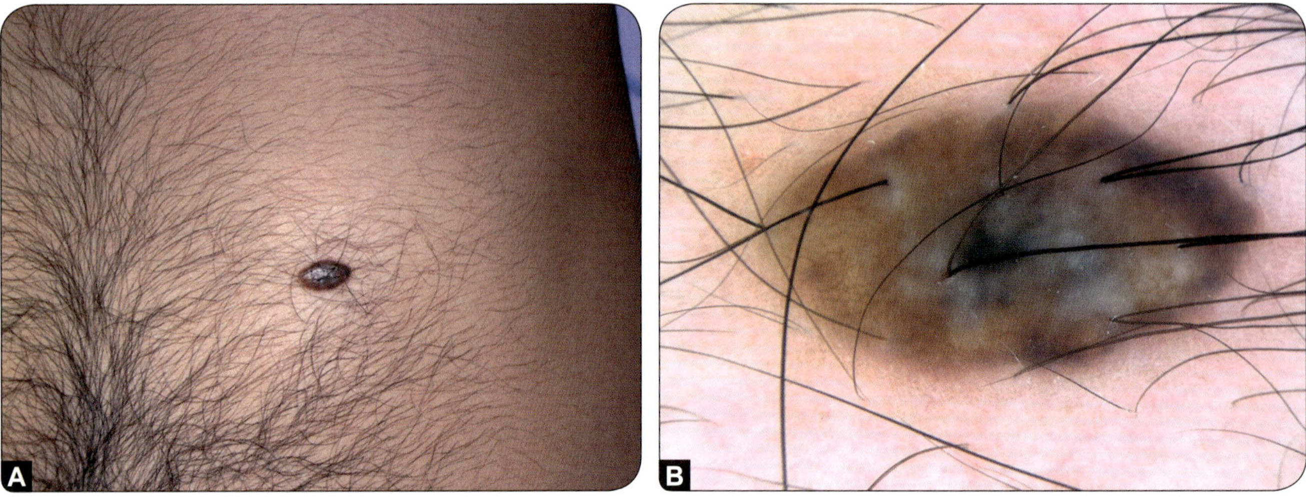

Figs. 7.15A and B: (A) Combined nevus; clinical view and (B) Combined nevus; dermoscopy view (blue nevus and compound nevus).

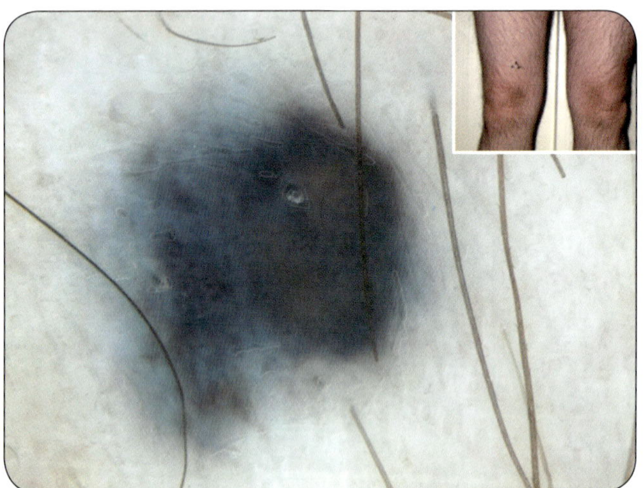

Fig. 7.16: Atypical blue nevus.

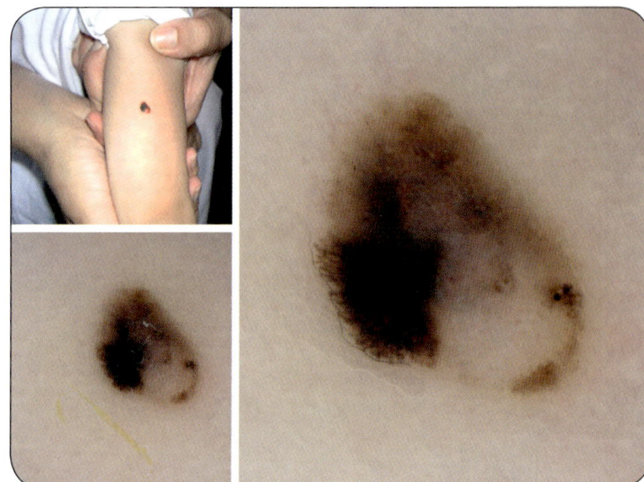

Fig. 7.17: Atypical Spitz nevus.

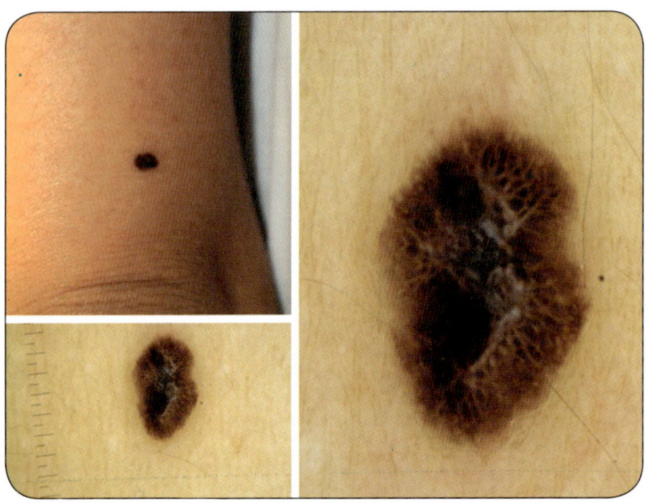

Figs. 7.18: Atypical Spitz nevus.

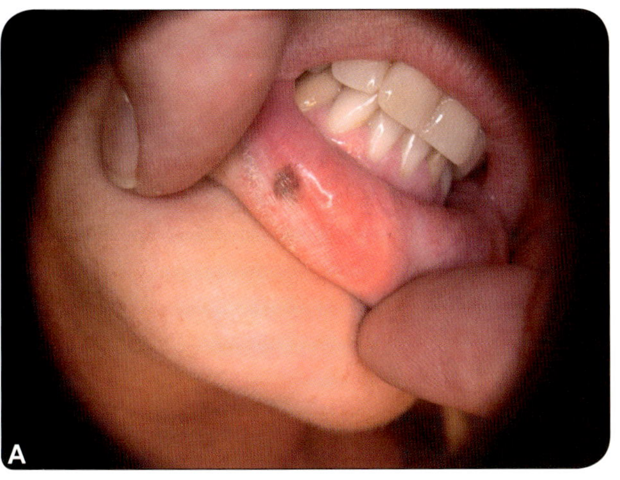

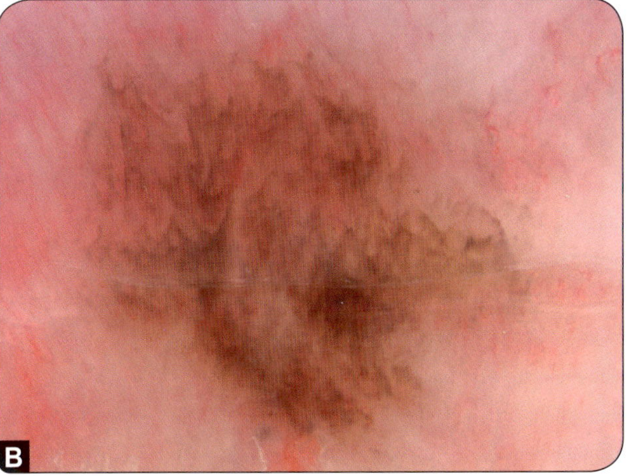

Figs. 7.19A and B: (A) Melanotic labial macule; clinical view and (B) Melanotic labial macule; dermoscopy view with the classical *"Fish scale-like pattern."*

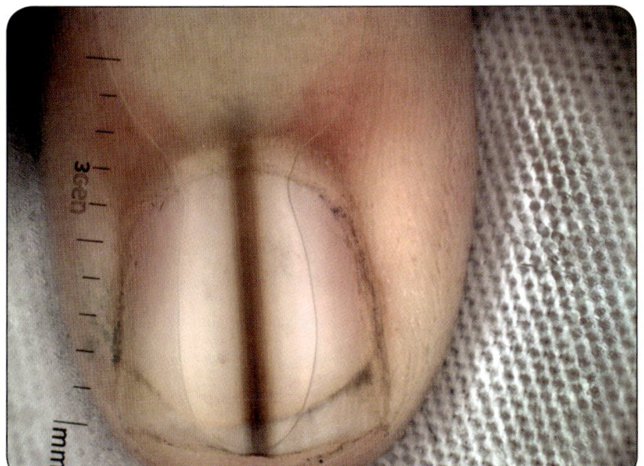

Fig. 7.20: Longitudinal melanonychia.

Table 7.1 Melanoma simulators.

Non melanocytics	*Melanocytics*
Basal cell carcinoma	Clark's nevus
Squamous cell carcinoma	Recurrent nevus
Actinic keratosis	Combined nevus
Ink spot lentigo	Blue nevus
Seborrheic keratosis	Spitz-Reed nevus
Dermatofibroma	Melanotic maculae
Thrombosed hemangioma	Longitudinal melanonychia
Hematomas	
Pyogenic granuloma	
Eccrine porome	
Collision tumors	

Even though these lesions have been described in previous chapters, we herein illustrate them with examples of the different cases (Table 7.1).

SUGGESTED READING

Argenziano G, Soyer P, De Giorgio V, et al. Interactive Atlas of Dermoscopy. Milán: EDRA Medical Publishing & New Media; 2000.

Cabo H. Dermatoscopia. Buenos Aires, Argentina: Weber Ferro; 2000.

Cabo H. Dermatoscopia, 2nd edition. Buenos Aires, Argentina: Ediciones Journal; 2012.

Johr R, Stolz W. Dermoscopy: An Illustrated Self-Assessment Guide, 2nd edition. New York: McGraw-Hill Education; 2015.

Jorh R, Soyer P, Argenziano G, et al. Dermoscopy. The Essentials (MOABT). New York: Elsevier Ltd; 2004.

Kittler H. Dermatoscopy. An Algorithmic Method Based on Pattern Analysis. facultas.wuvUniversitätsverlag, Austria www.facultas.wuv.at

Lallas A. Dermoscopy in general dermatology. Dermatol Clin. 2013;3:679-94.

Malvhey J, Puig S. Principles of dermoscopy. Barcelona: Creaciones Gráficas; 2009.

Marghoob A, Braun R, Kopf A. Atlas of dermoscopy. London: Taylor & Francis; 2005.

Menzies S, Crotty K, Ingvar C, et al. An atlas of surface microscopy of pigmented skin lesions. Sydney: McGraw-Hill Book Company; 1996.

Rabinovitz H, Kopf A. Dermoscopy: A Practical Guide. Miami: American Academy of Dermatology; 1999.

Soyer P, Argenziano G, Chimenti S, et al. Dermoscopy of Pigmented Skin Lesions. An Atlas Based on the Consensus Net Meeting on Dermoscopy. Milán: EDRA Medical Publishing & New Media; 2001.

Stolz W, Braun-Falco O, Bilek P, et al. Color Atlas of Dermatoscopy. USA: Blackwell Science; 1994.

Zalaudek I, Argenziano G, Giacomel J. Dermoscopy of Non-Pigmented Skin Tumors. Boca Raton, FL: CRC Press; 2016.

COMBINED LESIONS

8

Horacio A Cabo

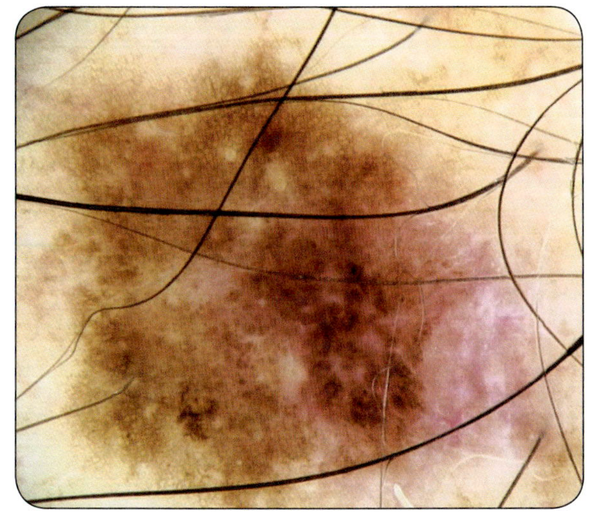

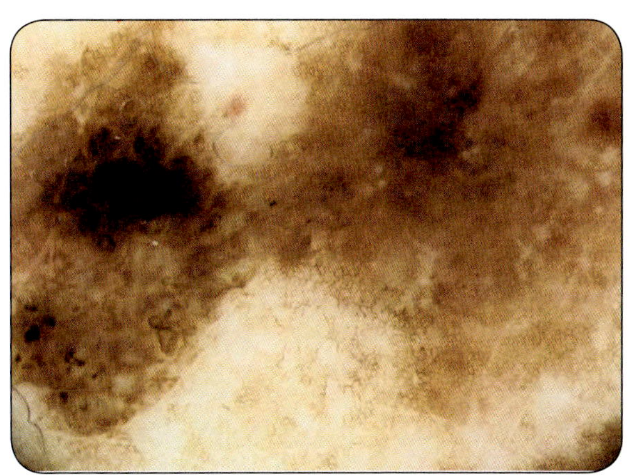

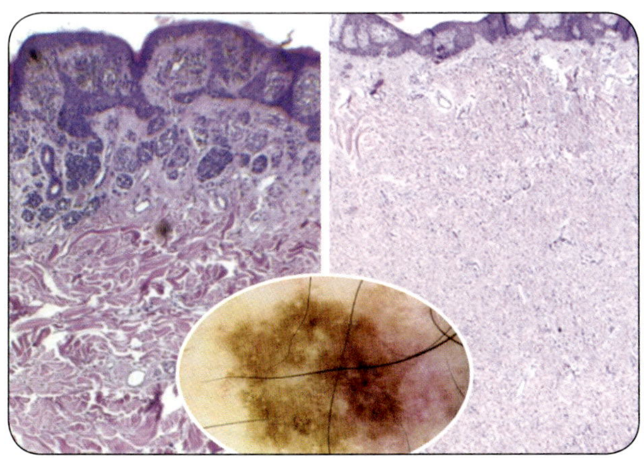

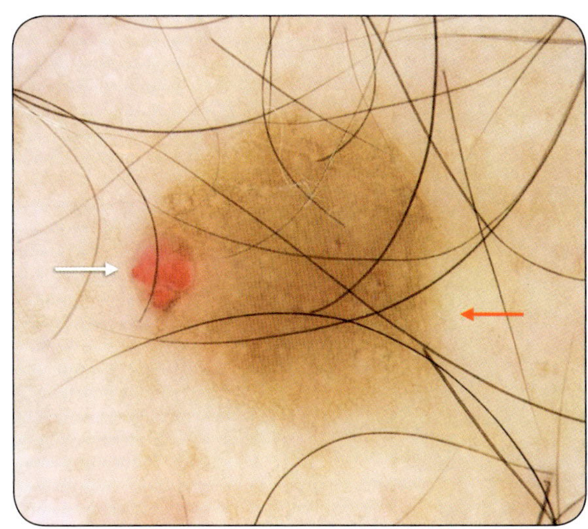

"Combined lesions are formed by two or more cutaneous lesions of different origin. These lesions do not include combined nevus developed on melanocytic nevus, due to their melanocytic origin. There is no association pattern between these lesions; in fact, in most cases,finding them is fortuitous and unexpected."

Combined lesions are formed by two or more cutaneous lesions of different origin. These lesions do not include combined nevus nonmelanoma developed on melanocytic nevus, due to their melanocytic origin.

There is no association pattern between these lesions; in fact, in most cases, finding them is fortuitous and unexpected.

According to the literature, the manifestation frequency is low: 0.06%. However, it is suspected to be higher.

Dermoscopy is very useful to diagnose combined lesions, since it makes it possible to observe the structures and patterns characteristic of each lesion, which have been described in detail in the different chapters of this book.

The combinations most frequently observed are between the following lesions:

- Hemangioma (H)
- Seborrheic keratosis (SK)
- Solar lentigo (SL)
- Lentigo (L)
- Basal cell carcinoma (BCC)
- Nevus (N)
- Melanoma (M)
- Squamous cell carcinoma (SCC)
- Dermatofibroma (D)
- Sebaceous hyperplasia (SH)

With reference to SK, it is important to take into account that, since this is the most frequent benign cutaneous tumor—which may combine with any of the previously described lesions—it is possible to find it in many of the observed combined lesions; even, on occasion, associated with more than one lesion.

Malignant tumors combined with SK are, in order of frequency, BCC, SCC, and M, and the most affected area is the back.

It is estimated that the frequency of combination of SK and BCC—considering the incidence of these tumors—is higher than the reported one. A possible explanation behind this could be that BCC might progressively destroy SK, or that residual SK may be overlooked in the histopathological examination.

In conclusion, in the face of a pigmented lesion presenting dermoscopic criteria corresponding to different lesions, whether melanocytic or nonmelanocytic, the possibility of a combined lesion must be considered (Figs. 8.1 to 8.14).

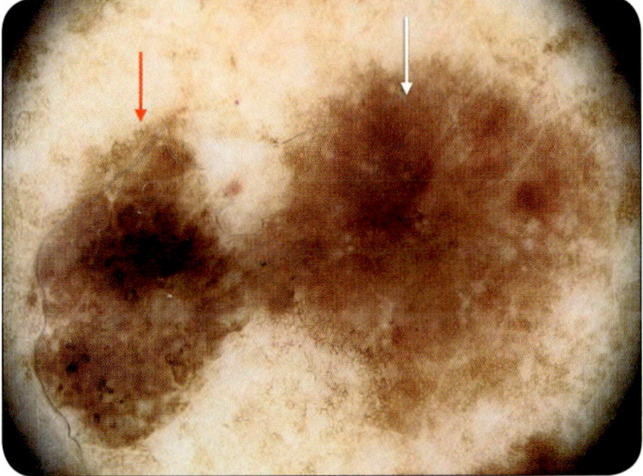

Fig. 8.1: Seborrheic keratosis (red arrow); junction nevus (white arrow).

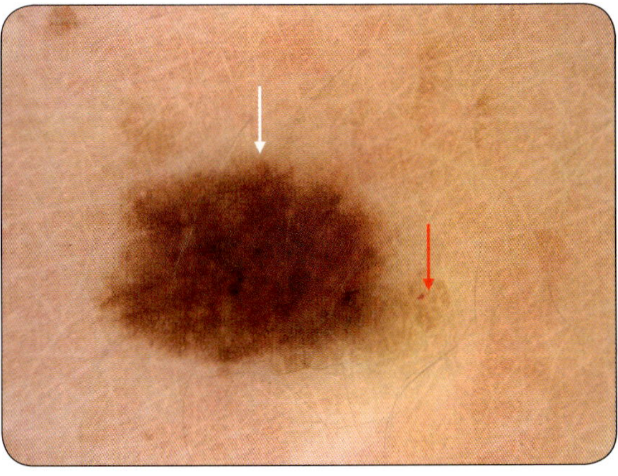

Fig. 8.2: Seborrheic keratosis (red arrow); junction nevus (white arrow).

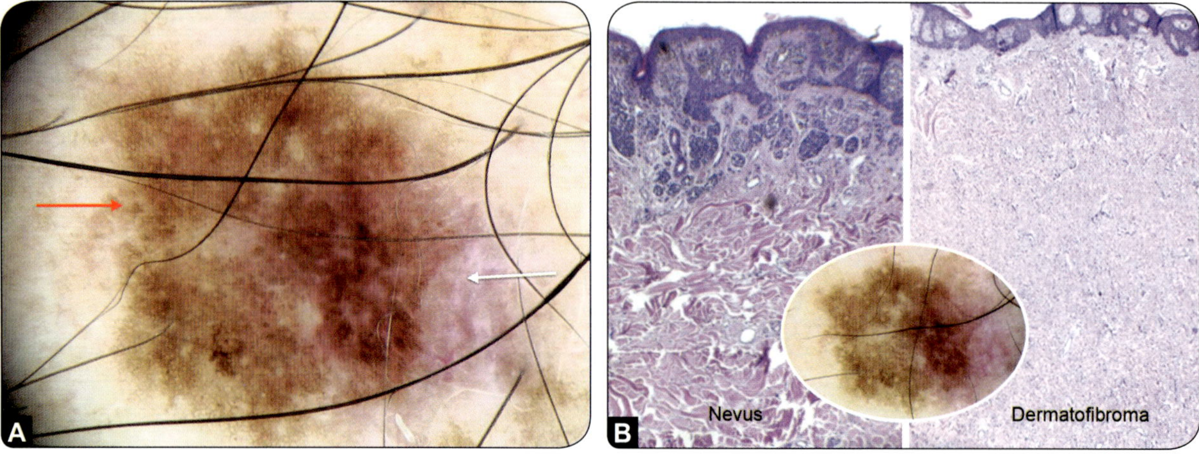

Figs. 8.3A and B: (A) Nevus (red arrow); dermatofibroma (white arrow) and (B) Nevus (left side); dermatofibroma (right side).

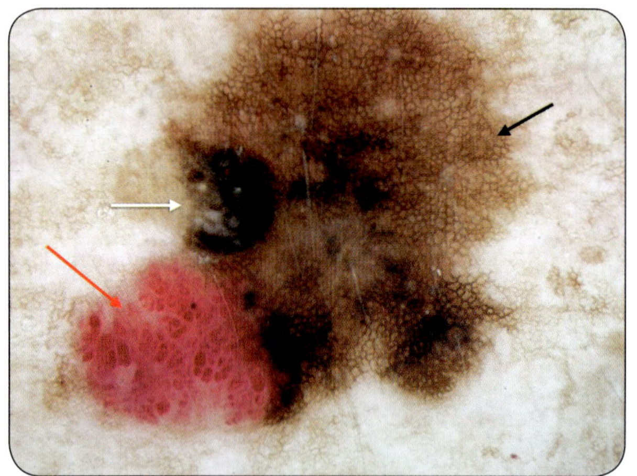

Fig. 8.4: Seborrheic keratosis (white arrow); angioma (red arrow); junction nevus (black arrow).

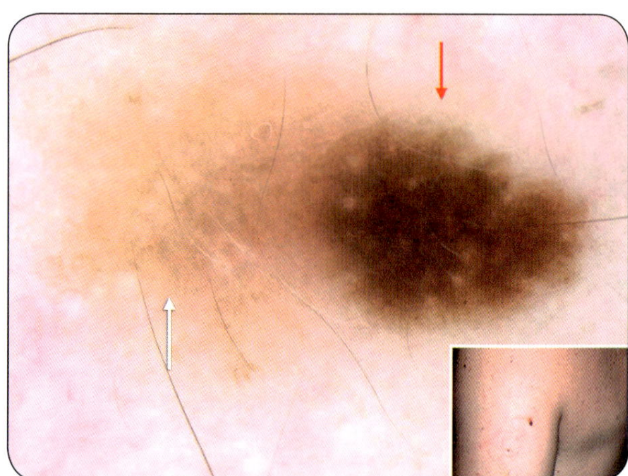

Fig. 8.5: Nevus (red arrow); dermatofibroma (white arrow).

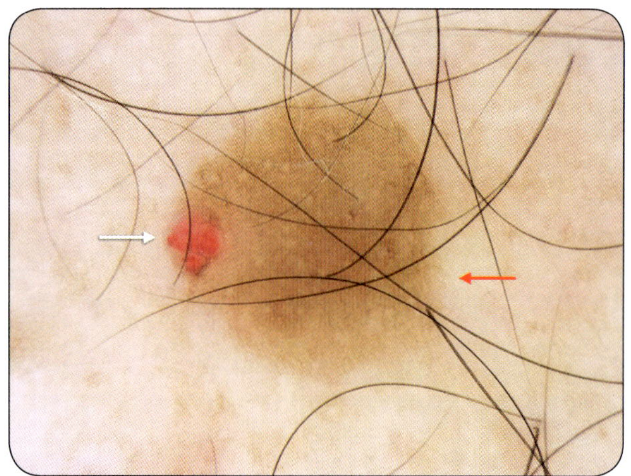

Fig. 8.6: Nevus (red arrow); angioma (white arrow).

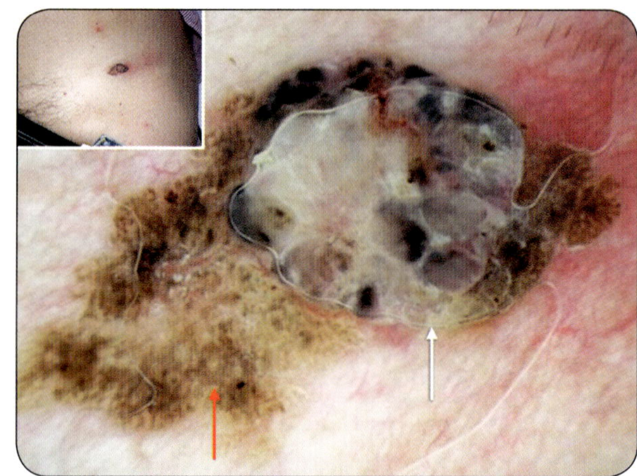

Fig. 8.7: Seborrheic keratosis (red arrow); basal cell carcinoma (white arrow).

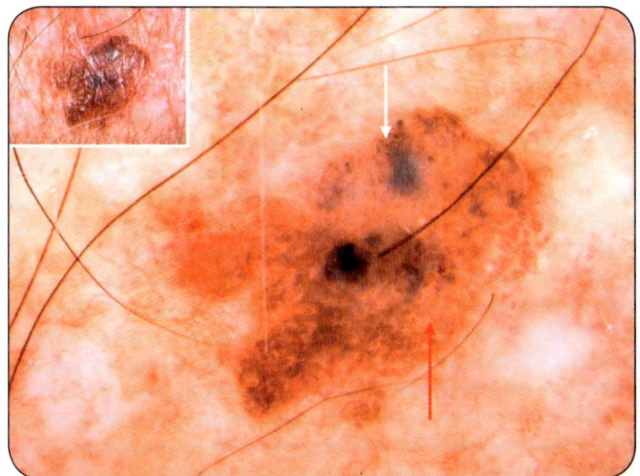

Fig. 8.8: Seborrheic keratosis (red arrow); basal cell carcinoma (white arrow).

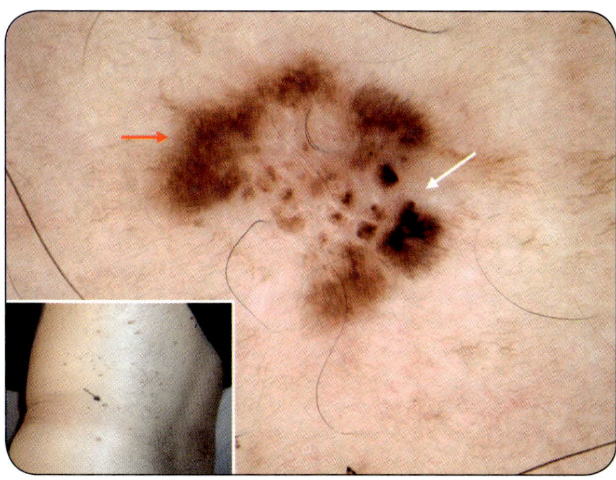

Fig. 8.9: Seborrheic keratosis (red arrow); basal cell carcinoma (white arrow) clinical view (black arrow).

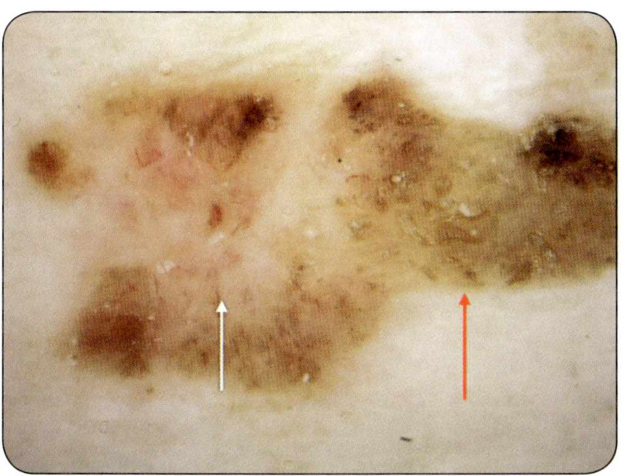

Fig. 8.10: Seborrheic keratosis (red arrow); basal cell carcinoma (white arrow).

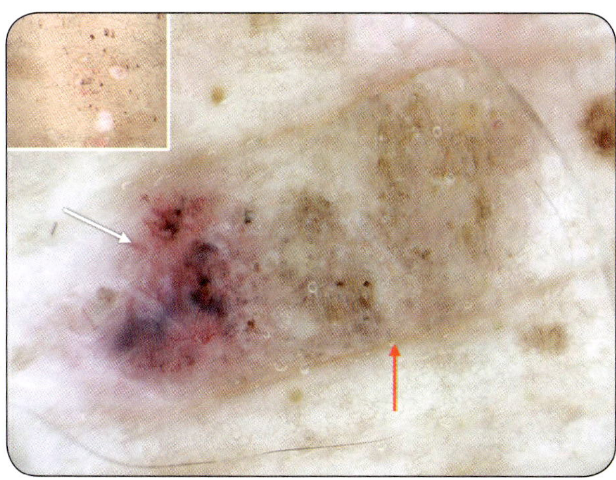

Fig. 8.11: Seborrheic keratosis (red arrow); basal cell carcinoma (white arrow).

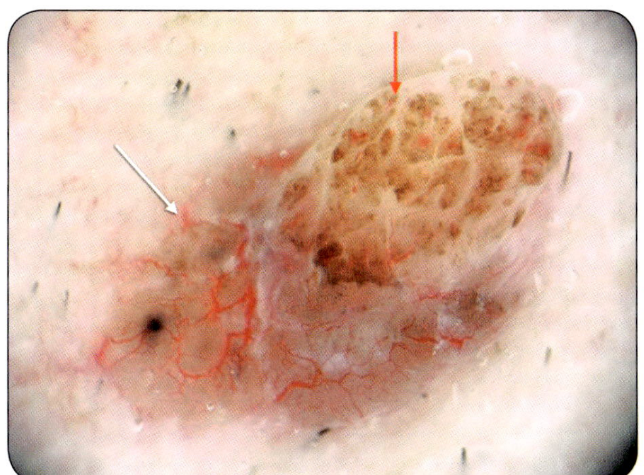

Fig. 8.12: Congenital nevus (red arrow); basal cell carcinoma (white arrow).

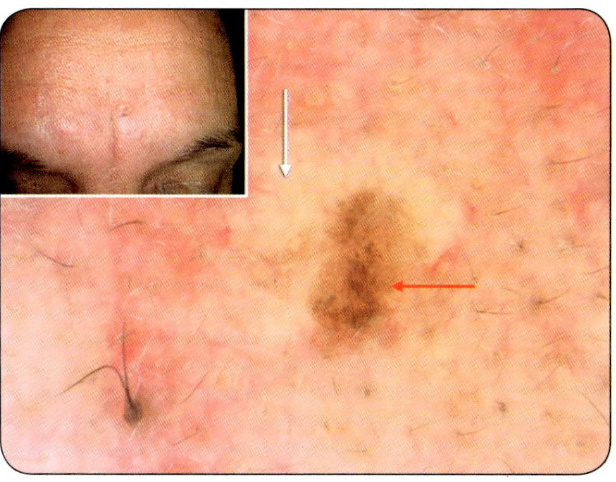

Fig. 8.13: Sebaceous hyperplasia (white arrow); seborrheic keratosis (red arrow).

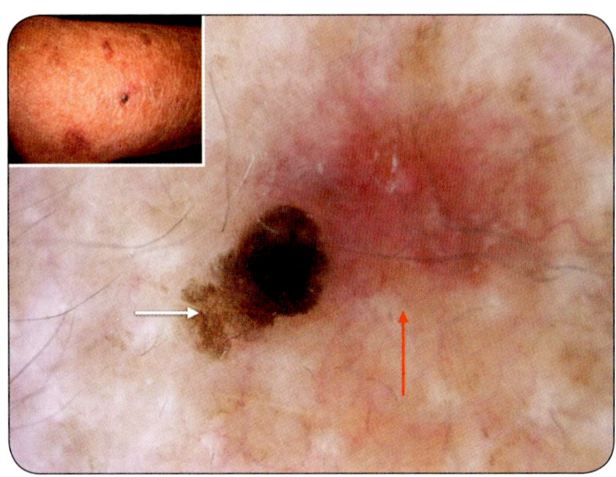

Fig. 8.14: Seborrheic keratosis (white arrow); senile purpura (red arrow).

SUGGESTED READING

Argenziano G, Soyer P, De Giorgio V, et al. Interactive Atlas of Dermoscopy. Milán: EDRA Medical Publishing & New Media; 2000.

Cabo H. Dermatoscopia. Buenos Aires, Argentina: Weber Ferro; 2000.

Cabo H. Dermatoscopia, 2nd edition. Buenos Aires, Argentina: Ediciones Journal; 2012.

Johr R, Stolz W. Dermoscopy: An Illustrated Self-Assessment Guide, 2nd edition. New York: McGraw-Hill Education; 2015.

Jorh R, Soyer P, Argenziano G, et al. Dermoscopy. The Essentials (MOABT). New York: Elsevier Ltd; 2004.

Kittler H. Dermatoscopy. An Algorithmic Method Based on Pattern Analysis 2011 Facultas Verlags- und Buchhandels AG facultas wuv Universitätsverlag, Austria www.facultas.wuv.at

Lallas A. Dermoscopy in General Dermatology. Dermatol Clin. 2013;3:679-94.

Malvhey J, Puig S. Principles of Dermoscopy. Barcelona: Creaciones Gráficas; 2009.

Marcucci C, Cohen Sabban E, Friedman P, et al. Dermoscopic findings in a collision tumor composed of a dermatofibroma and a melanocytic nevus mimicking melanoma. Dermatol Pract Concept. 2015;5(4):47-9.

Marghoob A, Braun R, Kopf A. Atlas of Dermoscopy. London: Taylor & Francis; 2005.

Menzies S, Crotty K, Ingvar C, et al. An Atlas of Surface Microscopy of Pigmented Skin Lesions. Sydney: McGraw-Hill Book Company; 1996.

Rabinovitz H, Kopf A. Dermoscopy: A Practical Guide. Miami: American Academy of Dermatology; 1999.

Soyer P, Argenziano G, Chimenti S, et al. Dermoscopy of Pigmented Skin Lesions. An Atlas Based on the Consensus Net Meeting on Dermoscopy. Milán: EDRA Medical Publishing & New Media; 2001.

Stolz W, Braun-Falco O, Bilek P, et al. Color Atlas of Dermatoscopy. USA: Blackwell Science; 1994.

Zaballos P, Bañuls J, Cabo H, et al. The usefulness of dermoscopy for the recognition of basal cell carcinoma-seborrhoeic keratosis compound tumors. Australas J Dermatol. 2013;54(3):208-12.

Zalaudek I, Argenziano G, Giacomel J. Dermoscopy of Non-Pigmented Skin Tumors. Boca Raton, FL: CRC Press; 2016.

SPECIAL LOCATIONS

9

Horacio A Cabo

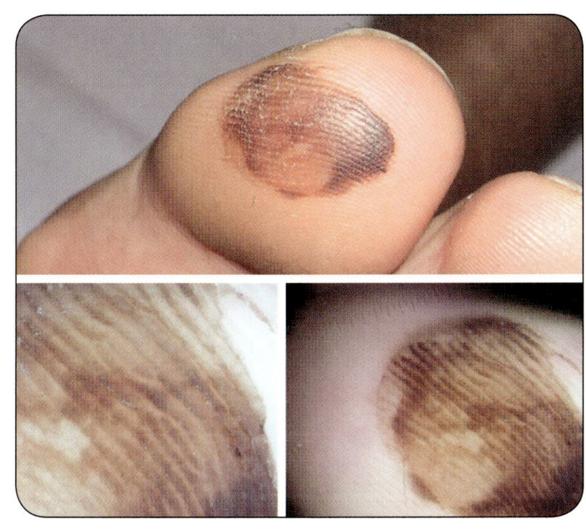

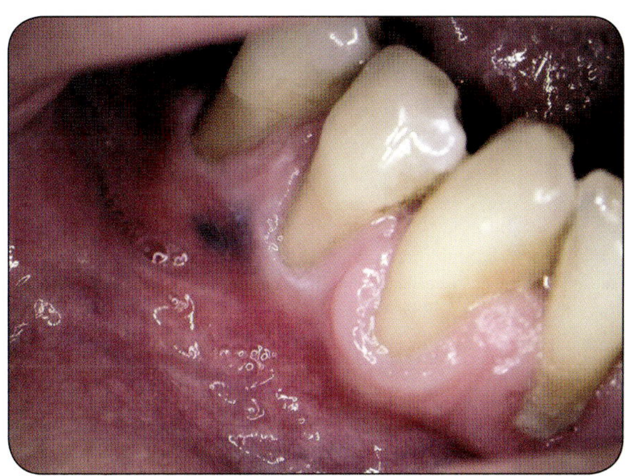

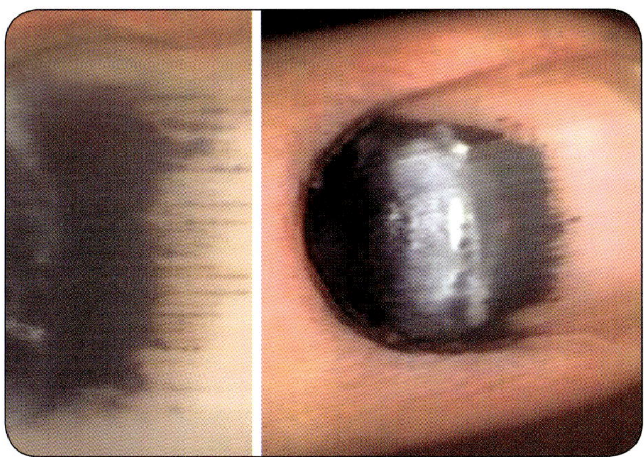

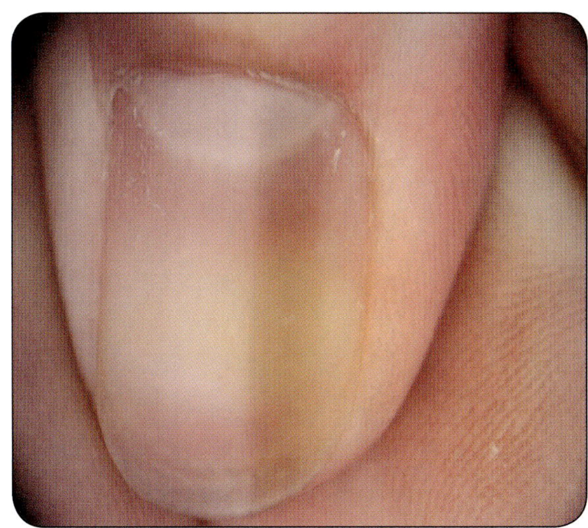

"The dermoscopy features in especial locations of pigmented and nonpigmented lesions are a very important issue.
Diagnosis and treatment of pigmented maculae on the face is one of the most difficult scenarios in the daily practice, even using a dermoscope.
To the acral site lesions, it is absolutely necessary to know the anatomy and histology of palms and soles that is different from the rest of the skin.
Dermoscopy have provided to improve the diagnosis of mucosa and nail lesions as well."

9.1 FACE

Horacio A Cabo

Diagnosis and treatment of pigmented maculae on the face is one of the most difficult scenarios in the daily practice, even using a dermoscope. The natural course and the prognosis are different in these pathologies, so that an accurate diagnosis is essential in order to guarantee a suitable management and treatment.

The face has a particular anatomic characteristic. In adult facial skin, the rete ridge is flattened or completely absent, which means that it is not possible to observe pigment network. The hair follicle opening, just like the sebaceous glands and sweat glands, has no pigment and presents a pseudonetwork formed by a thick mesh resulting from the skin color and whitish gaps, which correspond to the openings of the glands, since these areas lack melanin pigment. Therefore, this pseudonetwork is found in both melanocytic and nonmelanocytic lesions of the face, and consequently the pseudonetwork does not differentiate melanocytic from nonmelanocytic lesions in the case of the face, which makes it necessary to use other criteria (Figs. 9.1 to 9.3).

In the face, the most important differential diagnosis is between lentigo maligna melanoma (LMM), solar lentigo (SL), pigmented and nonpigmented actinic keratosis (PAK-AK) and lichen planus-like keratosis (Fig. 9.4).

Solar lentigo (Chapter 5, Part 5.2), PAK and AK (Chapter 5, Part 5.6), and LMM (Chapter 6, Part 6.9.3) have already been described, and therefore we will here discuss them in less detail.

Dermoscopic Criteria for SL (Fig. 9.5)

Fingerprint-Like Structures

These are brown structures, made up of fine parallel lines in fingerprint fashion. They are usually found in the peripheral part of the lesion.

Moth-Eaten Border

Concave edge of the lesion resembling the bite of a moth.

Jelly Sign

Light brown or yellowish in color; it resembles a very thin layer of jelly which has dried or a film covering the surface of the skin.

Dermoscopic Criteria for (AKs (Figs. 9.6 to 9.8)

Nonpigmented AK

- *Strawberry-like pattern*: It is possible to observe white or white-yellow follicular openings, in a reddish background resembling the surface of a strawberry.
- Vascular pattern with fine undulated vessels surrounding the hair follicle, dot-like vessels, and spiral-like vessels.

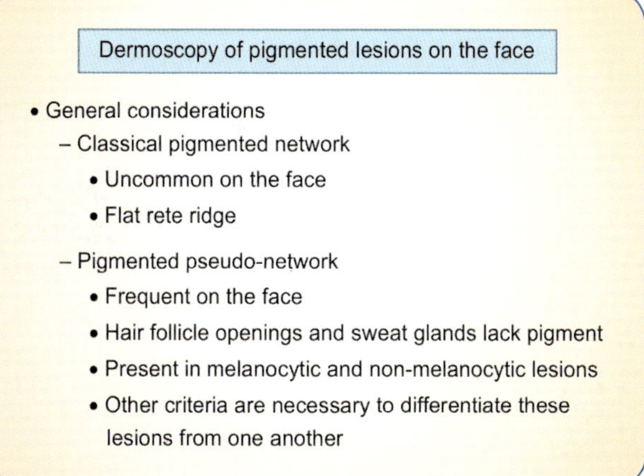

Fig. 9.1: Particular anatomic characteristic of the face.

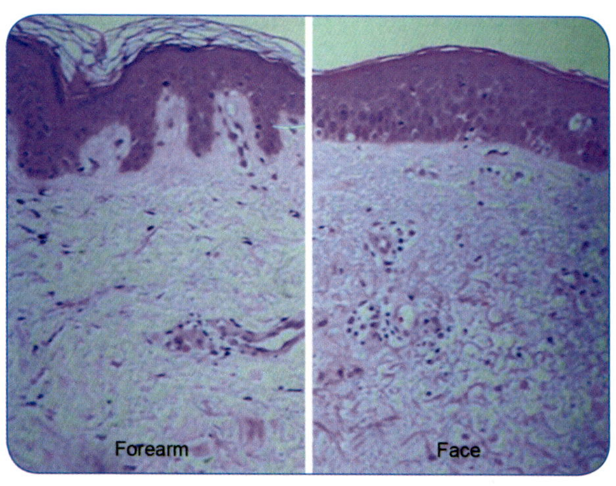

Fig. 9.2: Histologic differences between face and forearm skins.

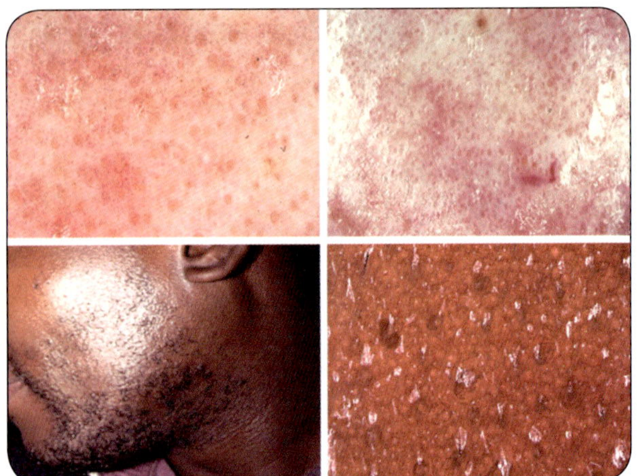

Fig. 9.3: Difference between light and dark skins. In dark skin, a physiologic pseudonetwork is clearly observed.

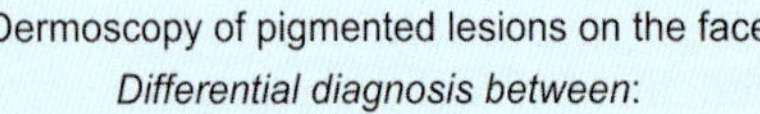

Fig. 9.4: The most important differential diagnosis in the face

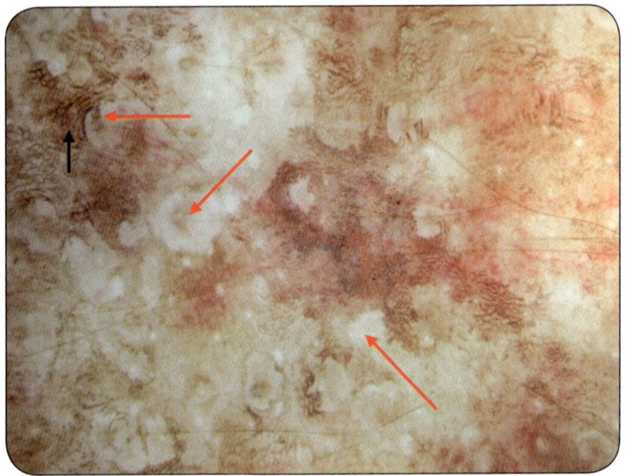

Fig. 9.5: Solar lentigo. Red arrows: Moth-eaten border. Black arrow: Fingerprint-like structures.

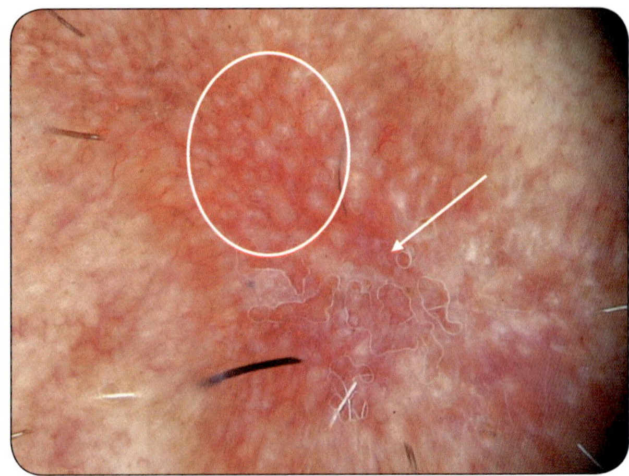

Fig. 9.6: Actinic keratosis: Strawberry pattern (white circle); Rosette-like structures (arrow).

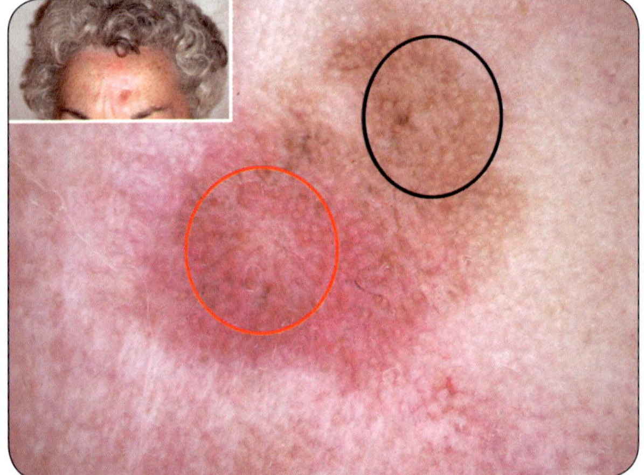

Fig. 9.7: Pigmented (black circle) and nonpigmented (red circle) actinic keratosis in the same lesion.

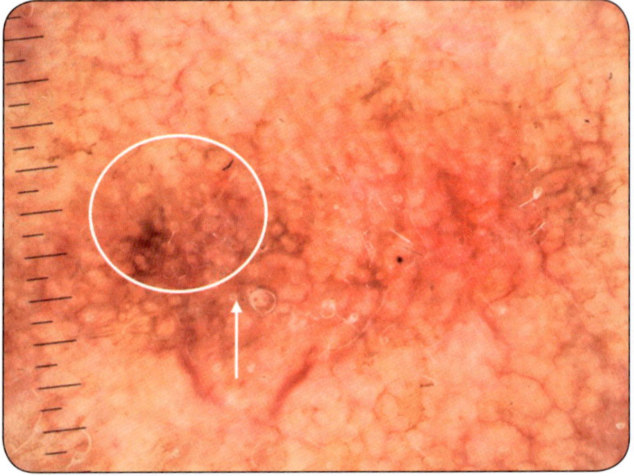

Fig. 9.8: Pigmented actinic keratosis: Pigmentation of the follicular openings (white circle); Rosette-like structures (arrow).

- Superficial yellowish-white scales.
- Hyperkeratotic follicles.
- *Rosettes*: They are observable with polarized light and correspond to four grouped white dots, resembling a four-leafed clover, located mainly within the follicular opening. They are nonspecific, and observable also in other tumors, especially keratinizing ones.

Pigmented AK

- Superficial brown color with the appearance of broken pseudonetwork.
- Hyperkeratotic follicles.
- *Inner gray halo*: Subtle homogeneous gray or light brown halo surrounding the follicular openings in the manner of an inner ring within the mesh of the brown pseudonetwork. It is the result of the pigmentation of the basal keratinocytes surrounding the hair follicle.
- Asymmetric pigmentation of the follicular opening [which can also be found in lentigo maligna (LM)].
- Rhomboidal structures (also found in LM).

Dermoscopic Criteria for Lichen Planus-Like Keratosis (Figs. 9.9 to 9.12)

- Lichen planus-like keratosis is a SL or seborrheic keratosis (SK) with regression which may simulate a LM. In lesions with incomplete regression, it is important to examine the areas of the pre-existing lesion (SK or SL). When regression is complete, there appear gray dots,

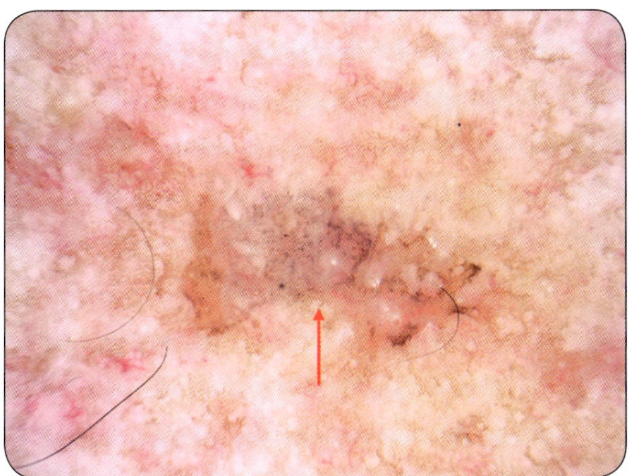

Fig. 9.9: Lichen planus-like keratosis: Seborrheic keratosis with regression (arrow).

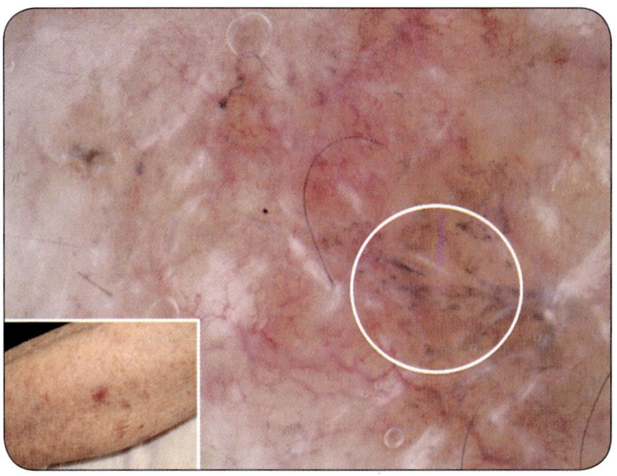

Fig. 9.10: Lichen planus-like keratosis: Actinic keratosis with regression (white circle).

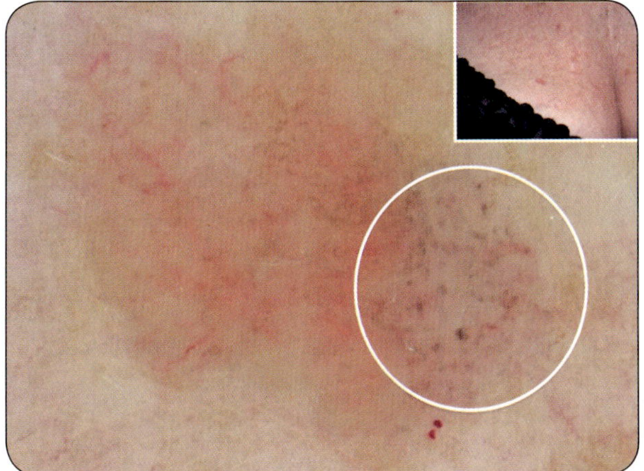

Fig. 9.11: Lichen planus-like keratosis: Actinic keratosis with regression (white circle).

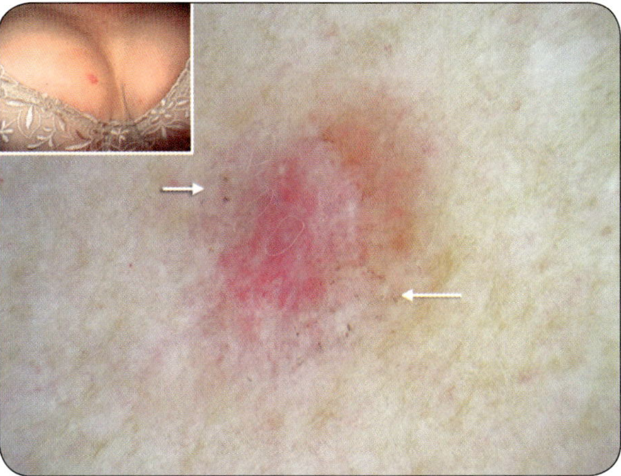

Fig. 9.12: Lichen planus-like keratosis: Actinic keratosis with regression (arrows).

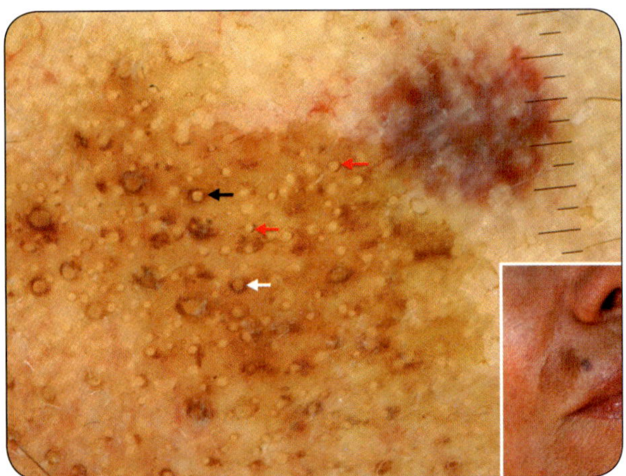

Fig. 9.13: Lentigo maligna: Blue-gray pigmented follicular openings (black arrow); asymmetric pigmentation of the follicular openings (red arrows); circle within a circle (white arrow).

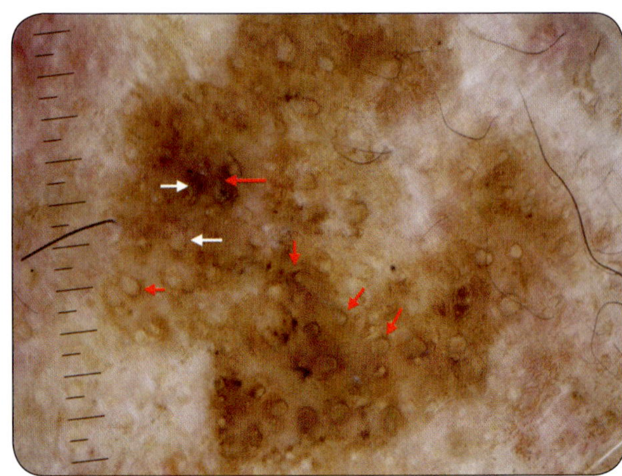

Fig. 9.14: Lentigo maligna: Asymmetric pigmentation of the follicular openings (red arrows); circle within a circle (white arrows).

globules, lines or even rhomboid structures. In these cases, a biopsy is recommended.

Dermoscopic Criteria for LM (Figs. 9.13 and 9.14)

Dermoscopic Features

- *Blue-gray color*: Sometimes, this color is the only clue to suspect a malignant lentigo.
- *Blue, gray, or black pigmented and asymmetrically pigmented follicular openings*: Dark brown or black in color, which indicates the irregular proliferation of atypical melanocytes within the follicles. In LM (melanoma in situ) and in LMM (invasive melanoma), if the follicles are close together, it is possible to perceive a second pseudonetwork characterized by a thin mesh, as opposed to the pseudonetwork which depends on location and which presents a thick mesh. These grid-like structures are pseudonetworks, since they do not arise from the pigmentation of the crests or ridges of the rete ridges but from the follicular openings in pigmented facial skin.
- *Two concentric circles (circle within a circle)*: This new criterion is highly useful and its significance, statistically undetermined yet, could be similar to that of the asymmetric pigmentation of the follicular openings.
- *Slate gray dots around the follicular openings*: It is an early sign of lentigo malignant and it is the beginning of *granular-annular pattern.*
- *Rhomboidal structures*: At a later stage, it is possible to detect dark brown or black lines or short streaks, highly specific around the follicles.
- *Homogeneous blue-gray areas* with the hair follicles spared or obliterated.

SUGGESTED READING

Argenziano G, Soyer P, De Giorgio V, et al. Interactive Atlas of Dermoscopy. Milán: EDRA Medical Publishing & New Media; 2000.

Cabo H. Dermatoscopia. Buenos Aires, Argentina: Weber Ferro; 2000.

Cabo H. Dermatoscopia, 2nd edition. Buenos Aires, Argentina: Ediciones Journal; 2012.

Johr R, Stolz W. Dermoscopy: An Illustrated Self-Assessment Guide, 2nd edition. New York: McGraw-Hill Education; 2015.

Jorh R, Soyer P, Argenziano G, et al. Dermoscopy. The Essentials (MOABT). New York: Elsevier Ltd; 2004.

Kittler H. Dermatoscopy. An Algorithmic Method Based on Pattern Analysis 2011 Facultas Verlags- und Buchhandels AG facultas wuv Universitätsverlag, Austria www.facultas.wuv.at

Lallas A. Dermoscopy in general dermatology. Dermatol Clin. 2013;3:679-94.

Malvhey J, Puig S. Principles of dermoscopy. Barcelona: Creaciones Gráficas; 2009.

Marghoob A, Braun R, Kopf A. Atlas of dermoscopy. London: Taylor & Francis; 2005.

Menzies S, Crotty K, Ingvar C, et al. An Atlas of Surface Microscopy of Pigmented Skin Lesions. Sydney: McGraw-Hill Book Company; 1996.

Rabinovitz H, Kopf A. Dermoscopy: A Practical Guide. Miami: American Academy of Dermatology; 1999.

Soyer P, Argenziano G, Chimenti S, et al. Dermoscopy of Pigmented Skin Lesions. An Atlas Based on the Consensus Net Meeting on Dermoscopy. Milán: EDRA Medical Publishing & New Media; 2001.

Stolz W, Braun-Falco O, Bilek P, et al. Color Atlas of Dermatoscopy. USA: Blackwell Science; 1994.

Zalaudek I, Argenziano G, Giacomel J. Dermoscopy of Nonpigmented Skin Tumors. Boca Raton, FL: CRC Press; 2016.

9.2 PALMS AND SOLES

Horacio A Cabo

In this chapter, we will talk about benign lesions in this location since the dermoscopic features of acral melanoma have been described in Chapter 6, Part 6.9.4.

It is absolutely necessary to know the anatomy and histology of palms and soles (Fig. 9.15).

The main anatomical feature is that the cutaneous surface presents dermatoglyphs composed of ridges and furrows, which are characteristic of each individual through genetic determination. Skin histology shows particular features due to the thickness of the corneum layer, the absence of hair follicles, the presence of eccrine glands, and the repetition of crista intermedia and crista limitans in the dermoepidermal junction, as shown in Figure 9.15.

Characteristically, eccrine glands are located in the crista intermedia; therefore, their eccrine ducts lead to the surface of the ridge.

In the case of benign melanocytic lesions, the nests of melanocytes tend to lie fundamentally in the crista limitans and this produces the pigmentation of the furrows.

This phenomenon, of unknown origin, gives rise to the dermoscopic patterns.

DERMOSCOPIC PATTERNS OF ACRAL NEVI

Parallel furrow pattern: It is the most frequent pattern in acral lesions, both in Asian and Caucasian races, and represents 50% of all melanocytic nevi. It consists in the presence of pigment, especially in the furrow, which configures a characteristic parallel pattern.

Variants:

- One line (Figs. 9.16 to 9.25)
- Double line (Figs. 9.26 to 9.33) (it probably corresponds to the congenital type acral nevus)
- Dotted line (Fig. 9.34)
- Double-dotted line (Figs. 9.35 to 9.37)

Lattice-like pattern: Variant of the parallel furrow pattern. It is the second most frequent pattern (14%). It is a parallel furrow pattern with lines crossing the crista from a furrow to the next (Figs. 9.38 to 9.43).

Fibrillar pattern: It is composed of usually delicate lines streaming from the sulcus and crossing many furrows and ridges in a discretely oblique fashion. This pigment pattern results from the optic effect of the fold of the ridges in higher pressure areas of palms and soles (Figs. 9.44 to 9.49).

Globular pattern: Similar to that observed in other melanocytic lesions (Fig. 9.50).

Homogeneous pattern: Some congenital nevi may show a homogeneous brown or blue pattern (Fig. 9.51).

Reticular pattern: Similar to nevi with reticular pattern (Figs. 9.52 to 9.55).

Atypical or uncharacteristic pattern: Those lesions that cannot be classified as corresponding to any of the previous patterns (Fig. 9.56).

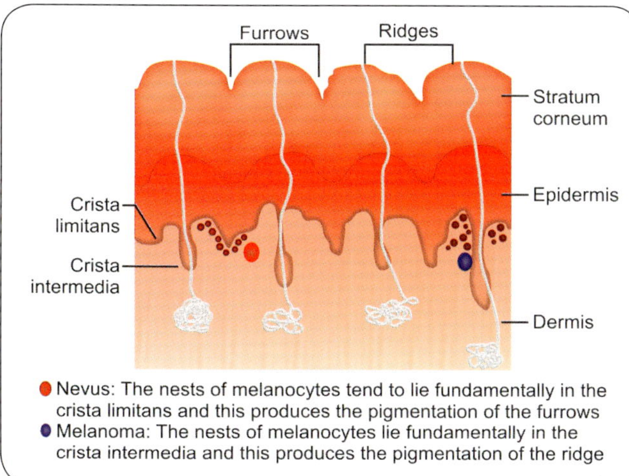

Fig. 9.15: Scheme of the skin anatomy in palms and soles.

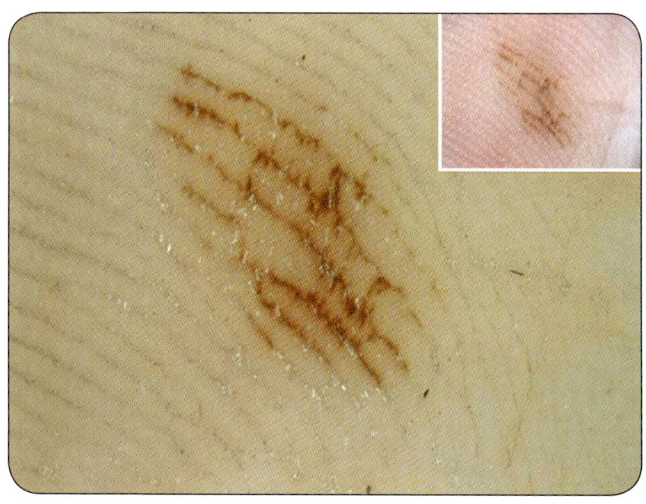

Fig. 9.16: Parallel furrow pattern: One line.

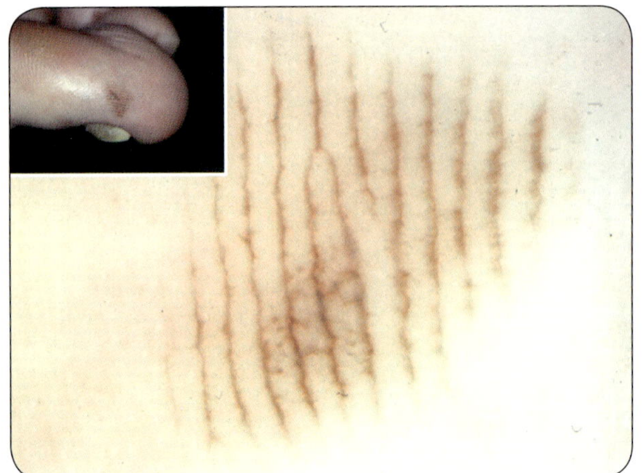

Fig. 9.17: Parallel furrow pattern: One line.

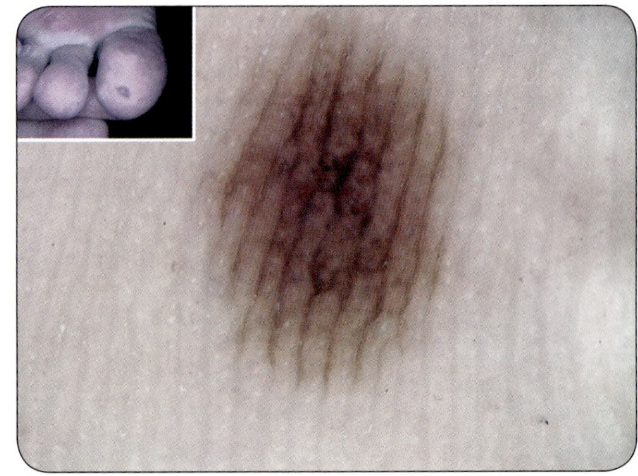

Fig. 9.18: Parallel furrow pattern: One line.

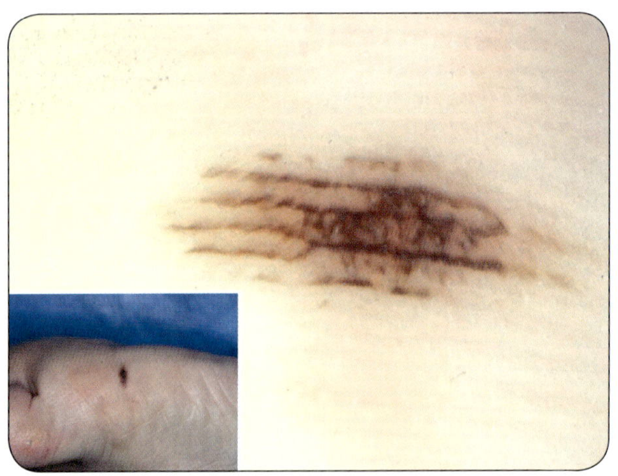

Fig. 9.19: Parallel furrow pattern: One line.

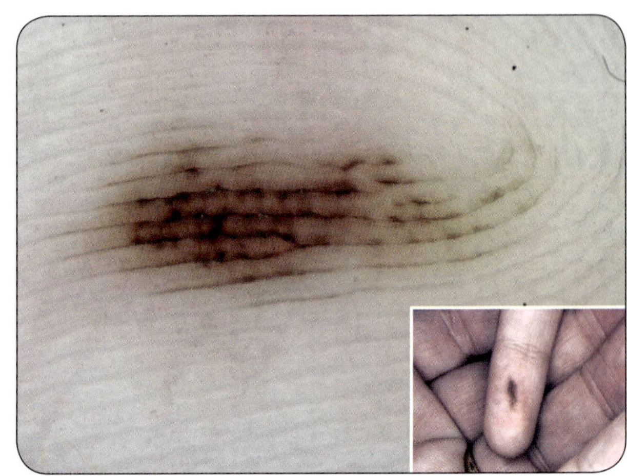

Fig. 9.20: Parallel furrow pattern: One line.

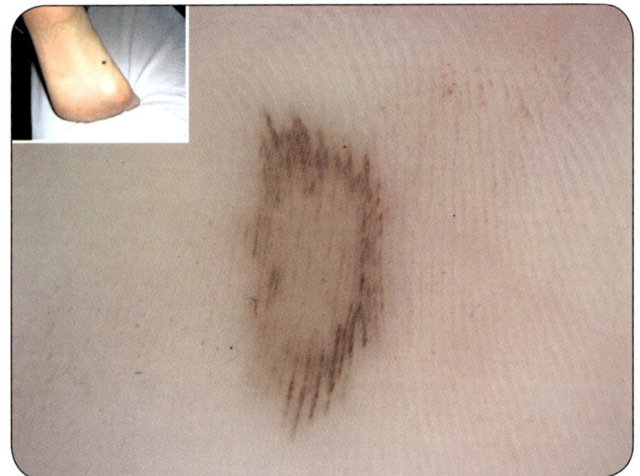

Fig. 9.21: Parallel furrow pattern: One line.

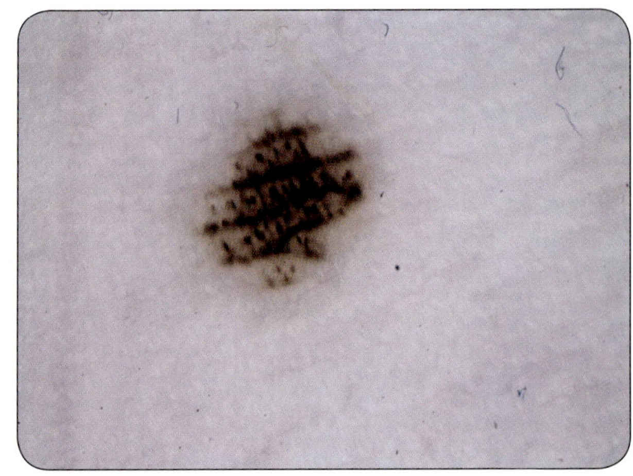

Fig. 9.22: Parallel furrow pattern: One line.

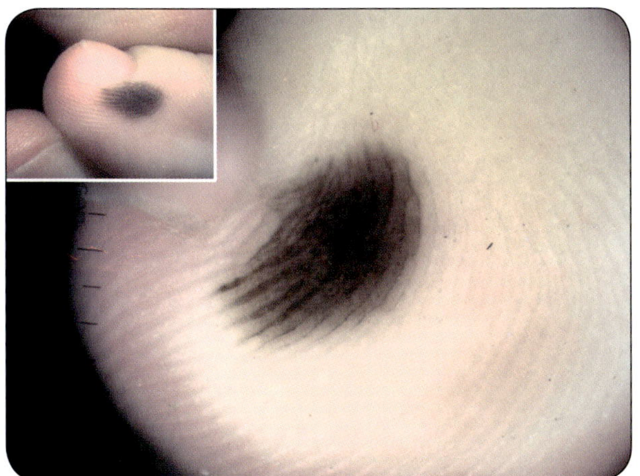

Fig. 9.23: Parallel furrow pattern: One line.

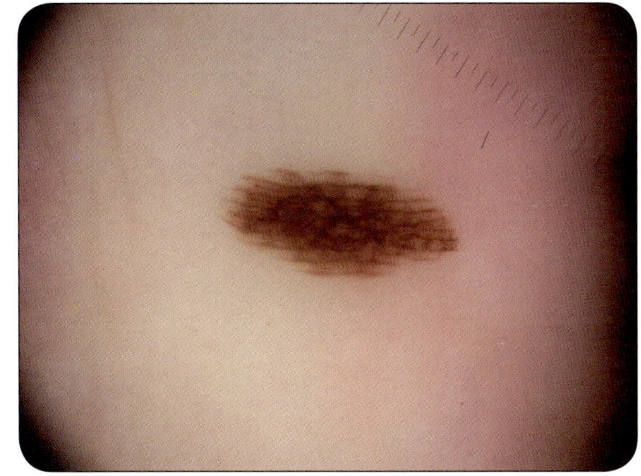

Fig. 9.24: Parallel furrow pattern: One line.

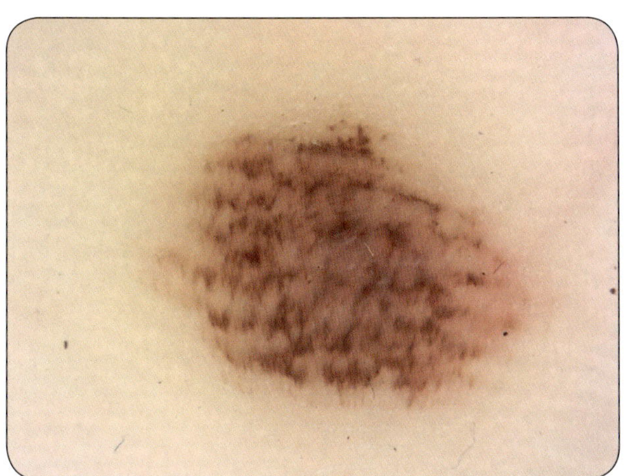

Fig. 9.25: Parallel furrow pattern: One line.

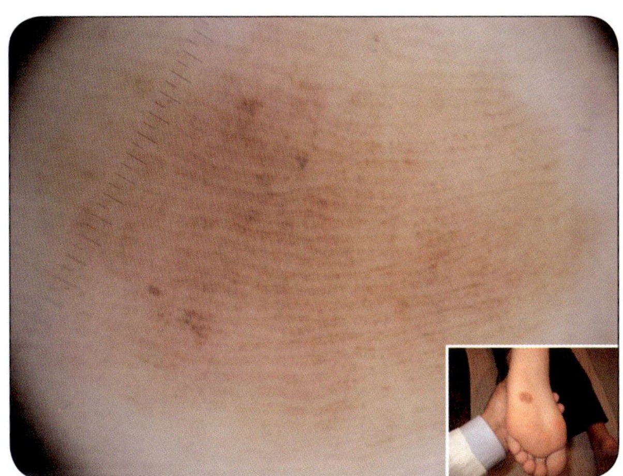

Fig. 9.26: Parallel furrow pattern: Double line.

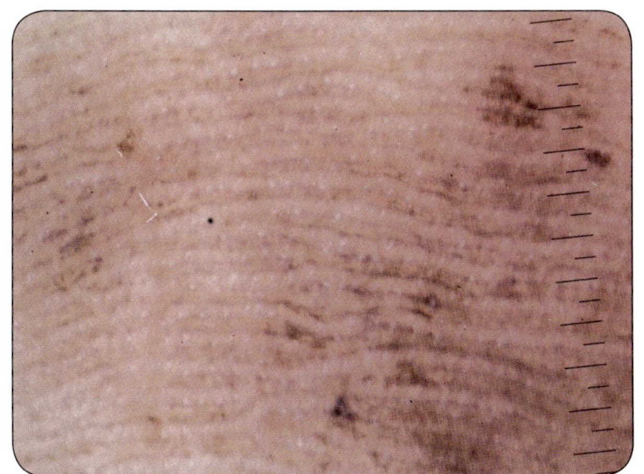

Fig. 9.27: Parallel furrow pattern: Double line.

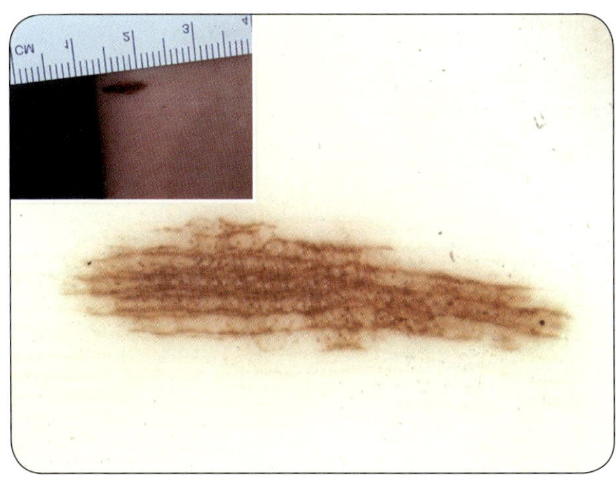

Fig. 9.28: Parallel furrow pattern: Double line.

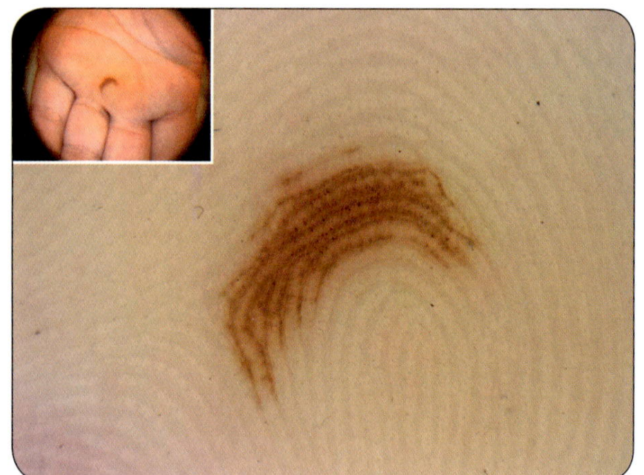

Fig. 9.29: Parallel furrow pattern: Double line.

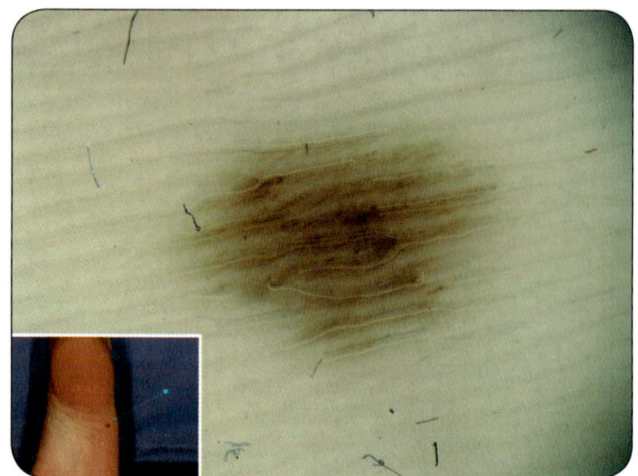

Fig. 9.30: Parallel furrow pattern: Double line.

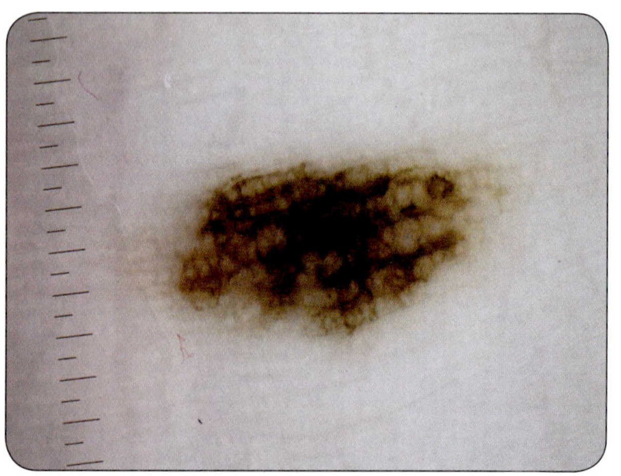

Fig. 9.31: Parallel furrow pattern: Double line.

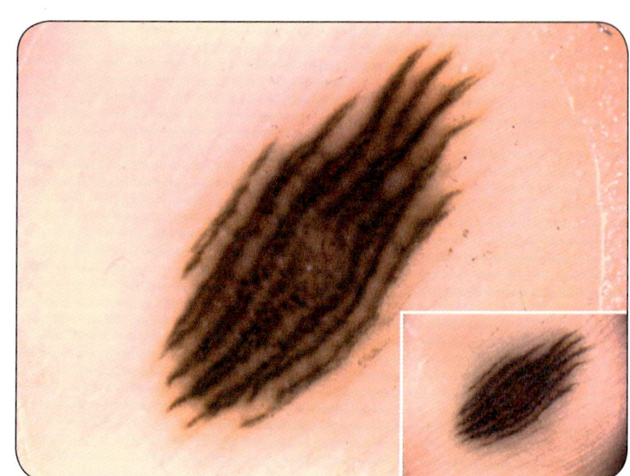

Fig. 9.32: Parallel furrow pattern: Double line.

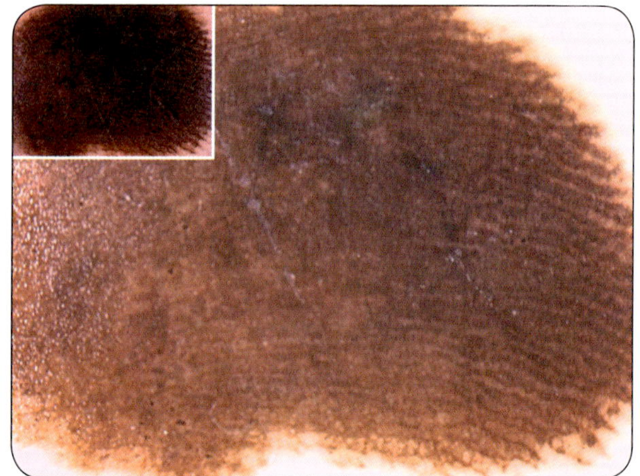

Fig. 9.33: Parallel furro pattern: Double line.

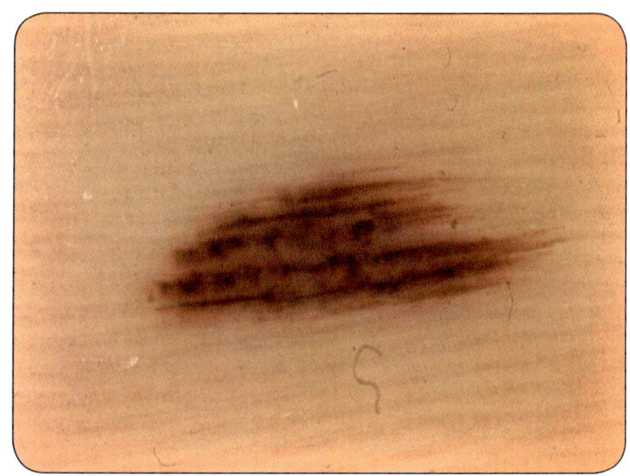

Fig. 9.34: Parallel furrow pattern: Dotted line.

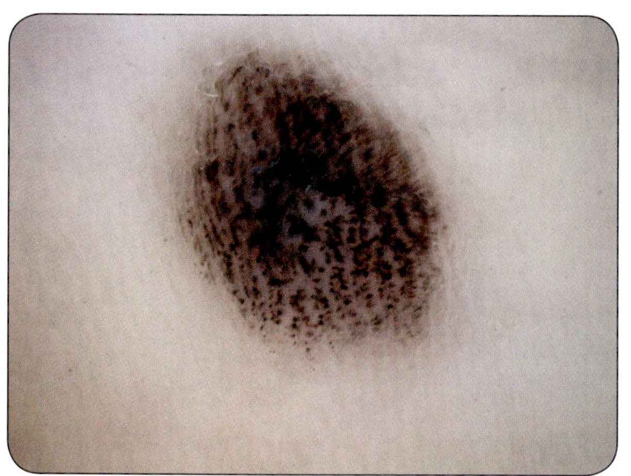

Fig. 9.35: Parallel furrow pattern: Double-dotted line.

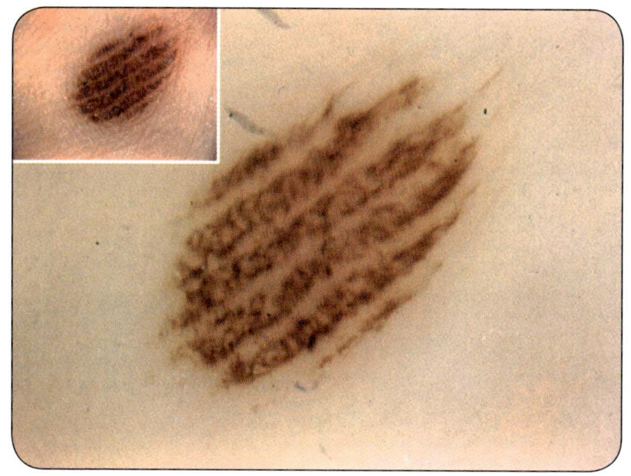

Fig. 9.36: Parallel furrow pattern: Double-dotted line.

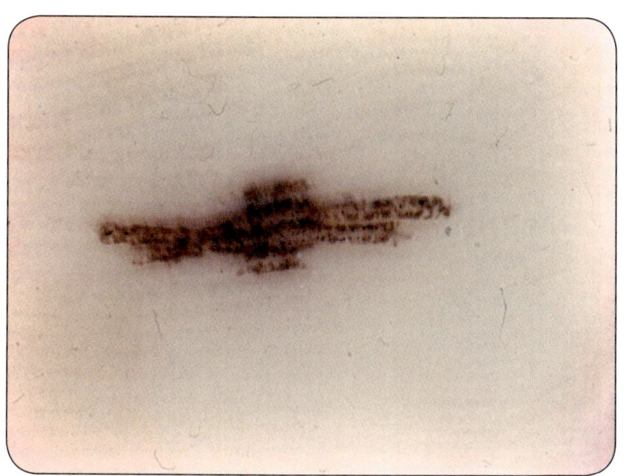

Fig. 9.37: Parallel furrow pattern: Double-dotted line.

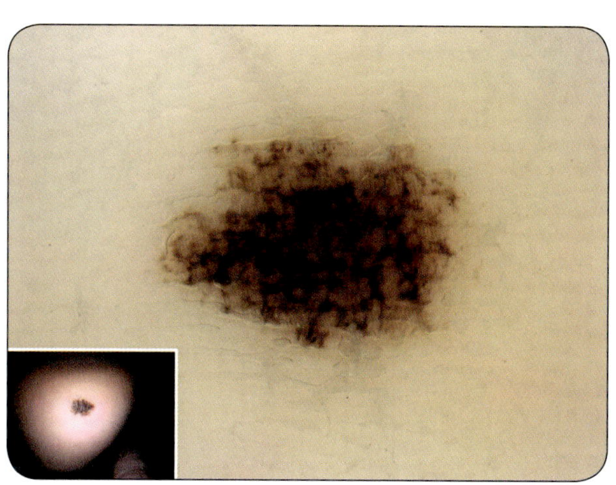

Fig. 9.38: Lattice-like pattern.

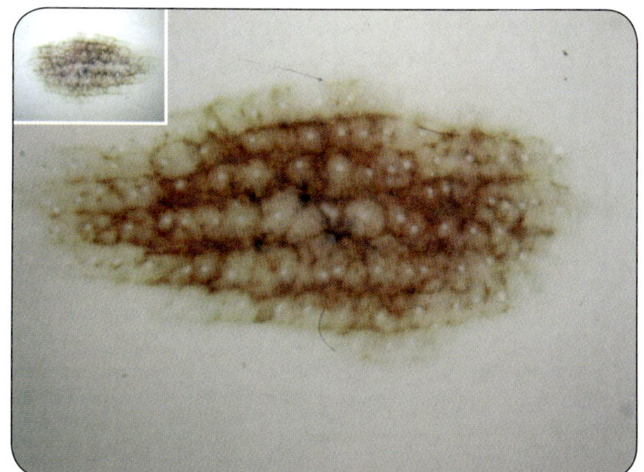

Fig. 9.39: Lattice-like pattern.

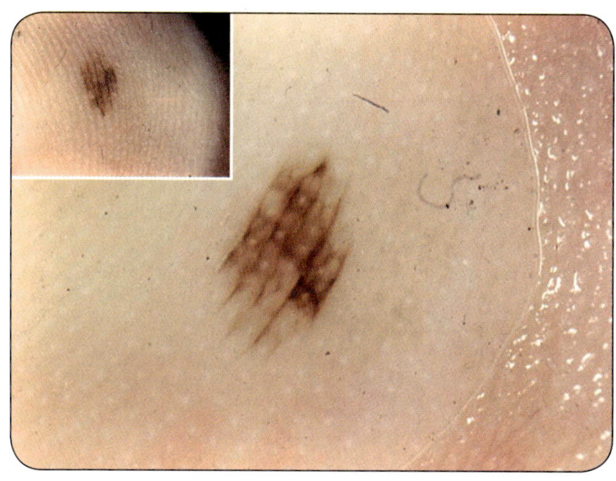

Fig. 9.40: Lattice-like pattern.

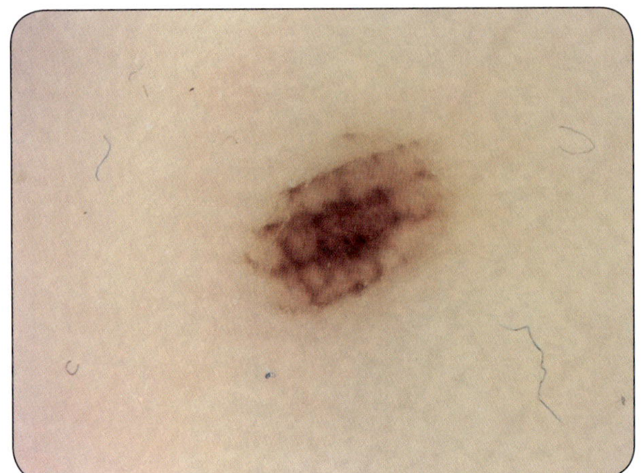

Fig. 9.41: Lattice-like pattern.

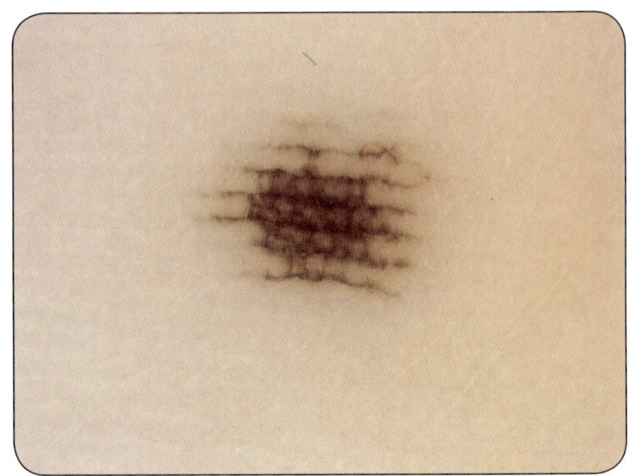

Fig. 9.42: Lattice-like pattern.

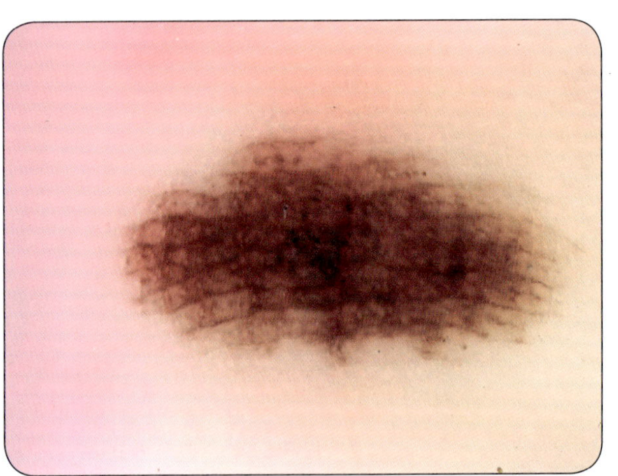

Fig. 9.43: Lattice-like pattern.

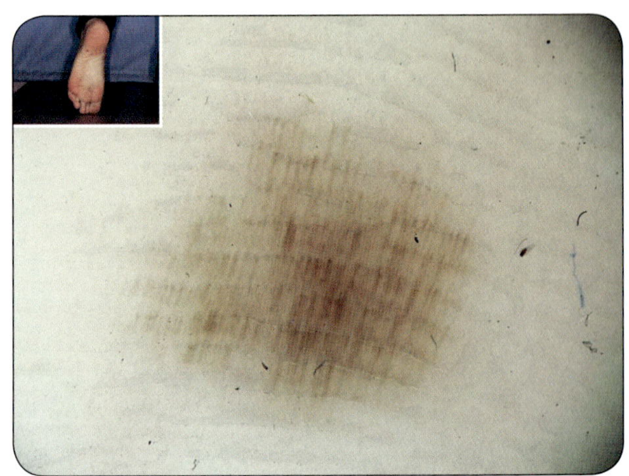

Fig. 9.44: Fibrillar pattern.

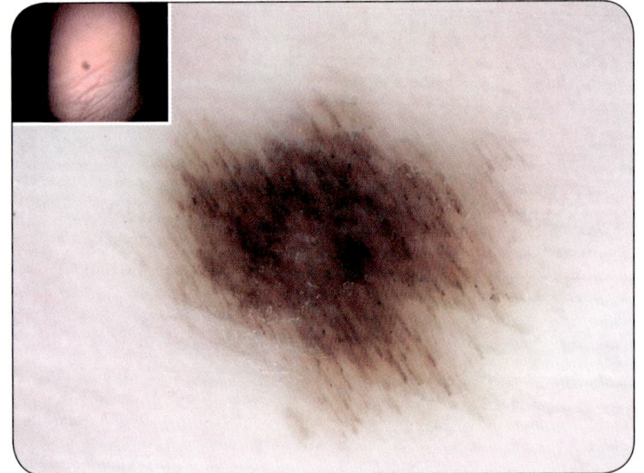

Fig. 9.45: Fibrillar pattern.

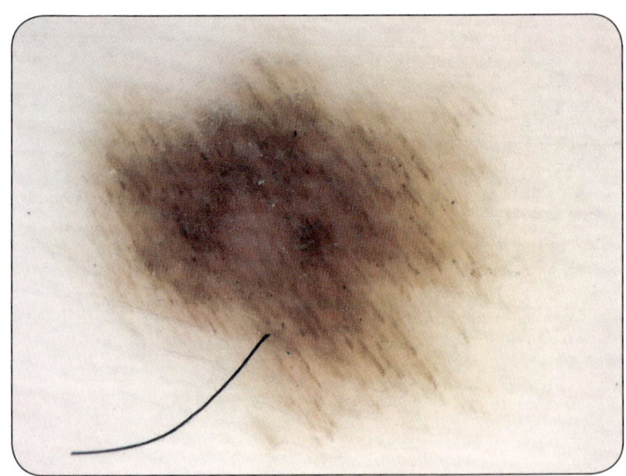

Fig. 9.46: Fibrillar pattern.

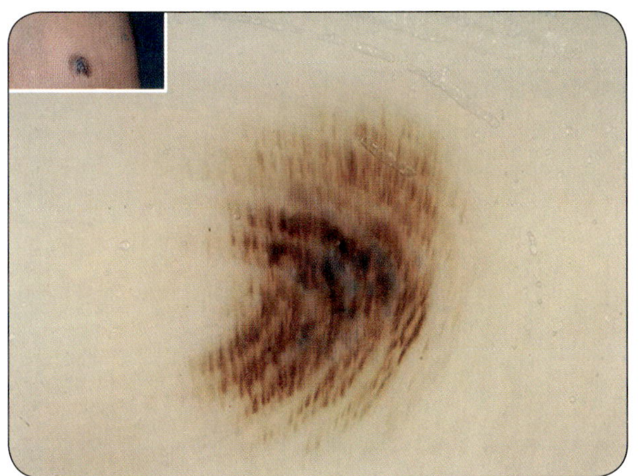

Fig. 9.47: Fibrillar pattern.

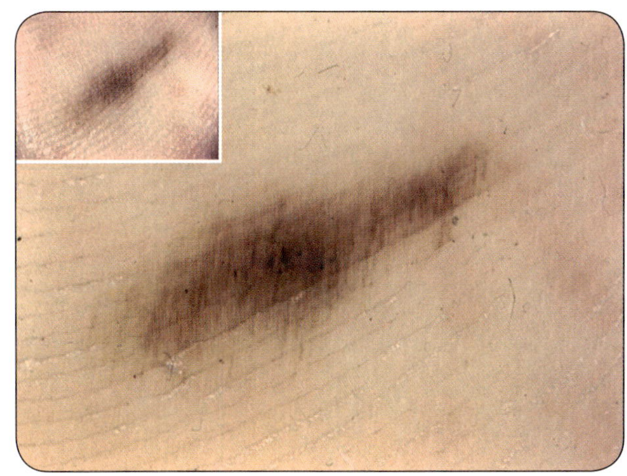

Fig. 9.48: Fibrillar pattern.

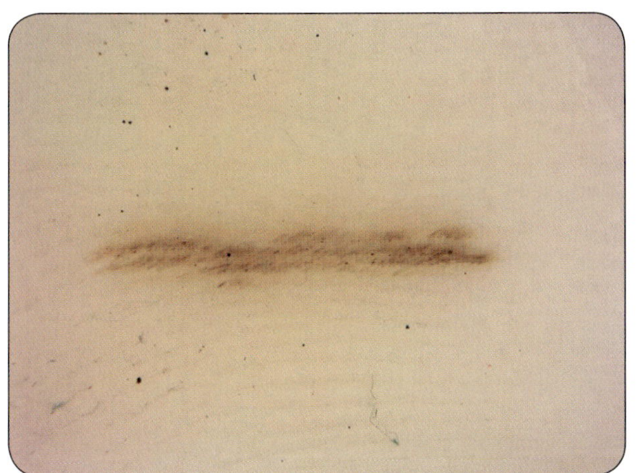

Fig. 9.49: Fibrillar pattern.

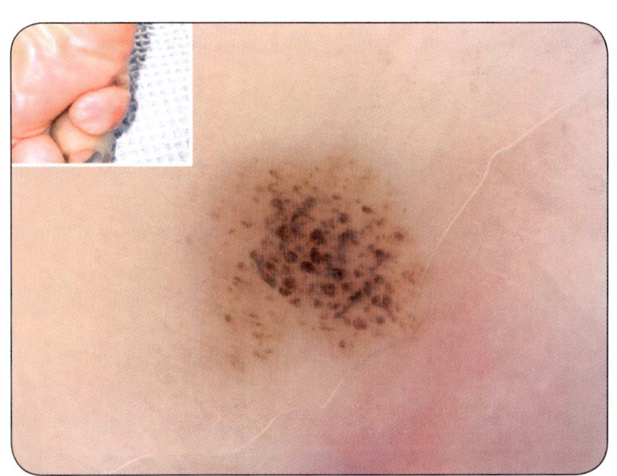

Fig. 9.50: Globular pattern.

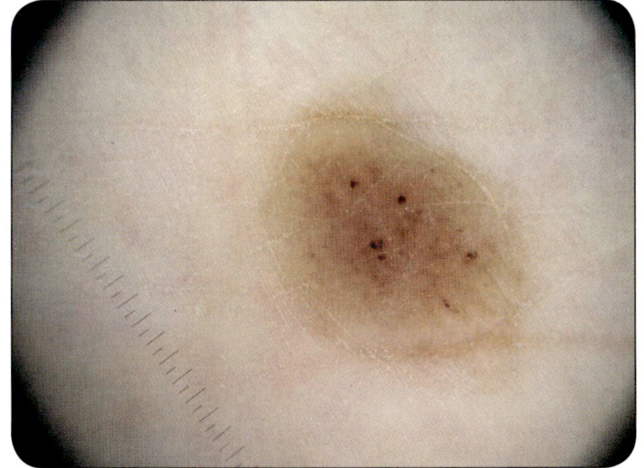

Fig. 9.51: Homogeneous pattern.

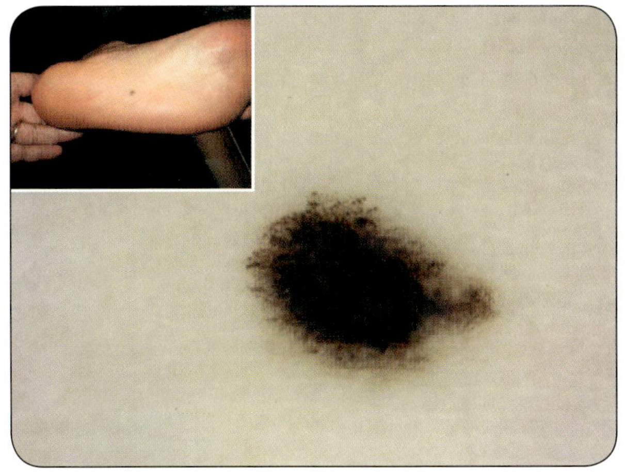

Fig. 9.52: Reticular pattern.

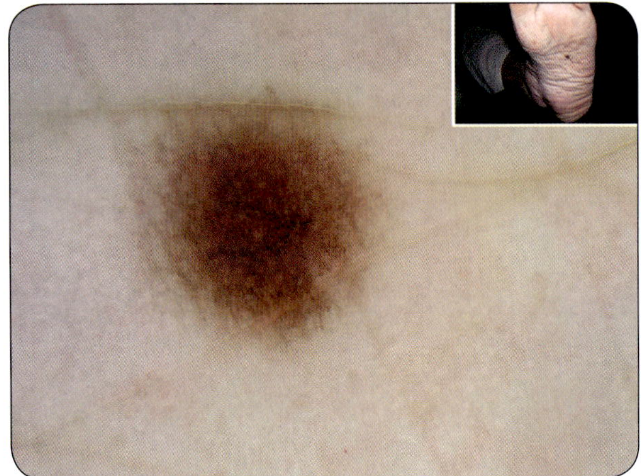

Fig. 9.53: Reticular pattern.

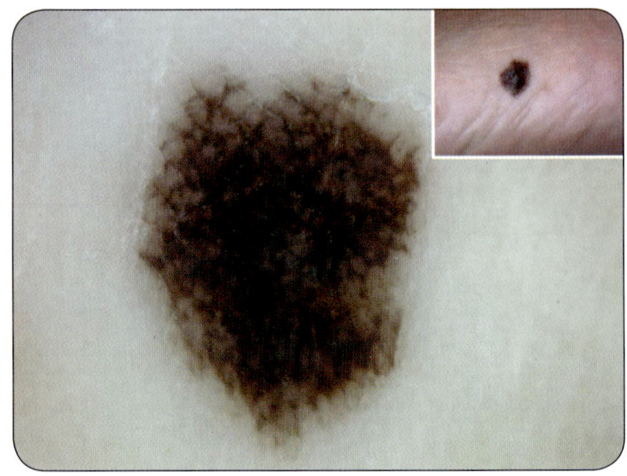

Fig. 9.54: Reticular pattern.

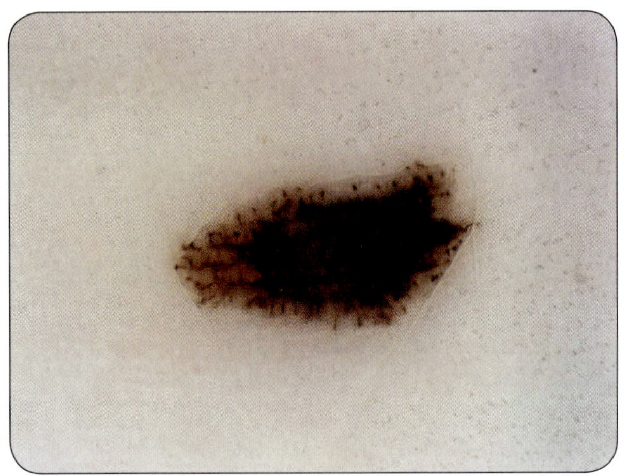

Fig. 9.55: Reticular pattern.

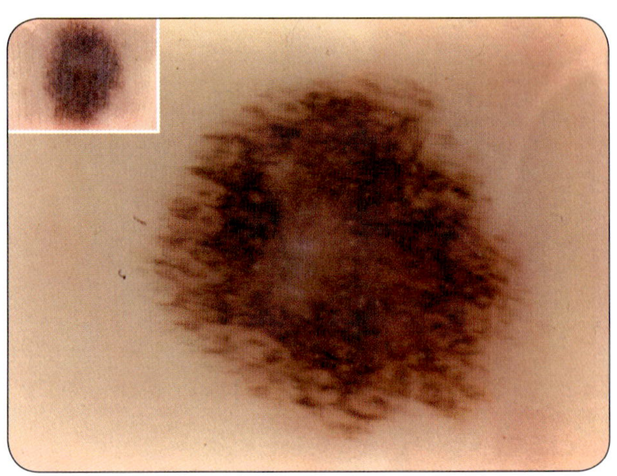

Fig. 9.56: Atypical or uncharacteristic pattern.

Transition pattern: In the case of localized lesions in the transition zone between volar skin and the back of hands and feet (Wallace line), there is a transition pattern combining benign parallel pattern and reticular pigmented pattern (Figs. 9.57 and 9.58).

Congenital nevus: Nevi showing crista dotted pattern and the double line variant (Figs. 9.26 to 9.59).

Pseudoparallel-ridge pattern: After trauma in palms and soles, the hemorrhage flows through the duct of the eccrine sweat gland and reaches the epidermis causing a pigmentation of the ridge due to hematic pigment (Figs. 9.60 to 9.64).

Main characteristics:

- Previous trauma history (not always remembered)

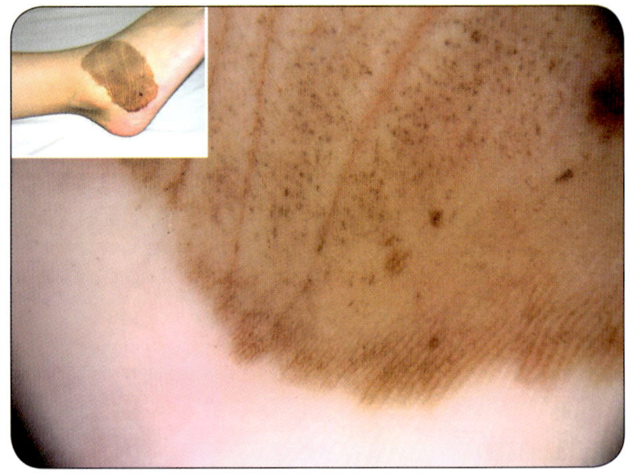

Fig. 9.57: Transition pattern.

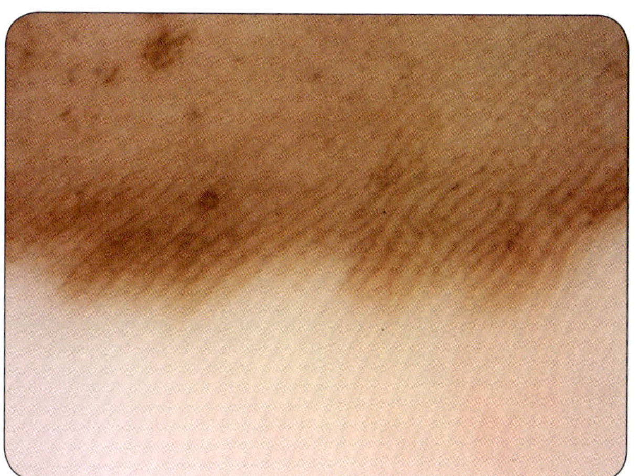

Fig. 9.58: Transition pattern.

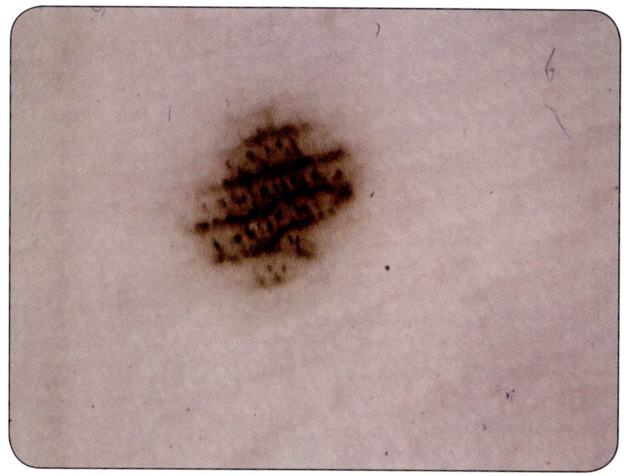

Fig. 9.59: Congenital nevus: Crista dotted pattern.

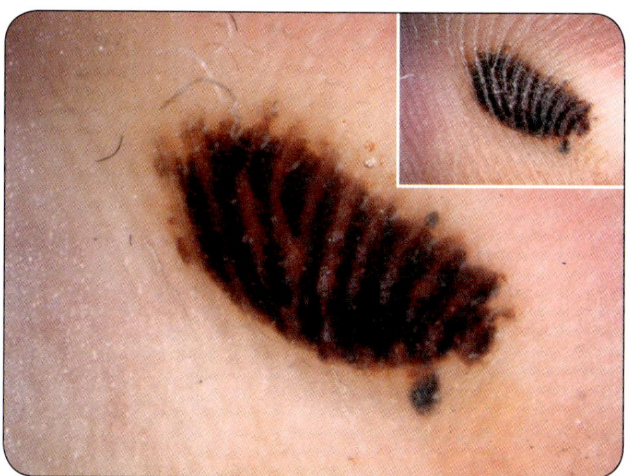

Fig. 9.60: Pseudoparallel-ridge pattern: After trauma in palms and soles, the hemorrhage flows through the duct of the eccrine sweat gland and reaches the epidermis causing a pigmentation of the ridge due to hematic pigment.

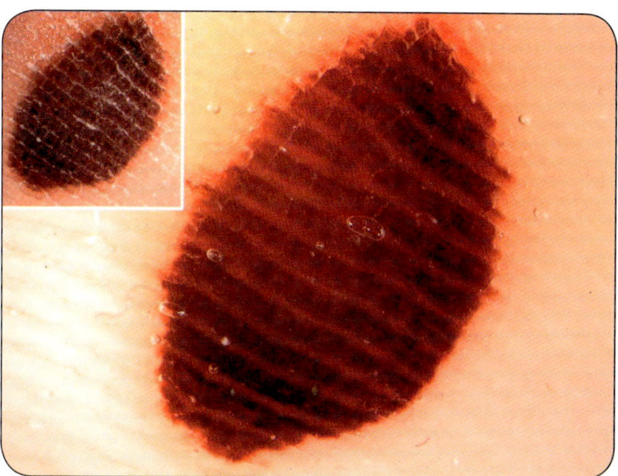

Fig. 9.61: Pseudoparallel-ridge pattern: After trauma in palms and soles, the hemorrhage flows through the duct of the eccrine sweat gland and reaches the epidermis causing a pigmentation of the ridge due to hematic pigment.

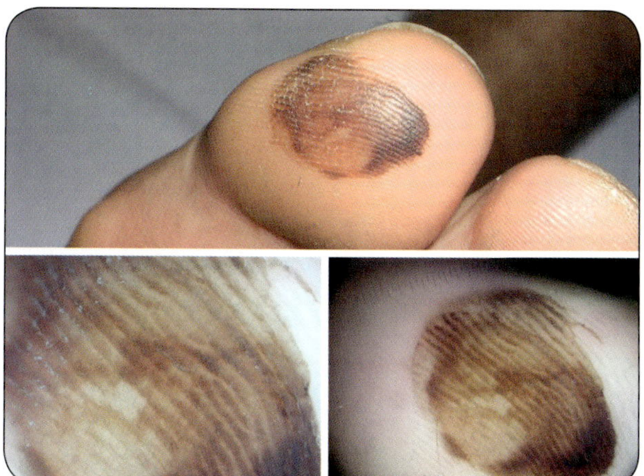

Fig. 9.62: Pseudoparallel-ridge pattern: After trauma in palms and soles, the hemorrhage flows through the duct of the eccrine sweat gland and reaches the epidermis causing a pigmentation of the ridge due to hematic pigment.

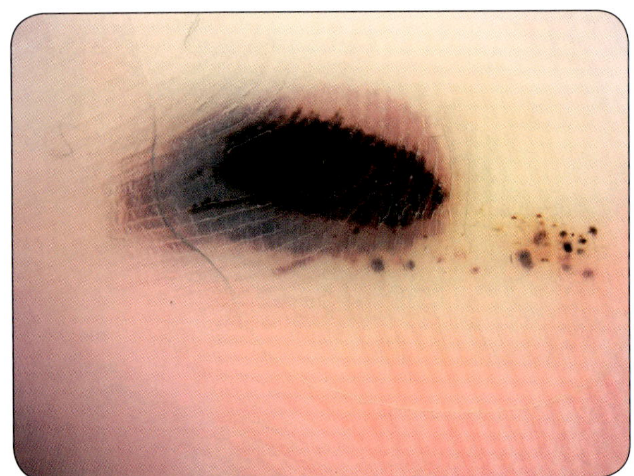

Fig. 9.63: Pseudoparallel-ridge pattern: After trauma in palms and soles, the hemorrhage flows through the duct of the eccrine sweat gland and reaches the epidermis causing a pigmentation of the ridge due to hematic pigment.

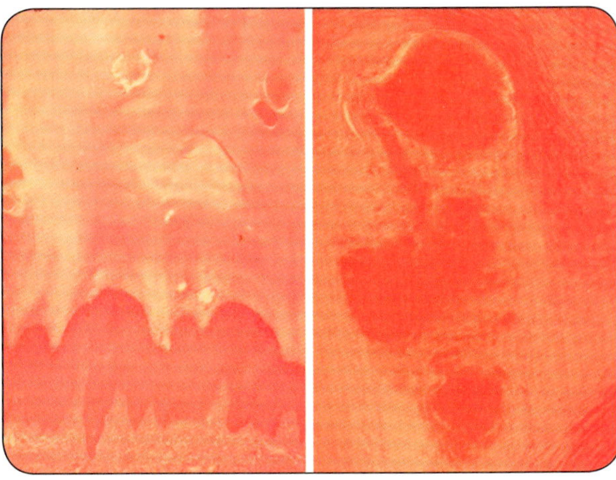

Fig. 9.64: Pseudoparallel-ridge pattern: After trauma in palms and soles, the hemorrhage flows through the duct of the eccrine sweat gland and reaches the epidermis causing a pigmentation of the ridge due to hematic pigment.

- Typical color
- Regularity
- Color changes accompanying hematoma resolution

SUGGESTED READING

Argenziano G, Soyer P, De Giorgio V, et al. Interactive Atlas of Dermoscopy. Milán: EDRA Medical Publishing & New Media; 2000.

Cabo H. Dermatoscopia. Buenos Aires, Argentina: Weber Ferro; 2000.

Cabo H. Dermatoscopia, 2nd edition. Buenos Aires, Argentina: Ediciones Journal; 2012.

Johr R, Stolz W. Dermoscopy: An Illustrated Self-Assessment Guide, 2nd edition. New York: Mc-Graw Hill Education; 2015.

Jorh R, Soyer P, Argenziano G, et al. Dermoscopy. The Essentials (MOABT). New York: Elsevier Ltd; 2004.

Kittler H. Dermatoscopy. An Algorithmic Method Based on Pattern Analysis 2011 Facultas Verlags- und Buchhandels AG facultas wuv Universitätsverlag, Austria www.facultas.wuv.at

Koga H, Saida T. Revised 3-step dermoscopic algorithm for the management of acral melanocytic lesions. Arch Dermatol. 2011;(6):741-2.

Lallas A. Dermoscopy in general dermatology. Dermatol Clin. 2013;3: 679-94.

Malvhey J, Puig S. Principles of Dermoscopy. Barcelona: Creaciones Gráficas; 2009.

Marghoob A, Braun R, Kopf A. Atlas of Dermoscopy. London: Taylor & Francis; 2005.

Menzies S, Crotty K, Ingvar C, et al. An Atlas of Surface Microscopy of Pigmented Skin Lesions. Sydney: McGraw-Hill Book Company; 1996.

Rabinovitz H, Kopf A. Dermoscopy: A Practical Guide. Miami: American Academy of Dermatology; 1999.

Soyer P, Argenziano G, Chimenti S, et al. Dermoscopy of Pigmented Skin Lesions. An Atlas Based on the Consensus Net Meeting on Dermoscopy. Milán: EDRA Medical Publishing & New Media; 2001.

Stolz W, Braun-Falco O, Bilek P, et al. Color Atlas of Dermatoscopy. USA: Blackwell Science; 1994.

Suzaki R, Ishizaki S, Iyatomi H, et al. Age-related prevalence of dermoscopic patterns of acral melanocytic nevi. Dermatol Pract Concept. 2013;4(1):53-7.

Zalaudek I, Argenziano G, Giacomel J. Dermoscopy of Non-pigmented Skin Tumors. Boca Raton, FL: CRC Press; 2016.

9.3 MUCOSA

Horacio A Cabo

The mucosa has a special epithelial type characterized by its thinness and being constantly lubricated. The horny layer or stratum corneum, granular layer, and sweat glands are absent, as opposed to what happens with the skin, which is why the observable dermoscopic criteria are different.

The pigmented lesions on the mucosae encompass a range of different entities which may have melanocytic origin or result from a precipitate of melanin pigment or of other substances with exogenous or endogenous origin.

The most frequent scenario is the melanocytic Macula, labial or genital, and has a typical dermatoscopy, but we think it is more useful to focus the dermatoscopy of mucous membranes (**on?**) recognizing patterns associated with benign lesions and others associated with malignant lesions, in order to make the decision **to biopsy or not the lesion. (whether to biopsy the lesion or not)**.

DERMOSCOPIC PATTERNS

Benign pigmented lesions

- *Dotted-globular pattern* (Figs. 9.65 to 9.69)
- *Homogeneous pattern* (Fig. 9.68)

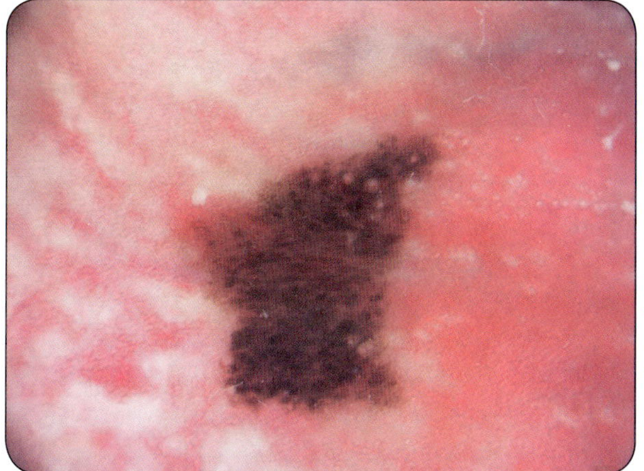

Fig. 9.65: Melanocytic nevus (lip): Dotted-globular pattern.

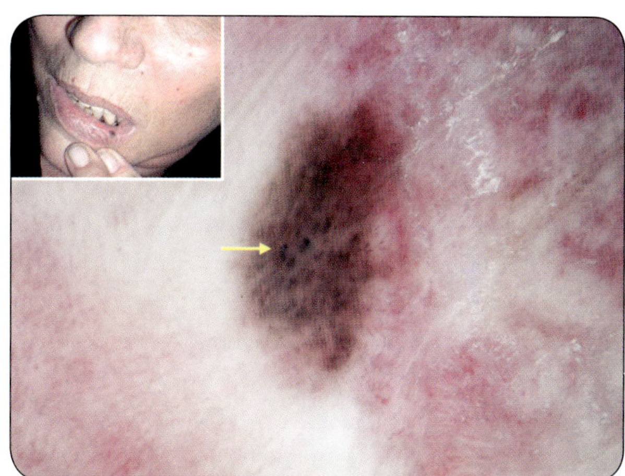

Fig. 9.66: Labial melanotic macule: dotted-globular pattern (arrow).

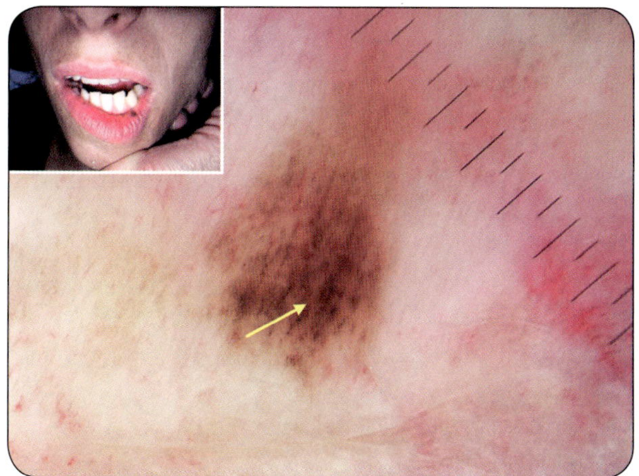

Fig. 9.67: Labial melanotic macule: Dotted-globular pattern (arrow).

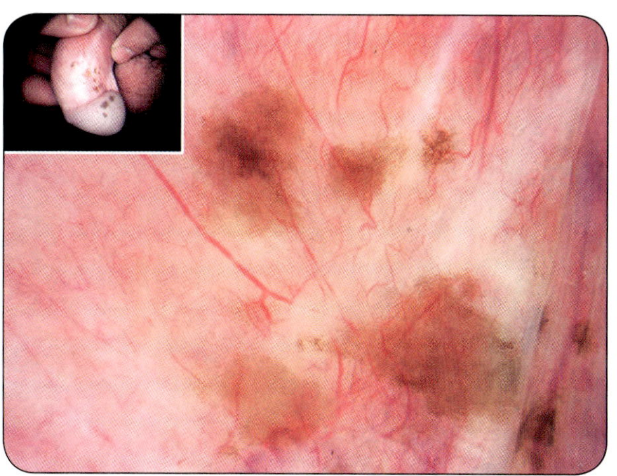

Fig. 9.68: Genital melanotic macule: Homogeneous pattern.

- *Fingerprint-like pattern* (Figs. 9.69 and 9.70)
- *Fish scale-like pattern*
- *Hyphal pattern* (Figs. 9.71 to 9.80)
- *Ring-like pattern*

Angioma (Fig. 9.81)

- Lichenoid chronic cheilitis (Figs. 9.82 and 9.83)
- Pigmented lichen planus (Fig. 9.84)
- Tattoos due to amalgama (Fig. 9.85)

Melanoma (Figs. 9.86 and 9.87)

- Multicomponent pattern and homogeneous pattern
  - Recently, we have found that the presence of structureless zones inside the lesions with blue, gray, or white color have:
    - For melanoma 100% sensitivity

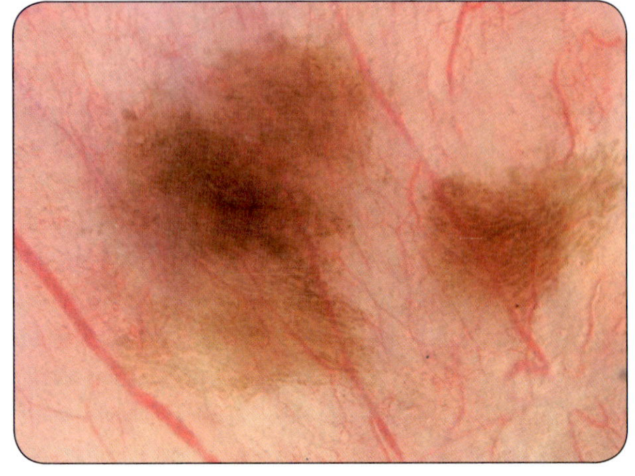

Fig. 9.69: Genital melanotic macule: Fingerprint-like pattern.

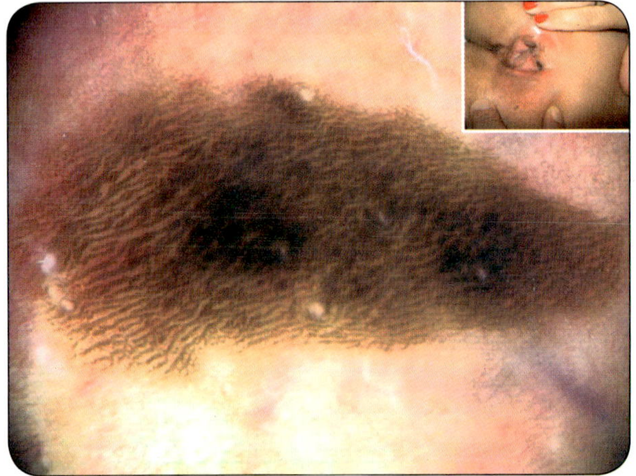

Fig. 9.70: Genital melanotic macule: Fingerprint-like pattern.

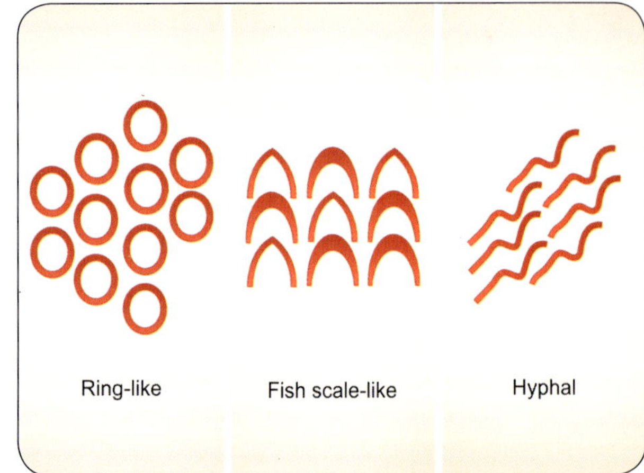

Fig. 9.71: Dermoscopic patterns associated with benign lesions.

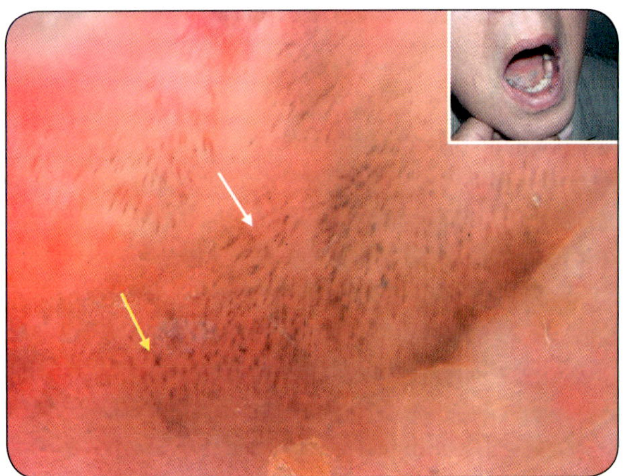

Fig. 9.72: Labial melanotic macule: Dotted-globular pattern (yellow arrow); fish scale-like pattern (white arrow).

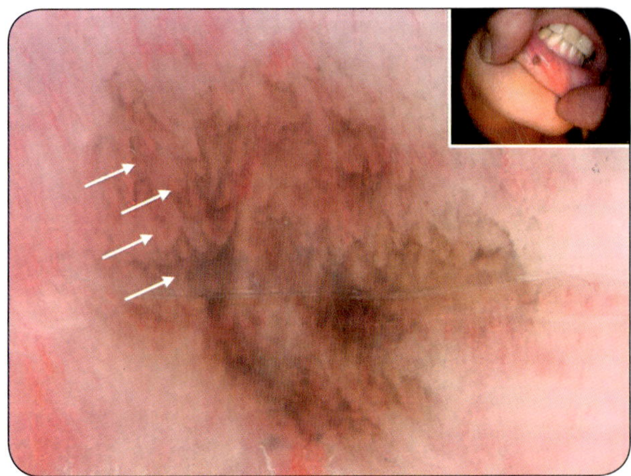

Fig. 9.73: Labial melanotic macule: Fish scale-like pattern (arrows).

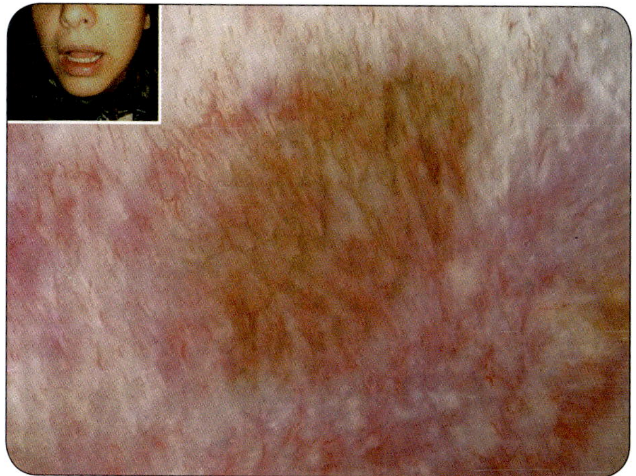

Fig. 9.74: Labial melanotic macule: Fish scale-like pattern.

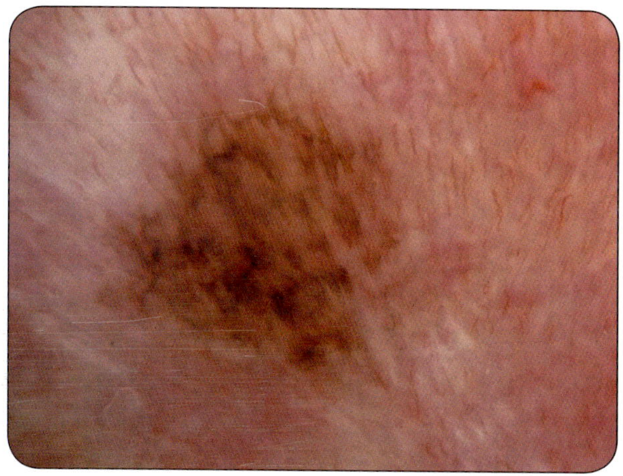

Fig. 9.75: Labial melanotic macule: Fish scale-like pattern.

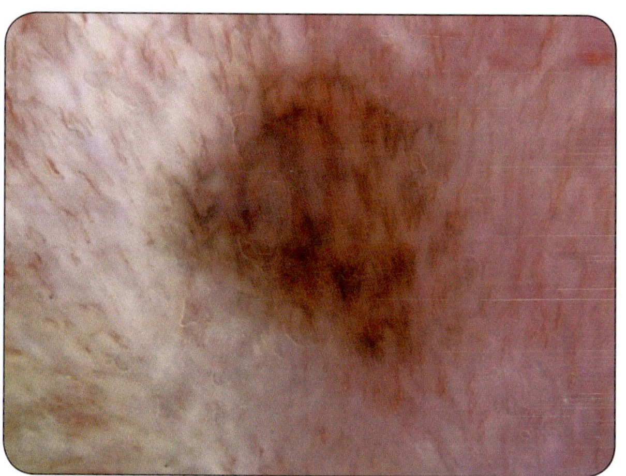

Fig. 9.76: Labial melanotic macule: Fish scale-like pattern.

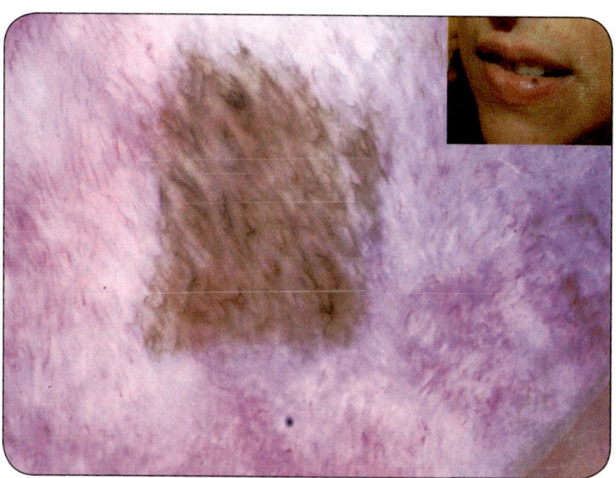

Fig. 9.77: Labial melanotic macule: Fish scale-like pattern.

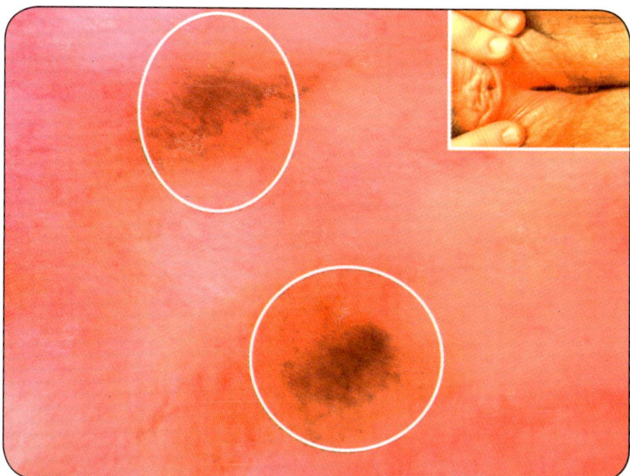

Fig. 9.78: Genital melanotic macule: Fish scale-like pattern (white circles).

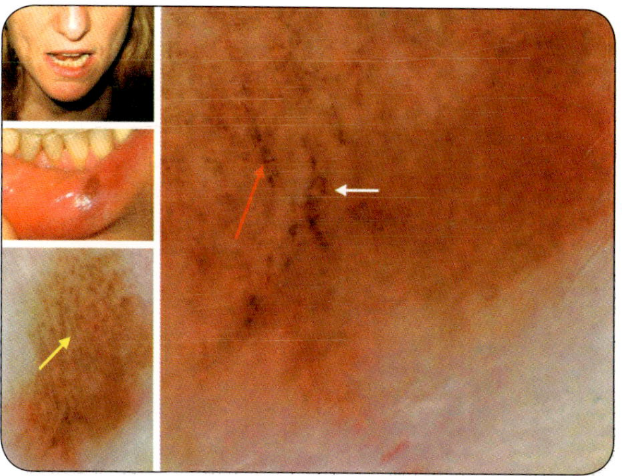

Fig. 9.79: Labial melanotic macule: Dotted-globular pattern (yellow arrow); hyphal pattern (white arrow); ring-like pattern (red arrow).

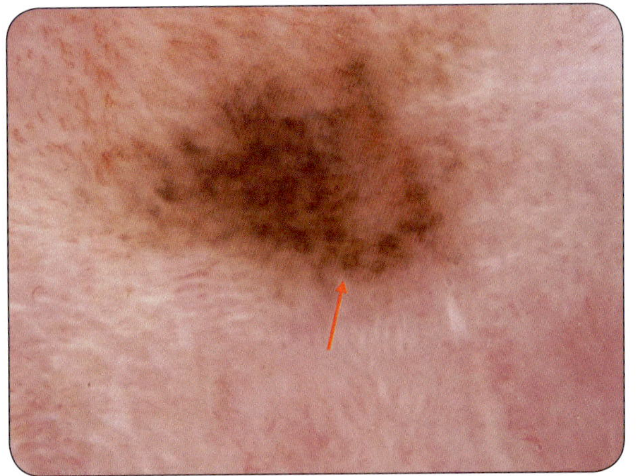

Fig. 9.80: Labial melanotic macule: Ring-like pattern (arrow).

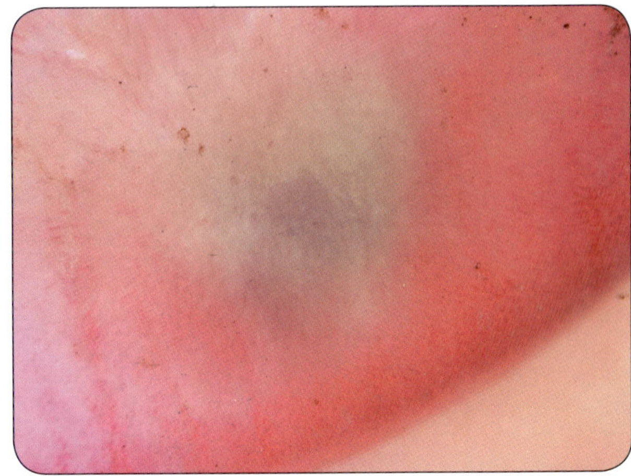

Fig. 9.81: Angioma (lip).

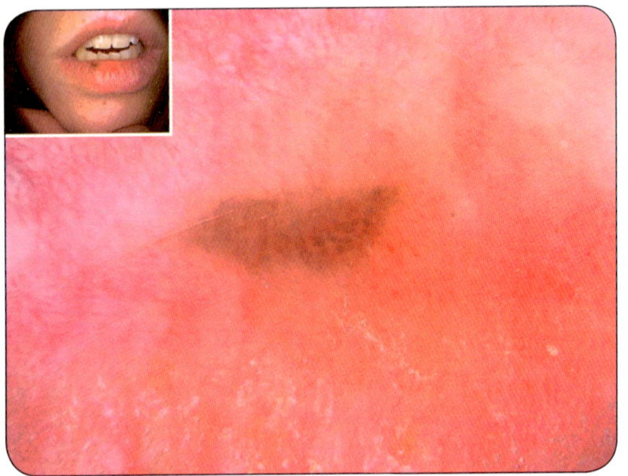

Fig. 9.82: Lichenoid chronic cheilitis.

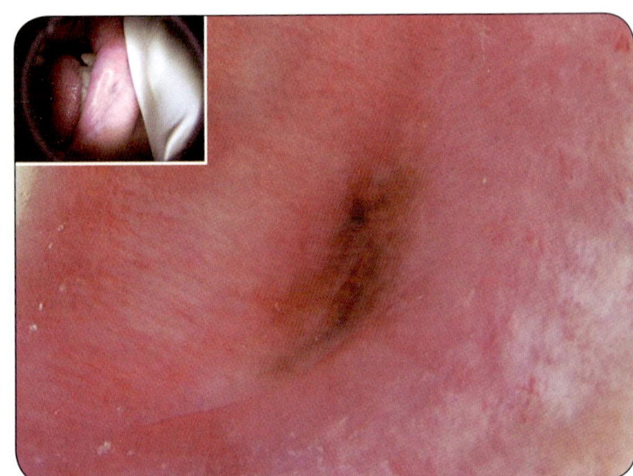

Fig. 9.83: Lichenoid chronic cheilitis.

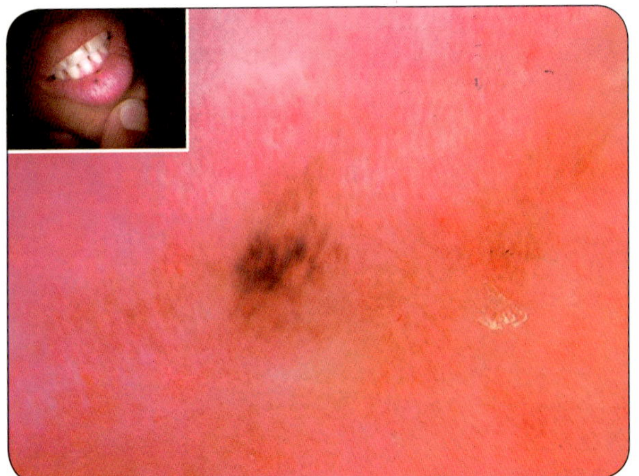

Fig. 9.84: Pigmented lichen planus.

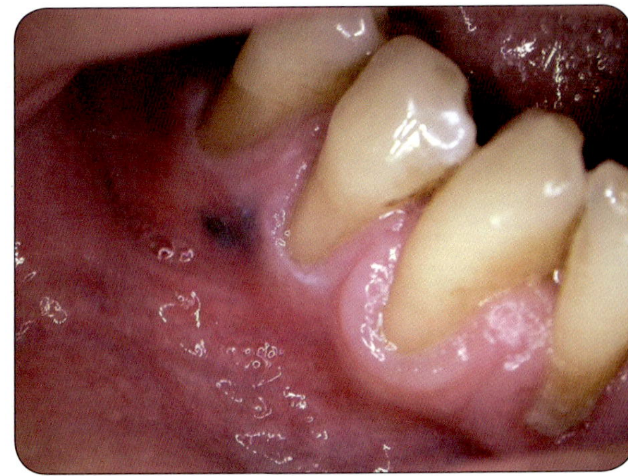

Fig. 9.85: Tattoos due to amalgama.

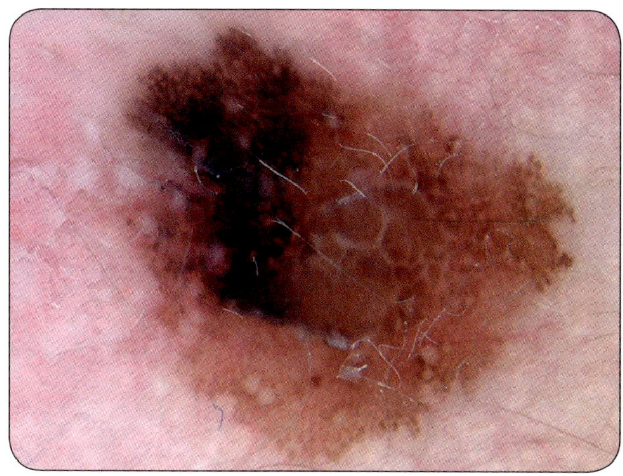

Fig. 9.86: Multicomponent pattern (melanoma).

Dermoscopy of pigmented lesions on the mucosa and the mucocutaneous junction

- ***Results:***
  - The presence of structureless zones inside the lesions with blue, gray, or white color
    - 100% sensitivity for melanoma
    - 82.2% specificity
    - 92.9% sensitivity for any malignant lesion
    - 83.3% specificity

Fig. 9.87: Dermoscopy of pigmented lesions of the mucosa and the mucocutaneous junction.

- 82.2% specificity
- For any malignant lesion 92.9% sensitivity
- 83.3% specificity (Fig. 9.87)

SUGGESTED READING

Blum A, Simionescu O, Argenziano G, et al. Dermoscopy of pigmented lesions of the mucosa and the mucocutaneous junction: results of a multicenter study by the International Dermoscopy Society (IDS). Arch Dermatol. 2011;147 (10):1181-7.

Ferrari, A, Zalaudek I, Argenziano G, et al. Dermoscopy of pigmented lesions of the vulva: A Retrospective Morphological Study. Dermatology. 2011;222:157-66.

Lin J, Koga H, Takata M, et al. Dermoscopy of pigmented lesions mucocutaneous junction and mucous membrane. BJD. 2009; 161:1255-61.

9.4 NAILS

Horacio A Cabo

The main objective is to recognize a melanoma in the nail apparatus with a high sensitivity when in the presence of a longitudinal melanonychia.

There are many other benign conditions which may present as a longitudinal melanonychia: nevi, lentigo, ethnic variation, subungual hemorrhages, and drug-induced pigmentation.

It is important to take into account that longitudinal biopsy is still the gold standard for a definite diagnosis, although the dermoscopic analysis of the lesion enables the identification of the most suspicious cases, avoiding a surgical biopsy, which is always technically difficult, painful and, on occasion, leading to a permanent dystrophy of the explored nail.

Nail dermoscopy may be performed by means of any model of handheld dermoscope and it is advisable to use a colorless ultrasound gel.

The clinical features are important:

- Suspicious features
  - The occurrence of melanonychia in adults
  - A single melanonychia
  - Heterogeneous pigmentation
  - Progressive melanonychia onset with the proximal area wider than the distal area
- Features usually associated with benign conditions
  - Manifestation during infancy
  - Stable over time
  - Homogeneous coloration
  - Multiple nails involvement

Different structures are recognizable

- Hemorrhagic spots
- Brown background
  - Regular parallel longitudinal lines
  - Irregular parallel longitudinal lines
- Gray background
  - Regular gray lines
- Micro-Hutchinson sign

HEMORRHAGIC SPOTS (FIGS. 9.88 TO 9.92)

Lesion color ranges between red, purple, and brown. It is blue-purple for recent lesions and black-brown for old lesions.

However, in all these lesions the proximal area remains polycyclic or round, while the distal area is elongated or lineal. (Parallel lineal pattern in splinter hemorrhages).

Follow up the lesion and rule out melanoma and SCC without history of trauma (Fig. 9.93).

BROWN BACKGROUND

This pattern corresponds to the association of regular or irregular pigmented lines on a homogeneous brown background, corresponding to the pigmented band.

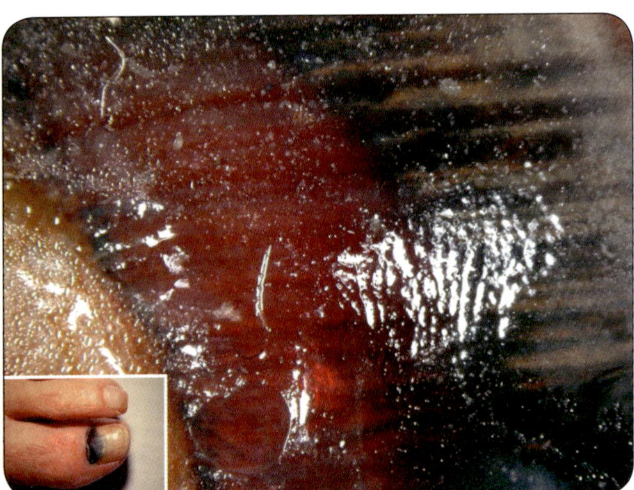

Fig. 9.88: Subungual hemorrhage: Blue-purple lesions with lineal distal area (parallel lineal pattern in splinter hemorrhages).

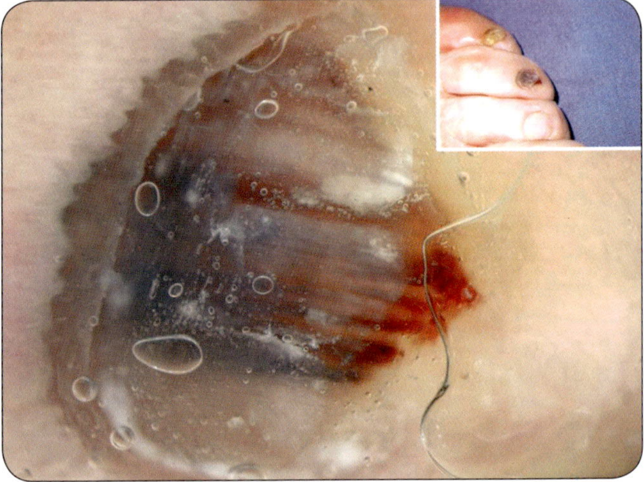

Fig. 9.89: Subungual hemorrhage: Blue-purple lesions with lineal distal area (parallel lineal pattern in splinter hemorrhages).

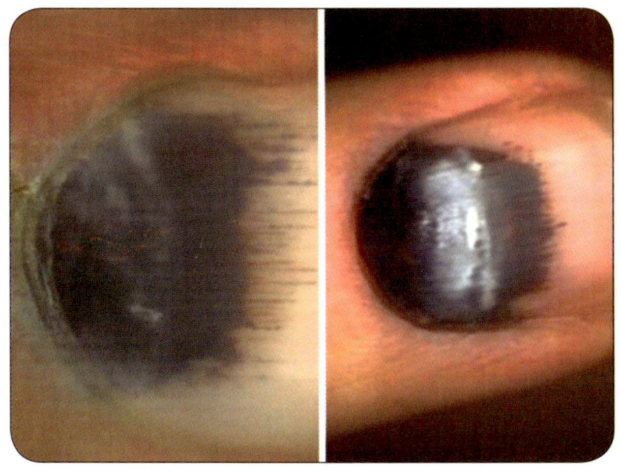

Fig. 9.90: Subungual hemorrhage: Blue-purple lesions with lineal distal area (parallel lineal pattern in splinter hemorrhages).

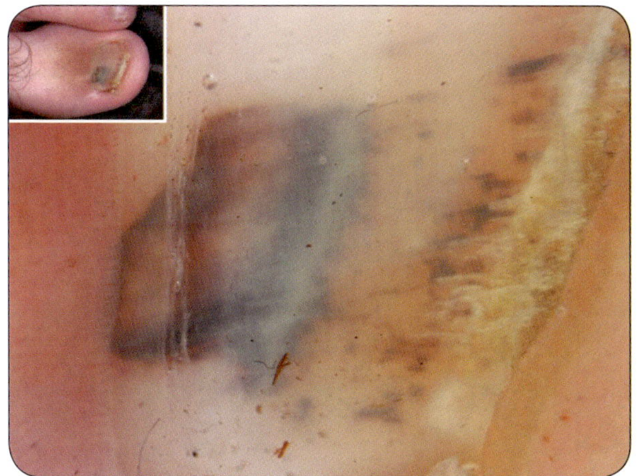

Fig. 9.91: Subungual hemorrhage: Brown color (old lesions).

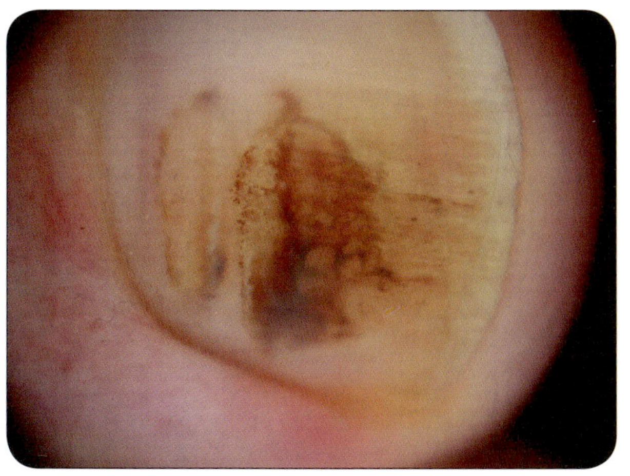

Fig. 9.92: Subungual hemorrhage: Brown color (old lesions).

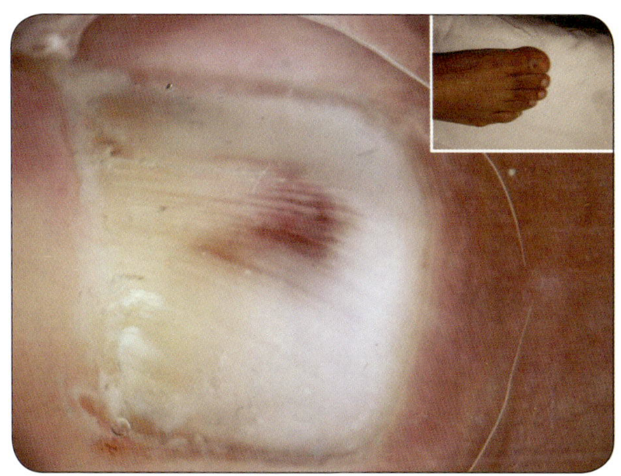

Fig. 9.93: Subungual hemorrhage due to squamous cell carcinoma.

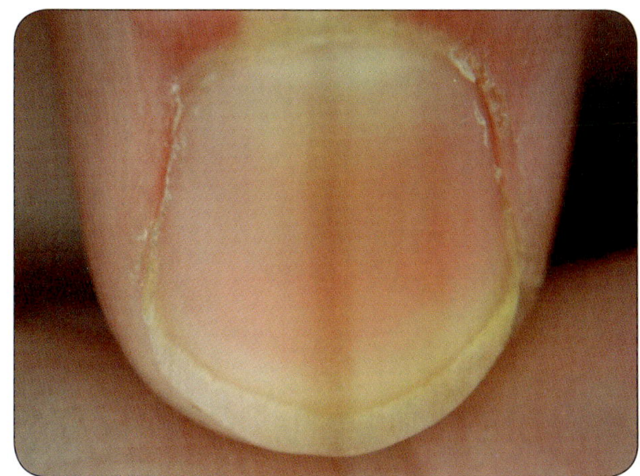

Fig. 9.94: Nevus: Brown background and regular parallel longitudinal lines.

Regular Parallel Longitudinal Lines (Figs. 9.94 to 9.98)

These appear overlapping the background homogeneous pattern.

The regular pattern points to a benign condition (nevi). It consists in:

- Regular spacing, width and coloration
- Absence of parallel disruption or no loss of parallelism
- All lines have the same shade and width
- Brown or black color points to melanocytic hyperplasia

Irregular Parallel Longitudinal Lines (Figs. 9.99 and 9.100)

The irregular pattern points to malignancy (melanoma). This pattern consists in:

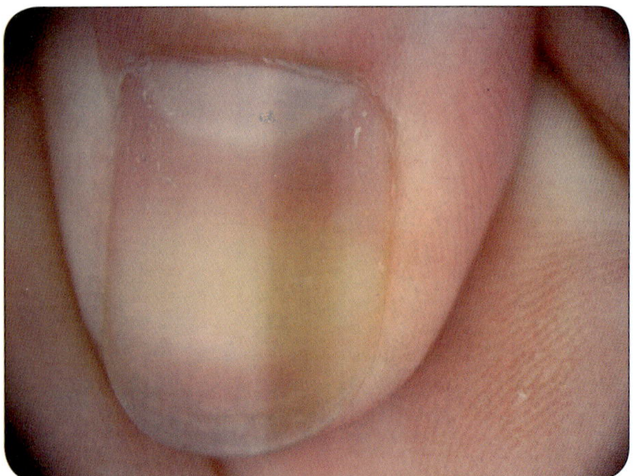

Fig. 9.95: Nevus: Brown background and regular parallel longitudinal lines.

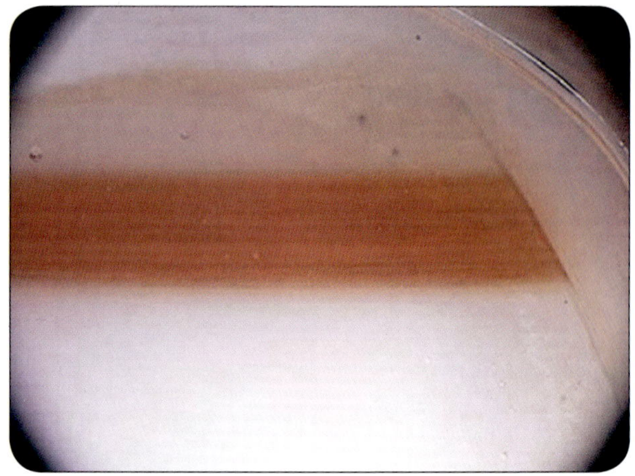

Fig. 9.96: Nevus: Brown background and regular parallel longitudinal lines.

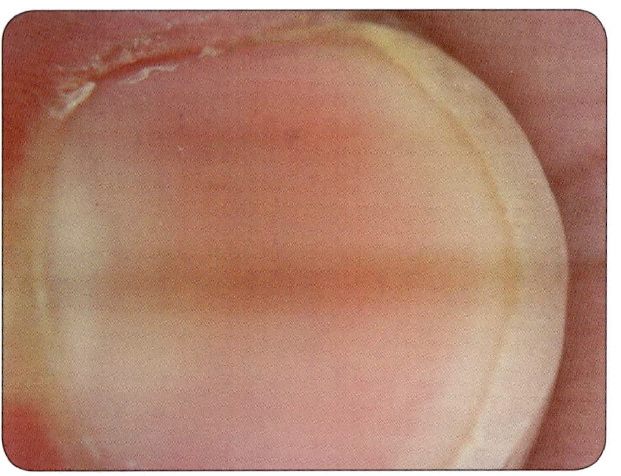

Fig. 9.97: Nevus: Brown background and regular parallel longitudinal lines.

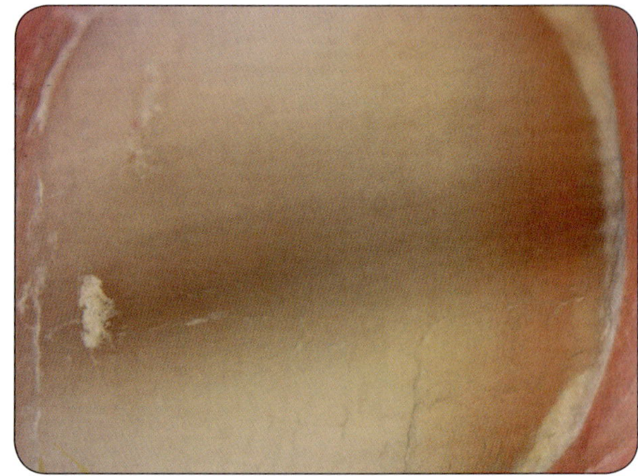

Fig. 9.98: Nevus: Brown background and regular parallel longitudinal lines.

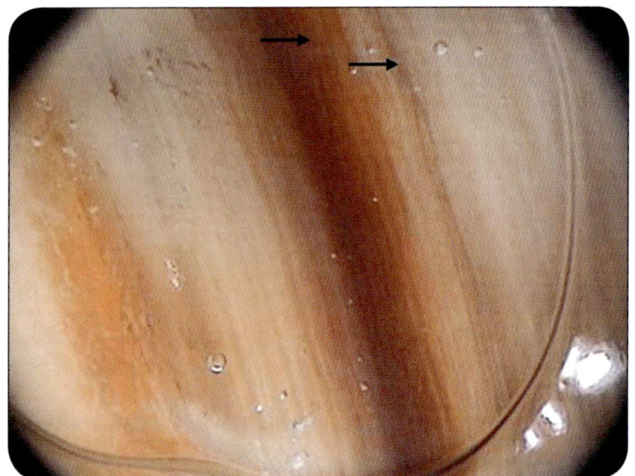

Fig. 9.99: Acral melanoma: Brown background with irregular pattern of the overlying lines in their thickness, color, and spacing (arrows).

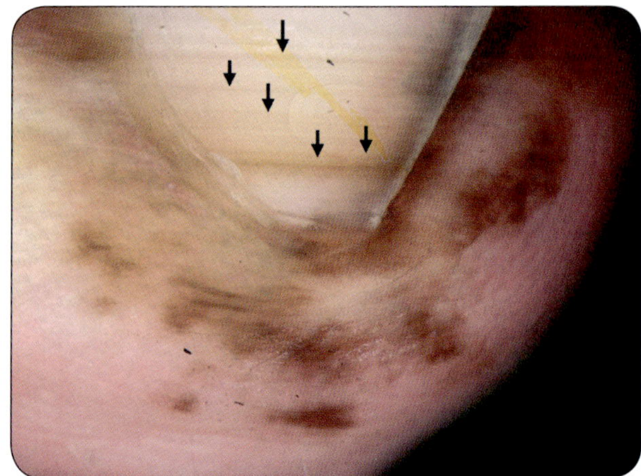

Fig. 9.100: Acral melanoma: Brown background with irregular pattern of the overlying lines in their thickness, color, and spacing (arrows).

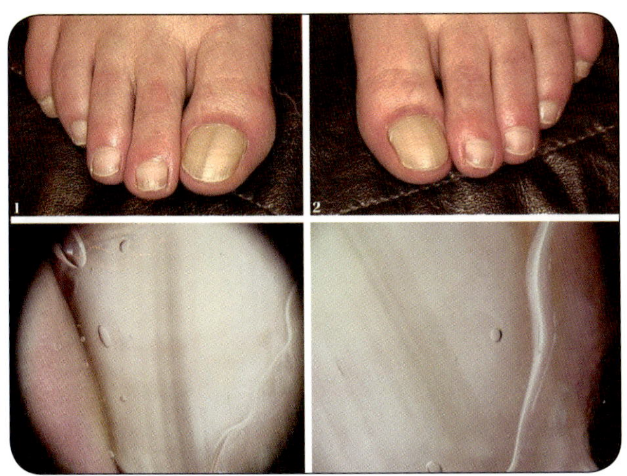

Fig. 9.101: Ethnic pigmentation: Clinical view (1-2) and dermoscopy view: regular gray lines.

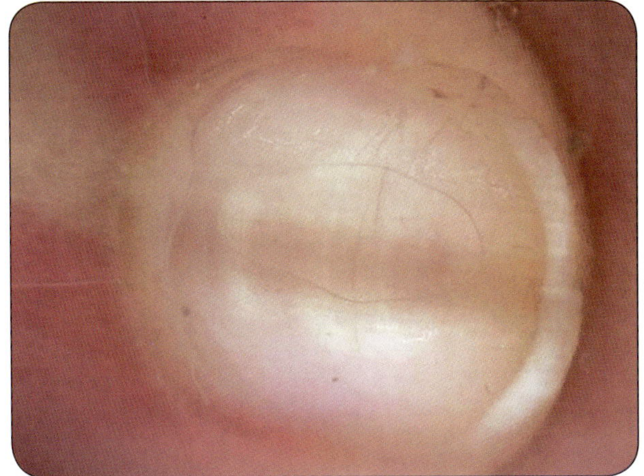
Fig. 9.102: Drug-induced pigmentation: Regular gray lines.

- Irregular spacing, width and coloration
- Loss of parallelism
- Lines with different shade and width
- Brown or black color points to melanocytic hyperplasia

GRAY BACKGROUND (FIGS. 9.101 AND 9.102)

Regular Gray Lines

Observable in:
- Ungual lentigo
- Ethnic pigmentation
- Laugier-Hunziker syndrome
- Drug-induced pigmentation

Consists in:
- Regular spacing, width and coloration
- No loss of parallelism
- All lines with the same shade and width
- Grey color points to epithelial hyperpigmentation without melanocyte hyperplasia

MICRO-HUTCHINSON SIGN

This refers to the pigmentation, observable only under dermoscopy but invisible to the naked eye, of the cuticle corresponding to a melanonychia extension. This kind of lesion is highly suspicious of melanoma.

CONCLUSION

Dermoscopy provides additional criteria to study nail pigmentation. These criteria will help the dermatologist to choose a longitudinal biopsy, were it necessary. When in doubt, perform a biopsy.

SUGGESTED READING

Argenziano G, Soyer P, De Giorgio V, et al. Interactive Atlas of Dermoscopy. Milán: EDRA Medical Publishing & New Media; 2000.

Cabo H. Dermatoscopia. Buenos Aires, Argentina: Weber Ferro; 2000.

Cabo H. Dermatoscopia, 2nd edition. Buenos Aires, Argentina: Ediciones Journal; 2012.

Johr R, Stolz, W. Dermoscopy: An Illustrated Self-Assessment Guide, 2nd edition. New York: Mc-Graw Hill Education; 2015.

Jorh R, Soyer P, Argenziano G, et al. Dermoscopy. The Essentials (MOABT). New York: Elsevier Ltd; 2004.

Kittler H. Dermatoscopy. An Algorithmic Method Based on Pattern Analysis 2011 Facultas Verlags- und Buchhandels AG facultas wuv Universitätsverlag, Austria www.facultas.wuv.at

Lallas A. Dermoscopy in general dermatology. Dermatol Clin. 2013;3:679-94.

Malvhey J, Puig S. Principles of Dermoscopy. Barcelona: Creaciones Gráficas; 2009.

Marghoob A, Braun R, Kopf A. Atlas of Dermoscopy. London: Taylor & Francis; 2005.

Menzies S, Crotty K, Ingvar C, et al. An Atlas of Surface Microscopy of Pigmented Skin Lesions. Sydney: McGraw-Hill Book Company; 1996.

Rabinovitz H, Kopf A. Dermoscopy: A Practical Guide. Miami: American Academy of Dermatology; 1999.

Soyer P, Argenziano G, Chimenti S, et al. Dermoscopy of Pigmented Skin Lesions. An Atlas Based on the Consensus Net Meeting on Dermoscopy. Milán: EDRA Medical Publishing & New Media; 2001.

Stolz W, Braun-Falco O, Bilek P, et al. Color Atlas of Dermatoscopy. USA: Blackwell Science; 1994.

Zalaudek I, Argenziano G, Giacomel, J. Dermoscopy of Non-pigmented Skin Tumors. Boca Raton, FL: CRC Press; 2016.

DIAGNOSTIC ALGORITHMS

10

Horacio A Cabo

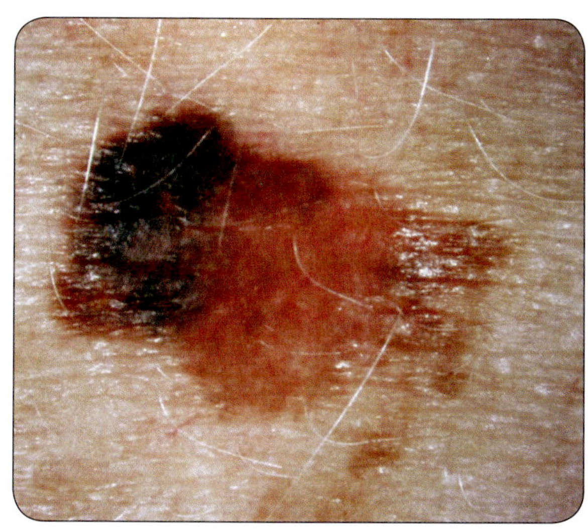

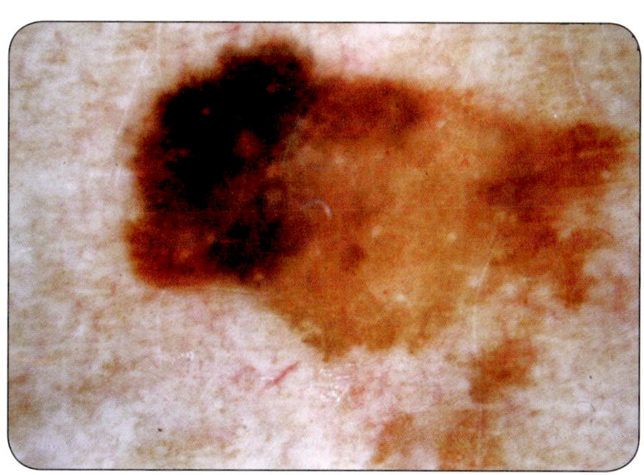

"There are different methods to evaluate pigmented lesions, especially melanoma.
The method most frequently used by experts is pattern analysis.
Although this is the one with highest sensitivity and specificity,
the difference between all the methods is very low.
The most used in addition to the pattern analysis are ABCD rule, 7-point chek-list,
11-point check-list and 3-point check-list between others."

There are different methods to evaluate pigmented lesions, especially melanoma. The method most frequently used by experts is pattern analysis. Although this is the one with highest sensitivity and specificity, the difference between all the methods is very low. During the internet Consensus in 2000, all the methods proved to be equally useful. We are going to describe the most used ones. All these algorithms have been elaborated on the basis of statistical studies (Graphs 10.1 and 10.2).

All these methods evaluate criteria and dermoscopic patterns that have already been described in other chapters, so here we will only describe the theoretical basis and analyze an example of melanoma with each of the different algorithms.

PATTERN ANALYSIS (TABLE 10.1, FIGS. 10.1 AND 10.2)

Pattern analysis is based on the qualitative assessment of several individual dermoscopic criteria. The difference between benign and malignant growth patterns is determined by the general appearance of the lesion and, in detail, by some structures suggesting malignancy. Therefore, pattern analysis consists in the general and local studies of pigmented lesions:

- *General features:* They enable or not a preliminary and quick analysis of a melanocytic lesion.
- *Local features:* They enable the detailed analysis of a melanocytic lesion.

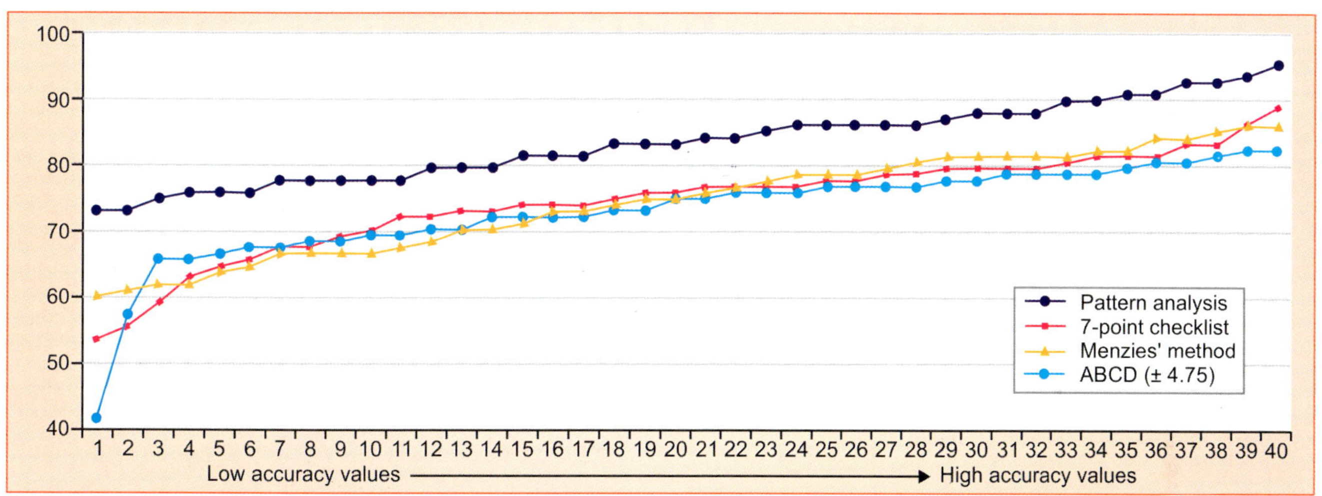

Graph 10.1: Diagnostic accuracy (%) for melanoma of 4 dermoscopic diagnostic methods.

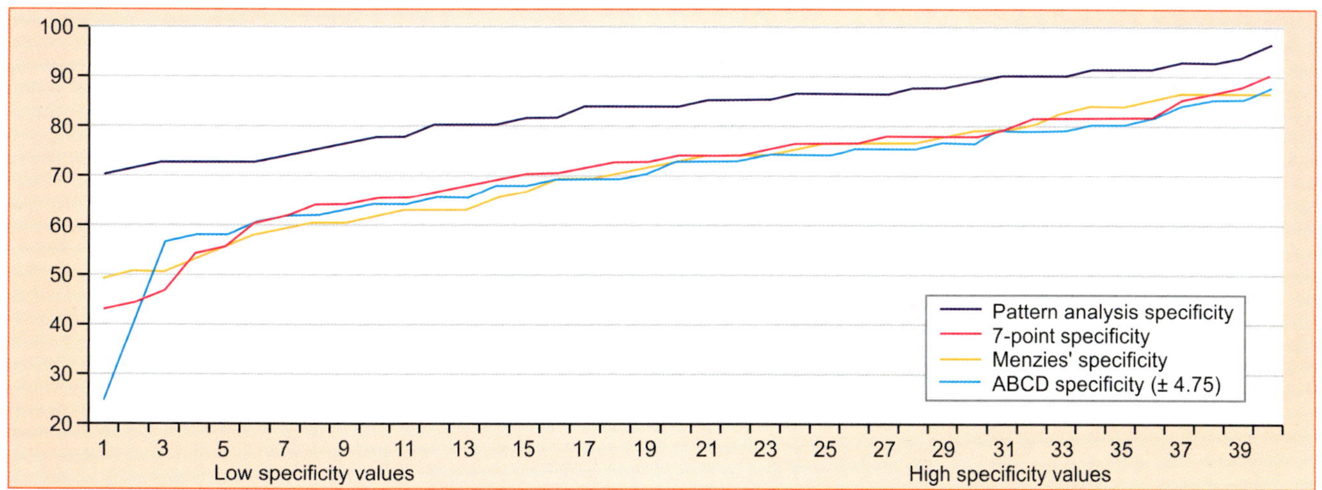

Graph 10.2: Specificity (%) for melanoma of 4 dermoscopic diagnostic methods.

Analyzing the *general features* means identifying the different structures that, because of repetition and covering an important part of the lesion, are known as patterns (Table 10.1):

- *Reticular pattern*: Pigment network covering most of a pigmented lesion
- *Globular pattern*: Round or oval structures of different sizes. They may be in different colors and shades (brown, gray, and black).
- *Cobblestone pattern*: Angulated globules resembling cobblestones, generally bigger than globules.
- *Homogeneous pattern*: Diffuse brown, gray, blue, or black pigmentation without the presence of any other criteria.
- *Starburst pattern*: Pigmented lines in radial arrangement from the edge of a pigmented lesion.
- *Parallel pattern*: In palms and soles. Pigmentation may follow the ridges or the furrows.
- *Multicomponent pattern*: This is a combination of three or more dermoscopic structures.
- *Nonspecific pattern*: Absence of definite dermoscopic structures or criteria.

Analyzing the *local features* means analyzing the lesion in detail and identifying some of the following structures:

- *Pigment network*: Typical or atypical
- *Streaks or projections*: Regular or irregular
- *Dots and globules*: With regular or irregular distribution
- Blue-white veil
- Asymmetric pigmentation
- Regression structures
- Vascular structures with atypical pattern

Table 10.1: Pattern analysis.

Global features	*Local features*
Reticular pattern	Pigment network
Globular pattern	Streaks
Cobblestone pattern	Dots and globules
Homogeneous pattern	Blue-whitish veil
Starburst pattern	Regression structures
Multicomponent pattern	Vascular structures
Unspecific pattern	Negative pigment network
	Shiny white structures

CONCLUSION

With the study of the general and local features of a given lesion, it is possible to make a diagnosis.

ABCD RULE (TABLES 10.2 AND 10.3, FIG.10.3)

ABCD rule is very useful to check if a melanocytic lesion is benign, suspicious, or malignant.

Through the use of a multiple variable analysis, it has been proved that there are *four criteria (asymmetry, border, color, and different dermoscopic criteria)* which are very important to recognize a malignant melanoma. In order to put them into practice, a system has been developed that aims at calculating a *total dermoscopy score* (TDS) by means of a linear equation. Total dermoscopy score enables the scoring of lesions regarding their

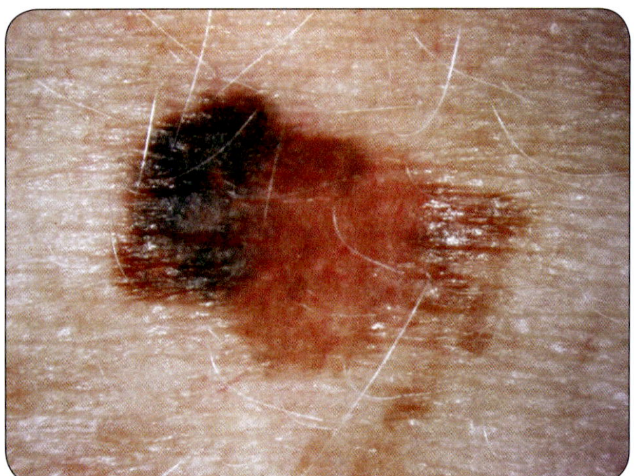

Fig. 10.1: Superficial spreading melanoma clinical image.

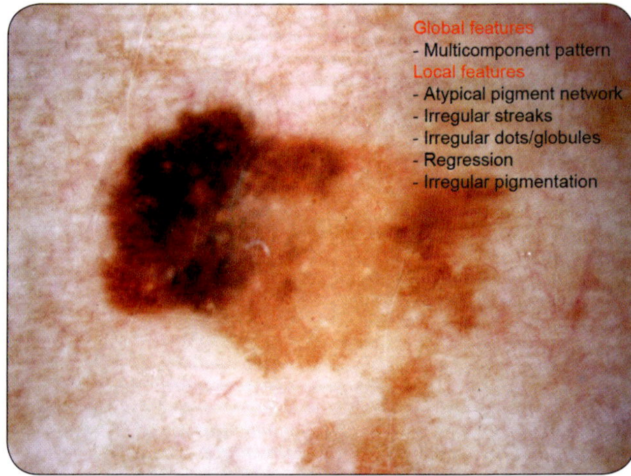

Fig. 10.2: Superficial spreading melanoma (Fig. 10.1) evaluated by pattern analysis.

Table 10.2: ABCD rule (Stolz).

- Asymmetry: in 0, 1, or 2 axes × 1.3
- Borders: 0–8 × 0.1
- Color: 1–6 × 0.5
  - Red, black, white, dark brown, light brown, and blue gray
- Different structures: 1–5 × 0.5
  - Pigment network, streaks, globules, dots, and structureless areas:
    - <4.75: Benign melanocytic lesion
    - 4.76–5.45: Suspicious lesion
    - >5.46: Melanoma

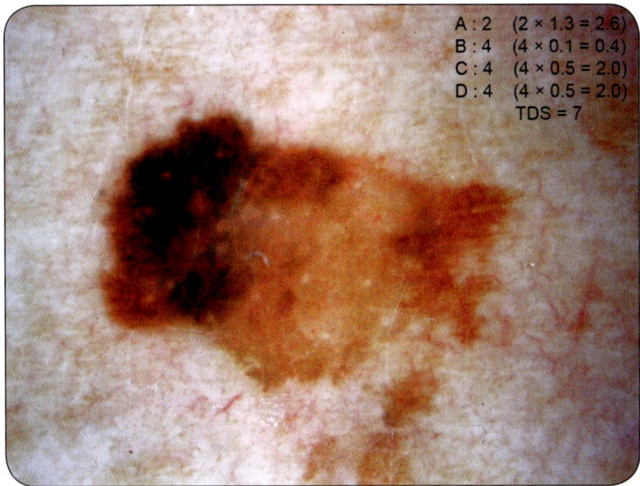

Fig. 10.3: SSM (Fig. 10.1) evaluated by the ABCD dermoscopy rule. (A: Asymmetry; B: Border; C: Color; D: Different structures; TDS: Total dermoscopy score.

potential malignancy. Before applying this rule it is necessary to rule out, through the identification of special patterns, several melanocytic lesions, such as globular, papillomatous, spindly cells (Reed), pigmented Spitz, congenital, recurrent, and "agminado" nevi, as well as spilus nevi.

Each criterion is assigned a value and multiplied by an established conversion factor, which yields the TDS, whose value indicates if the lesion is benign, suspicious, or malignant (Table 10.2).

Asymmetry (A)

To judge asymmetry, the lesion is bisected along two axes at 90°, positioned in such a way that they yield the lowest possible score. Asymmetry must be calculated according to the distribution of colors and structures on both sides of these axes and not just by the contour, as happens in the case of clinical ABCD rule. If there is no asymmetry with reference to both axes, the score is 0. If there is asymmetry with reference to only one axis, the score is 1; and in the case of asymmetry with reference to both axes, the score is 2.

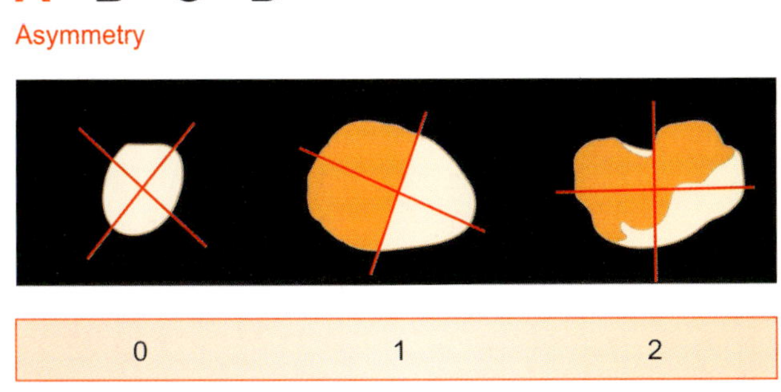

Border or Contour (B)

Evaluation of the border or contour was established on the basis of existence of either a sharp and abrupt ending of pigment at the periphery of the lesion or a gradual and blurred border. Based on this analysis, lesions are divided into octaves. In this manner, the maximum score for the border is 8, and the minimum score is 0. From the original description of this rule it is evident that on occasion reproducibility is low and the score of the border or contour only adds relevant information in very few lesions. Thus, in most lesions, it is possible to omit border score determination.

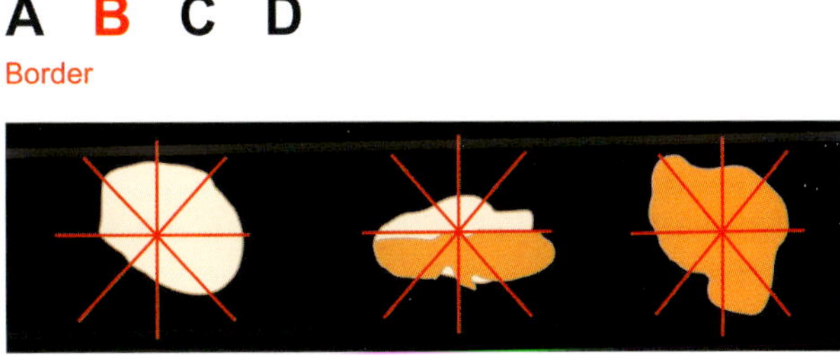

Color (C)

In order to determine the score for color, six hues can be identified with a dermatoscope: white, red, light brown, dark brown, blue-gray, and black. Four colors result from melanin distribution (light and dark brown, due to melanin in the dermoepidermal junction; black, resulting from melanin in the superior granular layer or stratum corneum; and blue-gray, owing to melanin in the papillary dermis). White is the consequence of regressive changes; and red is the consequence of inflammation or neovascularization. If the area is lighter than the adjacent normal skin, white is assigned to it. The values for color score go

Table 10.3: Additional criteria for malignancy.
Vascular pattern
Regression
Pseudopods

Table 10.4: 7-point checklist method (Argenziano).
• Major criteria (two point each)
– Atypical pigment network
– Blue-white veil
– Atypical vascular pattern
• Minor criteria (one point each)
– Irregular streaks
– Irregular dots and globules
– Irregular pigmentation
– Regression structures

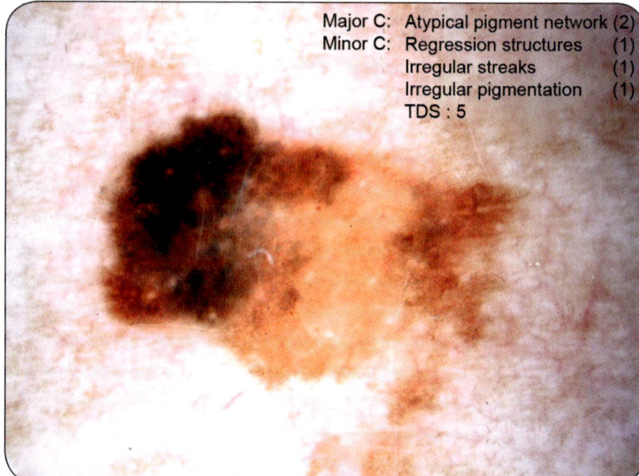

Fig. 10.4: SSM (Fig. 10.1) evaluated by the 7-point checklist method. (TDS: Total dermoscopy score).

from 1 to 6. As in asymmetry, the dermatoscope reveals a color range wider than that observed with the naked eye.

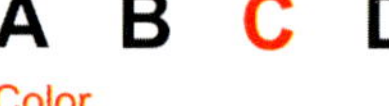

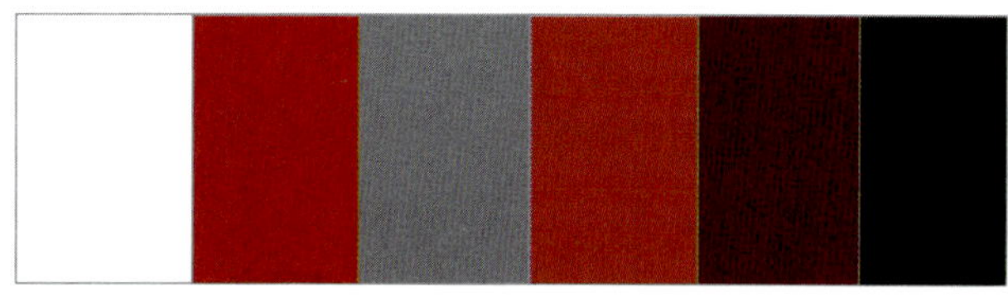

Different Structures (D)

To assess the different dermoscopic structures, five main features must be considered: structureless areas, pigment network, streaks or projections (branched streaks), dots, and globules.

ABCD Different Structures

- Pigment network
- Globulos
- Dots
- Streaks/branched streaks
- Structureless areas

If TDS falls within the benign or suspicious range, it is necessary at any rate to check if the additional malignancy criteria are present.

Three additional criteria have been identified: vascular pattern, regression, and pseudopods (Table 10.3).

7-POINT CHECKLIST (TABLE 10.4 AND FIG. 10.4)

The method of the 7-point checklist is a diagnostic algorithm that provides a quantitative scoring system and a simplification in comparison to the classical pattern analysis, since fewer features need to be identified. Because of its frequent association with melanoma, the features hereunder described were selected:

- Major criteria
  - Atypical pigment network
  - Blue-white veil
  - Atypical vascular pattern
- Minor criteria
  - Irregular streaks
  - Irregular dots and globules
  - Irregular pigmentation
  - Regression structures

The differences between melanomas and nevi have been evaluated through a statistical test. Using probability percentages, calculated by means of a multiple variable analysis, a score of 2 was assigned to three of the criteria with probability quotients >5, known as "major criteria," and a value of 1 to the four criteria with probability quotients <5, known as "minor criteria." By simply adding the individual scores, it was determined that *a score of 3 or more resulted in a melanoma diagnosis,* with 95% sensibility and 75% specificity (Table 10.4).

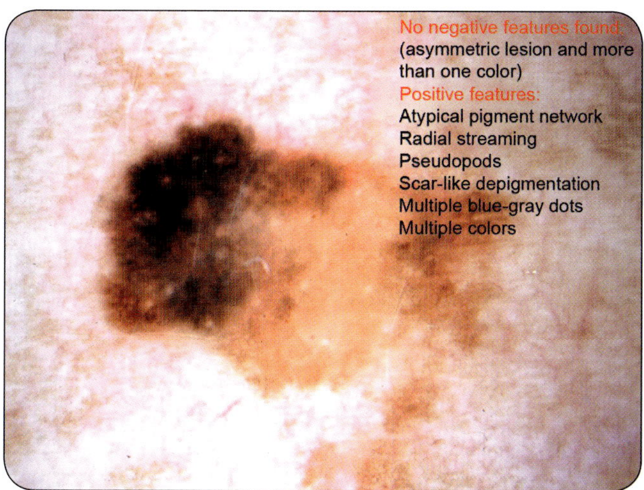

Fig. 10.5: SSM (Fig. 10.1) evaluated with the 11-point checklist method.

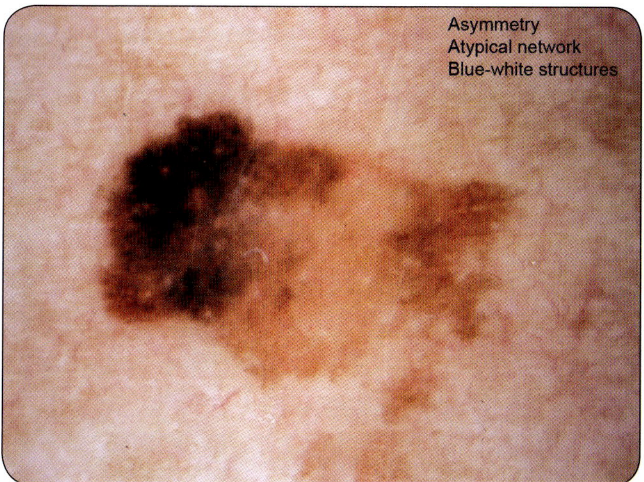

Fig. 10.6: SSM (Fig. 10.1) evaluated with the 3-point checklist method.

11-POINT CHECKLIST METHOD (FIG. 10.5)

This method has 92% sensibility and 71% specificity regarding melanoma diagnosis. This method works with positive and negative criteria or features. For a melanoma diagnosis, the *negative criteria*, with very low melanoma sensibility, must be *absent*, while at least one of the *positive criteria* must be *present*.

Negative Features

These are two features, lesion symmetry (symmetry of pattern) and single color, which must be absent.

Symmetry of Pattern

This feature refers to symmetry in all structures, including color, along any axis crossing through the center of the lesion. It does not require shape symmetry.

Single Color

The recorded colors are black, gray, blue, red, dark brown, and tan; white color is ignored. A single coloration excludes a melanoma diagnosis.

Positive Features

At least one of the following features must be present:

- Blue-white veil
- Multiple brown dots
- Streaks or radial streaming
- Pseudopods
- Scar-like whitish areas (regression)
- Peripheral black dots/globules
- Multiple colors (five or six colors)
- Multiple blue or gray dots
- Atypical pigment network

Table 10.5: 3-point checklist (Soyer).

Definition:
Asymmetry: in shape and/or color on one or two perpendicular axes
Atypical pigment network: irregular spaces and thick lines
White–blue structures: structureless areas (fibrosis, melanosis, or blue–gray globules)
The presence of two or more of these criteria points to a high probability of melanoma.

3-POINT CHECKLIST METHOD (TABLE 10.5 AND FIG. 10.6)

This method was devised for inexperienced dermoscopists (general practitioners, pediatricians, or beginner dermatologists) with a view to helping them make accurate diagnoses of melanomas while developing their skills. It was devised as a screening approach, which means that it is much more sensitive than specific. In this manner, the possibility of missing a melanoma is avoided.

It is an algorithm based on a simplified dermoscopic pattern, very useful to interpret, if a suspicious lesion must be excised.

Based on the results of the Dermoscopy Consensus Meeting of 2001, it was shown that there are three especially important criteria in order to make a diagnosis when assessing cutaneous pigmented lesions and, particularly, to differentiate benign pigmented lesions from melanoma.

These three criteria are *asymmetry, atypical pigment network, and the presence of blue-white structures*. In fact, these are the three points evaluated in this rule.

Color and/or structure asymmetry may locate on one or two perpendicular axes. The blue-white structures correspond to any shade of blue and/or white (a combination of the early changes of the blue-white veil and regression structures). Sensitivity for skin cancer (melanoma and basal cell carcinoma) was 91% and specificity was 71.9%. The three-point checklist is a simple, feasible, accurate, and reproducible method, which renders it an effective tool in skin cancer detection.

The presence of more than one criterion suggests that a lesion is suspicious. In general, only one criterion is found in early melanoma. Two criteria are found in melanoma and pigmented basal cell carcinoma. Therefore, excision is recommended for lesions with two or three positive points.

The advantage of this rule lies in its simplicity and its easy acquisition. By using it, it is possible to reach sensibility and specificity percentages for cancer detection comparable to those of the other algorithms that require higher training (Table 10.5).

SUGGESTED READING

Annesi G, Bono R, Sampogna F, et al. Sensitivity, specificity, and diagnostic accuracy of three dermoscopic algorithmic methods in the diagnosis of doubtful melanocytic lesions: the importance of light brown structureless areas in differentiating atypical melanocytic nevi from thin melanomas. J Am Acad Dermatol. 2007;56:759-67.

Argenziano G, Soyer HP, Chimenti S, et al. Dermoscopy of pigmented skin lesions: results of a consensus meeting via the Internet. J Am Acad Dermatol. 2003;48(5):679-93.

Argenziano G, Soyer P, De Giorgio V, et al. Interactive Atlas of Dermoscopy. Milán: EDRA Medical Publishing & New Media; 2000.

Cabo H. Dermatoscopia. Buenos Aires, Argentina: Weber Ferro; 2000.

Cabo H. Dermatoscopia, 2nd edition. Buenos Aires, Argentina: Ediciones Journal; 2012.

Jorh R, Soyer P, Argenziano G, et al. Dermoscopy. The Essentials (MOABT). New York: Elsevier Ltd; 2004.

Johr R, Stolz W. Dermoscopy: An Illustrated Self-Assessment Guide, 2nd edition. New York: McGraw-Hill Education; 2015.

Kittler H. Dermatoscopy. An Algorithmic Method Based on Pattern Analysis 2011 Facultas Verlags- und Buchhandels AG facultas wuv Universitätsverlag, Austria www.facultas.wuv.at

Lallas A. Dermoscopy in general dermatology. Dermatol Clin. 2013;3:679-94.

Malvhey J, Puig S. Principles of Dermoscopy. Barcelona: Creaciones Gráficas; 2009.

Marghoob A, Braun R, Kopf A. Atlas of Dermoscopy. London: Taylor & Francis; 2005.

Menzies S, Crotty K, Ingvar C, et al. An Atlas of Surface Microscopy of Pigmented Skin Lesions. Sydney: McGraw-Hill Book Company; 1996.

Rabinovitz H, Kopf A. Dermoscopy: A Practical Guide. Miami: American Academy of Dermatology; 1999.

Soyer P, Argenziano G, Chimenti S, et al. Dermoscopy of Pigmented Skin Lesions. An Atlas Based on the Consensus Net Meeting on Dermoscopy. Milán: EDRA Medical Publishing & New Media; 2001.

Stolz W, Braun-Falco O, Bilek P, et al. Color Atlas of Dermatoscopy. USA: Blackwell Science; 1994.

Zalaudek I, Argenziano G, Giacomel J. Dermoscopy of Non-Pigmented Skin Tumors. Boca Raton, FL: CRC Press; 2016.

TOTAL-BODY PHOTOGRAPHY AND SEQUENTIAL DIGITAL DERMOSCOPY IMAGES

11

Gabriel Salerni

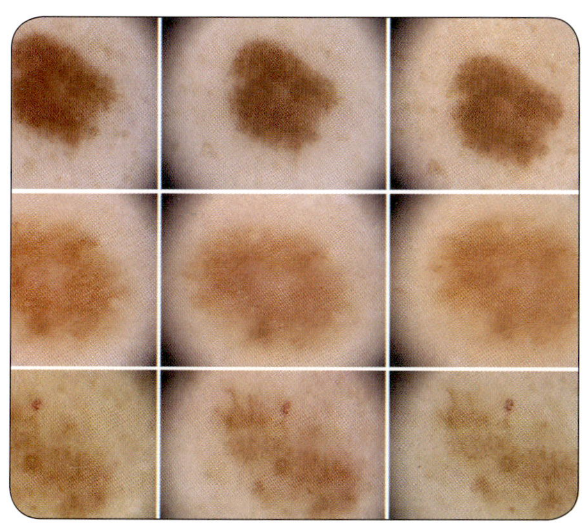

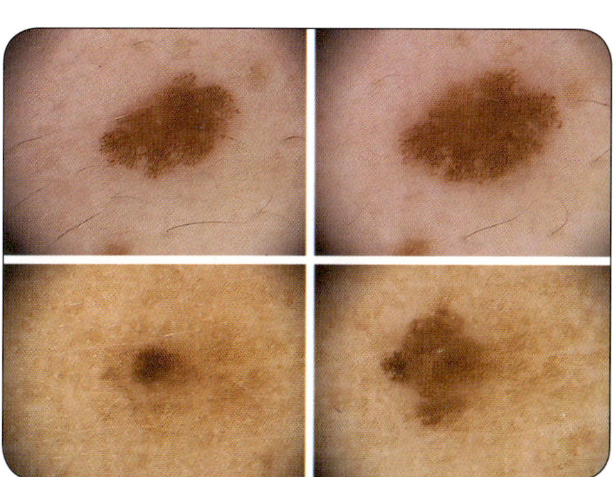

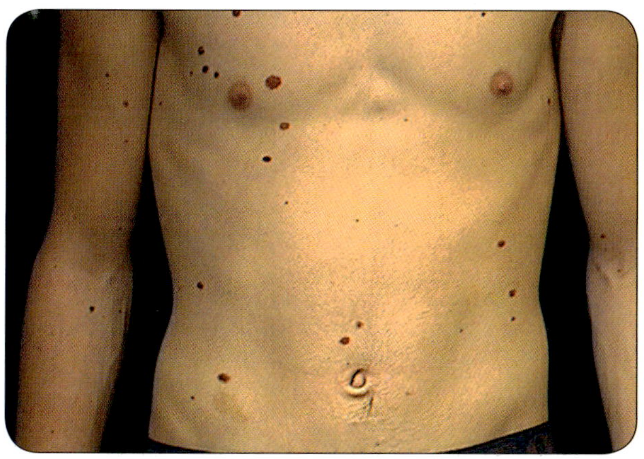

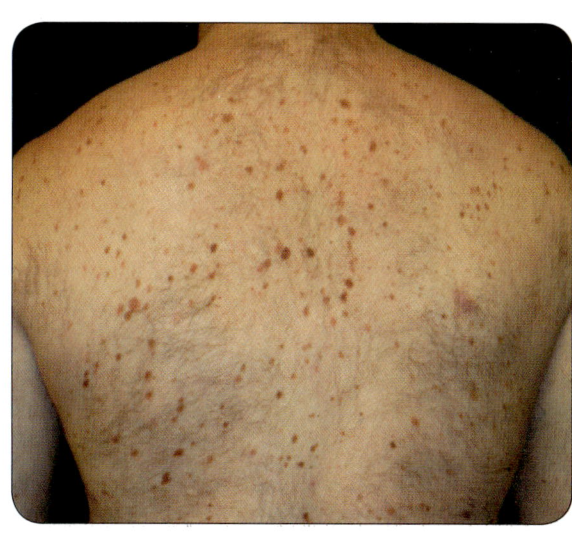

“Melanoma may be not only clinically but also dermoscopically indistinguishable from benign melanocytic lesions, especially in early stages. The overlap of dermoscopic criteria for melanoma and atypical nevi may lead to overlook melanomas and to excise a large number of benign lesions. Benign melanocytic lesions are usually stable, while melanomas tend to evolve and undergo changes over time, which are initially microscopic. Thus, comparison of sequential dermoscopy images of atypical melanocytic lesions has been proposed as a strategy to recognize incipient melanomas that may lack distinctive dermoscopic features“

Melanoma may be not only clinically but also dermoscopically indistinguishable from benign melanocytic lesions,[1-3] especially in early stages. The overlap of dermoscopic criteria for melanoma and atypical nevi may lead to overlook melanomas and to excise a large number of benign lesions.

Benign melanocytic lesions are usually stable, while melanomas tend to evolve and undergo changes over time, which are initially microscopic. Thus, comparison of sequential dermoscopy images of atypical melanocytic lesions has been proposed as a strategy to recognize incipient melanomas that may lack distinctive dermoscopic features (Fig. 11.1).[1]

The use of sequential dermoscopy images allows for an objective comparative analysis, which helps in the identification of subtle changes, otherwise not visible, adding useful information for the differentiation of early melanomas from benign melanocytic lesions. In a recent study,[4] melanomas diagnosed in patients enrolled in the digital follow-up program in a melanoma unit were compared with those diagnosed in patients referred for assessment with clinical suspicion of melanomas. It was demonstrated that melanomas diagnosed in patients under digital follow-up program had a low index of suspicion not only in the clinical but also in the dermoscopical evaluation (with almost 40% misclassified as benign according to the dermoscopic diagnostic algorithms).

EQUIPMENT

Several systems that allow for the record of clinical and dermoscopical images of skin lesions are currently available. These devices consist in a video and/or a photo camera adapted for dermoscopy, which is connected to a computer with special software for the storage and comparative analysis of sequential dermoscopy images.

Briefly, digital dermoscopy devices allow for the record of images by assigning a number and additional information such as location or other data of interest. More complex devices also allow for the total-body photograph registries or body mapping, which enables both the identification of the exact location of the lesions and the detection of new lesions by side-by-side comparison. The use of the latter is of radical importance in the management of patients with large numbers of melanocytic lesions, providing uniformity to the procedure and making the comparative analysis more reliable and objective.

FOLLOW-UP STRATEGY

The technique of digital dermoscopy follow-up includes two approaches: short-term follow-up and medium/long-term follow-up.

Short-term follow-up, usually in a period of 3 months, is used to make a clinical judgment on suspicious melanocytic lesions that are lack of specific dermoscopic criteria for melanoma.[5,6] In short-term follow-up, any significant morphological change requires the excision of the lesion.

Medium/long-term follow-up allows for the comparison of atypical nevi during standard periods, usually from 6 to 12 months.[7-9] This technique is generally restricted to patients with large numbers of atypical melanocytic lesions.

Both short- and medium/long-term follow-ups have demonstrated the improvement in the detection of melanomas with low index of suspicion, which can only be detected due to dermoscopic changes.[2]

CRITERIA FOR LESIONS SELECTION

Establishing which lesions are candidates for digital dermoscopy follow-up is a key requirement. These lesions should be those showing mild to moderate clinical and/or dermoscopical atypia. Suspicious lesions showing dermoscopic criteria for melanoma should be excised and submit for histopathology. Moreover, follow-up of lesions with clear-cut criteria for benignity is not justified in terms of cost efficiency.

SIGNIFICANT CHANGES DURING DIGITAL FOLLOW-UP

Significant changes during sequential dermoscopy have been defined by Kittler et al.[15] and adopted by different working groups in ulterior studies. Significant changes are as follow: (1) asymmetric enlargement; (2) changes in dermoscopic structures (expansion or decrease of pigment network; variation in the distribution or the number of dots/globules; modification of depigmented areas or regression structures; appearance of streaks, scar-like areas, blue-whitish veil, and atypical vessels); (3) increase in the number of colors; (4) regression features affecting >50% of the lesion; and (5) focal pigment modifications (Figs. 11.2A to I). In a recent study,[20] all types of changes

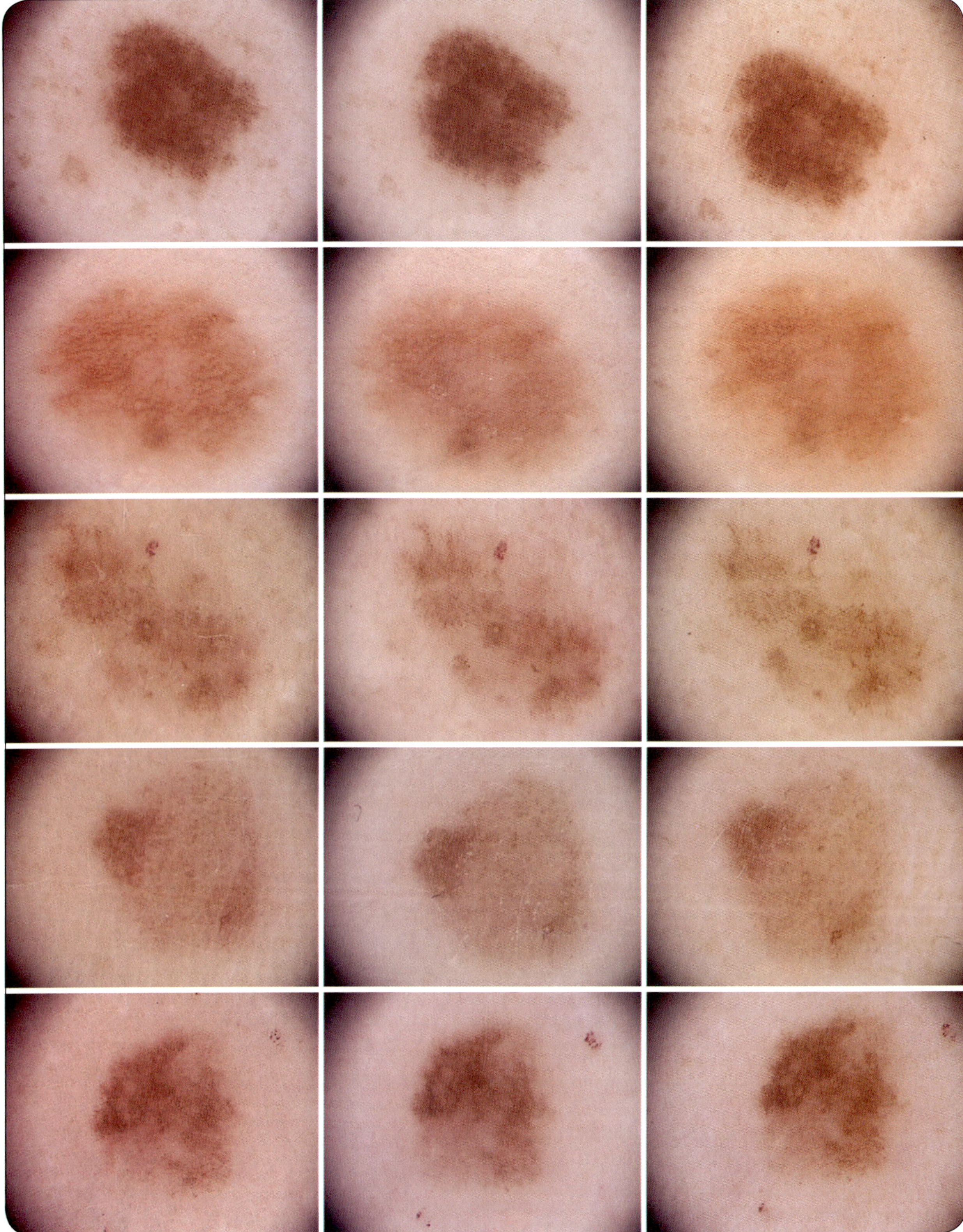

Fig. 11.1: Stable melanocytic lesions in a patient with a personal and familial history of melanoma. Although the lesions display signs of dermoscopic atypia, none has the criteria of malignancy.

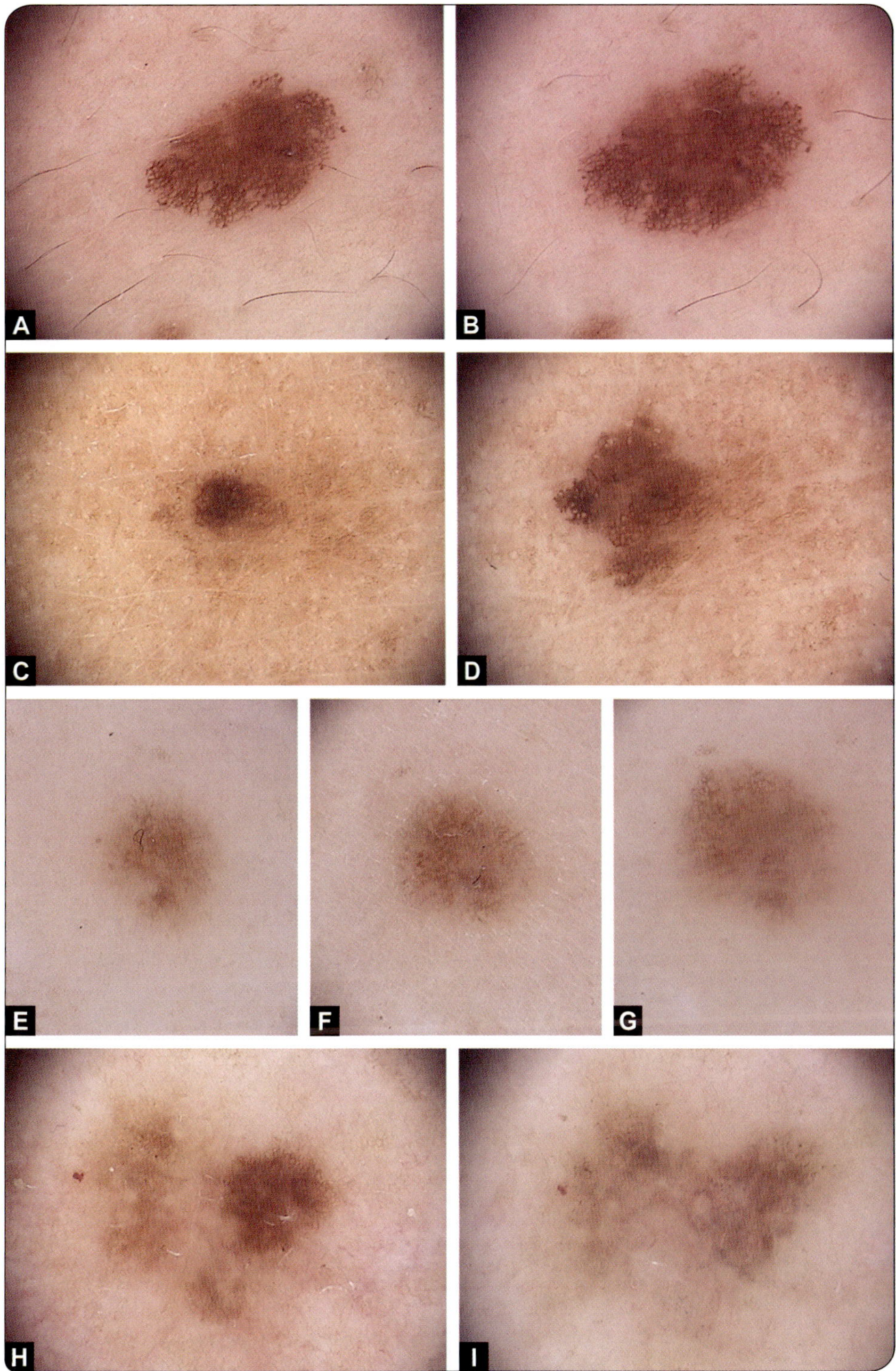

Figs. 11.2A to I: Melanomas detected due to changes during digital follow-up. (A and B) In situ melanoma in the back of a 63-year-old man, with atypical mole syndrome; the lesion showed asymmetric enlargement over a period of 9 months. (C and D) In situ melanoma in the leg of a 54-year-old woman, with a personal history of melanoma; asymmetric enlargement, changes in dermoscopic structures and focal pigment changes were observed after 18 months. (E to G) In situ melanoma detected due to asymmetric enlargement over a period of 20 months in the leg of a 36-year-old woman, carrier of mutation G101W in CDKN2A, a personal history of multiple melanoma and familial melanoma. (H and I) Invasive melanoma (Breslow 0.35 mm) in the back of a 65-year-old woman with a personal and a familial history of melanoma; the lesion showed regression features after 6 months.

considered significant during digital follow-up were more common in melanoma than in nevi. It was found that focal pigment changes and focal changes in the structure were significantly more common in melanoma than in nevi (with an odds ratio of 2.98 and 5.47, respectively), but no statistically significant differences were observed in terms of asymmetric enlargement, regression, or changes in the number of colors. In the same study, over a period of 10 years, 53 lesions were excised only due to symmetrical enlargement, a type of change that is considered not significant. Among these lesions, it was diagnosed one melanoma, Breslow 0.5 mm, which was classified as benign according to the ABCD rule of dermoscopy. Kittler et al.[15] reported that a melanoma initially diagnosed as an atypical nevus only showed symmetrical growth without dermoscopic structural modifications; the authors concluded that all atypical nevi with substantial changes in follow-up should be excised in order to not overlook a melanoma.

TOTAL-BODY PHOTOGRAPHY—BODY MAPPING

The detection of new or changing lesions in high-risk patients is difficult, especially in those patients with large numbers of melanocytic nevi, unless total-body photographs are available for comparison.[21]

Body mapping consists in the standardized record of body images in different positions in order to cover the entire body surface; these images are stored for the comparative study in successive controls (Figs. 11.3A to L). It is used in patients at high risk for melanoma, usually in the context of multiple dysplastic nevi, multiple nevi, prior melanoma, familial melanoma, or a history of multiple primary melanomas.[22-24]

It has been suggested that a monitoring strategy that focuses solely on sequential digital dermoscopy of those atypical nevi registered in a first visit will probably overlook melanomas that arise as new lesions or corresponding to lesions that have not been considered for follow-up initially.[9,25]

TOTAL-BODY PHOTOGRAPHY AND DIGITAL DERMATOSCOPY (TWO-STEP METHOD OF DIGITAL FOLLOW-UP)

The "two-step method of digital follow-up"[7] consists of the combined use of total-body photographs and sequential digital dermoscopy images of atypical lesions in every visit. Thus, through the comparative analysis of body mapping, one can objectively determine the appearance of new lesions during the follow-up and, by comparing dermoscopy records, detect microscopic changes, not visible to the naked eye in lesions selected for monitoring.

The baseline examinations consist of two steps: the first step is total-body photography, for clinical examination of the patient and body mapping; and the second step is digital dermoscopy, for clinical and dermoscopic examinations in real time of all individual lesions. Digital storage of dermoscopy images of each lesion showing atypical features is performed.

The follow-up examinations include two steps: the first step is body mapping, for comparison of total-body images with previous registries to detect any changes in shape, color, or surface eventually occurring in any pigmented skin lesions, and for identification of new lesions; and the second step is sequential digital dermoscopy, for the dermoscopic comparison and storage of lesions with atypical features, and for the clinical and dermoscopic examinations of eventual new lesions not previously registered.

The "two-step method of digital follow-up"[7] has been proposed as an approach for the assessment of individuals at high risk, being potentially more accurate than the two strategies separately. A recent series of studies[8,20] analyzed the 10-year experience of follow-up with total-body photography and sequential digital dermoscopy in a unit melanoma, the authors found that almost 40% of melanomas diagnosed in patients under surveillance corresponded to new lesions detected by the comparison of body maps, or lesions that are already present have not been initially considered for follow-up with dermoscopy.

BENEFITS OF DIGITAL FOLLOW-UP

In the last years, multiple studies have shown the benefits of monitoring high-risk patients with sequential digital dermoscopy, basically, the early diagnosis of melanoma with a low rate of excisions.[7-20]

Of the 98 melanomas diagnosed over 10 years using the "two-step method of digital follow-up" in the melanoma unit of the Hospital Clinic in Barcelona, Spain,[8] 53 melanomas were in situ, and the rest 45 invasive melanomas corresponded entirely to stage IA. These findings are consistent with those from the main working groups in this issue. Fuller et al.[9] reported six melanomas diagnosed during follow-up (although only one was diagnosed due to dermoscopic changes); two were in situ and the tumor

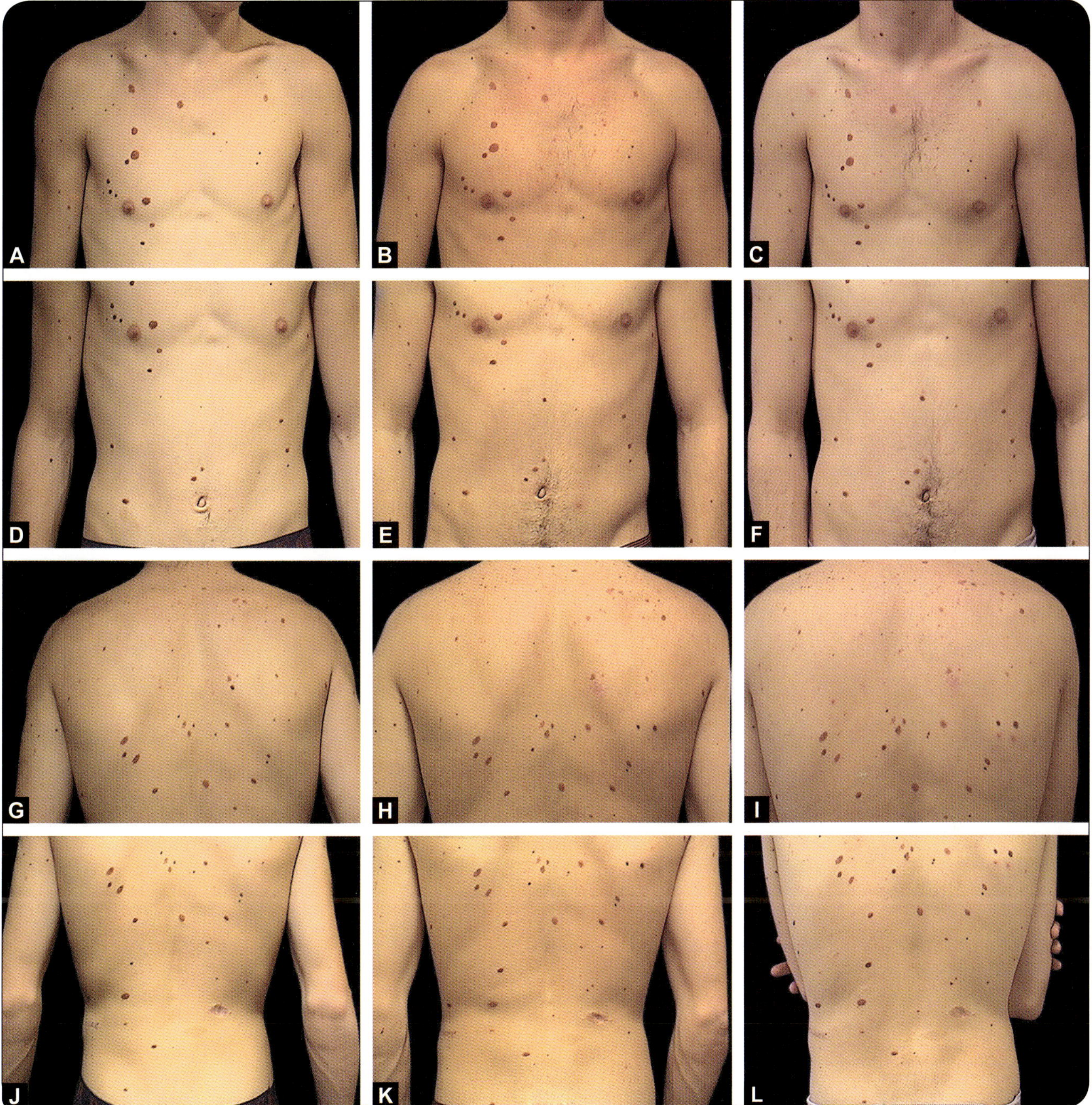

Figs. 11.3A to L: Body mapping comparison of the trunk of a 20-year-old patient with atypical mole syndrome and a familial history of melanoma over a period of 3 years.

thickness of invasive melanomas ranged between 0.23 and 0.35 mm. Bauer et al.[12] diagnosed two melanomas, and Robinson and Nickoloff[13] diagnosed four melanomas, all in situ. In 2000, Kittler et al.[16] diagnosed eight melanomas during follow-up, five in situ, and the rest three invasive with a tumor thickness of <0.75 mm. Similar results were reported by Menzies et al.[5] who diagnosed five in situ and two invasive melanomas (0.25 and 0.28 mm). In 2002, Malvehy and Puig[7] reported eight melanomas diagnosed during follow-up, of which two were in situ and six invasive with a tumor thickness of <0.75 mm. Argenziano et al.[17] diagnosed 12 melanomas in their study, 6 in situ and 6 invasive with a mean tumor thickness of 0.52 mm. Altamura et al.,[6] in 2008, reported 81 digital melanomas diagnosed during follow-up, 55 in situ and the rest 26 invasive, all with a tumor thickness of <1 mm. Haenssle et al. reported their experience over 10 years in monitoring patients at risk for melanoma with digital dermoscopy;[14,18] 87 melanomas were detected during follow-up, 38 were in situ, and 49 invasive, with a mean thickness of 0.57 mm. According to these publications, more than half of melanomas diagnosed during follow-up were in situ, and among invasive none had a thickness of >1 mm, confirming that sequential digital dermoscopy is an effective strategy for early diagnosis.

In late 2012, a meta-analysis of sequential digital dermoscopy was published on behalf of the International Dermoscopy Society.[26] This analysis showed that monitoring melanocytic lesions with sequential digital dermoscopy allows for the detection of incipient melanomas with a low rate of excisions. With this approach, the proportion of in situ and thin melanomas are higher than expected in general population. It was also demonstrated that chances to detect a melanoma during surveillance increase as the length of follow-up extends, so surveillance must be maintained over time in high-risk population.

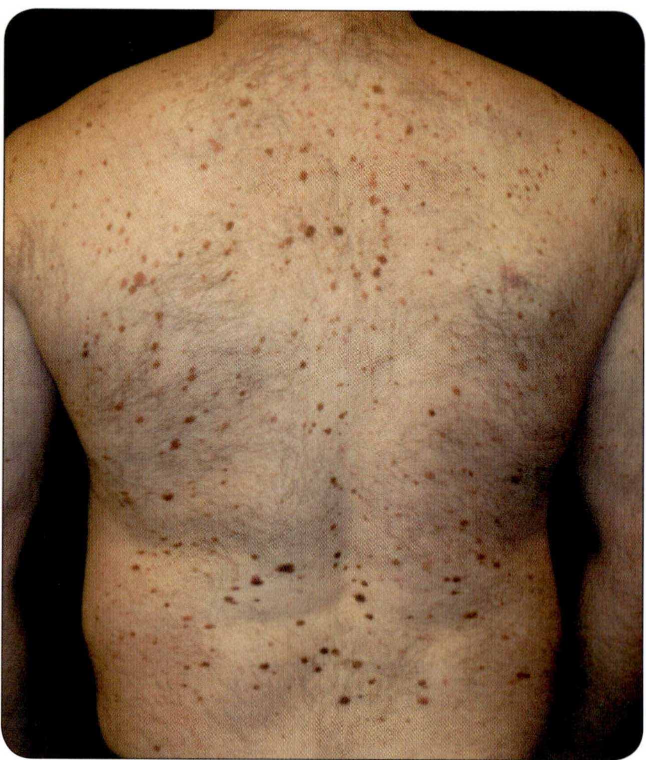

Fig. 11.4: Patient eligible for digital follow-up. The patient has a personal history of melanoma and atypical mole syndrome, with large numbers of melanocytic lesions, both typical and atypical.

INDICATIONS OF DIGITAL FOLLOW-UP

Already in 2007, Carli questioned the use of sequential digital dermoscopy in terms of cost effectiveness; highlighting the overwhelming burden that digital follow-up implicates.[27]

Chances of success in digital follow-up depend mainly on the proper selection of patients. Even though any patient can benefit from this approach, the fact that it is time consuming and expensive in terms of training and equipment makes its use justified only in individuals at high risk for melanoma (Fig. 11.4). The presence of large numbers of melanocytic lesions, both clinical and atypical nevi, is associated with a risk of melanoma 7–10 times higher than general population.[28-30] Although some nevi may be melanoma precursors, they are mostly markers of an increased risk.[30] History of previous melanoma is associated with an increased risk of a second primary melanoma.[28,29] Patients with a strong familial history of melanoma and multiple clinically atypical nevi represent the population at highest risk for melanoma (35–1,000 times).[28,29] In the context of these families, the presence of mutations in *CDKN2A* and *CDK4* genes implies a disease penetrance from 35% to 90% at the age of 80, depending on the country.[31]

In a recent study,[8] 12.6% of the patients included in the digital dermoscopy follow-up program (approximately one out of seven) were diagnosed with a new melanoma during surveillance. Furthermore, the percentage of patients who were diagnosed with melanoma during follow-up increased from 7% in patients without a history of melanoma to 18% and 23% in patients with a history of single and multiple primary melanomas, respectively, prior to the beginning of monitoring. This implies that including only patients at high risk of developing melanoma is a key requirement, since melanoma incidence among these patients was almost 1,500 times higher than the normal population.

LIMITATIONS

Sequential digital dermoscopy is a reliable strategy for the care of patients at high risk for melanoma, and its use is recommended in the main worldwide clinical guidelines for the recognition of early melanomas without specific dermoscopic features. However, this technique does not lack limitations, and some points are worthy of consideration.

The possibility of monitoring may lead to choose a suspicious lesion that should be removed. Facing the decision to follow-up, the patient might not attend to the next control with the consequent risk that a lesion, which could be a melanoma, is not removed promptly. The indiscriminate use of image registries is not recommended, since the utility of this strategy depends on the physician's experience in the interpretation of the images (it is basically an operator-dependent technique) and compliance by the patient.

CONCLUSION

The inclusion of patients who are at high risk for melanoma in follow-up programs with digital dermoscopy has proven to be a useful approach in early melanoma detection, enabling the diagnosis of lesions with a low rate of suspicious not only clinically but also dermoscopically, while minimizing the excision of benign lesions. The chances of success during follow-up depend mainly on the proper selection of patients and lesions to monitor. Experience in the interpretation of the images by the physician and patient compliance are key requirements.

REFERENCES

1. Puig S, Argenziano G, Zalaudek I, et al. Melanomas that failed dermoscopic detection: a combined clinicodermoscopic approach for not missing melanoma. Dermatol Surg. 2007;33: 1262-73.
2. Kittler H, Guitera P, Riedl E, et al. Identification of clinically featureless incipient melanoma using sequential dermoscopy imaging. Arch Dermatol. 2006;142:1113-9.
3. Stolz W, Schiffner R, Pillet L, et al. Improvement of monitoring of melanocytic skin lesions with the use of a computerized acquisition and surveillance unit with a skin surface microscopic television camera. J Am Acad Dermatol. 1996;35:202-7.
4. Salerni G, Lovatto L, Carrera C, et al. Melanomas detected in a follow-up program compared with melanomas referred to a melanoma unit. Arch Dermatol. 2011;147:549-55.
5. Menzies SW, Gutenev A, Avramidis M, et al. Short-term digital surface microscopic monitoring of atypical or changing melanocytic lesions. Arch Dermatol. 2001;137:1583.
6. Altamura D, Avramidis M, Menzies SW. Assessment of the optimal interval for and sensitivity of short-term sequential digital dermoscopy monitoring for the diagnosis of melanoma. Arch Dermatol. 2008;144(4):502-6.
7. Malvehy J, Puig S. Follow-up of melanocytic skin lesions with digital total-body photography and digital dermoscopy: a two-step method. Clin Dermatol. 2002;20:297-304.
8. Salerni G, Carrera C, Lovatto L, et al. Benefits of total body photography and digital dermoscopy ("two-step method of digital follow-up") in the early diagnosis of melanoma in high-risk patients. J Am Acad Dermatol. 2012;67(1):e17-27.
9. Fuller SR, Bowen GM, Tanner B, et al. Digital dermoscopic monitoring of atypical nevi in patients at risk for melanoma. Dermatol Surg. 2007;33:1198-206.
10. Schiffner R, Schiffner-Rohe J, Landthaler M, et al. Long-term dermoscopic follow-up of melanocytic naevi: clinical outcome and patient compliance. Br J Dermatol. 2003;149:79-86.
11. Haenssle HA, Krueger U, Vente C, et al. Results from an observational trial: digital epiluminescence microscopy follow-up of atypical nevi increases the sensitivity and the chance of success of conventional dermoscopy in detecting melanoma. J Invest Dermatol. 2006;126:980-5.
12. Bauer J, Blum A, Strohhacker U, et al. Surveillance of patients at high risk for cutaneous malignant melanoma using digital dermoscopy. Br J Dermatol. 2005;152:87-92.
13. Robinson JK, Nickoloff BJ. Digital epiluminescence microscopy monitoring of high-risk patients. Arch Dermatol. 2004;140:49-56.
14. Haenssle HA, Korpas B, Hansen-Hagge C, et al. Selection of patients for long-term surveillance with digital dermoscopy by assessment of melanoma risk factors. Arch Dermatol. 2010;146:257-64.
15. Kittler H, Pehamberger H, Wolff K, et al. Follow-up of melanocytic skin lesions with digital epiluminescence microscopy: patterns of modifications observed in early melanoma, atypical nevi, and common nevi. J Am Acad Dermatol. 2000;43:467-76.
16. Kittler H, Seltenheim M, Dawid M, et al. Frequency and characteristics of enlarging common melanocytic nevi. Arch Dermatol. 2000;136:316-20.
17. Argenziano G, Mordente I, Ferrara G, et al. Dermoscopic monitoring of melanocytic skin lesions: clinical outcome and patient compliance vary according to follow-up protocols. Br J Dermatol. 2008;159(2):331-6.
18. Haenssle HA, Korpas B, Hansen-Hagge C, et al. Seven-point checklist for dermatoscopy: performance during 10 years of prospective surveillance of patients at increased melanoma risk. J Am Acad Dermatol. 2010;62(5):785-93.
19. Haenssle HA, Vente C, Bertsch HP, et al. Results of a surveillance programme for patients at high risk of malignant melanoma using digital and conventional dermoscopy. Eur J Cancer Prev. 2004;13(2):133-8.
20. Salerni G, Carrera C, Lovatto L, et al. Characterization of 1152 lesions excised over 10 years using total-body photography and digital dermatoscopy in the surveillance of patients at high risk for melanoma. J Am Acad Dermatol. 2012;67(5):836-45.
21. Menzies S. Cutaneous melanoma: making a clinical diagnosis, present and future. Dermatol Ther. 2006;19:32-9.
22. Halpern AC. Total body skin imaging as an aid to melanoma detection. Semin Cutan Med Surg. 2003;22:2-8.
23. Banky JP, Kelly JW, English DR, et al. Incidence of new and changed nevi and melanomas detected using baseline images and dermoscopy in patients at high risk for melanoma. Arch Dermatol. 2005;141:998-1006.

24. Wang SQ, Kopf AW, Koenig K, et al. Detection of melanomas in patients followed up with total cutaneous examinations, total cutaneous photography, and dermoscopy. J Am Acad Dermatol. 2004;50:15-20.
25. Goodson AG, Florell SR, Hyde M, et al. Comparative analysis of total body and dermoscopic photographic monitoring of nevi in similar patient populations at risk for cutaneous melanoma. Dermatol Surg. 2010;36(7): 1087-98.
26. Salerni G, Terán T, Puig S, et al. Meta-analysis of digital dermoscopy follow-up of melanocytic skin lesions: a study on behalf of the international dermoscopy society. J Eur Acad Dermatol Venereol. 2013;27(7):805-14.
27. Carli P. Identification of incipient tumors by means of sequential dermoscopy imaging: a new way to inflate the "epidemic" of melanoma? Arch Dermatol. 2007;143(6):805; author reply 805-6.
28. Bataille V, de Vries E. Melanoma—Part 1: epidemiology, risk factors, and prevention. BMJ. 2008;337:a2249.
29. Gandini S, Sera F, Cattaruzza MS, et al. Meta-analysis of risk factors for cutaneous melanoma: III. Family history, actinic damage and phenotypic factors. Eur J Cancer. 2005;41: 2040-59.
30. Cho E, Rosner BA, Feskanich D, et al. Risk factors and individual probabilities of melanoma for whites. J Clin Oncol. 2005;23:2669-75.
31. Tsao H, Atkins MB, Sober A. Management of cutaneous melanoma. N Engl J Med. 2004;351:998-1012.

REVISED PATTERN ANALYSIS

12

Cliff Rosendahl, Harald Kittler

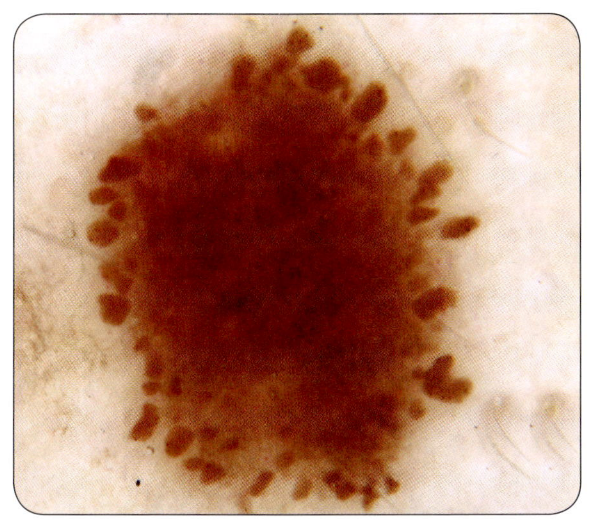

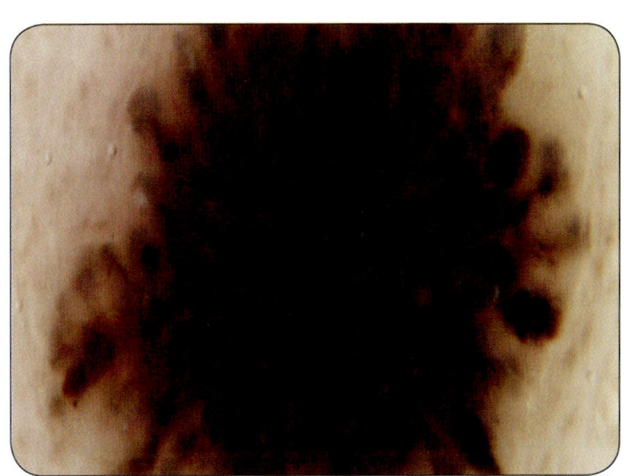

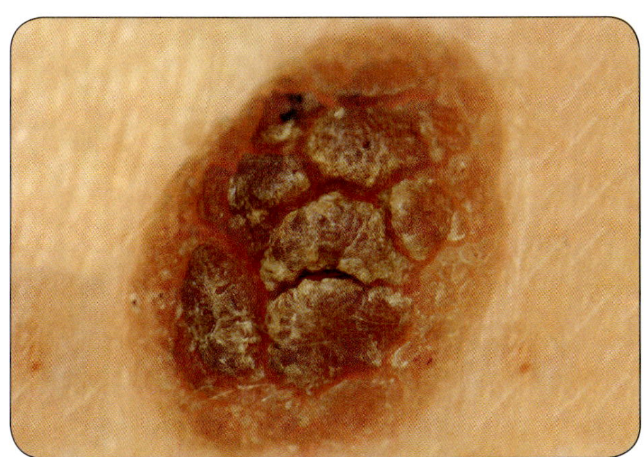

"Revised pattern analysis is a stepwise algorithmic method for the diagnosis of pigmented skin lesions, pigmented by melanin, significant blood pigment (as in structureless blood or red clots), or discolored keratin. The method of pattern analysis was first published in 1987 and no method has since been shown to be more accurate, but there was no stepwise process and the language of dermatoscopy evolved with a myriad of poorly defined or undefined metaphorical terms that in many cases carried preconceived diagnostic implications.

Revised pattern analysis uses a limited number of clearly defined geometric terms and provides a clear stepwise process of analysis, assessing patterns then colors and finally clues, leading the clinician to a specific provisional diagnosis or alternatively a limited differential diagnosis. "

Revised pattern analysis (RPA) is a stepwise algorithmic method for the diagnosis of pigmented skin lesions, pigmented by melanin, significant blood pigment (as in structureless blood or red clods), or discolored keratin.[1,2] The method of pattern analysis was first published in 1987 by Pehamberger et al.[3] and no method has since been shown to be more accurate, but there was no stepwise process and the language of dermatoscopy evolved with a myriad of poorly defined or undefined metaphorical terms that in many cases carried preconceived diagnostic implications. Revised pattern analysis uses a limited number of clearly defined geometric terms and provides a clear stepwise process of analysis, assessing patterns then colors and finally clues, leading the clinician to a specific provisional diagnosis or alternatively a limited differential diagnosis (Fig. 12.1).

In the language of RPA, there are five basic structures: lines, pseudopods, circles, clods, and dots (Fig. 12.1, vertical). Because lines are a very specific structure, they are further subdivided into five different types: reticular, branched, parallel, radial, and curved (Fig. 12.1, horizontal). A pattern is an area made up of multiple repetitions of a basic structure. The terms used are clearly defined:

- A *line* is a structure with length greatly exceeding width.
- A *pseudopod* is a line with a bulbous end.
- A *circle* is a curved line sensibly equidistant from a central point (this includes ellipses).
- A *clod* is a well-defined, solid object larger than a dot and it can be of any color and any shape.
- A *dot* is an object too small to have a discernable shape (at 10 times magnification).
- A *structureless* area is an area covering a significant portion of a lesion with no basic structure predominating.

A pattern is formed by multiple repetitions of a basic structure and it must cover a significant portion of a lesion to be regarded as a pattern. For example, a few lines covering 5–10% of a lesion with an otherwise structureless pattern would constitute a clue rather than a pattern. If however reticular lines covered 30% of an otherwise structureless lesion, then the lesion would be regarded as having two patterns (Fig. 12.2). In Figure 12.2, the right-hand side of the lesion has a pattern of lines reticular. There are a few lines and dots on the left side but as none of these structures predominate, this portion of the lesion is termed structureless. Note that structureless does not necessarily equate with featureless.

Patterns should be assessed as such and a few structures out of synchrony do not destroy a pattern. For example, looking at the right side of Figure 12.2 you may recognize a few circles but that does not interfere with the description of a pattern of reticular lines. It must be remembered that we are describing biological material rather than an architect's design and it is appropriate to tolerate reasonable variation.

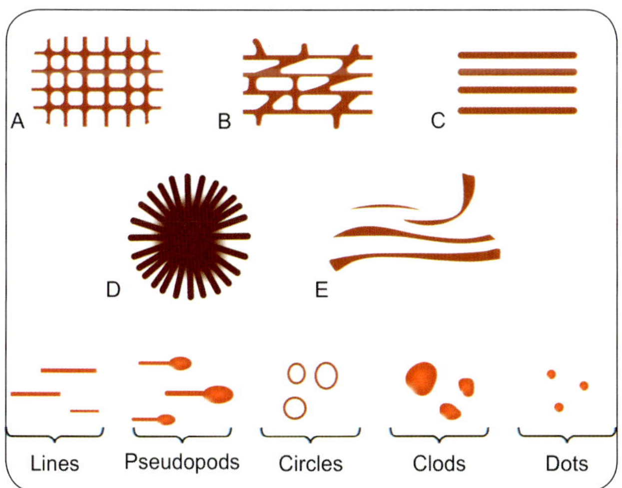

Fig. 12.1: There are five basic structures in revised pattern analysis: Lines (A: Reticular; B: Branched; C: Parallel; D: Radial; and E: Curved), pseudopods, circles, clods, and dots.

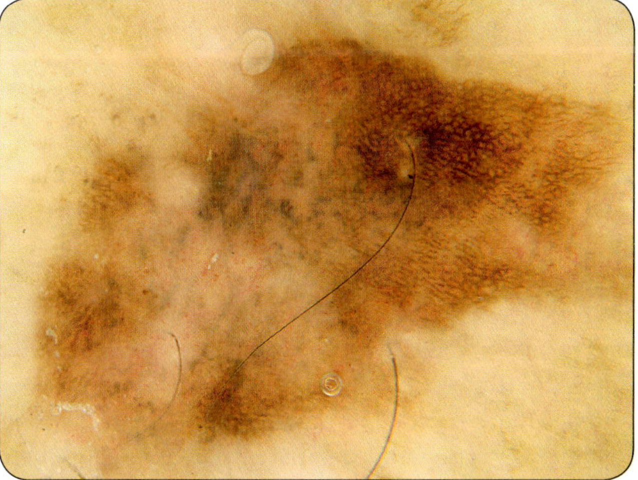

Fig. 12.2: A pigmented skin lesion with a pattern of lines reticular on the right. Although there are some lines and dots on the left, none of these predominate so the pattern is structureless. This is a solar lentigo on the right-hand side in collision with a pigmented squamous cell carcinoma on the left-hand side.

WHY THE TWO-STEP METHOD OF DERMATOSCOPY IS NOT USED IN REVISED PATTERN ANALYSIS

The two-step method of dermatoscopy requires that melanocytic status be determined by dermatoscopy as a first step before the lesion is assessed for clues to melanoma as a second step.[4,5] The so-called melanocytic criteria (network, pseudonetwork, aggregated brown globules, radial streaming, pseudopods, homogeneous blue pigmentation, and parallel ridge pattern) are not melanocytic criteria at all. They are just melanotic criteria and can occur in any pigmented lesion whether it has a proliferation of melanocytes or not. The lesion in Figure 12.2 has clear pigment network but it is a solar lentigo in collision with a pigmented squamous cell carcinoma (pSCC) in situ, neither of which are melanocytic. The so-called pseudonetwork is commonly seen in solar lentigo and pigmented actinic keratosis (pAK), neither of which are melanocytic. Lines radial segmental are seen in a basal cell carcinoma (BCC) (*see* Fig. 12.20) and in SCC in situ (*see* Fig. 12.22), neither of which are melanocytic. The sensitivity and specificity of the first step of the two-step process were evaluated in a study on consecutive lesion in a practice in Europe, compared to a practice in Australia.[6] The specificity was found to be 67.9% in Europe and 33.6% in Australia.

APPLYING REVISED PATTERN ANALYSIS

The three fundamental steps in pattern analysis—patterns, colors, and clues—are shown in Figure 12.3.[2]

Before RPA is applied, a lesion must be identified as pigmented. Although pigmentation may be obvious, it is important to understand that the presence of any visible pigment at all should, as a rule, lead to the lesion being assessed as a pigmented lesion. Pigmented structures are far more specific as diagnostic clues than nonpigmented structures such as blood vessels, and should always be given priority when present.[1]

Step 1: Once a lesion is recognized as pigmented, the first step is to assess the pattern(s) with a decision made as to whether there is *one pattern or more than one pattern*. Defining a precise number of patterns does not additionally assist the diagnostic process and so the simple decision on whether there is one pattern or more than one is adequate. In the case of one pattern, the assessment proceeds in a stepwise fashion, which will be described, and if there is more than one pattern, the primary pattern will

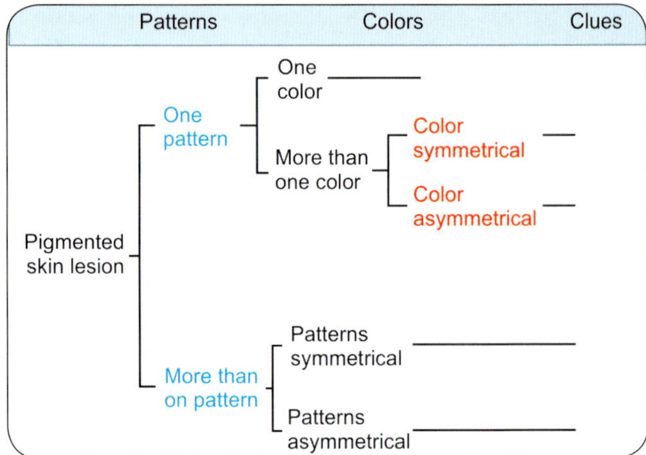

Fig. 12.3: The three basic steps in revised pattern analysis: a stepwise assessment of patterns, colors, and clues.

determine the stepwise assessment. The primary pattern is the first pattern encountered in the order lines (reticular, branched, parallel, radial, and curved), pseudopods, circles, clods, dots, and structureless, regardless of whether it is the pattern that covers the greatest area.

Step 2: After deciding what pattern is present, or in the case that there is more than one pattern—what the primary pattern is—a decision must be made as to whether the lesion is *symmetrical or not*. Symmetry is decided on the basis of structure and color, regardless of the shape.

In the case of only one pattern, symmetry is decided on the basis of color. If there is one pattern and one color, then by definition the lesion is symmetrical. If there is one pattern but more than one color and the colors are combined asymmetrically, the lesion is asymmetrical (Fig. 12.4).

In Figure 12.4, the lesion on the left has a pattern of yellow clods. There is one pattern and one color. The background does not constitute a structureless pattern because it is overlaid by the pattern of yellow clods. A couple of white clods have no impact on the *pattern* although they are additional *clues* to the diagnosis of seborrheic keratosis. With one pattern and one color the lesion is symmetrical.

In the case of more than one pattern, symmetry is determined by the structures, and color is disregarded in the assessment of symmetry (Fig. 12.3). The lesion in the right of Figure 12.4 has two patterns, a central structureless pattern and peripheral clods combined symmetrically in a concentric arrangement. It does not matter that there are a few clods missing at the top. Such variation is acceptable

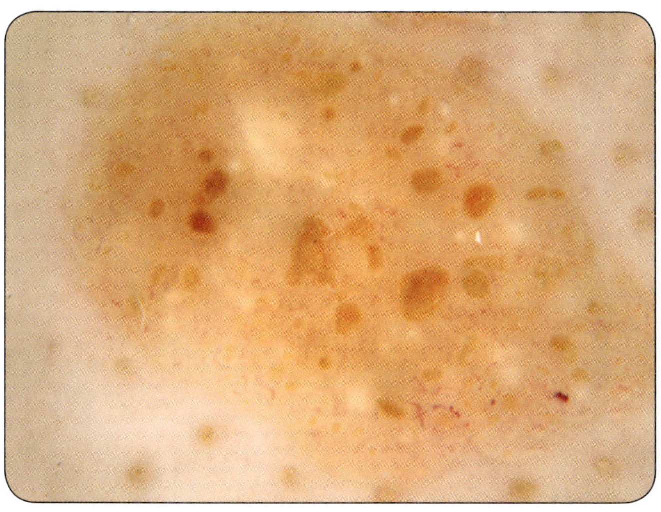
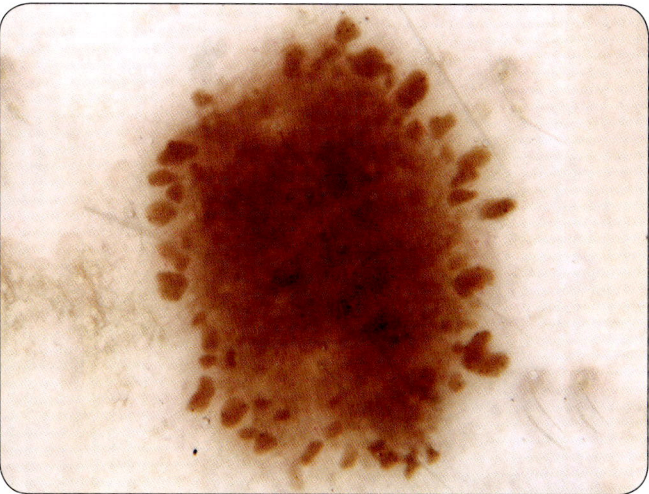

Fig. 12.4: The lesion on the left has one pattern clods and one color yellow. By definition, it is symmetrical. The lesion on the right has two patterns: central structureless and peripheral clods, combined in a symmetrical concentric pattern.

in biological tissue. Another way of understanding this is to realize that such a degree of variation is not consistent with the disorganized behavior of malignant tissue.

Step 3: Having assessed the patterns and symmetry of a pigmented skin lesion, RPA then proceeds in a stepwise fashion according to *clues* (*see* Fig. 12.3). This stepwise process is illustrated for lesions with one pattern, clods, in Figure 12.5 and with more than one pattern including a primary pattern of clods in Figure 12.6.

AN AIDE MEMOIRE FOR REVISED PATTERN ANALYSIS

This stepwise process permits assessment of lesions in a logical progression starting with an assessment of the patterns, colors, and finally the clues (*see* Fig. 12.3). Patterns and colors are assessed as if from a distance, actually avoiding attention to subtle details, and when that assessment discovers biological symmetry, the likelihood of malignancy is very low. On the other hand, the discovery of patterns and/or colors combined asymmetrically raises the possibility of malignancy and should lead to a careful examination for clues that may support that suspicion. Such an assessment can proceed in the stepwise manner illustrated for the pattern of clods in Figure 12.5 or 12.6. Alternatively, a simpler method should use the primary pattern to provide *a limited differential diagnosis* that is then sorted according to specific clues to the defined alternatives. This simplified approach is presented as an "Aide Memoire" for RPA (Fig. 12.7).

USING THE AIDE MEMOIRE FOR REVISED PATTERN ANALYSIS

Using the aide memoire presented in Figure 12.7, the lesions relevant to pattern analysis have been conveniently subdivided into just six groups.

The sixth group includes lesions pigmented by pigments other than melanin and only needs to be considered when that is evident.

The fifth group is for dermatofibroma (DF) and its inclusion ensures that this diagnosis is considered even when not obvious. The diagnosis of DF can usually be confirmed confidently by a symmetrical combination of virtually any dermoscopic pattern peripherally combined with a central hypopigmented structureless area. Commonly, polarizing-specific white lines are seen in the central hypopigmented area. A history of stability of a clinical palpable nodule that characteristically retracts when the lesion is laterally compressed is usually compelling additional support for the diagnosis of DF.

Considering that the groups "DF" and "other" generally do not provide a diagnostic challenge, the application of RPA can concentrate primarily on the use of clues to establish a provisional diagnosis of lesions in the first four categories defined in the RPA aide memoire: melanocytic lesions, benign keratinocytic lesions, BCC, and SCC including AK and SCC in situ (Fig. 12.8).

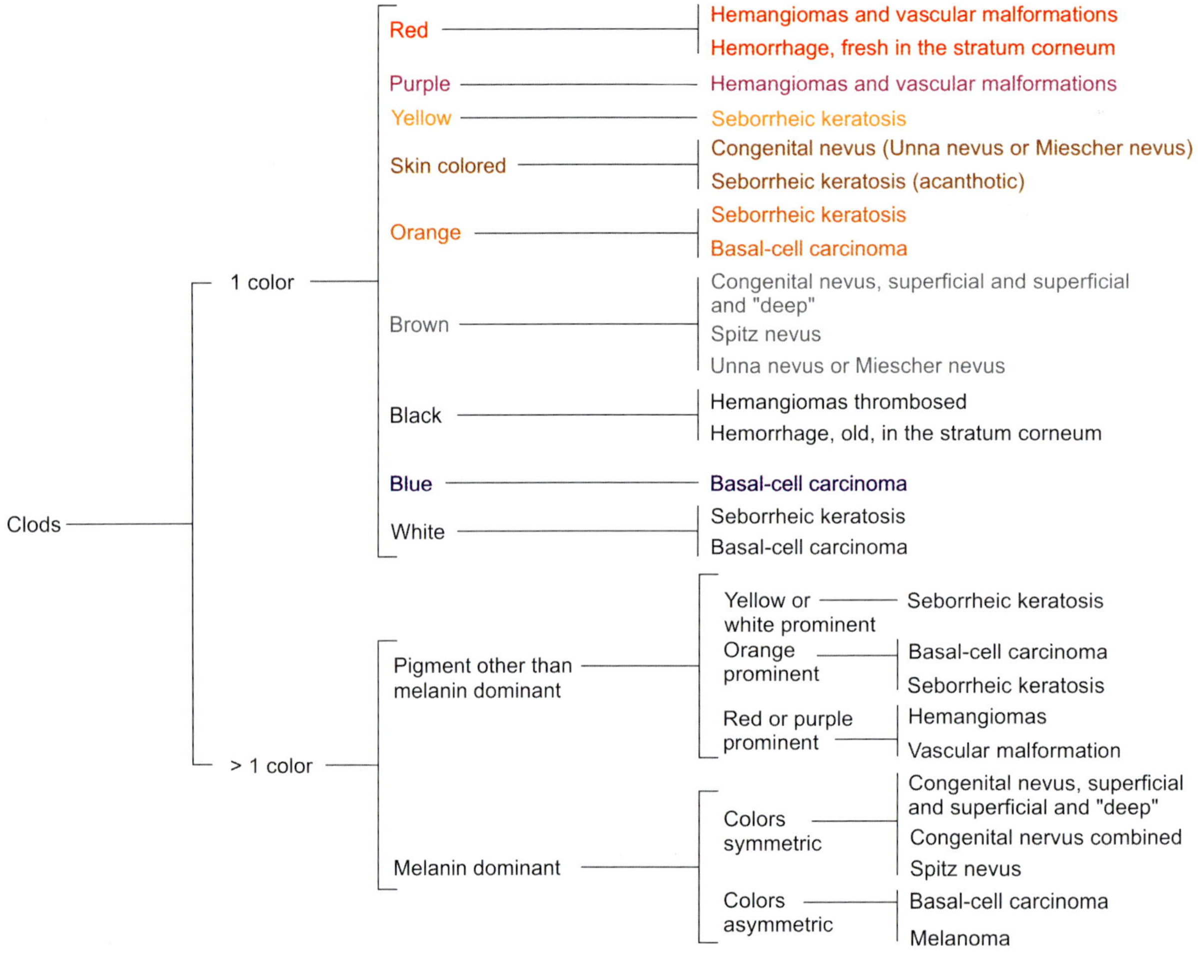

- Clods
  - 1 color
    - Red
      - Hemangiomas and vascular malformations
      - Hemorrhage, fresh in the stratum corneum
    - Purple
      - Hemangiomas and vascular malformations
    - Yellow
      - Seborrheic keratosis
    - Skin colored
      - Congenital nevus (Unna nevus or Miescher nevus)
      - Seborrheic keratosis (acanthotic)
    - Orange
      - Seborrheic keratosis
      - Basal-cell carcinoma
    - Brown
      - Congenital nevus, superficial and superficial and "deep"
      - Spitz nevus
      - Unna nevus or Miescher nevus
    - Black
      - Hemangiomas thrombosed
      - Hemorrhage, old, in the stratum corneum
    - Blue
      - Basal-cell carcinoma
    - White
      - Seborrheic keratosis
      - Basal-cell carcinoma
  - > 1 color
    - Pigment other than melanin dominant
      - Yellow or white prominent
        - Seborrheic keratosis
      - Orange prominent
        - Basal-cell carcinoma
        - Seborrheic keratosis
      - Red or purple prominent
        - Hemangiomas
        - Vascular malformation
    - Melanin dominant
      - Colors symmetric
        - Congenital nevus, superficial and superficial and "deep"
        - Congenital nervus combined
        - Spitz nevus
      - Colors asymmetric
        - Basal-cell carcinoma
        - Melanoma

Fig. 12.5: The stepwise assessment of clues in lesions with one pattern, clods.

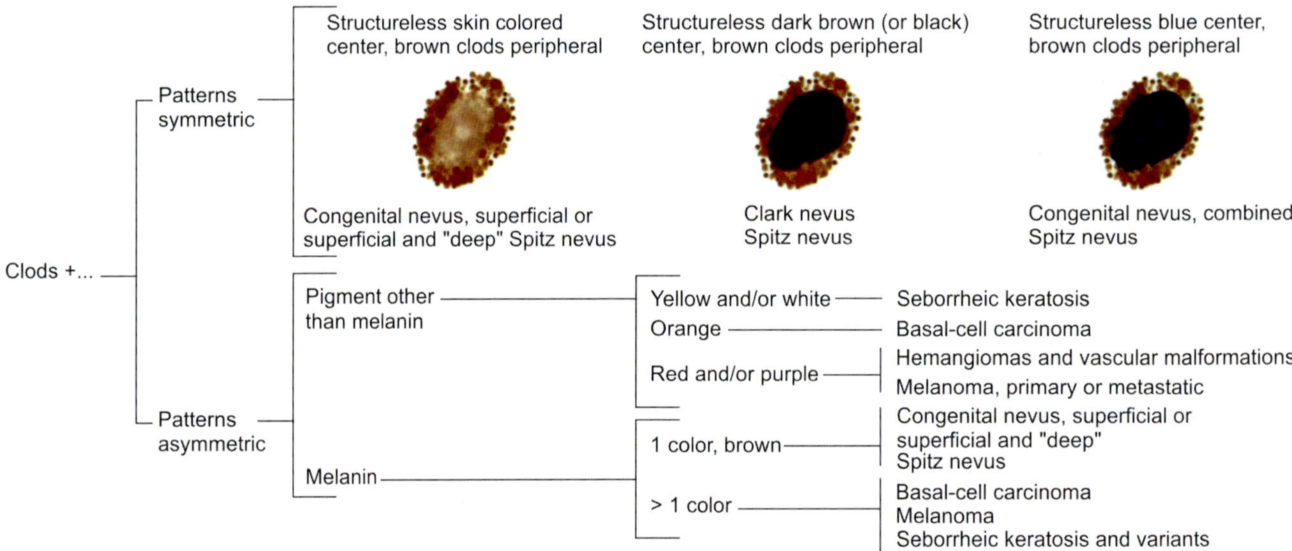

Fig. 12.6: The stepwise assessment of clues in lesions with a primary pattern of clods combined with any secondary pattern (dots or structureless).

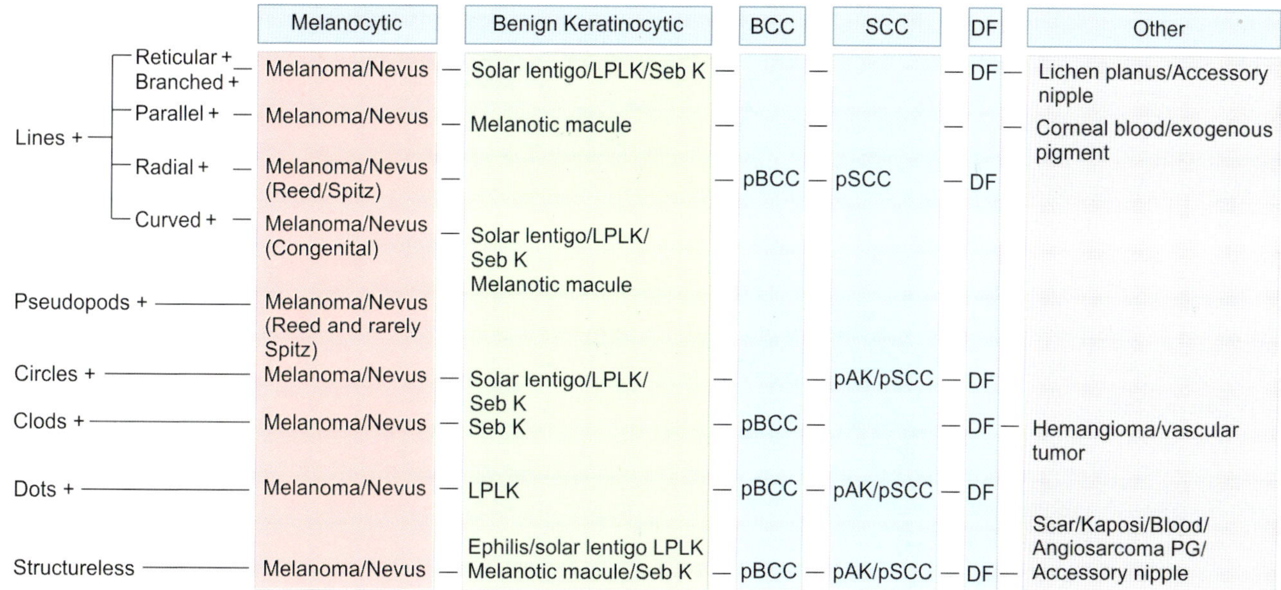

Pattern		Melanocytic	Benign Keratinocytic	BCC	SCC	DF	Other
Lines +	Reticular + / Branched +	Melanoma/Nevus	Solar lentigo/LPLK/Seb K			DF	Lichen planus/Accessory nipple
	Parallel +	Melanoma/Nevus	Melanotic macule				Corneal blood/exogenous pigment
	Radial +	Melanoma/Nevus (Reed/Spitz)		pBCC	pSCC	DF	
	Curved +	Melanoma/Nevus (Congenital)	Solar lentigo/LPLK/ Seb K Melanotic macule				
Pseudopods +		Melanoma/Nevus (Reed and rarely Spitz)					
Circles +		Melanoma/Nevus	Solar lentigo/LPLK/ Seb K		pAK/pSCC	DF	
Clods +		Melanoma/Nevus	Seb K	pBCC		DF	Hemangioma/vascular tumor
Dots +		Melanoma/Nevus	LPLK	pBCC	pAK/pSCC	DF	
Structureless		Melanoma/Nevus	Ephilis/solar lentigo LPLK Melanotic macule/Seb K	pBCC	pAK/pSCC	DF	Scar/Kaposi/Blood/ Angiosarcoma PG/ Accessory nipple

Fig. 12.7: The use of an aide memoire to provide a limited list of diagnostic categories in revised pattern analysis. The patterns are listed in order of specificity and the list of categories is smaller for more specific patterns. A lesion is examined for patterns and the first pattern encountered in the order shown above is the primary pattern. The differential diagnosis will be limited to the categories populated for that primary pattern. (LPLK: Lichen planus like keratosis; pBCC: Pigmented basal cell carcinoma; pSCC: Pigmented squamous cell carcinoma; DF: Dermatofibroma; Seb K: Seborrheic keratosis; pAK: Pigmented actinic keratosis; Kaposi: Kaposi's sacrcoma).

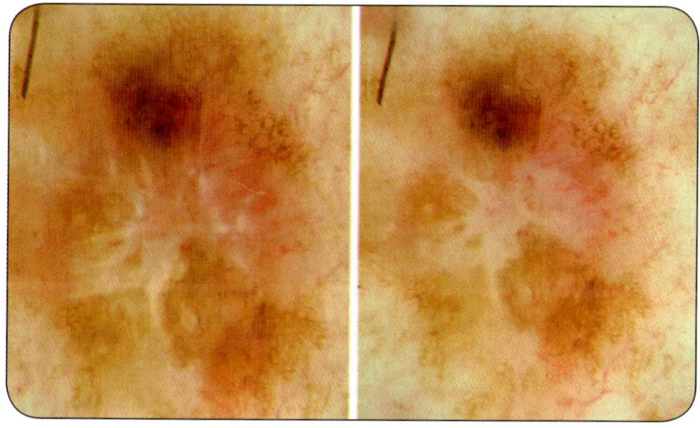

Fig. 12.8: This lesion had more than one pattern—structureless centrally and lines reticular (or circles—such variations of perception do no alter the outcome of revised pattern analysis) peripherally, with asymmetry produced by a small eccentric structureless gray area superiorly, and the additional clue to malignancy of polarizing-specific white lines (left). Palpation and lateral compression by squeezing suggested the diagnosis of dermatofibroma that was consistent with a history of stability over >20 years.

THE PATTERN OF LINES RETICULAR OR BRANCHED

Lines reticular and branched are very similar and while the presence of branched lines can be a useful clue to ink-spot lentigo, as patterns, the two will be considered together.

A lesion with one pattern, lines reticular/branched, or a lesion with more than one pattern but with a primary pattern of lines reticular/branched, and which is not an *accessory nipple* or *DF* will be limited to only two categories: *melanocytic or benign keratinocytic.*

A lesion with one pattern, thin lines reticular and one color, brown can be either a solar lentigo or a Clark nevus. A solar lentigo may have the clues of a sharply demarcated (abrupt) scalloped border whereas a Clark nevus usually has a gradual border over the entire periphery without scalloped areas. In reality, the distinction cannot always be made. This must be acknowledged as a limitation of the method but as both lesions are benign, it has no relevance to any necessity of a biopsy.

If the reticular lines are thick and brown, then superficial congenital nevus and early seborrheic keratosis can be considered along with Clark nevus.

If the lines are black, this is consistent with ink-spot lentigo with additional clues being branched as well as reticular lines and a very abrupt border.

A symmetrical lesion with only reticular lines but more than one color can be a solar lentigo (clues as described above, seborrheic keratosis (clues of multiple white clods, multiple orange/yellow clods, well demarcated border, thick curved lines and vessels as loops, or coils), Clark nevus (clues as above), congenital nevus or in situ melanoma (clues including an asymmetrical combination of the colors, gray or blue structures, eccentric structureless area other than skin colored, thick reticular lines, peripheral black dots/clods, segmental radial lines/pseudopods, white lines, polymorphous vessels, or polygons.

A symmetrical reticular-pattern lesion with a darker center is most likely a Clark nevus. If the colors are combined in a variegate pattern and there are no clues to melanoma then it is likely to be either a Clark nevus or a congenital nevus. If one or more of the clues to melanoma mentioned above are present, this diagnosis must be seriously considered.

A symmetrical reticular-pattern lesion with hyperpigmentation peripherally can be a Clark nevus or a melanoma (if a clue to a melanoma is present).

A lesion with a primary pattern of lines reticular/branched can be combined with any of the other patterns (lines parallel, radial, or curved; pseudopods; circles; clods; dots; or structureless) and if the combination is symmetrical for practical purposes there are five combinations to consider. First, a pattern with central clods and peripheral reticular lines is most consistent with a congenital or more rarely a Clark nevus. Second, a lesion with central reticular lines and peripheral clods/dots will be a growing nevus, either Clark or congenital. Third, reticular lines and clods/dots combined in a variegate pattern can be seen in either Clark or congenital nevus. Fourth, a peripheral reticular pattern can be combined with a central structureless pattern. In this case, a skin colored center points to congenital nevus or accessory nipple; a dark brown or black center points to a Clark or Reed nevus; a blue center is consistent with a combined congenital nevus; and a white center makes the diagnosis of DF most likely—subject to the other clues to DF mentioned above. Finally, a symmetrical combination of central reticular lines with either radial lines or pseudopods (or both) peripherally is consistent with the diagnosis of Reed nevus. After puberty such lesions should be excised as melanoma can sometimes present in this way.

Any asymmetrical combination of reticular lines with another pattern must be assessed very carefully for clues to melanoma, and if none are present then the differential diagnosis includes both Clark and congenital nevi.

CLUES TO MELANOMA[2,7,8]

With respect to color these clues depend on the fact that melanin appears as different colors depending on its depth in the skin.[9] Melanin, being a very efficient pigment, absorbs all light and, therefore, it appears black at the level of the stratum corneum. At the dermoepidermal junction and the epidermis, the normal location of melanin in healthy skin, some light is reflected back by cells in the epidermis so it appears near-black, which is brown. Because of the fact that the collagen particles of the dermis scatter back short wavelength (blue) light preferentially to long wavelength (red) light, while blocking the color of heme from below, melanin in the superficial and deep dermis appears gray and black, respectively.

Gray or blue structures correlate with melanin in the superficial and deep dermis, respectively. In melanomas, blue correlates with immature nested pigmented melanocytes in the deep dermis, and in an asymmetrical lesion it is a strong clue to invasive melanoma. In melanomas, gray dots usually correlate with melanophages in the papillary dermis and they are a common finding in the majority of in situ melanomas as well as being common in invasive melanomas.

An eccentric structureless area must cover a sufficient portion of the lesion to form a pattern; it must be contrasted to a structured pattern within the lesion and it must be a color other than skin colored. In melanomas, if colored with the colors of melanin, it is produced by the chaotic behavior of malignant melanocytes; if pink, it is caused by increased blood flow; and if white, it may correlate with fibrosis after regression.

Thick lines reticular are defined when the lines are thicker than the holes that they surround. They correlate with rete ridges that are widened by pigment-laden malignant melanocytes.

Peripheral black dots and clods correlate with pigmented pagetoid melanocytes and nests of melanocytes close to the stratum corneum where melanin is expected to appear black.

White lines must be whiter than normal surrounding skin and may be polarizing-specific, or alternatively, white lines that are seen in both modalities. Polarizing-specific white lines are shiny white lines orientated perpendicularly to each other but not crossing. They are only seen with polarizing dermatoscopy but they may correlate with reticular white lines seen with nonpolarized dermatoscopy. Polarizing-specific white line can also be seen commonly in BCC as well as DF and Spitz nevus. They are not specific to these lesions but their presence is not expected in any other type of nevus or in seborrheic keratoses. If they are seen in such lesions, they should be excised to rule out malignancy even if there is a history of preceding

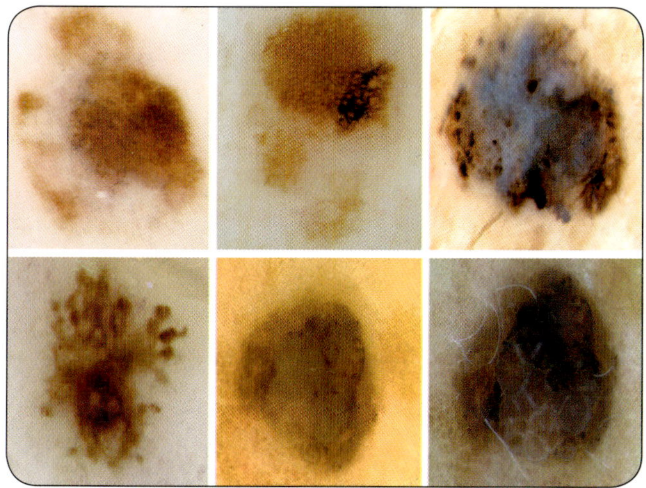

Fig. 12.9: Clues to melanoma—asymmetry plus: "gray dots" (upper left); "thick lines reticular" and "eccentric structureless area light brown" (upper center); "eccentric structureless blue" and "black clods peripheral" (upper right); "lines radial and pseudopods, segmental" (lower left); "polarizing-specific white lines" (lower right with non-polarized dermatoscopy—lower center).

trauma. Polarizing-specific "white" lines appear blue in some lesions and these polarizing-specific lines, with the same perpendicular morphology and only seen in polarizing-specific mode, have the same diagnostic significance.

Lines radial or pseudopods segmental correlate with fascicles of pigmented melanocytes extending from the periphery of a lesion and they signify radial growth. In melanomas, they should be distributed asymmetrically and should extend from reticular lines, clods, or structureless areas of equivalent pigmentation to the radial lines or pseudopods. This can distinguish them from the radial lines seen in BCCs.

Polymorphous vessels in melanomas are expected to include various types of linear vessels in raised portions and patterns of dot vessel as well as any pattern of linear vessel in macular portions. Generally, other clues apart from polymorphous vessels (pigment clues and/or white lines) are expected in a melanoma and the vessel clues are then useful in differentiating melanoma from pigmented basal cell carcinoma (pBCC) and pSCC in situ.

Polygons[10] are defined as geometric polygonal shapes, complete or incomplete, bounded by straight lines, or by a straight pigment interface, meeting at angles and larger than the holes caused by individual follicles and larger by far than the holes bounded by reticular lines (Figs. 12.9 and 12.10).[11,12]

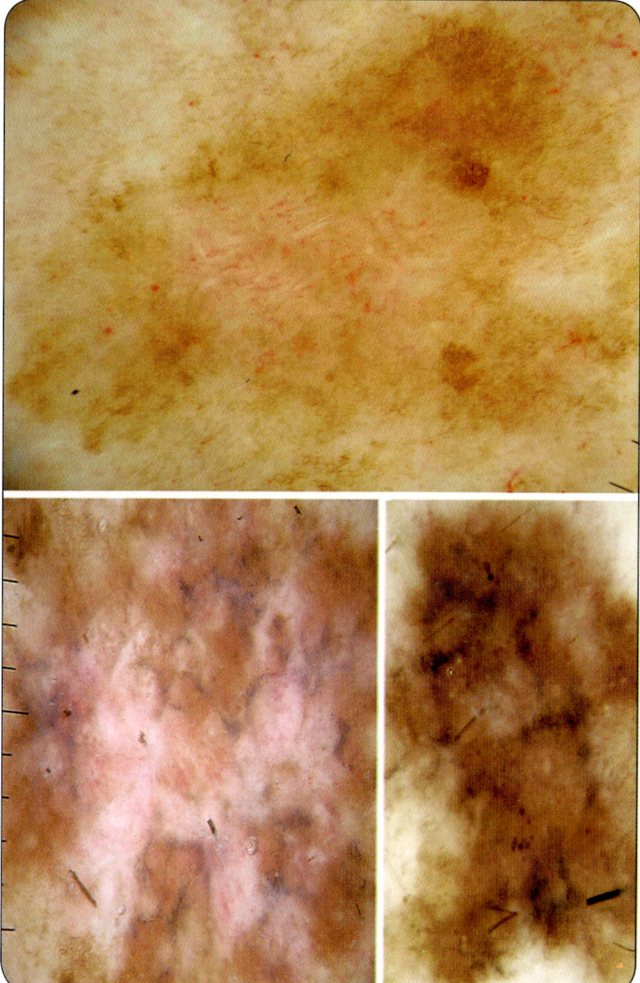

Fig. 12.10: Clues to melanoma—asymmetry plus: polymorphous vessels and polarizing-specific white lines (upper), polygons (both lesions lower).

THE PATTERN OF LINES PARALLEL

A lesion with one pattern, lines parallel, or a lesion with more than one pattern but with a primary pattern of lines parallel and that is pigmented by melanin, will be restricted to the melanocytic *or benign keratinocytic category.*

A pattern of lines parallel only, on acral skin, in which the lines, pigmented by melanin, are located on the dermatoglyphic ridges, is a clue to melanoma but can also rarely be seen with any type of acral nevus. Clues to nevus include onset in youth combined with long-term stability but the index of suspicion should be high and evidence of the onset at mature age and/or change should lead to an appropriate biopsy. Of course, very large size or variations in pigment density in poorly defined lesions may be additional clues to melanoma. It should be remembered that melanomas in these locations may be very lightly pigmented but with small areas of subtle ridge-pattern pigmentation.

A pattern of lines parallel only, on acral skin, pigmented by blood products, is due to intracorneal hemorrhage and additional clues include satellite clods. Exogenous pigment like that caused by silver nitrate therapy to warts can also cause a ridge pattern.

A pattern of lines parallel only, on acral skin, in the dermatoglyphic furrows and pigmented by melanin, is consistent with the diagnosis of nevus.

A crossing pattern as pattern of lines parallel only, on acral skin, with lines crossing both ridges and furrows should be resolved into a parallel furrow or ridge pattern by tilting the dermatoscope, to facilitate assessment as described above.

A primary pattern of lines parallel, combined with any other pattern, should be examined very carefully for clues to melanoma. Clues to melanoma include those described above for the assessment of reticular-pattern lesions with the addition of the clue of a pattern of parallel lines in the dermatoglyphic ridges seen in any part of the lesion.

A primary pattern of lines parallel, in the furrows, may be consistent with a diagnosis of nevus if the lesion is symmetrical and there are no clues to melanoma, but if the lesion is asymmetrical and there are any of the described clues to melanoma, then the possibility of melanoma arising in association with a nevus must be considered (Fig. 12.11).

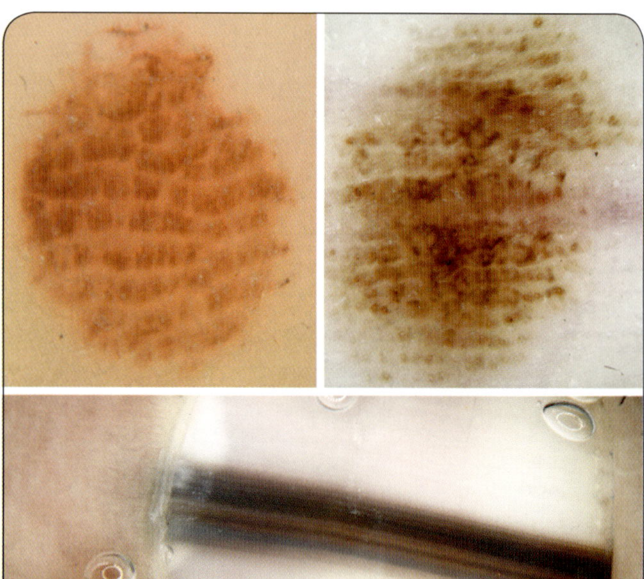

Fig. 12.11: Clues to melanoma on acral skin and the nail matrix. The upper images are patterns of parallel lines on the dermatoglyphic ridges on acral skin. Although the lesion on the upper left was a corneal hemorrhage, there were no satellite clods as a clue to that. The lesion had almost cleared after 2 weeks. The lesion on the upper right was a small acral melanoma. The broad ridge pattern is best appreciated at the edges of the lesion, which is symmetrical. The lower lesion displays lines parallel varying in width, interval, and color (lines parallel chaotic) in the nail plate of a thumb and nail-matrix biopsy conformed the diagnosis on melanoma in situ.

THE PATTERN OF LINES RADIAL

A lesion with one pattern, lines radial, or a lesion with more than one pattern but with a primary pattern of lines radial, which is not a *DF*, will be restricted to the *melanocytic*, *BCC*, and *SCC* categories.

The pattern of radial lines always occurs in combination with another pattern.

If the lesion is symmetrical, the radial lines must be peripheral and circumferential. If in such a lesion the center is structureless and white, the provisional diagnosis is DF. If the center is structureless and brown, black, or gray, then Reed nevus is the likely diagnosis. If the center has a pattern of dark clods, then Reed nevus is also likely.

If the lesion is asymmetrical, then the radial lines must be segmental and this is a clue to malignancy, either melanoma, pBCC, or pSCC in situ.

In melanoma, the radial lines will be connected to either lines reticular or to a pigmented structureless area, or pigmented clods, as heavily pigmented as the radial lines.

In BCC the radial lines will often converge together, and this convergence may or may not be to a central clod, a dot, or a line. Radial lines, converging to a central point within a lesion, rather than at the periphery are highly specific for BCC. Also in BCC in contrast to melanoma, the radial lines may project from a hypopigmented area.

In pigmented Bowen's disease, radial lines peripheral segmental are usually comprised of dots in linear arrangement.

THE PATTERN OF LINES CURVED

A lesion with one pattern, lines curved, or a lesion with more than one pattern but with a primary pattern of lines curved will be restricted to the *melanocytic and benign keratinocytic* categories.

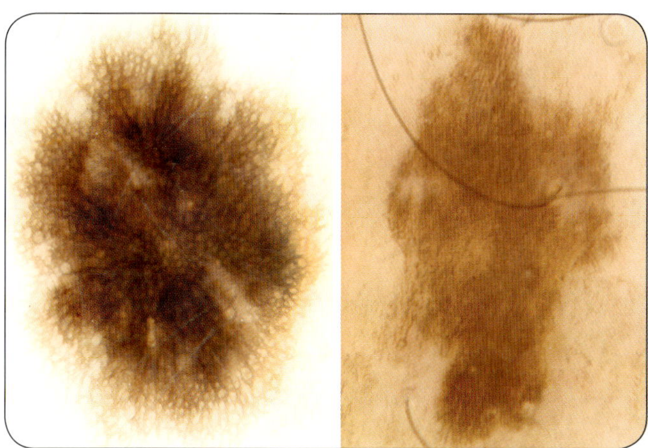

Fig. 12.12: The lesion on the left has one pattern lines reticular and one color brown. The gradual (nonabrupt) border points to a diagnosis of Clark nevus. The lesion on the right has one pattern lines curved and with an abrupt border this is most consistent with the diagnosis of solar lentigo.

A lesion with one pattern, lines curved can be either a solar lentigo or a seborrheic keratosis, and these can be distinguished according to specific clues as described above.

A primary pattern of lines curved, combined with a secondary pattern, can be combined with any of the other patterns, and if it has only one color brown, it is also likely to be a solar lentigo or a seborrheic keratosis whether symmetrical or not. If any other colors of melanin are present, a careful search for clues to melanoma is necessary before making a diagnosis of either seborrheic keratosis or lichen planus like keratosis (LPLK) (Figs. 12.12 and 12.13).

THE PATTERN OF PSEUDOPODS

A lesion with a pattern of pseudopods will always have this pattern in combination with another pattern and its diagnosis is restricted to the *melanocytic category* only. This is the most specific of all patterns.

A pattern of pseudopods, which can only occur peripherally, will occur in combination with a central pattern, which may be structureless, less often clods, and rarely lines reticular. In all cases, the differential diagnosis includes melanoma and Reed or, rarely, Spitz nevus.

The dermoscopic description should be independent of factors such as age but such factors are relevant to treatment decisions. After puberty all such lesions, whether symmetrical or not, should be excised (Fig. 12.14).

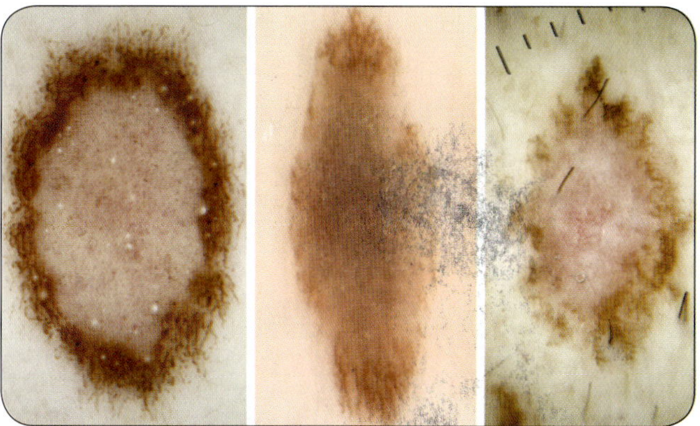

Fig. 12.13: Each of these three lesions has a pattern of lines peripherally combined in the lesions in the left and right with a central structureless area and in the lesion in the middle with a central pattern of clods. The lesion on the left is symmetrical and has the clue of white dots to support a diagnosis of congenital nevus. The lesion in the middle is also symmetrical, and the pattern of peripheral lines combined with central clods is also consistent with congenital nevus. The fact that the lines at one end are branched and at the other end curved (or as the clinician thought radial) leads to excision but in retrospect this variation was not consistent with the chaotic behavior of malignant tissue. The lesion on the right is asymmetrical, the central pink structureless area extending to the periphery on one side but not the other. In addition to the clue of an eccentric structureless area (not skin colored), there is the clue of lines radial segmental at the upper border of the dermoscopic image. The asymmetry of this lesion, although it has a central structureless area and a peripheral pattern of lines like the other two lesions, is due to a degree of disorganization, which is quite consistent with the chaotic behavior of malignant tissue. It was an invasive melanoma.

THE PATTERN OF CIRCLES

A lesion with one pattern, circles, or a lesion with more than one pattern but with a primary pattern of circles, in which the circles are one of the colors of melanin and that is not a *DF*, will be restricted to the *melanocytic, benign keratinocytic, and SCC* categories.

A pattern of circles pigmented by melanin can be caused by either pigment in follicular epithelium or, alternatively, by basal hyperpigmentation in the presence of acanthosis that causes the individual units of the rete-ridge reticular pattern to be separated from each other and appear as circles.

A pattern of pigmented circles only, which define follicles on the head or neck, is a significant clue to melanoma regardless of color,[13] the differential diagnosis being solar lentigo if they are brown and pSCC in situ and LPLK if they are gray. Biopsy may be necessary to resolve the diagnosis. Unlike a pattern of pigmented *circles* on facial skin, the pattern of structureless pigment on facial skin *interrupted*

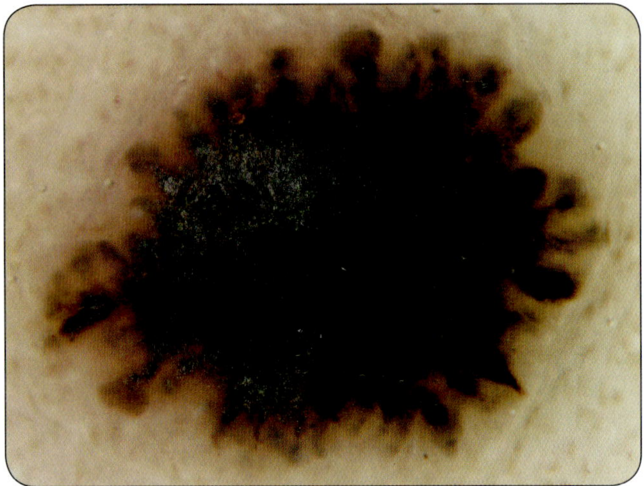

Fig. 12.14: This lesion on the forearm of a 9-year-old child has a peripheral circumferential pattern of lines radial and pseudopods combined symmetrically with a pattern of clods of equally dark pigmentation. When radial lines and pseudopods are combined in a concentric pattern, they are regarded as one pattern, defaulting to the more specific structure of pseudopods. The differential diagnosis includes Reed nevus and melanoma. Histology confirmed this as a Reed nevus, which was the expected diagnosis in a child.

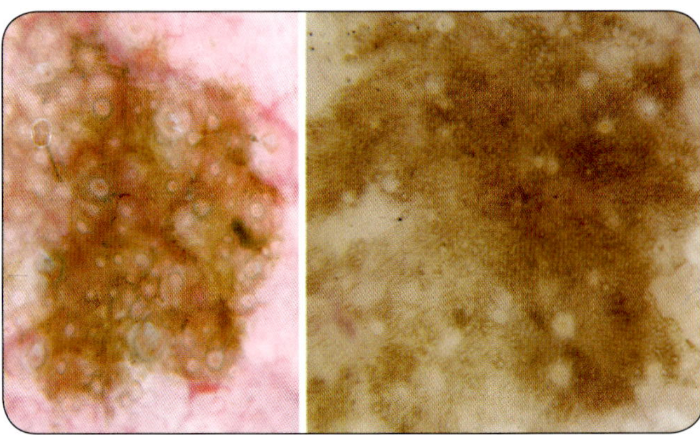

Fig. 12.15: Both of these pigmented lesions are located on facial skin so as predicted, the pigment is interrupted by follicular openings. On the left, a pattern of gray circles is a compelling clue to melanoma while on the right a pattern of curved lines interrupted by follicular openings is simply assessed as one pattern lines curved, one color brown with a sharply demarcated scalloped border as an additional clue to solar lentigo. Follicular opening does not rate as either a pattern or a clue and, unless defined by a circular line, they should be ignored.

by follicular openings has no diagnostic significance at all apart from being a clue that the lesion is on facial skin.

Although pigmented circles defining follicles are occasionally seen in melanomas on the trunk and extremities, they are not regarded as a clue to melanoma at these locations as they commonly occur in benign lesions.

A pattern of pigmented circles only that do not surround follicles should be regarded in the same way as reticular lines and as they caused by acanthosis they are a compelling clue to seborrheic keratosis.

A primary pattern of pigmented circles can be combined symmetrically as a peripheral pattern with a central structureless or polarizing-specific white-line pattern in a DF. For practical purposes there are no other symmetrical combinations of a pattern of circles with clod, dot, or structureless patterns.

For asymmetrical patterns that include a primary pattern of pigmented circles defining follicles, on the head or neck, the diagnosis of melanoma must be very strongly suspected.[13] Such a pattern on the body should be assessed according to previously defined clues to melanoma, which means the pigmented circles would be regarded as a clue to melanoma only if they were gray.

Asymmetrical patterns with a primary pattern of pigmented circles that do *not* define follicles should be assessed as if the circles were reticular lines.

A pattern of white circles (whiter than the surrounding skin), combined symmetrically or asymmetrically with a pattern of gray dots on the head or neck, is a clue to pAK or pSCC in situ. These dots may be randomly distributed between the white circles or they may surround them as gray circles, concentrically located around the white circles (Figs. 12.15 and 12.16).

THE PATTERN OF CLODS

A lesion with one pattern clods or a lesion with more than one pattern but with a primary pattern of clods and which is not a *DF* will be restricted to the *melanocytic, benign keratinocytic, and BCC* categories.

In the case of one pattern clods, the differential diagnosis is sorted according to the color of the clods as detailed in Figure 12.5.

The differential diagnosis, if there is a single color, includes BCC if the color is orange (caused by ulceration and serum) or blue; congenital nevus, if they are skin colored or brown; seborrheic keratosis, if they are skin colored, yellow, orange, or white; hemangioma if they are red, purple, or black; and blood, if they are red or black.

If there is more than one color with melanin pigment dominant and the colors being symmetrically combined, the differential diagnosis includes congenital and Spitz nevi. If the colors are combined asymmetrically, then melanoma and BCC must be distinguished by specific clues. Clues to melanoma have been described. Specific clues

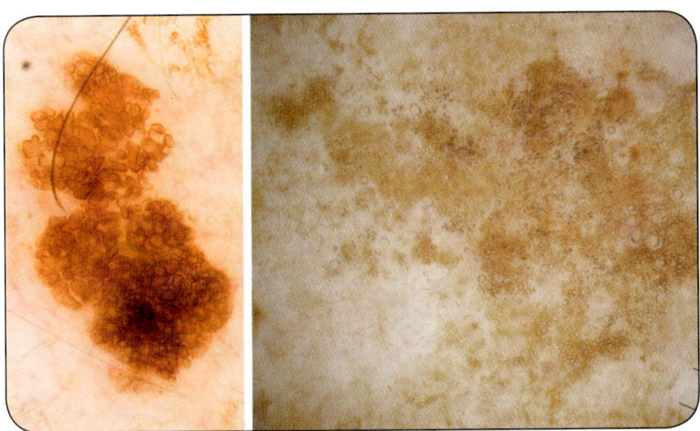

Fig. 12.16: Both of these lesions on the torso contain pigmented circles. The lesion on the left consists of one pattern circles (they are not clods because the center is lightly pigmented compared to the periphery), one color brown (the degree of color variation is not significant and certainly not consistent with the disorganized behavior expected of malignant tissue). The circles are not related to follicles and are caused by basal hyperpigmentation of acanthotic rete ridges. Such a lesion is predictably a seborrheic keratosis and the sharply demarcated border is an additional clue to that diagnosis. The lesion on the right has a pattern of short curved lines interrupted by a few pigmented circles that are related to follicles. Although there is some gray color and the lesion is not perfectly symmetrical the diagnosis of seborrheic keratosis was made with confidence due to the very regular pattern of the short curved lines. The lesion also had a palpably rough surface texture uniformly over its surface as an additional clue to seborrheic keratosis.

to BCC are described at the end of this section on the pattern of clods.

If there is more than one color, with nonmelanin pigment dominant, the lesion may be an ulcerated BCC (orange prominent), a seborrheic keratosis (yellow, white, or orange prominent), or a hemangioma/vascular malformation (red or purple prominent) (Figs. 12.17 and 12.18).

A primary pattern of clods, combined with a secondary pattern (dots or structureless), can be symmetrical or asymmetrical and the differential diagnoses are shown in Figure 12.6.

For practical purposes the only symmetrical patterns with a primary pattern of clods will have brown clods peripherally located around a central structureless area. A skin-colored central structureless area points to the diagnosis of congenital nevus or Spitz nevus; a dark brown or black central structureless area is consistent with the diagnosis of Clark nevus or Spitz nevus; and a blue structureless center makes combined congenital nevus more likely than the differential diagnosis of Spitz nevus. Although peripheral clods are expected in a growing nevus, such a pattern should raise suspicion at the mature age when nevi are not expected to either appear as new lesions or grow (Fig. 12.19).[11]

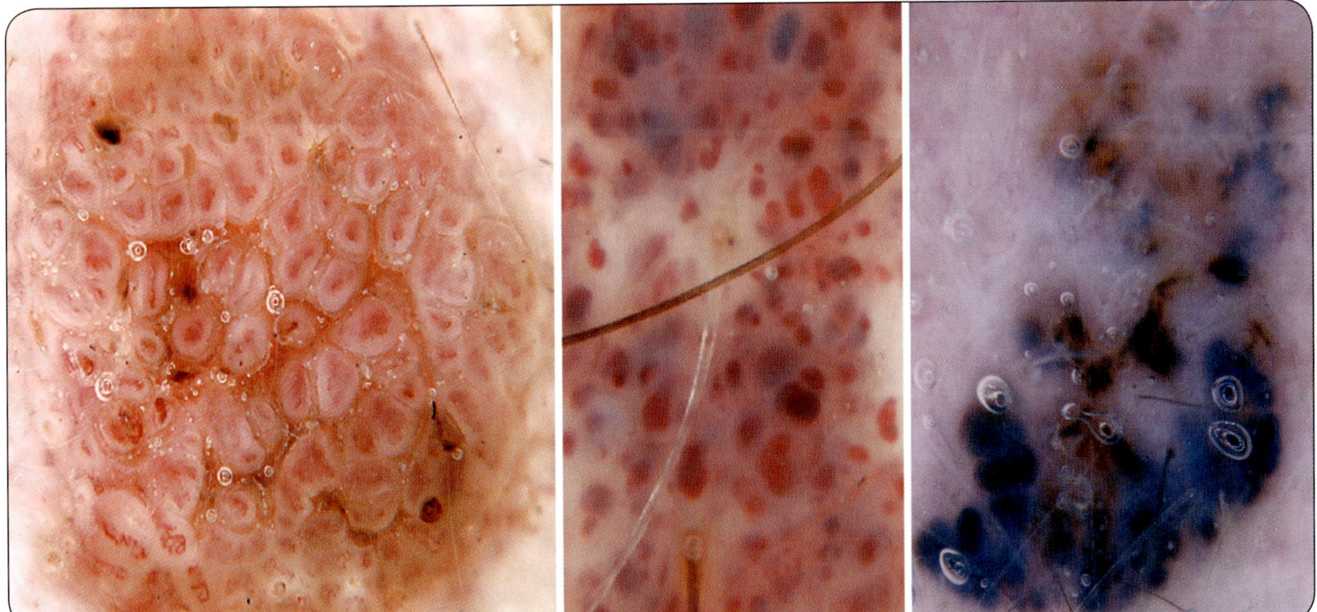

Fig. 12.17: All these three lesions have one pattern clods. On the left, a pattern of skin-colored clods with centered vessels is consistent with either a seborrheic keratosis or congenital nevus. In the center, a pattern of red and purple clods, with no linear vessels, is consistent with a hemangioma. On the right, a pattern of blue clods points confidently to the diagnosis of basal cell carcinoma.

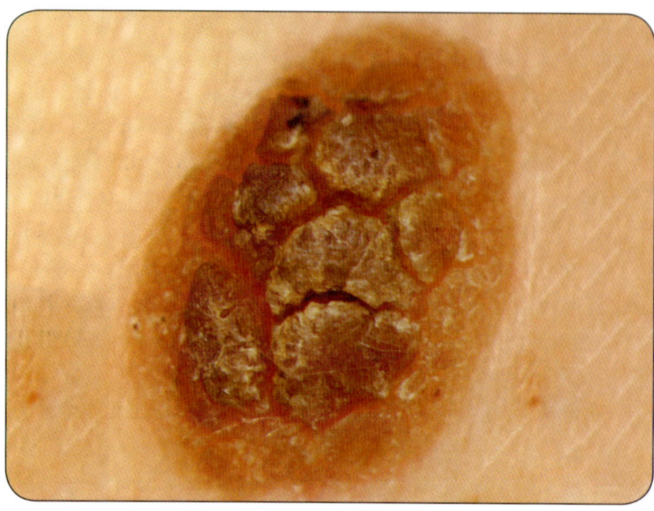
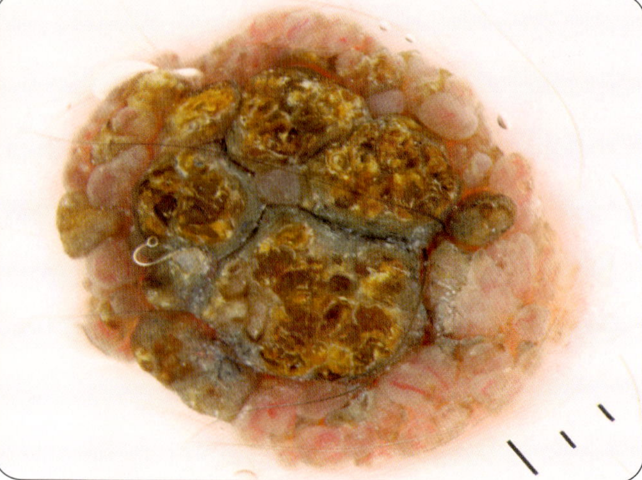

Fig. 12.18: The lesion on the left has a pattern of orange keratin clods only, this being compelling evidence for seborrheic keratosis. The lesion on the right also has a pattern of clods only, including a symmetrical combination of both central keratin clods (both orange and gray) and peripheral skin-colored clods. Terminal hair is a clue that this is in fact a congenital nevus. It had been present since childhood.

If a pattern of clods is combined asymmetrically with a secondary pattern of dots or structureless, the differential diagnosis is sorted according to whether melanin or non-melanin pigments are present. If the pigment is not melanin, the differential includes seborrheic keratosis (white, yellow, or orange), BCC (orange), hemangioma (red and/or purple), and melanoma, primary or metastatic (red and/or purple). If the pigment is melanin and there is one color brown, the prediction will be nevus, congenital or Spitz. In the case that there is more than one color, the differential diagnosis includes melanoma, BCC, and seborrheic keratosis, and these alternatives should be sorted according to specific clues, discussed in detail above for melanoma and seborrheic keratosis and in the following section for BCC.

CLUES TO BCC

Clues to BCC include lack of reticular lines plus one or more of ulceration, blue clods, radial lines (as described in the above section for a primary pattern of lines radial), and monomorphous serpentine or serpentine branched vessels. Polarizing-specific white lines can support the diagnosis of both BCC and melanoma but they are more frequently encountered in BCC (Fig. 12.20).

THE PATTERN OF DOTS

As dots are the least specific pattern apart from the structureless pattern, a lesion with one pattern, dots, or a lesion with a pattern of dots combined with a structureless pattern can fall into any of the defined categories.

A solo pattern of dots can only be sorted on the basis of color. A pattern of brown dots may be seen in a Clark nevus or pSCC in situ. A pattern of gray dots may occur in an LPLK, pAK, pSCC in situ, or a melanoma, and on the face a melanoma may have only one pattern and one color—in other words, it may be symmetrical. A further clue to pSCC in situ is that the dots may be in a linear arrangement.

A pattern of dots combined with the only possible secondary pattern, structureless, is also sorted according to the color of the dots. If the dots are brown, then solar lentigo and congenital nevus are added to the differential diagnoses of Clark nevus and pSCC in situ. If the dots are gray, the options are the same as for a solo pattern of gray dots with the addition of BCC. If there are blue dots, the likely diagnosis is BCC. The occurrence of black dots is a clue to melanoma, if they are peripheral, with a differential diagnosis of Clark nevus (Fig. 12.21).[13]

CLUES TO PIGMENTED SCC IN SITU

In a study of 52 consecutive cases of pSCC in situ (pigmented Bowen's disease), the lesions were typified by the absence of a pattern of reticular lines and by the presence of a pattern of dots and/or structureless zones.[14] A single pattern was present in 53.8% with 48.1% being only structureless. Hypopigmented (pink, skin colored, or white) structureless areas were present in 67.3%. The presence of

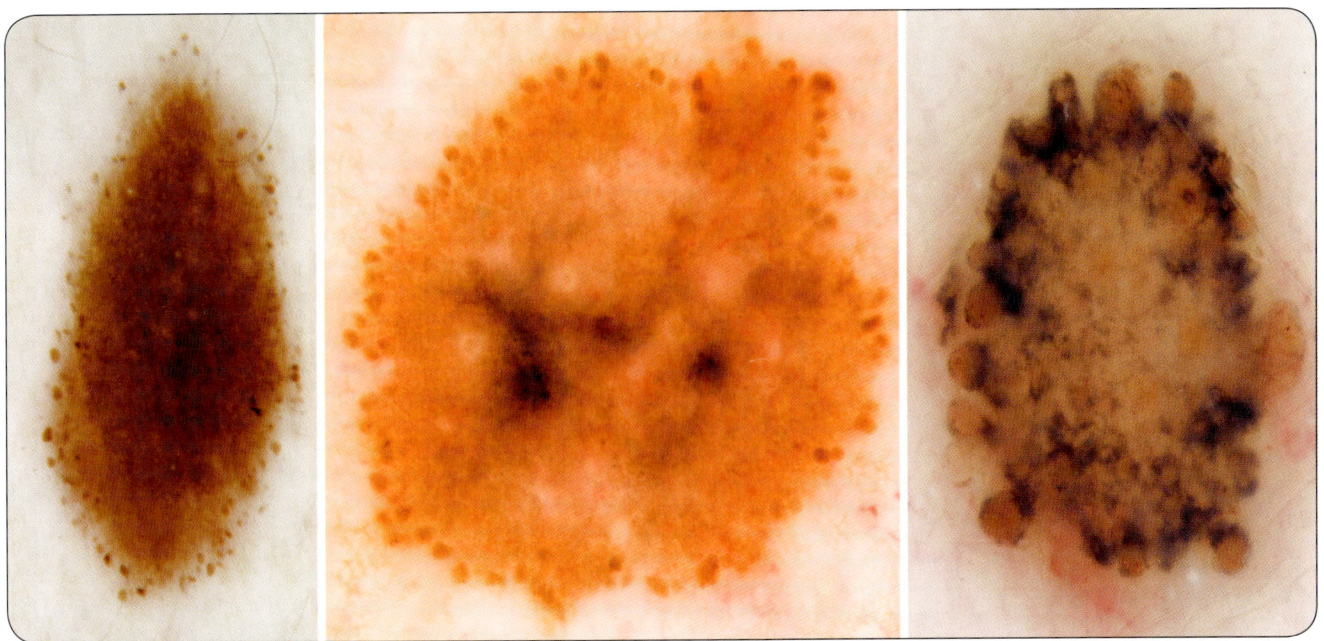

Fig. 12.19: On the left, a symmetrical lesion with a central pattern of reticular lines and peripheral pattern of clods (or dots depending on perception), on a 30-year-old man is predictably a growing Clark nevus. The middle lesion may appear similar but the central structureless area has an asymmetrical distribution of colors and one of these colors, gray, is a clue to melanoma. In this case, on the chest of a 50-year-old man the peripheral clods or dots are not a clue to a growing nevus but to a growing melanoma in situ. Similarly, the lesion on the right, on the chest of a 60-year-old lady, with peripheral clods surrounding a structureless center is not a nevus but is in fact a nodular melanoma, 3 mm in diameter and 1 mm thick.

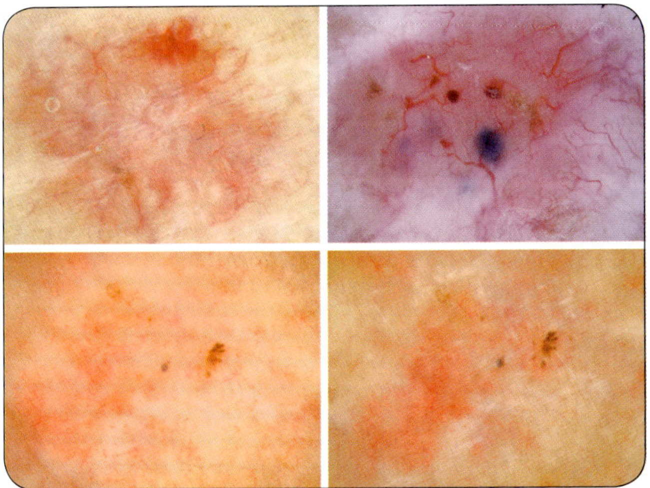

Fig. 12.20: Clues to basal cell carcinoma (BCC) include the absence of reticular lines and ulceration, polarizing-specific white lines, and linear serpentine vessels (upper left: a small cluster of gray dots in the lower left of the lesion makes this BCC pigmented for the purpose of analysis); blue clods; and linear serpentine vessels in a branched arrangement with branches projecting from progressively thinner branches (upper right); lines radial segmental converging that originate from a hypopigmented structureless area (lower left) with the addition of polarizing-specific white lines in the image lower right of the same lesion taken with the dermatoscope in polarizing mode.

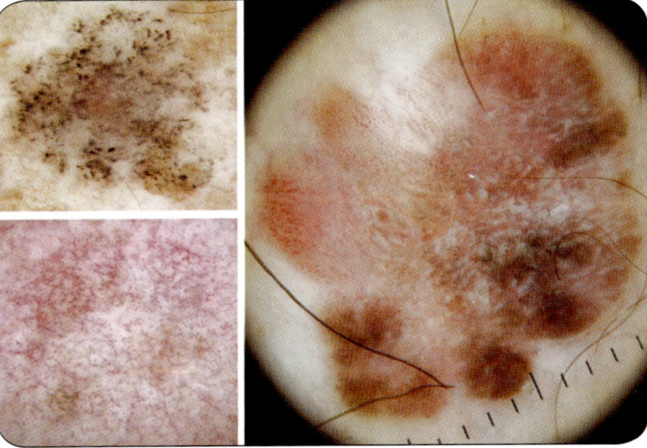

Fig. 12.21: Both lesions on the left have on pattern dots and one color gray. The upper lesion is located on the back and this pattern on the torso or limbs is consistent with lichen planus like keratosis, which this was. The lower lesion is on the face; at this location any lesion with dermoscopic gray will have melanoma in the differential diagnosis. This lesion was an in situ melanoma. The lesion on the right has a pattern of dots (left side of the image) combined asymmetrically with a structureless pattern on the right side. Red dots (not on their own constituting a pattern in revised pattern analysis) merge into brown dots. The linear arrangement of the dots was consistent with the confirmed diagnosis of squamous cell carcinoma in situ.

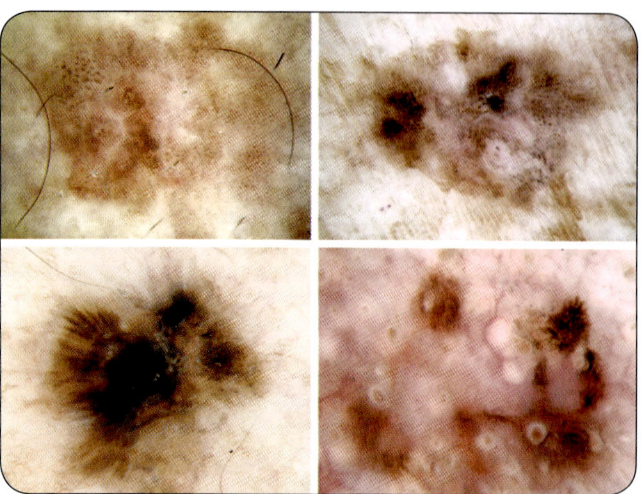

Fig. 12.22: Four cases of pigmented squamous cell carcinoma (SCC) in situ: a pattern of brown dots in linear arrangement combined asymmetrically with a structureless area in the lower left of the lesion (upper left); a pattern of brown dots in linear arrangement combined asymmetrically with a structureless area in the lower half of the lesion (upper right); a pattern of lines radial segmental composed of dots in linear arrangement combined asymmetrically with a structureless area, partly hyperpigmented and partly hypopigmented (lower left); a structureless pigmented lesion on the face with the clue of lines radial segmental on the upper right of the lesion and the additional clues to SCC in situ on the face, of white circles, whiter than surrounding skin (lower right).

brown or gray dots in a linear arrangement was present in 21.2% and the presence of a linear arrangement of coiled vessels was present in 11.5% (Fig. 12.22).

THE STRUCTURELESS PATTERN

A structureless pattern is the least specific of all, and as with a pattern of dots; any lesion with a structureless-only pattern can fall into any of the defined categories. The possibilities are numerous and they can only be sorted by colors and the arrangement of these colors, plus the clues seen due to pigmented structures, which, although not sufficient to form a pattern, may provide valuable clues. In lightly pigmented structureless lesions, vessels may be seen and, although they do not contribute to any pattern of pigmented structures, these vessels may provide clues to the diagnosis. For example, a structureless lesion may display a polymorphic pattern of vessels including a dot pattern as a clue to the diagnosis of melanoma. Small fragments of reticular lines, if also present, could add additional weight to this evidence.

The differential diagnoses of structureless lesions according to color are shown in Figure 12.23.

A structureless pattern with one color black is usually caused by an old hemorrhage into or onto the skin, or thrombosis of a hemangioma, and structureless red is most consistent with a fresh hemorrhage into the stratum corneum. Very rarely a Clark nevus, a Reed nevus, or a melanoma can be structureless and black. A structureless blue lesion is consistent with a blue nevus unless there is a history that raises the likelihood of melanoma metastases. A structureless brown lesion can be an ephelis, solar lentigo, or pSCC in situ.

A structureless pattern with more than one color is sorted according to whether the dominant pigment is melanin or not. If white, yellow, or orange pigment is dominant, the possibilities include seborrheic keratosis, BCC, and amelanotic melanoma. If red color dominates then the likely diagnosis is a fresh hemorrhage in the stratum corneum. If melanin pigment is dominant and the colors are combined symmetrically, then a diagnosis of nevus is expected (congenital, congenital combined, blue, Clark, Spitz, or Reed). If melanin pigment is dominant and the colors are combined asymmetrically, then the differential diagnosis includes melanoma, primary, or metastatic and pSCC in situ (Fig. 12.24).[15]

CHAOS AND CLUES: A DECISION ALGORITHM FOR PIGMENTED LESIONS BASED ON REVISED PATTERN ANALYSIS

Revised pattern analysis is designed to lead to a provisional diagnosis in a logical stepwise process. Chaos and clues is an algorithmic method that uses pattern analysis to guide the clinician in a stepwise process to the decision about whether a biopsy is indicated.[8]

The flowchart for the chaos and clues algorithm is shown in Figure 12.25.

Chaos

Chaos is defined as the presence of dermoscopic asymmetry of pattern and/or color and it is assessed by the method described for RPA. Although natural laws (gravity, electrical and magnetic fields, surface tension, and feedback mechanisms) favor symmetry, malignant tissue defies natural laws and this is the basis for both dermatopathological and dermoscopic chaos in malignant tissue.[8] Another feature that is an additional property of many malignant chaotic lesions is chaos of border abruptness [chaos of border abruptness was first recognized and described by Francis Drugge, the 12-year-old son of a dermatologist, Rhett Drugge (Stanford, CT, USA)]. Although

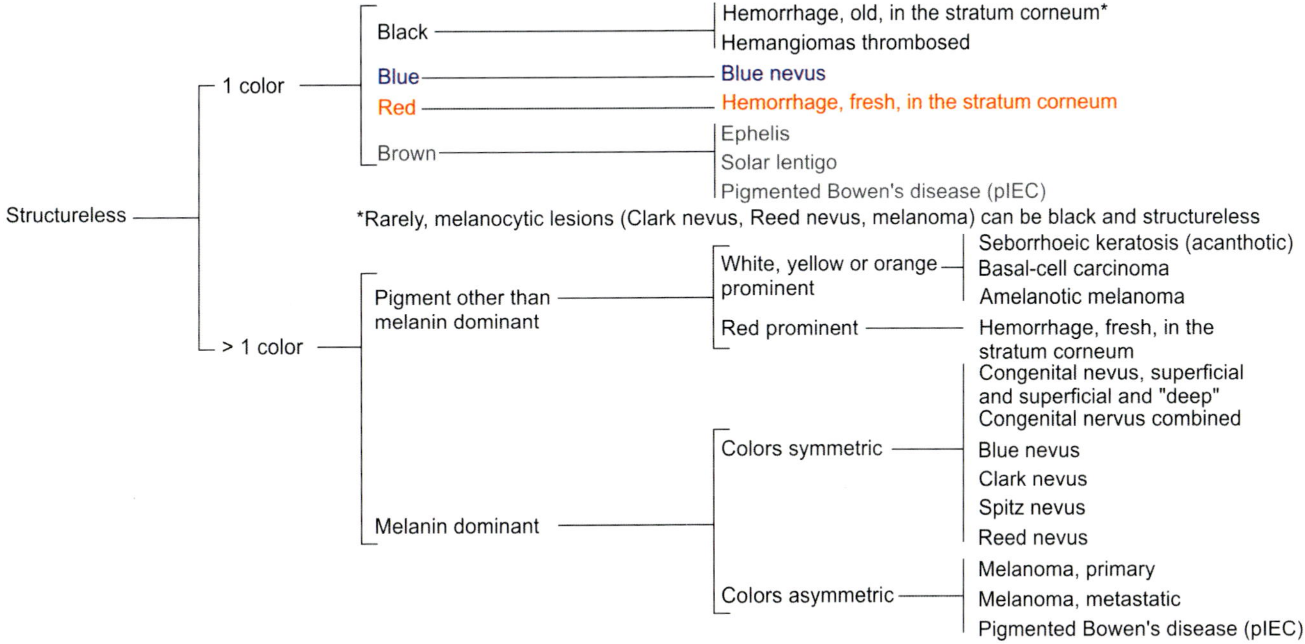

Fig. 12.23: The stepwise analysis of clues for pigmented lesions with one pattern structureless.

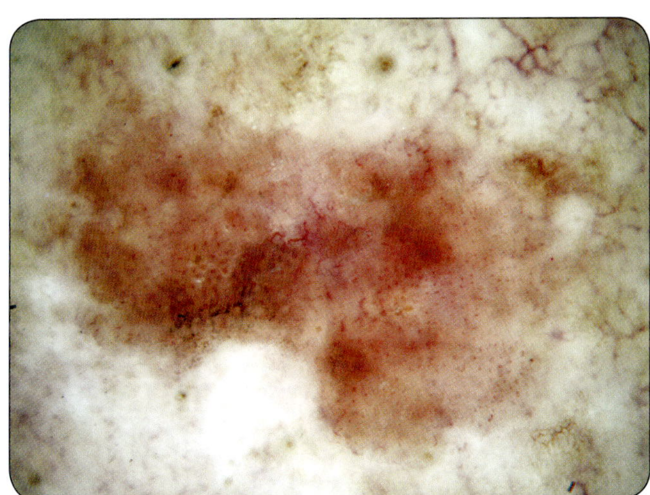

Fig. 12.24: This lightly pigmented lesion has one pattern structureless, the small area of gray dots constituting a clue to malignancy although being insufficient for a pattern. In addition to the clues of asymmetry of color (brown, gray, pink, and white), this lesion has polymorphous vessels including patterns of both linear (serpentine) and dot vessels, pointing correctly to the diagnosis of melanoma. Note the feature of peripheral structureless brown, this being reported as a clue to hypopigmented melanoma. It should be noted that a significant proportion of melanomas, like this one, do not have any reticular lines.

border abruptness is assessed in the ABCD method of dermatoscopy, this is given most significance in that method when the total border is abrupt. The ABCD method would therefore allocate the highest score for border abruptness to an ink-spot lentigo or solar lentigo (*see* Fig. 12.12, right). Chaos of border abruptness is seen when parts of the border are abrupt and parts gradual (see all of the melanomas in Figure 12.9, top row) (Fig. 12.26).

Clues

1. *Gray or blue structures* (including structureless): This clue, in a chaotic lesion, applies to both melanocytic and nonmelanocytic malignancies. Gray color is the most sensitive clue to malignancy and is seen in most in situ melanomas and many pBCC and pSCC; *see* Figure 12.2; Figure 12.9, upper left and upper right; Figure 12.10 lower images, Figure 12.11 lower image, Figure 12.15 left image, Figure 12.17 right image, Figure 12.19 middle and right images, Figure 12.20, Figure 12.21 right side, and Figure 12.24. Blue color correlates with pigment in the deep dermis, most commonly in melanocytes or nests of BCC.
2. *An eccentric structureless area* must cover a sufficient portion of the lesion to form a pattern; it must be contrasted to a structured pattern that is also within the lesion and it must be a color other than skin colored. If colored with the colors of melanin, it is produced by the chaotic behavior of malignant melanocytes; if pink, it is caused by increased blood flow; and if white, it may correlate with fibrosis after regression. This clue also applies to both melanocytic and nonmelanocytic

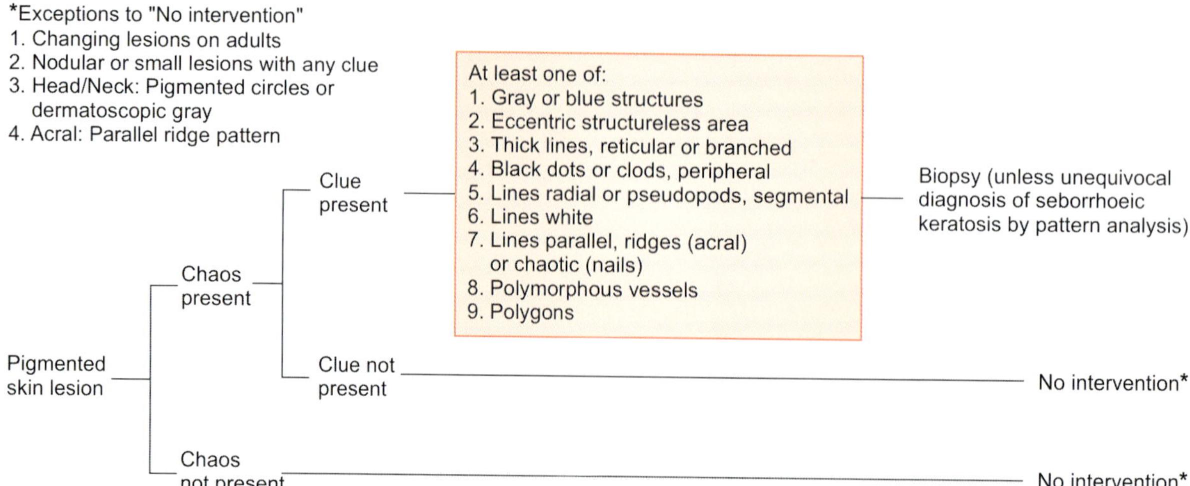

Fig. 12.25: The chaos and clues algorithm. Pigmented lesions are first assessed for the presence of chaos (defined as dermoscopic asymmetry of pattern and/or color) and if chaos is present they are examined or any one or more of nine clues to malignancy. If a clue is present, an adequate biopsy is considered unless an unequivocal diagnosis of seborrheic keratosis can be made by pattern analysis. There are four exceptions in which biopsy is considered even for nonchaotic lesions: any changing lesion on an adult, a nodular or a small (<6 mm) lesion which has any clue to malignancy, any lesion on the head or neck with either pigmented circles or dermoscopic gray color and any acral lesion with a parallel ridge pattern.

malignancies; *see* Figure 12.2, Figure 12.9 upper row, Figure 12.13 right, Figure 12.21 right, Figure 12.22 upper row and bottom left.

3. *Thick lines reticular* are defined when the lines are thicker than the holes that they surround and they correlate with rete ridges, which are widened by pigment-laden malignant melanocytes. This clue is specific to melanoma as the presence of reticular lines rules out the diagnosis of BCC or SCC; *see* Figure 12.9 upper middle.
4. *Black dots and clods, peripheral,* correlate with pigmented pagetoid melanocytes and nests of melanocytes in melanomas and therefore this clue should be specific to melanomas. In reality, because dots are common in both pBCC and pSCC in situ, and because gray may be perceived as black, this clue can also be seen in those lesions. The reason for the designation that they be peripherally located is because central black dots can be seen centrally in nevi that have been traumatized, correlating with pigment in ascending keratinocytes. Pagetoid spread can occur anywhere in a melanoma, so when black dots or clods are seen peripherally they are regarded as a clue to malignancy.
5. *Lines radial or pseudopods segmental* are clues to malignancy, pseudopods being specific to melanoma and lines radial segmental being found in all three pigmented malignancies. In melanomas, these structures correlate with fascicles of pigmented melanocytes extending from the periphery of a lesion and they signify growth. In melanomas, they should be distributed asymmetrically and should extend from reticular lines, clods, or structureless areas of equivalent pigmentation to the radial lines or pseudopods (*see* Fig. 12.9 bottom left and Fig. 12.26 bottom right). This can distinguish them from the radial lines seen on BCCs, which may project from hypopigmented structureless areas (*see* Fig. 12.20 bottom row). Lines radial segmental are also seen in pSCC in situ and they are usually created by dots in a linear arrangement (*see* Fig. 12.22 upper right and lower row).
6. *White lines* must be whiter than normal surrounding skin and they may be polarizing-specific, or alternatively, white lines that are seen with both modalities. Polarizing-specific white lines are shiny white lines orientated perpendicularly to each other but not crossing. They are only seen with polarizing dermatoscopy but they may correlate with reticular white lines seen with nonpolarized dermatoscopy. Polarizing-specific white lines can be seen very commonly in BCC (pigmented or nonpigmented) and they are not unusual in melanoma (pigmented or nonpigmented). They are only rarely seen in pSCC in situ. They are also commonly seen in both DF and Spitz nevi but their

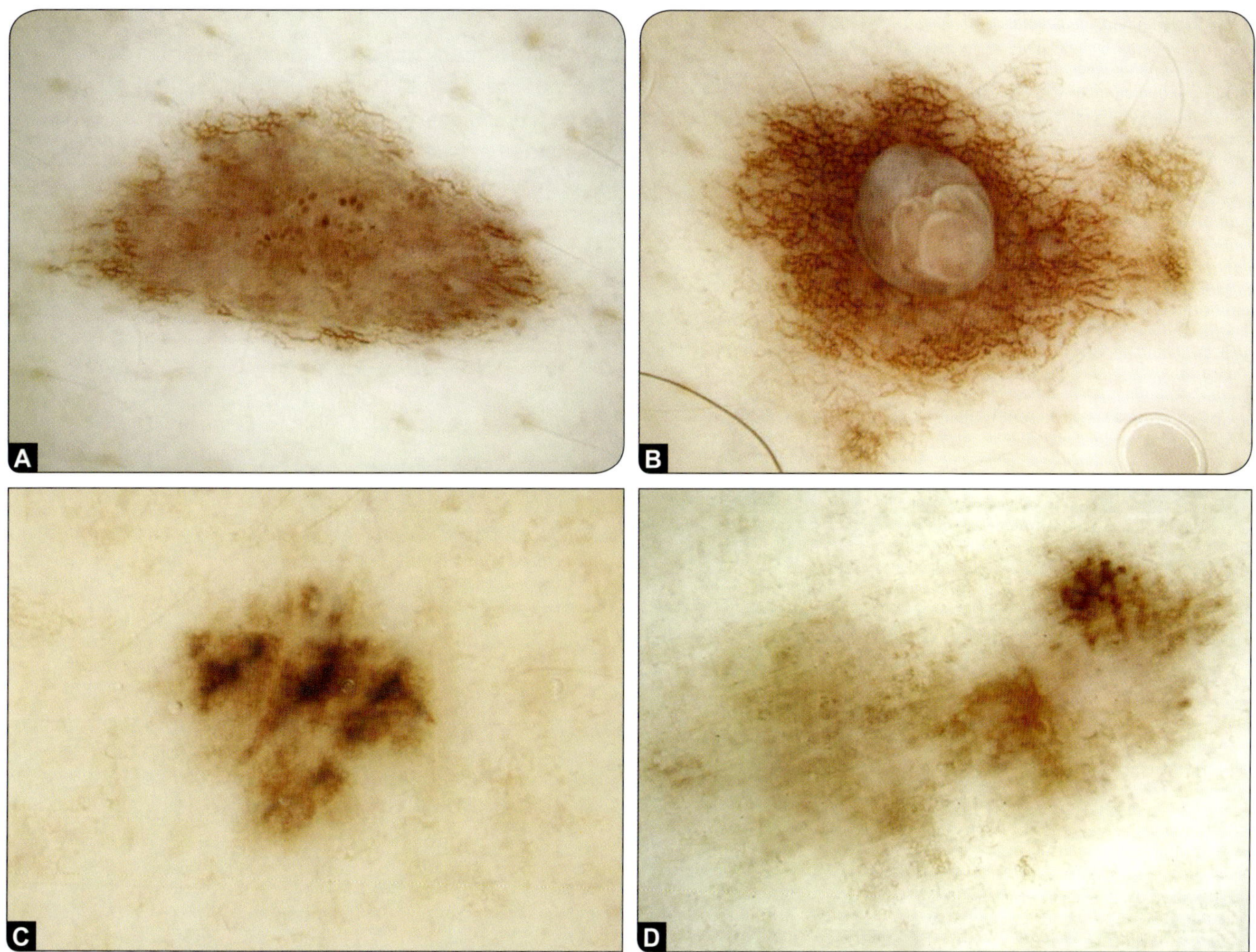

Figs. 12.26A to D: Assessment for the presence of chaos of four different lesions on the same patient: (A) a concentric nonchaotic pattern with clods centrally surrounded by a structureless area that is surrounded by a pattern of lines; (B) a concentric nonchaotic pattern with skin-colored clods centrally and reticular lines peripherally. The shape of the lesion is irrelevant; (C) a nonchaotic structureless pattern, hyperpigmented centrally with relatively hypopigmented areas at the upper and lower extremities; (D) a chaotic lesion, in this case by all parameters—pattern, color, and border abruptness. Lesions A to C have not been excised but they have the morphology of congenital nevi. Lesion D, being chaotic and with the clue of pseudopods, was a melanoma in situ.

presence is not expected in any other type of nevus (unless traumatized) or in seborrheic keratoses.

7. *Polymorphous vessels* are a clue to both melanomas and pBCC but not to pSCC in situ. Pigmented BCC often has a monomorphous pattern of serpentine or serpentine branched vessels but it may have a pattern of polymorphous linear vessels, especially on the lower limb. A pattern of dot vessels is not expected in pBCC but ulceration, commonly present in BCC, and associated keratinization may produce polymorphous vessels including looped vessels in radial arrangement and even dot vessels. In melanomas, polymorphous vessels may include various types of linear vessels in raised portions, and a pattern of dot vessel as well as any pattern of linear vessel in macular portions. Generally, other clues apart from polymorphous vessels (pigment clues and/or white lines) are expected in a melanoma and the vessel clues are then useful in differentiating melanoma from pBCC and pSCC in situ. Pigmented SCC in situ is expected to have a monomorphous pattern of coiled vessels, which may resolve as dots depending on visual acuity.
8. *Polygons* are defined as geometric polygonal shapes, complete or incomplete, bounded by straight lines, or by a straight pigment interface, meeting at angles and larger than the holes caused by individual follicles and

larger by far than the holes bounded by reticular lines. This clue, in a chaotic lesion, is not only a valuable clue to melanoma but may also rarely be seen in pBCC.

9. *Lines parallel on the ridges (acral) or lines parallel chaotic on the nails* are a clue to melanoma, specifically, on acral skin or in nail matrix, respectively. This is the only one of the listed clues to malignancy that is specific to a particular anatomical site. It is important to remember that the longer an acral or nail-matrix melanoma remains untreated; the more likely it is to develop any of the other clues to melanoma. Melanoma may also arise in an acral nevus in which case any of the other eight clues will override a benign parallel furrow pattern, which may be present; *see* Figure 12.11 upper right and lower image.

EXCEPTIONS

Chaos and clues was tested on a consecutive series of pigmented lesions, the majority of melanomas in the series being in situ, and was found to have a diagnostic sensitivity of 90.6% (BCC: 98.5%, SCC: 86.5%, and melanoma: 79.3%) with a specificity of 62.7% for the diagnosis of malignancy, of any type.[7] In an attempt to move the sensitivity closer to 100% the following exceptions are included, to select lesions for biopsy, even if not chaotic:

1. Any changing lesion on an adult. This includes a lesion with a history of change, lesions with monitored change, and lesions with dermoscopic clues to change such as the presence of peripheral clods (*see* Fig. 12.19 middle and right).
2. A nodular or small lesion that has any of the clues to malignancy. We define small, arbitrarily, as <6 mm in diameter, this being the size cited in the clinical ABCD method of dermatoscopy (*see* Fig. 12.19 right: this 3-mm diameter nodular melanoma was arguably symmetrical but in addition to peripheral clods as a dermoscopic clue to change, it had the clue of gray color).
3. Any lesion on the head or neck with pigmented circles and/or any dermoscopic gray. This clue acknowledges the fact that young melanomas at these locations, possibly related to a physical barrier effect of numerous follicles, may be symmetrical (*see* Fig. 12.15 left).
4. Any lesion on acral skin with a parallel ridge pattern. This clue acknowledges the fact that young melanomas at these locations, possibly related to a physical barrier effect of numerous eccrine ducts, may be symmetrical (*see* Fig. 12.11 upper right).

Chaos and clues are not a method designed for robots and it should not be regarded as an ultimate method, set in stone. It has been designed as a useful tool, avoiding tedious mathematical calculations, unburdened by a language of innumerable poorly defined metaphorical terms carrying preconceived diagnostic implications, and suitable for seamless integration into routine practice. Individuals are encouraged to use it as a framework on which they organize their accumulated experience as they individualize the method for their own style and practice.

REFERENCES

1. Kittler H. Dermatoscopy: Introduction of a new algorithmic method based on pattern analysis for diagnosis of pigmented skin lesions. Dermatol Pract Concept. 2007;13(1):3.
2. Kittler H, Rosendahl C, Cameron A, et al. Dermatoscopy. Austria: Facultas; 2011.
3. Pehamberger H, Steiner A, Wolff K. In vivo epiluminescence microscopy of pigmented skin lesions. I. Pattern analysis of pigmented skin lesions. J Am Acad Dermatol. 1987;17(4):571-83.
4. Argenziano G, Soyer HP, Chimenti S, et al. Dermoscopy of pigmented skin lesions: results of a consensus meeting via the Internet. J Am Acad Dermatol. 2003;48(5):679-93.
5. Marghoob AA, Braun R. Proposal for a revised 2-step algorithm for the classification of lesions of the skin using dermoscopy. Arch Dermatol. 2010;146(4):426-8.
6. Tschandl P, Rosendahl C, Kittler H. Accuracy of the first step of the dermoscopic 2-step algorithm for pigmented skin lesions. Dermatol Pract Concept. 2012;2(3):203a08.
7. Rosendahl C, Tschandl P, Cameron A, et al. Diagnostic accuracy of dermatoscopy for melanocytic and nonmelanocytic pigmented lesions. J Am Acad Dermatol. 2011;64(6):1068-73.
8. Rosendahl C, Cameron A, McColl I, et al. Dermatoscopy in routine practice—"chaos and clues." Aust Fam Physician. 2012;41(7):482-7.
9. Weismann K, Lorentzen HF. Dermoscopic color perspective. Arch Dermatol. 2006;142:1250.
10. Keir J. Dermoscopic features of cutaneous non-facial non-acral lentiginous growth pattern melanomas. Dermatol Pract Concept. 2014;4:77-82.
11. Rosendahl C, Hishon M, Cameron A, et al. Nodular melanoma: five consecutive cases in a general practice with polarized and non-polarized dermatoscopy and dermatopathology. Dermatol Pract Concept. 2014;4(2):15.
12. Cohen YK, Elpern DJ, Wolpowitz D, et al. Glowing in the dark: case report of a clue-poor melanoma unmasked by polarized dermatoscopy. Dermatol Pract Concept. 2014;4(1):14. [online] Available from http://dx.doi.org/10.5826/dpc.0401a14
13. Tschandl P, Rosendahl C, Kittler H. Dermatoscopy of flat pigmented facial lesions. J Eur Acad Dermatol Venereol. 2015;29(1):120-7.
14. Cameron A, Rosendahl C, Tschandl P, et al. Dermatoscopy of pigmented Bowen's disease. J Am Acad Dermatol. 2010;62(4):597-604.
15. Menzies SW, Kreusch J, Byth K, et al. Dermoscopic evaluation of amelanotic and hypomelanotic melanoma. Arch Dermatol. 2008;144(9):1120-7.

13

ENTOMODERMOSCOPY

Renato Marchiori Bakos

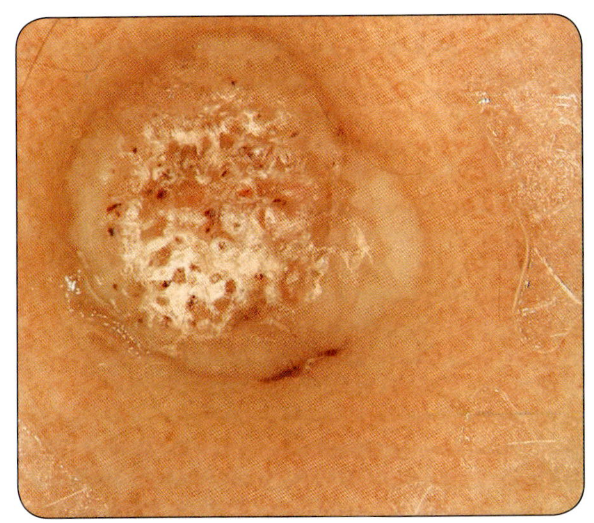

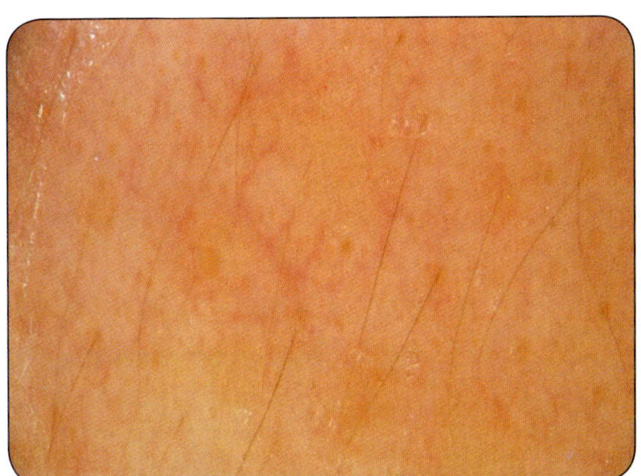

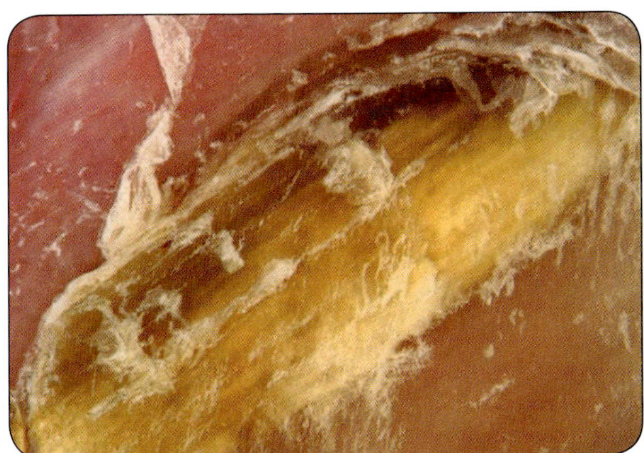

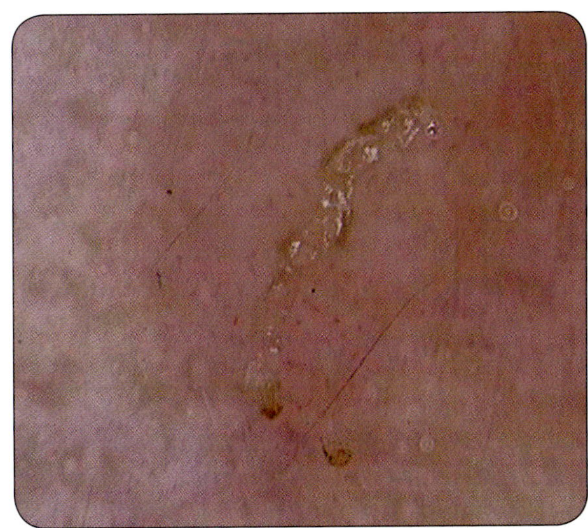

Entomology refers to the study of insects and their environment. Consequently, entomodermoscopy would lead to the description of dermoscopic aspects of insect-related diseases. Actually, the term involves not only the evaluation of insect reactions under dermoscopy but also of infectious diseases (viral and fungal) and also parasitic infestations. Clearly some of these skin conditions have a well- defined dermoscopic pattern, and eventually the offending agent might also be visualized.

Dermoscopy has been used for improving accuracy in the diagnosis of pigmented and nonpigmented skin tumors. Additionally, it has been proven to help in the daily dermatological practice when evaluating a sort of different clinical scenarios permitting the identification of infestation agents and of other infectious diseases.

Entomology refers to the study of insects and their environment. Consequently, entomodermoscopy would lead to the description of dermoscopic aspects of insect-related diseases. Actually, the term involves not only the evaluating of insect reactions under dermoscopy but also of infectious diseases (viral and fungal) and also parasitic infestations.[1,2]

Clearly some of these skin conditions have a well-defined dermoscopic pattern, and eventually the offending agent might also be visualized. The major descriptions of entomodermatoscopy will be mentioned below.

VIRAL INFECTIONS

Warts

Viral warts are benign skin lesions caused by *human papillomavirus* (HPV). Diagnosis is usually made in a clinical basis but dermoscopy might be helpful to reveal equivocal lesions. On dermoscopy they present as hyperkeratotic papules with homogeneously distributed dotted vessels some presenting with hemorrhages (Figs. 13.1A and B). Histopathological dotted vessels correspond to dilated capillaries on papillary dermis and some might be thrombosed leading to the hemorrhages.[2-4]

Common warts are more keratotic and present more frequently with hemorrhagic structures. In contrast, flat warts usually show the well-distributed dotted vessels (Fig. 13.2).[2] Vascular pattern of flat warts might be especially important to differentiate them from other micropapular eruptions on the face like acneiform and comedonic lesions or milia cysts. Plantar warts also present hemorrhagic dotted or linear vessels that allow us to rule out acral amelanotic melanoma or callus (Fig. 13.3).[3] Genital warts also demonstrate a similar vascular pattern. The occurrence of hyperkeratotic papules with dotted vessels on the genital area is highly suspicious of HPV infection and helps the clinician to differentiate them from pearly penile papules.[1]

Finally, dermoscopy is extremely important to monitor warts' treatment. Some series of patients demonstrated that naked eye evaluation was less accurate to define persistent warts after cryotherapy than dermoscopy; therefore, it should be used to optimize therapies.[5]

Molluscum Contagiosum

Molluscum contagiosum is a cutaneous infection caused by a poxvirus. It is more common among children, especially with atopy and immunosuppressed individuals. It can be clinically diagnosed presenting as normochromic to erythematous papules with umbilicated center. Some cases might be challenging and dermoscopy can also lead to a correct evaluation.[6]

Dermoscopic aspects of molluscum contagiosum are composed of whitish or yellowish polylobulated amorphous

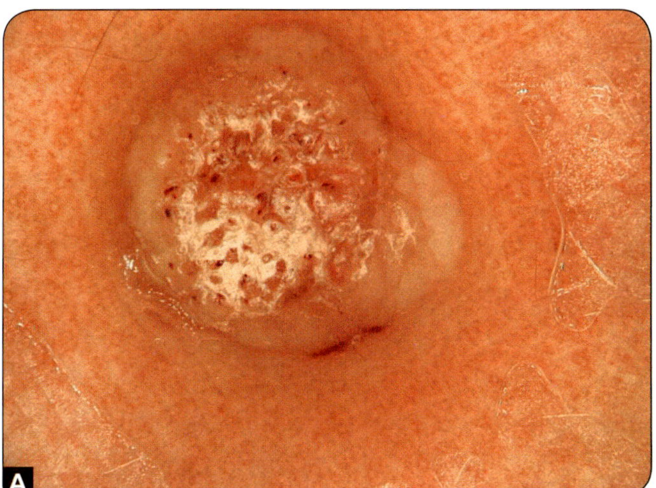

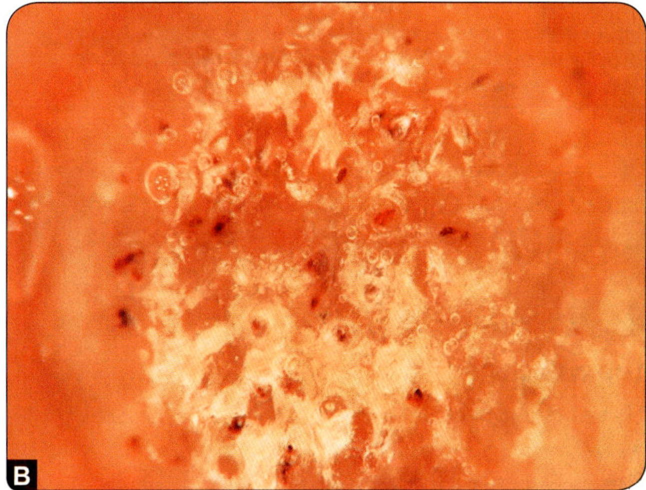

Figs. 13.1A and B: (A) Multiple thrombosed vessels in viral wart (Fotofinder Systems, Germany, 20× original magnification). (B) Multiple thrombosed vessels in viral wart (Fotofinder Systems, Germany, 40× original magnification).

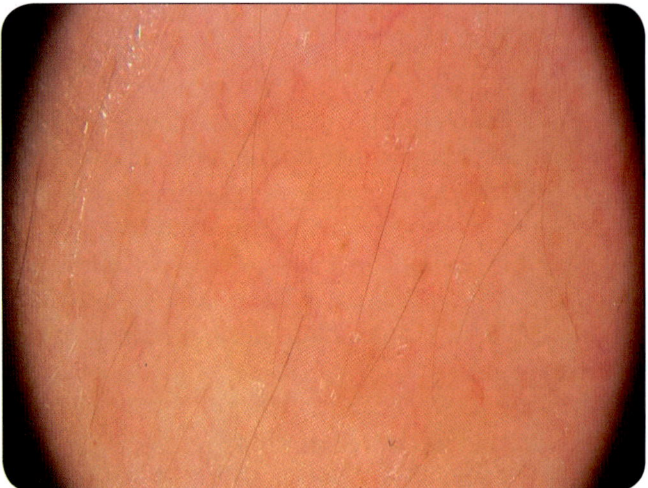

Fig. 13.2: Small well-distributed dotted vessels in flat warts (Fotofinder Systems, Germany, 20× original magnification).

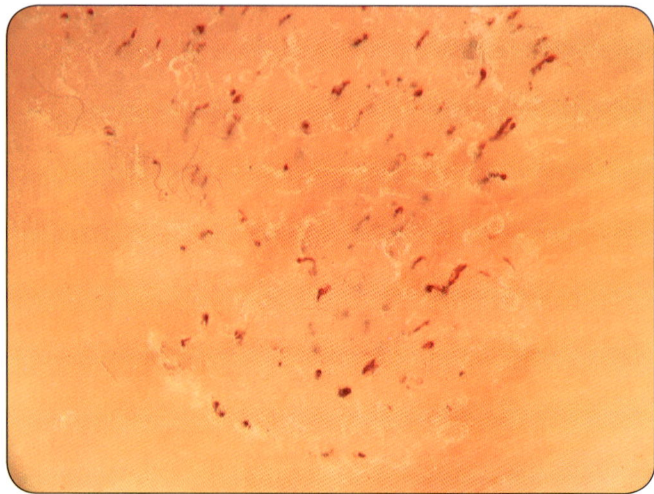

Fig. 13.3: Multiple thrombosed dotted and linear vessels in plantar wart (Fotofinder Systems, Germany, 40× original magnification).

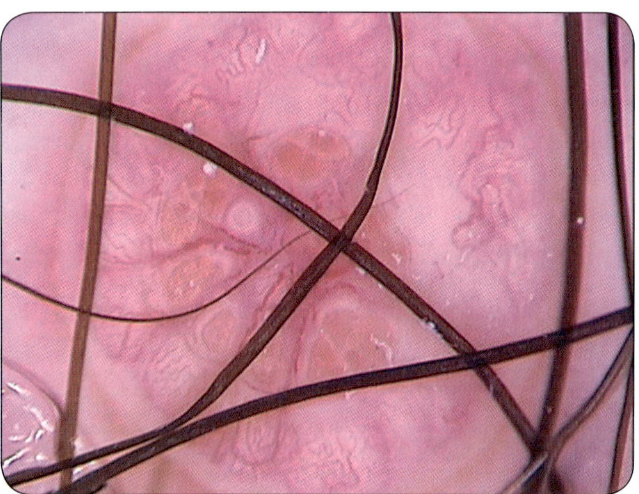

Fig. 13.4: Amorphous structures centrally distributed with peripheral telangiectatic vessels in molluscum contagiosum (Fotofinder Systems, Germany, 20× original magnification).

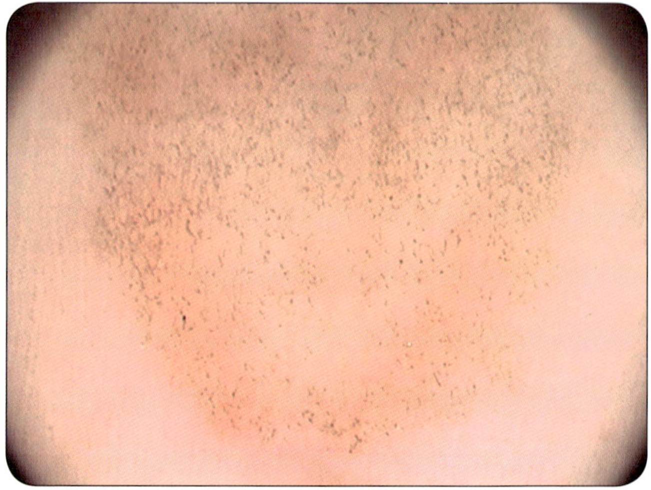

Fig. 13.5: Multiple dark linear structures in tinea nigra (Fotofinder Systems, Germany, 20× original magnification).

structures centrally distributed surrounded by telangiectatic vessels that do not cross the center of the lesion (Fig. 13.4).[6]

FUNGAL INFECTIONS

Tinea Nigra

Tinea nigra is caused by the dematiaceous fungus *Phaeoannellomyces werneckii*, also called *Exophiala werneckii*, *Exophiala phaeoannellomyces* or *Cladosporium werneckii*. It usually occurs on the plantar and palmar aspects of children and young adults.[2] It might mimic malignant melanoma and dermoscopy easily leads to the recognition of tinea nigra. It is characterized by the presence of light-brown linear structures crossing and tangled (Fig. 13.5).[1]

Tinea Capitis

Tinea *capitis* is caused by different species of dermatophytes. It is more common among children and present clinically as a patch of alopecia with tonsured hair. Erythema and scales are frequent as well as have itchy sensation. Definitive diagnosis is performed by culture but dermoscopy might be of great value for the initial suspiciousness. Comma-like hair is frequently seen in tinea

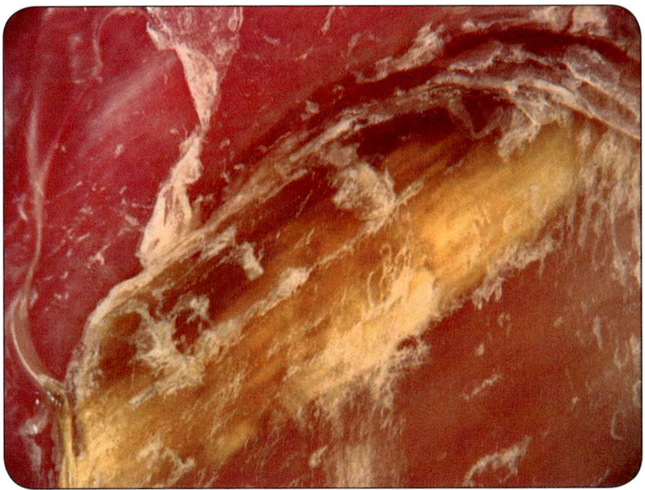

Fig. 13.6: Longitudinal striae of different colors in onychomycosis (Fotofinder Systems, Germany, 20× original magnification).

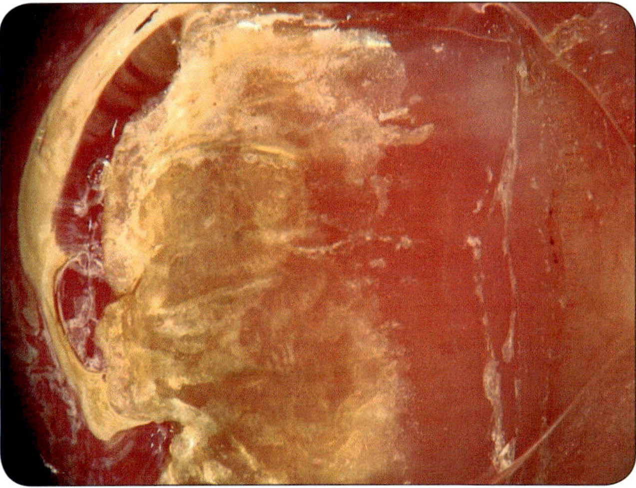

Fig. 13.7: Spiked pattern in onychomycosis (Fotofinder Systems, Germany, 20× original magnification).

capitis as well as tonsured hair.[7] Darker-skin-type individuals might also present with corkscrew-like hair.

Onychomycosis

Fungal infection of the nail plate is very common being responsible for 50% of the nail disorders. Clinical inspection and cultural examination are usually sufficient to diagnose the offending agent. Some cases might also be challenging, especially in pigmented onychomycosis. Some dermoscopic patterns have been reported in onychomycosis patients like the spiked pattern, the longitudinal striae pattern, and the linear edge pattern (Figs. 13.6 and 13.7).[8]

PARASITIC INFESTATIONS

Scabies

Scabies is caused by *Sarcoptes scabiei* variant *hominis*. It is common and might also occur in an epidemic pattern. Clinical manifestations may vary substantially but it usually occurs as erythematous excoriated papules on the axillae, wrists, interdigital spaces, and genital area.

Although skin scrapping and observation of epithelial material under an optic microscope is the gold standard method for the identification of the mite, dermoscopy might play a major role in the evaluation of suspicious cases. Dermoscopy is less invasive, faster, and more practical to evaluate every necessary lesion and shows good accuracy for scabies diagnosis.[9]

Dermoscopic aspects of scabies were initially described by Argenziano et al. In their report, they found 93% of the cases to show a small brown triangular structure localized on the final portion of a linear scaly structure that was called "jet with contrail" (Fig. 13.8). These structures correspond, respectively, to the anterior aspect of the mite and to the scabiotic furrow.[10] Higher magnification dermatoscopes (50–70) facilitate the mite observation.

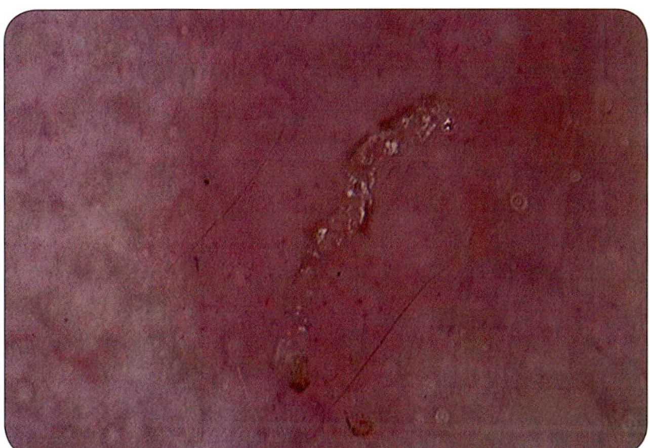

Fig. 13.8: "Jet with contrail" structure in scabies (Fotofinder Systems, Germany, 20× original magnification).

One clinical trial compared dermoscopy to skin scrapping for the diagnosis of scabies. They found, respectively, sensitivities of 91% and 90% and accuracies of 89% and 95% for the methods. Interestingly, patients preferred to have dermoscopy performed as it is a painless noninvasive tool. Moreover, time to evaluate the patients was significantly less also for dermoscopy corroborating that it is a fast method for this purpose.[9]

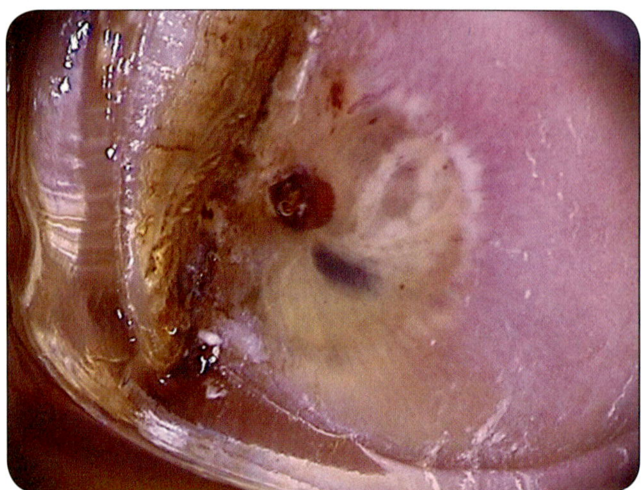

Fig. 13.9: Dark-brown opening, violaceous structure and whitish chains in tungiasis (Fotofinder Systems, Germany, 20× original magnification).

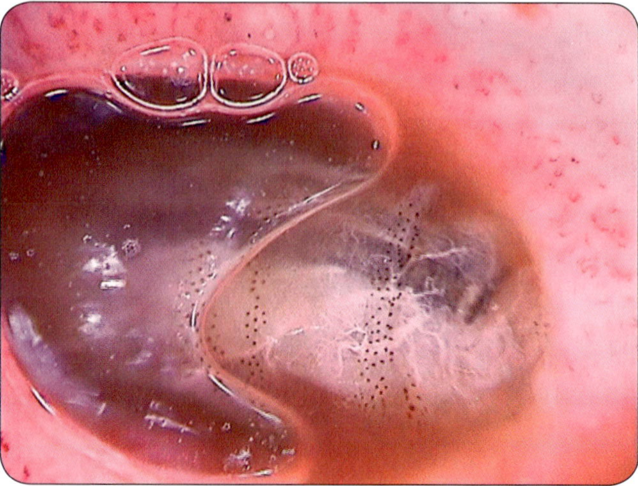

Fig. 13.10: *Dermatobia hominis* maggot in a furuncular myiasis (Fotofinder Systems, Germany, 20× original magnification).

Tungiasis

Tungiasis is caused after skin infestation by the flea *Tunga penetrans*. It affects most commonly the lower extremities, like the plantar region, the periungual tissue or the toes. It is usually self-limited but in some cases, if not recognized early, the infestation might lead to pain and secondary infection.

The dermoscopic is very characteristic.[11,12] It is possible to observe a central pigmented ring, which corresponds to the chitin portion that covers the posterior aspect of the flea exoesqueletum. Violaceous globules and whitish chains of globules are also seen (Fig. 13.9).[11] The latter structure corresponds to the eggs of the flea that will be expelled and can sometimes be visualized on the skin.[11,12]

Furuncular Myiasis

Furuncular myiasis occurs after infestation of the skin by *Dermatobia hominis* maggots. Clinically, it is characterized by a painful inflammatory nodule with a central opening that does not relieve after topical or systemic antibiotics. A single lesion is usually observed but infestations by multiple maggots and consequently a variable number of lesions might be seen. Therefore, its diagnosis might not be initially thought.

Dermoscopy can be extremely important in these cases for early observation of the maggot. It is visualized better with contact dermoscopy closing the nodule opening for some minutes. The maggot necessarily needs to breath and will appear at the surface of the opening (Fig. 13.10). If the opening is not occluded by the dermatoscope lens, the visualization of the maggot might take longer. In order to avoid contamination of the dermatoscope, it is recommended to use a protective plaster on the lens when touching ulcerated skin. The maggot appears with a whitish to yellowish color with small black spines. The maggot is removed easily after death. It is recommended to occlude the opening for 24 hours. On the next day, one should check again for breathing movements with dermoscopy. If they do not occur, it can be safely removed only by holding the maggot with tweezers and gently pulling out.[1,13]

Lice

Head lice are most frequent among children and are caused by infestation by *Pediculus humanis capitis*. Direct transmission is very common, and prompt recognition and treatment are recommended. It is usually characterized by pruritus and by the visualization of the louse on the scalp and nits attached to the hair shafts.

Polarized light dermoscopes allow in vivo observation of the louse and the nits. It is also possible to monitor treatment efficacy as empty or filled nits might be seen.[1] Nonpolarized contact dermoscopy might also be used for nits observation after cutting some of the affected hair and attaching them with to the lens with a tape.[14]

Other lice like *Phthirus pubis* in the genital might also be better visualized by dermoscopy.

Larva Migrans

Larva migrans is caused by the worm *Ancylostoma braziliense*. It is typically transmitted after barefoot walk on contaminated soil with dogs and cats feces. Clinical history

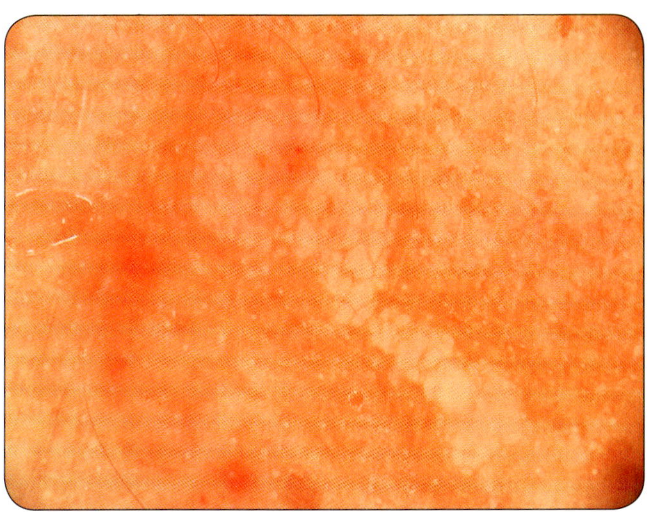

Fig. 13.11: Amorphous translucent light brown structures in a linear pattern in larva migrans (Fotofinder Systems, Germany, 20× original magnification).

and physical examination are very characteristic and correspond to an itchy sensation on a linear erythematous plaque on the feet or eventually buttocks (by seating on the contaminated soil). The lesion tends to increase in length making a serpiginous pathway until the worm dies. Amorphous translucent light brown structures in a linear pattern were described in larva migrans although in the majority of the cases clinical aspects might be sufficient to the correct diagnosis (Fig. 13.11).[1,15]

MISCELLANEOUS

Irritative Dermatitis by Spider Spine

Tarantulas are large spiders that reach 30 cm in size and are not offensive for humans. Some individuals handle those animals as a hobby. A case report of an irritative dermatitis with erythematous papules on interdigital areas and wrists mimicking scabies was reported. The visualization of the small black spicules instead of a potential scabies infestation reveals the correct origin of the reaction.[16]

Ixodes ricinus

Ixodes ricinus is potentially the vector for a series of infectious conditions as Lyme disease. If they are small (≤1 mm), it might be confounded with a pigmented lesion, even melanocytic nevi. Dermoscopy easily facilitates the differentiation and also permits us to observe remaining portions of the tick after mechanical removal.[1]

Lupus Vulgaris

Lupus vulgaris is a variant of cutaneous tuberculosis and may present with distinct clinical forms ranging from isolated or multiple nodules to large plaques with "apple jelly" aspect. On dermoscopy it is possible to observe orange to golden structures and linear vessels as well as whitish streaks.[1]

Leishmaniosis

Leishmaniosis is caused by protozoan of the genus *Leishmania*. Clinical aspects are variable depending on the agent and might be confounded with other skin conditions. Dermoscopy of *Leishmania infantum* demonstrates an erythema and other vascular structures in 100% of the cases. Additionally, yellowish tears and a whitish starbust-like pattern that correspond, respectively, to follicular plugs and parakeratosis were also described.[17]

REFERENCES

1. Tschandl P, Argenziano G, Bakos R, et al. Dermoscopy and entomology (entomodermoscopy). J Dtsch Dermatol Ges. 2009;7(7):589-96.
2. Zalaudek I, Giacomel J, Cabo H, et al. Entodermoscopy: a new tool for diagnosing skin infections and infestations. Dermatology. 2008;216(1):14-23.
3. Teoli M, Di Stefani A, Botti E, et al. Dermoscopy for treatment monitoring of viral warts. Dermatology. 2006;212:318.
4. Vazquez-Lopez F, Kreusch J, Marghoob AA. Dermoscopic semiology: further insights into vascular features by screening a large spectrum of nontumoral skin lesions. Br J Dermatol. 2004;150:226-31.
5. Bae JM, Kang H, Kim HO, et al. Differential diagnosis of plantar wart from corn, callus and healed wart with the aid of dermoscopy. Br J Dermatol. 2009;160(1):220-2.
6. Zaballos P, Ara M, Puig S, et al. Dermoscopy of molluscum contagiosum: a useful tool for clinical diagnosis in adulthood. J Eur Acad Dermatol Venereol. 2006;20(4):482-3.
7. Slowinska M, Rudnicka L, Schwartz RA, et al. Comma hairs: a dermoscopic marker for tinea capitis: a rapid diagnostic method. J Am Acad Dermatol. 2008;59(5 Suppl):S77-9.
8. Jesús-Silva MA, Fernández-Martínez R, Roldán-Marín R, et al. Dermoscopic patterns in patients with a clinical diagnosis of onychomycosis-results of a prospective study including data of potassium hydroxide (KOH) and culture examination. Dermatol Pract Concept. 2015;5(2):39-44.
9. Dupuy A, Dehen L, Bourrat E, et al. Accuracy of standard dermoscopy for diagnosing scabies. J Am Acad Dermatol. 2007;56(1):53-62.
10. Argenziano G, Fabroccini G, Delfino M. Epiluminescence microscopy: a new approach to in vivo detection of Sarcoptes scabiei. Arch Dermatol. 1997;133(6):751-3.

11. Bakos RM, Bakos L. "Whitish chains": a remarkable in vivo dermoscopic finding of tungiasis. Br J Dermatol. 2008; 159(4):991-2.
12. Cabrera R, Daza F. Dermoscopy in the diagnosis of tungiasis. Br J Dermatol. 2009;160(5):1136-7.
13. Bakos RM, Bakos L. Dermoscopic diagnosis of furuncular myiasis. Arch Dermatol. 2007;143(1):123-4.
14. Bakos RM, Bakos L. Dermoscopy for diagnosis of pediculosis capitis. J Am Acad Dermatol. 2007;57(4):727-8.
15. Lallas A, Zalaudek I, Argenziano G, et al. Dermoscopy in general dermatology. Dermatol Clin. 2013;31(4):679-94.
16. Bakos RM, Rezende RL, Bakos L, et al. Spider spines detected by dermoscopy. Arch Dermatol. 2006;142:1517-8.
17. Llambrich A, Zaballos P, Terrasa F, et al. Dermoscopy of cutaneous leishmaniasis. Br J Dermatol. 2009;160(4):756-61.

14

INFLAMMATOSCOPY

Renato Marchiori Bakos

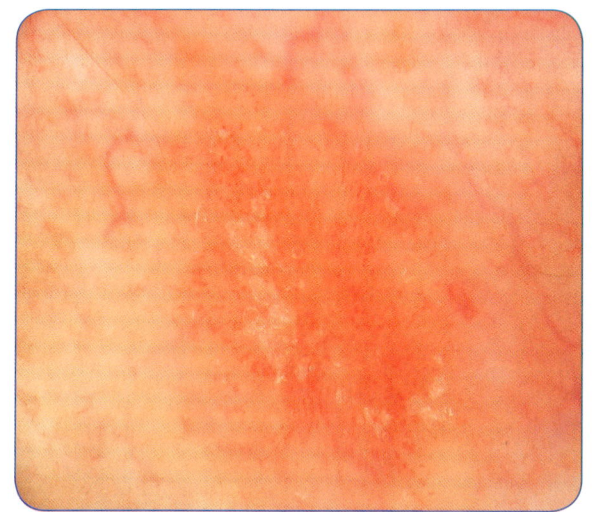

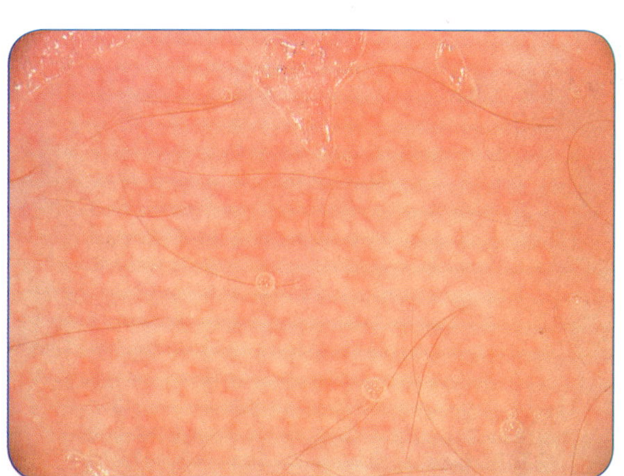

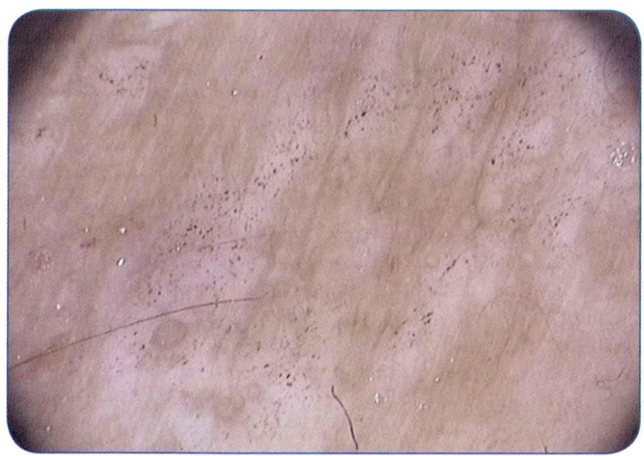

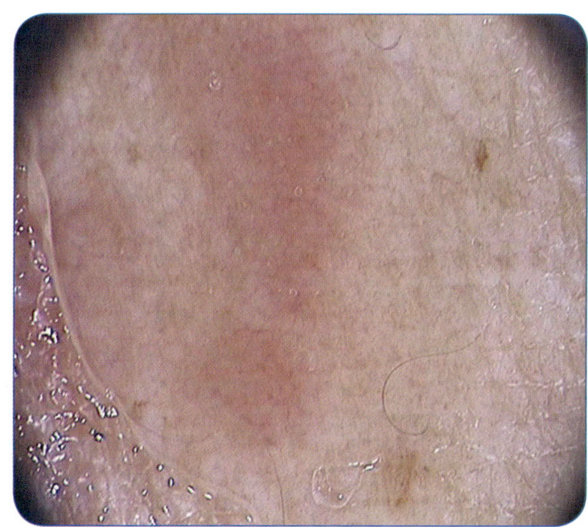

"It is always important to stress that clinical history and physical examination findings remain highly necessary in this scenario.

Characteristic symptoms and signs added to a particular dermoscopic pattern or structures then increase the level of suspiciousness of these groups of diseases. Nevertheless, histopathologic examination should be performed in equivocal clinicodermatoscopic lesions.

Although the majority of the inflammatory cutaneous diseases might not show a pathognomonic dermoscopic pattern, the observation of several structures or also the absence of others may help in characterizing them. As they show few pigmented structures, the observation of vascular patterns and colors are generally of great help."

Dermoscopy is probably the most important noninvasive diagnostic tool for dermatologic practice, being considered the "dermatologist stethoscope."[1] Inflammatory processes may occur secondarily in ordinary lesions and change their usual clinical aspects. This phenomenon is seen, for example, in some melanocytic nevi (Meyerson nevus) or irritated seborrheic keratosis. Especially, the current chapter will present dermoscopic patterns and aspects of different major cutaneous inflammatory diseases that have been reported.[2,3]

Dermoscopy may facilitate inflammatory dermatoses recognition, differentiate them from skin tumors like basal cell carcinoma, Bowen's disease, and amelanotic melanoma and also help in monitoring therapeutic actions, although it might sometimes give little information alone. It is always important to stress that clinical history and physical examination findings remain highly necessary in this scenario. Characteristic symptoms and signs added to a particular dermoscopic pattern or structures then increase the level of suspiciousness of these groups of diseases. Nevertheless, histopathologic examination should be performed in equivocal clinicodermatoscopic lesions.

Although the majority of the inflammatory cutaneous diseases might not show a pathognomonic dermoscopic pattern, the observation of several structures or also the absence of others may help in characterizing them. As they show few pigmented structures, the observation of vascular patterns and colors are generally of great help.[2,3]

Distinct dermoscopic aspects of cutaneous inflammatory diseases are described below.

PSORIASIS

Psoriasis is usually diagnosed on the clinical basis. Histologically, it is characterized by hyperkeratosis, acanthosis, and parakeratosis; elongated rete ridges; and capillary loop dilatation. It is possible to recognize a characteristic dermoscopic pattern in psoriasis. It corresponds to the presence of multiple dotted vessels homogeneously and symmetrically distributed over the lesion (Fig. 14.1).[4,5] These vascular structures correspond to the dilated papillary vessels associated with the epidermic changes. It is the dermoscopic representation of the Auspitz sign. Scales are also seen in dermoscopy and their quantity may be used as a parameter for treatment.[2] Other variants, not in psoriasis vulgaris, may present this pattern. Dotted vessels may be found in several skin conditions, also in melanocytic diseases. The clinicodermoscopic information of a homogeneous and symmetric vascular pattern occurring in an erythematosquamous reaction suggests the diagnosis of psoriasis.

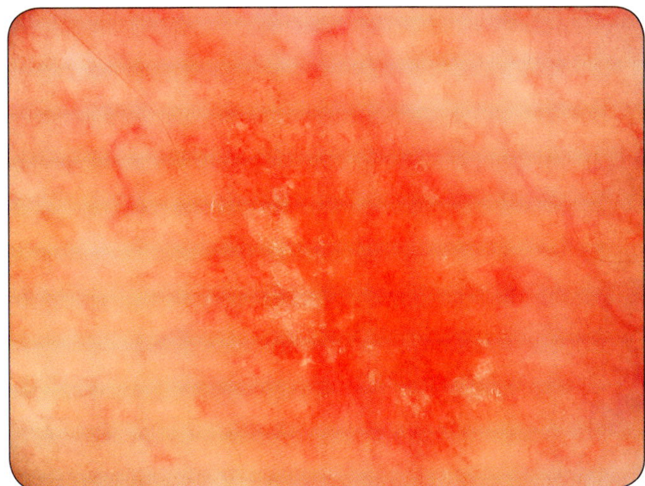

Fig. 14.1: Homogeneous and symmetrically distributed dotted vessels in plaque psoriasis. (Fotofinder Systems, Germany, 20× original magnification)

PITYRIASIS ROSEA

Pityriasis might clinically resemble guttate psoriasis. It is characterized by the absence of the homogeneous dotted vessels and the presence of a collarette-like peripherally distributed white scale and yellow background (Fig. 14.2).[6] Dotted vessels may also be present in the plaques, but distributed irregularly.[2]

LICHEN PLANUS

Dermoscopy is especially helpful for the clinical diagnosis of lichen planus. It is possible to visualize in the majority of the cases White streaks (92% of the cases), which correspond to the Wickham streaks, that can be observed frequently with the naked eye. Small linear vessels as well as some dotted vessels are also seen in 80% of the cases (Fig. 14.3).[4,5] Darker skin type patients present hyperpigmented plaques that show dark-brown structures surrounding the white streaks which may be confounded with dermatofibromas.[7]

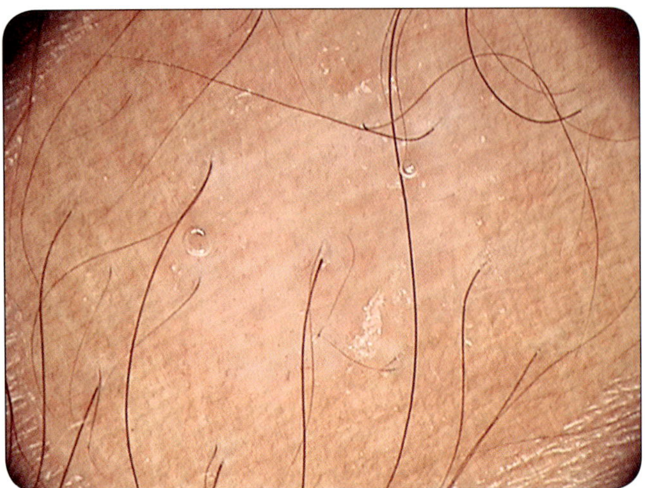

Fig. 14.2: Collarette scale in pityriasis rosea. (Fotofinder Systems, Germany, 20× original magnification)

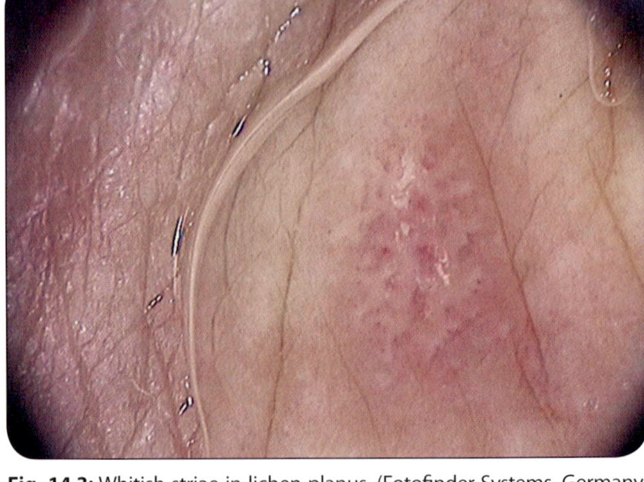

Fig. 14.3: Whitish striae in lichen planus. (Fotofinder Systems, Germany, 20× original magnification)

ECZEMAS

Eczemas do not have a characteristic dermoscopic aspect. Acute forms may show a generalized erythema with vesiculation observed with the dermatoscope. Some vascular structures such as linear vessels may also be seen.[2] Chronic plaques might resemble psoriasis but dotted vessels are irregularly distributed and yellow scales also might be present.[8] It can help at least to rule out other conditions that might occur in this clinical scenario.

URTICARIA

Clinically, urticaria is characterized by erythemato-edematous lesions. On dermoscopy, it is possible to observe erythema and dilated vessels that disappear with contact dermoscopy (Fig. 14.4). It is particularly interesting to differentiate them from urticarial vasculitis that generally shows small hemorrhagic structures (Fig. 14.7).[9]

DISCHOID LUPUS

Dischoid lupus occurs most frequently in sun-exposed areas. It might be confounded with other dermatoses and dermoscopy can also help in its recognition. Moreover, recent report demonstrated different structures that may occur in early-onset lesions (perifollicular whitish halo, follicular plugging, and white scales) (Fig. 14.5) and other structures seen in long-standing lesions (telangiectatic vessels, pigmented structures, and whitish structureless areas)(Fig. 14.6).[2,10,11] Lupus scalp lesions are described elsewhere.[12,13]

LICHEN SCLEROSUS AND MORPHEA

Both lichen sclerosus and morphea appear dermoscopically with white-yellow structures. Genital lichen sclerosus lesions usually have linear vessels while extragenital lesions show keratotic plugs. Scattered black dots that correspond to melanophages might also be seen (Fig. 14.7). Morphea also show linear vessels and a lilac ring and keratotic plugs are not observed.[2,8] Capillaroscopy with a dermoscope might also be helpful in evaluating some inflammatory diseases.[14]

NONINFECTIOUS GRANULOMAS

Immunologic granulomas have also been investigated with dermoscopy. Generally, it is possible to observe a yellow to orange background, sometimes whitish. In necrobiosis lipoidica, there is a rich vascular network with arborizing telangiectasias, mimicking basal cell carcinoma vascular structures that correspond to reticular dermis vessels and small tortuous or linear vessels in the papillary dermis (Figs. 14.8A and B).[15] Granuloma annulare presents with linear vessels in the papular aspect of the lesion (Fig. 14.9).[2] In sarcoidosis, the lesions present in homogeneous or structureless orange areas with linear vessels (Fig. 14.10).[16-18]

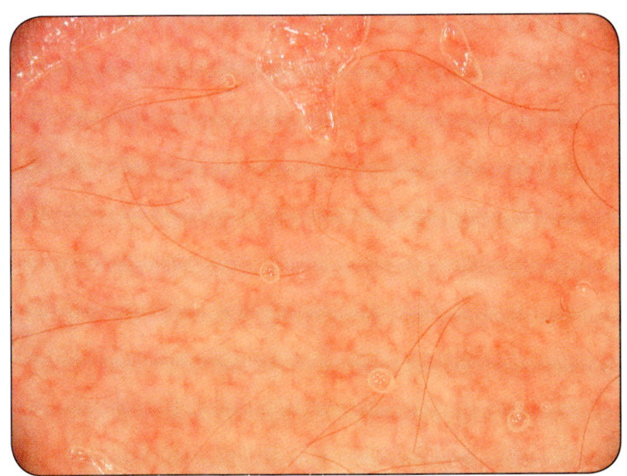

Fig. 14.4: Telangiectatic vessels in urticaria. (Fotofinder Systems, Germany, 20× original magnification)

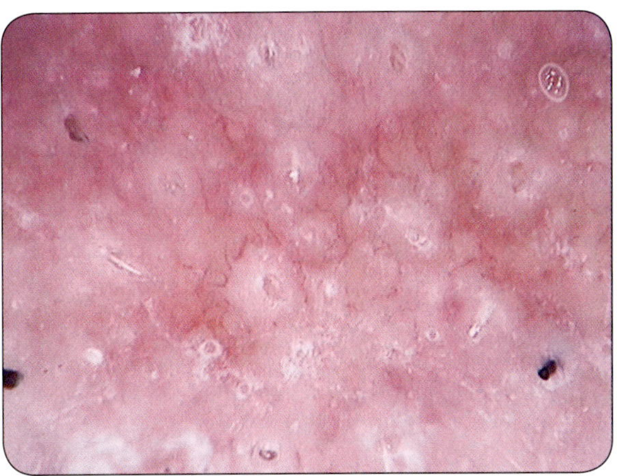

Fig. 14.5: Perifollicular whitish halo, follicular plugging and white scales in an early-onset dischoid lupus plaque. (Fotofinder Systems, Germany, 20× original magnification)

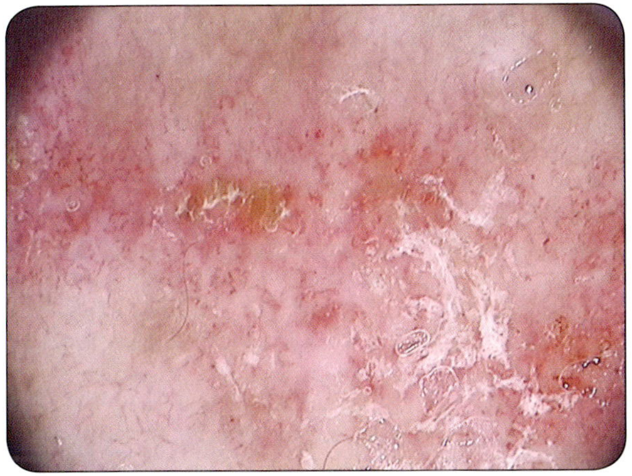

Fig. 14.6: Telangiectatic vessels and whitish structureless areas in long-standing dischoid lupus lesions. (Fotofinder Systems, Germany, 20× original magnification)

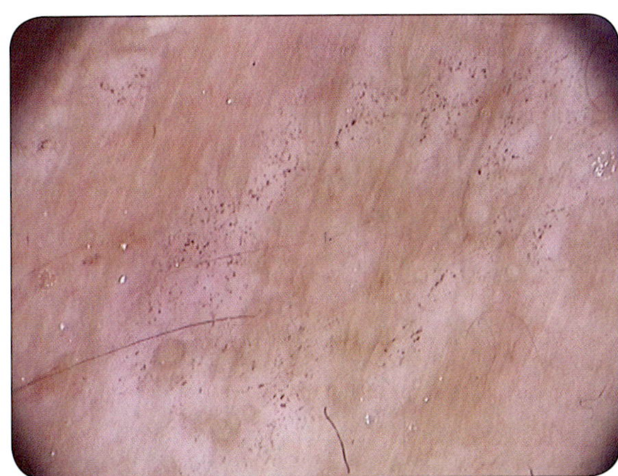

Fig. 14.7: Whitish area with keratotic plug and scattered black dots in lichen sclerosus. (Fotofinder Systems, Germany, 20× original magnification)

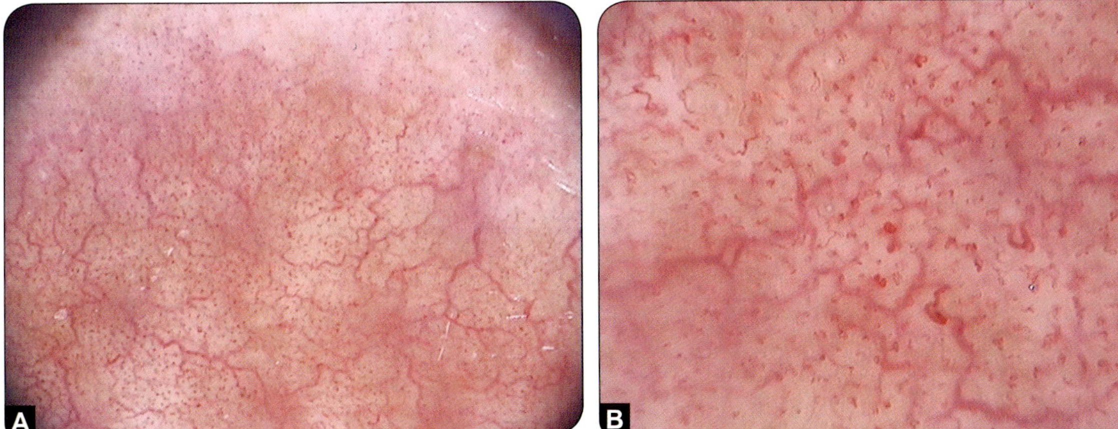

Figs. 14.8A and B: Arborizing telangiectasias and yellow-orange background in necrobiosis lipoidica. (Fotofinder Systems, Germany, 20× original magnification)

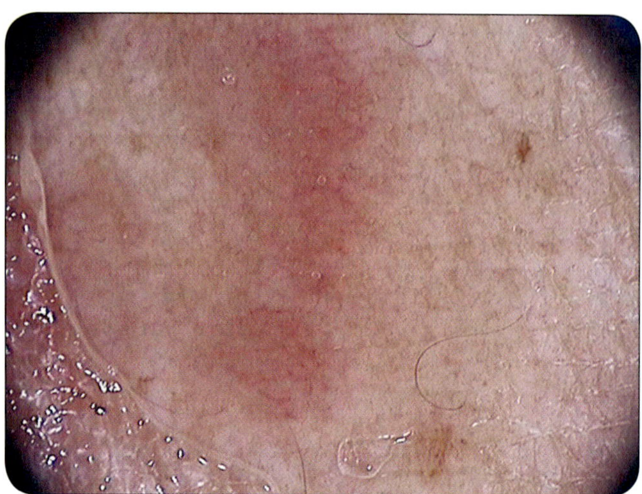

Fig. 14.9: Linear vessels in granuloma annulare. (Fotofinder Systems, Germany, 20× original magnification).

Fig. 14.10: Orange background and linear vessels in sarcoidosis. (Fotofinder Systems, Germany, 20× original magnification)

REFERENCES

1. Tschandl P, Argenziano G, Bakos R, et al. Dermoscopy and entomology (entomodermoscopy). J Dtsch Dermatol Ges. 2009;7:589-96.
2. Vázquez-López F, Kreusch J, Marghoob AA. Dermoscopic semiology: further insights into vascular features by screening a large spectrum of nontumoral skin lesions. Br J Dermatol. 2004;150:226-31.
3. Zalaudek I, Argenziano G, Di Stefani A, et al. Dermoscopy in General Dermatology. Dermatology. 2006;212:7-18.
4. Vázquez-López F, Manjón-Haces JA, Maldonado-Seral C, et al. Dermoscopic features of plaque psoriasis and lichen planus: new observations. Dermatology. 2003;207:151-6.
5. Zalaudek I, Argenziano G. Dermoscopy subpatterns of inflammatory skin disorders. Arch Dermatol. 2006;142:808.
6. Chuh AAT. Collarette scaling in pityriasis rosea demonstrated by digital epiluminescence dermatoscopy. Australas J Dermatol. 2001;42:288-90.
7. Vázquez-López F, Maldonado-Seral C, López-Escobar M, et al. Dermoscopy of pigmented lichen planus lesions. Clin Exp Dermatol. 2003;28:554-64.
8. Lallas A, Zalaudek I, Argenziano G, et al. Dermoscopy in general dermatology. Dermatol Clin. 2013;31(4):679-94.
9. Vázquez-López F, Fueyo A, Sánchez-Martin J, et al. Dermoscopy for the screening of common urticaria and urticaria vasculitis. Arch Dermatol. 2008;144:568
10. Lopez-Tintos BO, Garcia-Hidalgo L, Orozco-Topete R. Dermoscopy in active discoid lupus. Arch Dermatol. 2009;145:358.
11. Lallas A, Apalla Z, Lefaki I, et al. Dermoscopy of discoid lupus erythematosus. Br J Dermatol. 2012;168:284-8.
12. Abraham LS, Piñeiro-Maceira J, Duque-Estrada B, et al. Pinpoint white dots in the scalp: dermoscopic and histopathologic correlation. J Am Acad Dermatol. 2010;63:721-2.
13. Duque-Estrada B, Tamler C, Sodré CT, et al. Dermoscopy patterns of cicatricial alopecia resulting from discoid lupus erythematosus and lichen planopilaris. An Bras Dermatol. 2010;85:179-83.
14. Hasegawa M. Dermoscopy findings of nail fold capillaries in connective tissue diseases. J Dermatol. 2011;38(1):66-70.
15. Bakos RM, Cartell A, Bakos L. Dermoscopy of early-onset necrobiosis lipoidica. J Am Acad Dermatol. 2012;66(4):e143-4.
16. Pellicano R, Tiodorovic-Zivkovic D, Gourhant JY, et al. Dermoscopy of cutaneous sarcoidosis. Dermatology. 2010;221:51-4.
17. Brasiello M, Zalaudek I, Ferrara G, et al. Lupus vulgaris: a new look at an old symptom—the lupoma observed with dermoscopy. Dermatology. 2009;218:172-4.
18. Lallas A, Zaballos P, Zalaudek I, et al. Dermoscopic patterns of granuloma annulare and necrobiosis lipoidica. Clin Exp Dermatol. 2013;38:424-9.

15

TRICHOSCOPY

Lidia Rudnicka

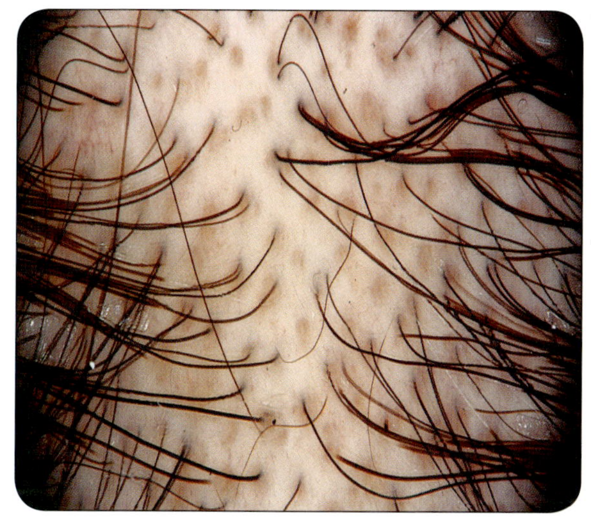

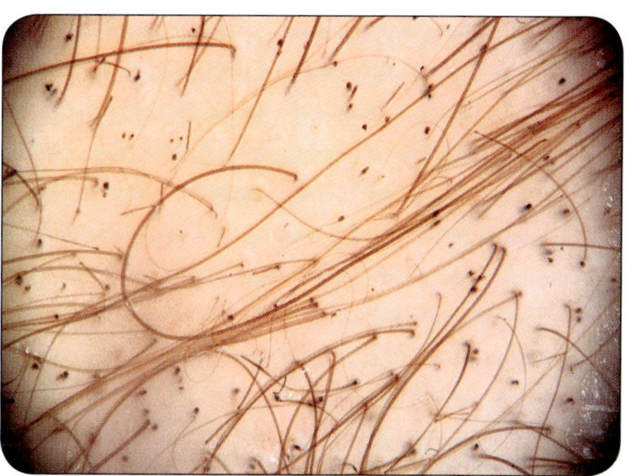

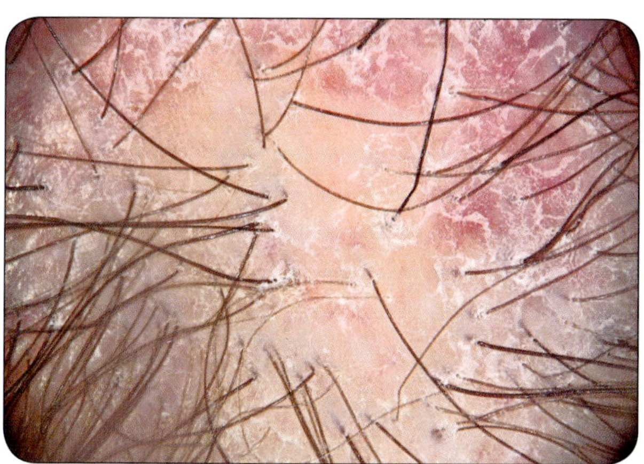

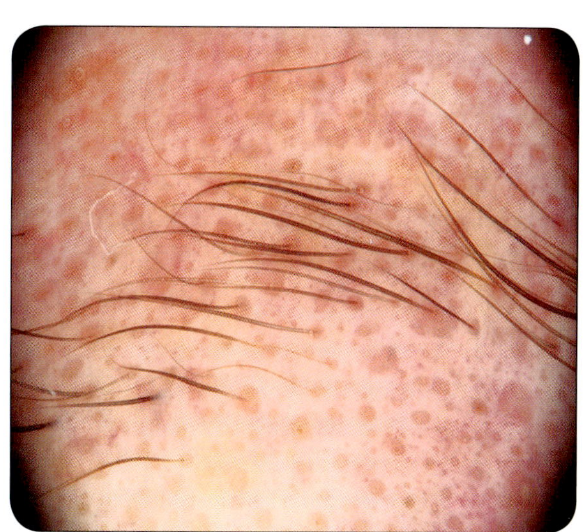

"The term "trichoscopy" refers to dermoscopy or videodermoscopy of hair and scalp.
Trichoscopy is used for differential diagnosis of hair and scalp diseases,
monitoring treatment efficacy in individual patients and evaluation of therapeutic
or cosmetic products in clinical trials and animal experiments.
Any hand-held dermoscope or videodermoscope may be used to perform trichoscopy."

The term "trichoscopy" was first used in literature in 2008[1] and it refers to dermoscopy or videodermoscopy of hair and scalp.[2] Trichoscopy is used for differential diagnosis of hair and scalp diseases,[3] monitoring treatment efficacy in individual patients[2] and evaluation of therapeutic or cosmetic products in clinical trials and animal experiments.[4]

Any handheld dermoscope or videodermoscope may be used to perform trichoscopy. Among handheld dermoscopes, there are devices that require immersion fluid and that use polarized light to cancel out reflections from the stratum corneum. Polarized light dermoscopes may have a contact or noncontact lens. Devices that combine contact and noncontact lenses (hybrid dermoscopes) also are available. The choice of a particular device to perform trichoscopy is a matter of individual's preference.

A normal terminal hair is uniform in thickness and color throughout its length.[5,6] Up to 10% of normal human scalp hairs are vellus hairs that appear short, thin, and hypopigmented on trichoscopy. Abnormalities in hair shaft structure or color may be indicative of several hair and scalp diseases. Hair follicle openings appear in trichoscopy as small round structures, called "dots". The following types of dots may be distinguished: yellow dots (follicular openings filled with sebum and keratotic material), black dots (follicular openings filled with pigmented hair residues), white dots (follicular openings replaced by fibrotic tissue), and pinpoint white dots (normal follicular openings that appear lighter on dark background of sun-exposed skin or in patients with dark skin phototypes).[7,8] The shape of scalp blood vessels, scaling, or exudates may also provide some diagnostic information.[2]

NONCICATRICIAL ALOPECIA

Androgenetic Alopecia

Androgenetic alopecia in men and women shares similar trichoscopy features. The most typical, almost pathognomonic, trichoscopy feature of androgenetic alopecia is the simultaneous presence of thick, intermediate, thin vellus hairs in one field of view of a dermoscope, also called hair shaft thickness heterogeneity. This exemplifies the ongoing process of hair follicle miniaturization.[9] Vellus hairs may be present in a healthy person, but their proportion usually does not exceed 10%.[5] A higher proportion of vellus hairs are indicative of androgenetic alopecia. Another typical trichoscopy feature is a decreased number of hairs per follicular. A healthy follicular unit contains two or three (sometimes four) hairs. In patients with androgenetic alopecia follicular units with only one hair will usually predominate. Empty hair follicles present as yellow dots, usually sparsely distributed between the normal and thinned hairs. The presence of yellow dots appears to be a variable feature of androgenetic alopecia. In various studies, yellow dots were observed in 7–66% of women with androgenetic alopecia, depending on the study.[2] Brown perifollicular discoloration (the peripilar sign) is observed in 20–66% of patients (Fig. 15.1).

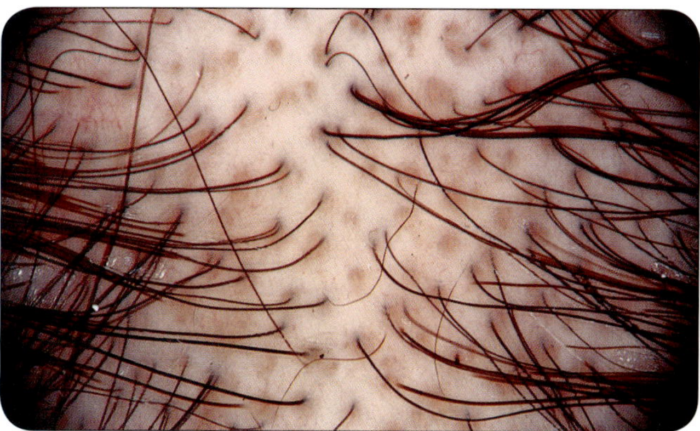

Fig. 15.1: Female androgenetic alopecia. Hair shaft heterogeneity, predominance of follicular units with only one hair shaft, yellow dots.

Alopecia Areata

The trichoscopy presentation of alopecia areata differs depending on disease activity. The hallmark features of active disease are exclamation mark hairs and black dots.[3,10] Other less frequent manifestations of active alopecia areata are trichorrhexis nodosa (3–16%), monilethrix-like hairs, and zigzag hairs. Zigzag hairs may also be present in tinea capitis, so this feature may be misleading, if not associated with other trichoscopy features of alopecia areata.[11] Nonactive, long-lasting disease is usually characterized by multiple, regularly distributed yellow dots.[12] Some authors indicate that yellow dots are not present in childhood alopecia areata.[13]

In the regrowth phase, multiple upright regrowing hairs may be visible (Figs. 15.2A and B).

Trichotillomania

The most characteristic trichoscopy feature of trichotillomania is the chaotic arrangement of hairs broken at different lengths. The distal ends of the broken hairs may be classified as transverse fractures, fractures with trichoptilosis (split ends), coiled hairs with a ragged ends, and flame hairs.[14] Black dots may develop when hair brake at

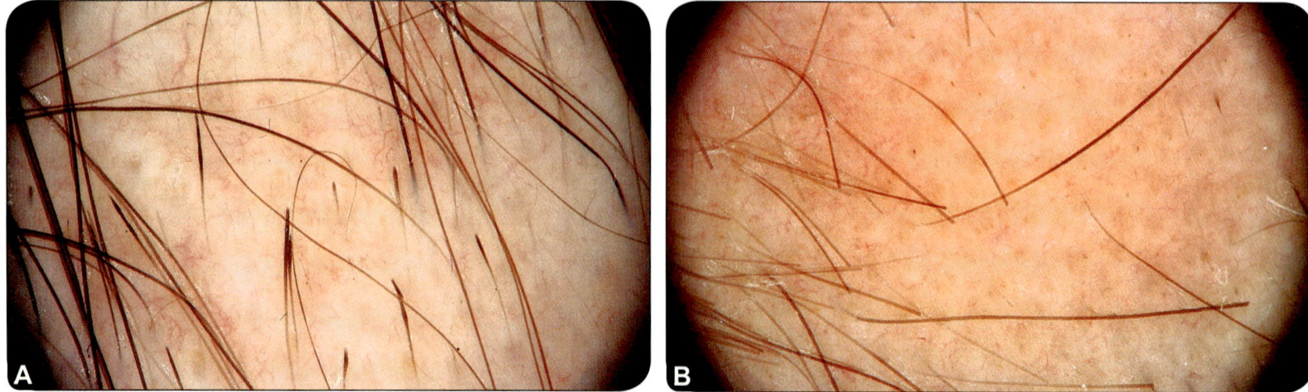

Figs. 15.2A and B: Alopecia areata. (A) Multiple exclamation mark hairs and black dots are a marker of high disease activity. (B) Regularly distributed yellow dots in a stable disease.

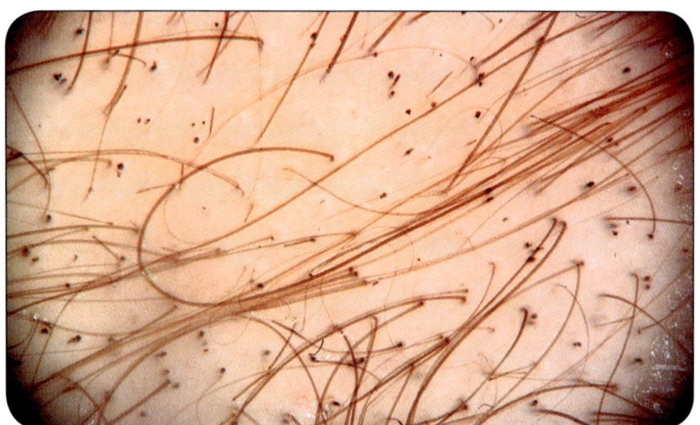

Fig. 15.3: Trichotillomania. Hairs broken at different lengths and black dots.

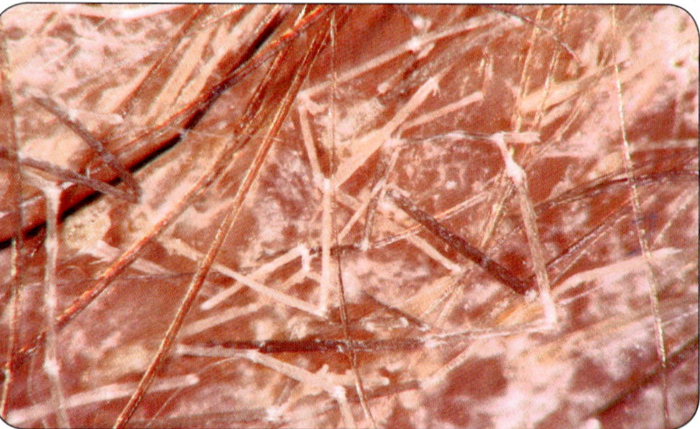

Fig. 15.4: Tinea capitis. Zigzag hairs (hairs bend at sharp angles) may also be observed in the initial phase of alopecia areata.

the scalp level.[15-17] Yellow dots are generally not observed in trichotillomania.[15] Inui et al.[18] and later Rudnicka et al.[2] observed yellow dots in one patient with this condition. These dots differ from yellow dots in other diseases by containing a black peppering in their central part.[18] Exclamation mark hairs are rare in trichotillomania,[19,20] but they may be a diagnostic pitfall and cause misdiagnosis of alopecia areata. It should be kept in mind that these two diseases, trichotillomania and alopecia areata, relatively commonly coexist,[21] what makes trichoscopic differential diagnosis even more challenging (Fig. 15.3).

Tinea Capitis

Trichoscopy has a major benefit over mycological culture in that it gives immediate results. The typical trichoscopy features of tinea capitis are comma hairs[22] and corkscrew hairs,[23] the latter being more common in patients with dark skin phototypes.[24] These typical hair shaft structure abnormalities are commonly accompanied by scaling, diffuse, or perifollicular.[25] It was documented that the typical trichoscopy abnormalities are associated with both ectothrix and endothrix types of fungal invasion.[26] Other less common features of tinea capitis include block hairs, i-hairs, and zigzag hairs. Tinea capitis may present with tufted folliculitis (Fig. 15.4).[27,28]

Ultraviolet-enhanced trichoscopy, first described in 2011,[20] is a new method, which may aid in the identification of tinea capitis. The method is based on the combination of Wood's light and trichoscopy (Fig. 15.5).[20]

CICATRICIAL ALOPECIA

Lichen Planopilaris

Trichoscopy of lichen planopilaris depends on the stage of disease. In the active, inflammatory phase of the disease, the predominant trichoscopy feature is perifollicular

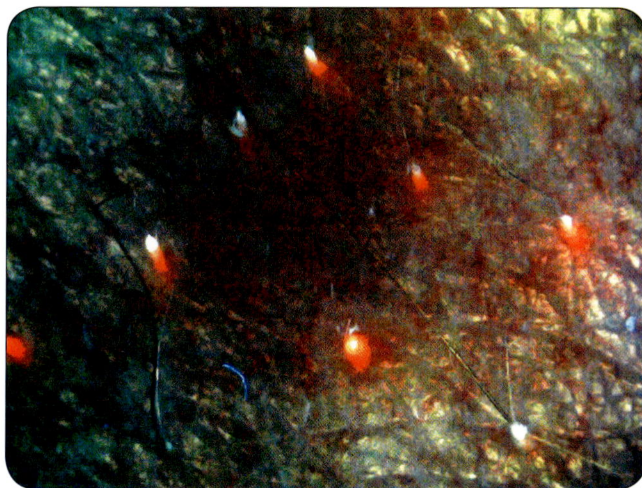

Fig. 15.5: Ultraviolet (UV)-enhanced trichoscopy is performed with a dermoscope equipped with a UV light source, which overlaps with Wood's lamp wavelength.

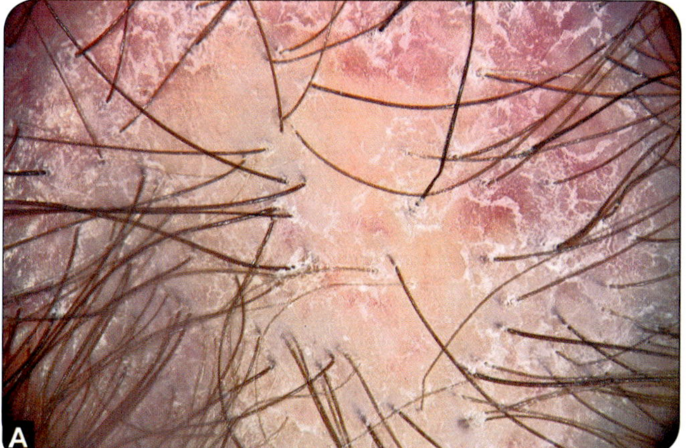

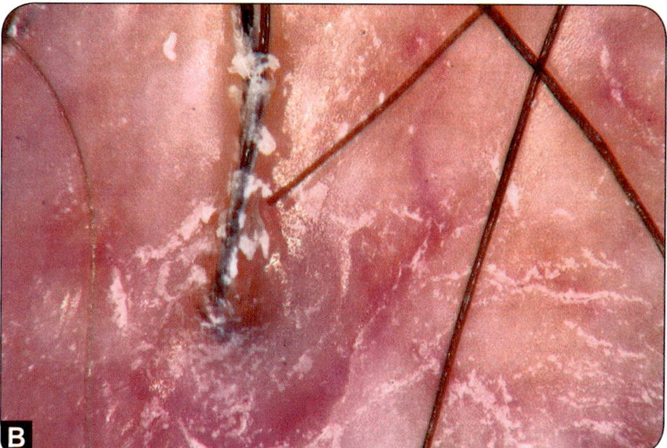

Figs. 15.6A and B: Lichen planopilaris. (A) Perifollicular scaling (20-fold magnification). (B) The scales entangle the hair shaft up to a few millimeters above the hair follicle opening—"tubular scaling" (70-fold magnification).

scaling. Scales migrate along the hair shaft and form a tubular structure, which covers the proximal portion of the emerging hair shaft (tubular scaling or tubular perifollicular hyperkeratosis).[7,29] This feature is a characteristic, but not pathognomonic, of Lichen plano pilaris (LPP). It may also be observed in other folliculocentric alopecias, in particular, in folliculitis decalvans. Round, perifollicular, blue-gray, or violaceous areas surrounding empty hair follicle openings in a targetoid pattern were described in patients with dark phototypes.[30] Elongated perifollicular blood vessels may be a manifestation of the ongoing inflammatory process.

In the late fibrotic stage of the disease, the dominating trichoscopy presentations are white dots, milky-white areas, and white areas. White dots in lichen planopilaris are considered a residue of conduced perifollicular fibrosis.[31] These are irregularly shaped, small whitish areas. These are slightly bigger compared to yellow and black dots and have a tendency to merge and form milky-red areas (fibrosis of the recent onset) and white areas (late-stage fibrosis). These white dots have to be distinguished from small pinpoint white dots, which represent empty follicular ostia in patients with dark skin phototypes (Figs. 15.6A and B).[32]

Frontal Fibrosing Alopecia

Frontal fibrosing alopecia is considered a subtype of lichen planopilaris. Thus, these two diseases share some common trichoscopy features. The main trichoscopy findings in frontal fibrosing alopecia include lack of follicular

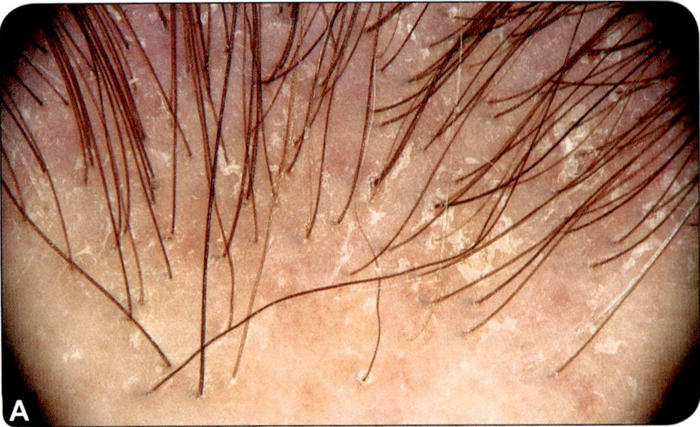

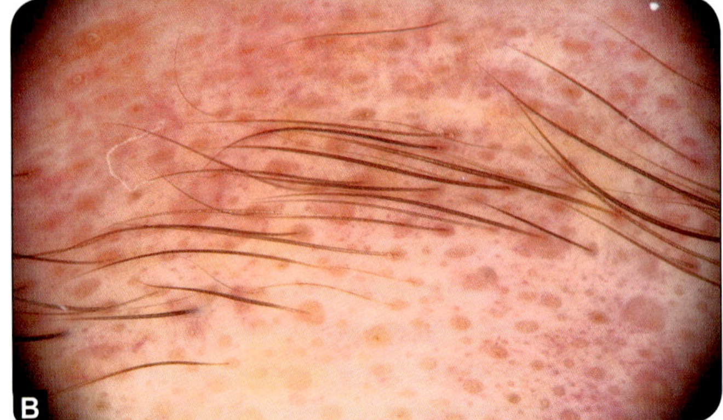

Figs. 15.7A and B: (A) Frontal fibrosing alopecia. Mild perifollicular scaling, lonely hair, and areas with no follicular openings in the frontal scalp. (B) Trichoscopy of the eyebrow area shows multiple hair follicle openings (brownish dots).

openings and minor perifollicular scaling. Perifollicular erythema is not common and is considered a feature of active disease.[33] There is a strong predominance of follicular openings with only one hair at the hair-baring margin. Lonely hair, defined as single terminal hairs surrounded by cicatricial alopecia, may be observed clinically as well as in trichoscopy.[34]

In the eyebrow area, trichoscopy shows regularly distributed reddish or gray dots (early disease) or an area lacking follicular openings (late disease) (Figs. 15.7A and B).[2]

Folliculitis Decalvans

As in all other types of cicatricial alopecia, trichoscopy will depend on the stage of disease. In early, active disease, trichoscopy shows tufts of five or more hairs emerging from one follicular opening. The hair tufts are surrounded by tubular perifollicular scaling. Unlike lichen planopilaris, where the scales are usually white, in folliculitis decalvans, the tubular scaly structures appear yellowish. This results from the purulent content in these structures.

The tufts may be surrounded by perifollicular epidermal hyperplasia, which may be arranged in a starburst pattern (starburst sign).[35] Other trichoscopy features of active folliculitis decalvans are follicular pustules, yellow discharge, and perifollicular arrangement of blood vessels.[29] In long-lasting lesions, white, fibrotic areas predominate in trichoscopy images (Fig. 15.8).[29]

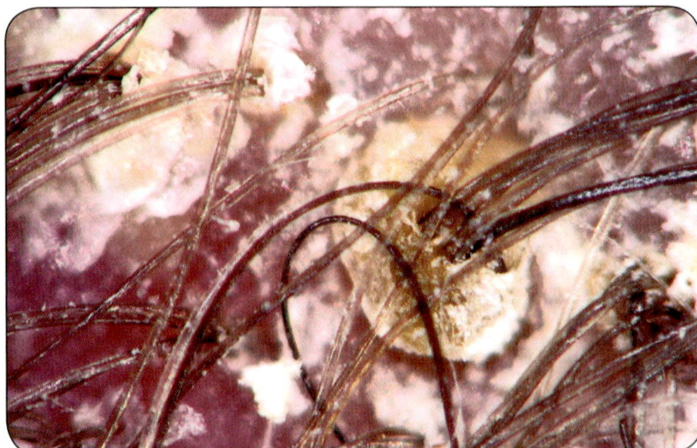

Fig. 15.8: Folliculitis decalvans. Hair tufts surrounded by yellowish scales.

Discoid Lupus Erythematosus

Despite being categorized as primary cicatricial alopecia, discoid lupus erythematosus is not a "true" folliculocentric disease. Thus, the trichoscopy abnormalities do not seem to be strictly associated with follicular openings. The most characteristic trichoscopy features of active discoid lupus erythematosus are thick arborizing vessels, large yellow dots (keratotic plugs), scattered dark-brown discoloration, and blue-gray dots.[29,36] Large yellow dots in DLE are darker compared to other diseases, usually dark yellow to yellow brown in color. Yellow dots with radial, thin arborizing vessels emerging from the dots are considered highly characteristic of late discoid lupus erythematosus (DLE) lesions and were called "red spider in yellow dot" by Rakowska et al.[29]

Long-lasting, inactive DLE lesions differ from active lesions. They are characterized by the presence of structureless milky-red or white areas and lack of follicular openings (Figs. 15.9A and B).

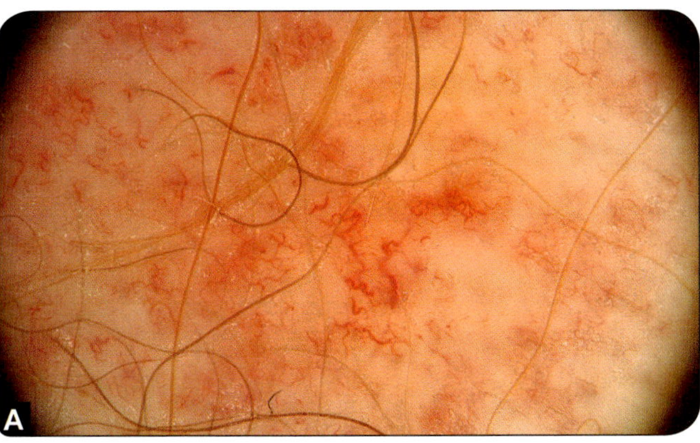

Figs. 15.9A and B: Discoid lupus erythematosus. (A) Thick arborizing vessels. (B) In the eyebrow area, the disease may present with a strawberry pattern.

REFERENCES

1. Rudnicka L, Olszewska M, Rakowska A, et al. Trichoscopy: a new method for diagnosing hair loss. J Drugs Dermatol. 2008;7(7):651-4.
2. Rudnicka L, Olszewska M, Rakowska A. Atlas of Trichoscopy: Dermoscopy in Hair and Scalp Disease. London: Springer; 2012. pp. xiv, 507.
3. Mubki T, Rudnicka L, Olszewska M, et al. Evaluation and diagnosis of the hair loss patient: part II. Trichoscopic and laboratory evaluations. J Am Acad Dermatol. 2014;71(3):431e1-11.
4. Orasan MS, Bolfa P, Coneac A, et al. Topical products for human hair regeneration: a comparative study on an animal model. Ann Dermatol. 2016;28(1):65-73.
5. Rakowska A. Trichoscopy (hair and scalp videodermoscopy) in the healthy female. Method standardization and norms for measurable parameters. J Dermatol Case Rep. 2009;3(1):14-9.
6. Vogt A, McElwee K, Blume-Peytavi U. Biology of the hair follicle. In: Blume-Peytavi U, Tosti A, Whiting D, Trüeb R (Eds). Hair; from Basic Science to Clinical Application. Berlin, Germany: Springer-Verlag; 2008. pp. 1-22.
7. Rudnicka L, Olszewska M, Rakowska A, et al. Trichoscopy update 2011. J Dermatol Case Rep. 2011;5(4):82-8.
8. Torres F, Tosti A. Trichoscopy: an update. G Ital Dermatol Venereol. 2014;149(1):83-91.
9. Olszewska M, Warszawik O, Rakowska A, et al. Methods of hair loss evaluation in patients with endocrine disorders. Endokrynol Pol. 2010;61(4):406-11.
10. Lacarrubba F, Dall'Oglio F, Rita Nasca M, et al. Videodermatoscopy enhances diagnostic capability in some forms of hair loss. Am J Clin Dermatol. 2004;5(3):205-8.
11. Rudnicka L, Rakowska A, Kerzeja M, et al. Hair shafts in trichoscopy: clues for diagnosis of hair and scalp diseases. Dermatol Clin. 2013;31(4):695-708, x.
12. Ross EK, Vincenzi C, Tosti A. Videodermoscopy in the evaluation of hair and scalp disorders. J Am Acad Dermatol. 2006;55(5):799-806.
13. Miteva M, Tosti A. Hair and scalp dermatoscopy. J Am Acad Dermatol. 2012;67(5):1040-8.
14. Rakowska A, Slowinska M, Olszewska M, et al. New trichoscopy findings in trichotillomania: flame hairs, V-sign, hook hairs, hair powder, tulip hairs. Acta Derm Venereol. 2014;94(3):303-6.
15. Abraham LS, Torres FN, Azulay-Abulafia L. Dermoscopic clues to distinguish trichotillomania from patchy alopecia areata. An Bras Dermatol. 2010;85(5):723-6.
16. Gallouj S, Rabhi S, Baybay H, et al. [Trichotemnomania associated to trichotillomania: a case report with emphasis on the diagnostic value of dermoscopy]. Ann Dermatol Venereol. 2011;138(2):140-1.
17. Lee DY, Lee JH, Yang JM, et al. The use of dermoscopy for the diagnosis of trichotillomania. J Eur Acad Dermatol Venereol. 2009;23(6):731-2.
18. Inui S, Nakajima T, Nakagawa K, et al. Clinical significance of dermoscopy in alopecia areata: analysis of 300 cases. Int J Dermatol. 2008;47(7):688-93.
19. Ihm CW, Han JH. Diagnostic value of exclamation mark hairs. Dermatology. 1993;186(2):99-102.
20. Rudnicka L, Olszewska M, Rakowska A, et al. Trichoscopy update 2011. J Dermatol Case Rep. 2011;5(4):82-8.
21. Sah DE, Koo J, Price VH. Trichotillomania. Dermatol Ther. 2008;21(1):13-21.
22. Slowinska M, Rudnicka L, Schwartz RA, et al. Comma hairs: a dermoscopic marker for tinea capitis: a rapid diagnostic method. J Am Acad Dermatol. 2008;59(5 Suppl):S77-9.
23. Pinheiro AM, Lobato LA, Varella TC. Dermoscopy findings in tinea capitis: case report and literature review. An Bras Dermatol. 2012;87(2):313-4.
24. Hughes R, Chiaverini C, Bahadoran P, et al. Corkscrew hair: a new dermoscopic sign for diagnosis of tinea capitis in black children. Arch Dermatol. 2011;147(3):355-6.
25. Brasileiro A, Campos S, Cabete J, et al. Trichoscopy as an additional tool for the differential diagnosis of tinea capitis. Br J Dermatol. 2016; 175:113-21.
26. Sandoval AB, Ortiz JA, Rodriguez JM, et al. [Dermoscopic pattern in tinea capitis]. Rev Iberoam Micol. 2010;27(3):151-2.
27. Baroni A, Ruocco E, Aiello FS, et al. Tinea capitis mimicking tufted hair folliculitis. Clin Exp Dermatol. 2009;34(8): e699-701.

28. Tangjaturonrusamee C, Piraccini BM, Vincenzi C, et al. Tinea capitis mimicking folliculitis decalvans. Mycoses. 2011;54(1):87-8.
29. Rakowska A, Slowinska M, Kowalska-Oledzka E, et al. Trichoscopy of cicatricial alopecia. J Drugs Dermatol. 2012;11(6):753-8.
30. Duque-Estrada B, Tamler C, Sodre CT, et al. Dermoscopy patterns of cicatricial alopecia resulting from discoid lupus erythematosus and lichen planopilaris. An Bras Dermatol. 2010;85(2):179-83.
31. Miteva M, Tosti A. Dermoscopy-guided scalp biopsy in cicatricial alopecia. J Eur Acad Dermatol Venereol. 2013; 27(10):1299-303.
32. Abraham LS, Pineiro-Maceira J, Duque-Estrada B, et al. Pinpoint white dots in the scalp: dermoscopic and histopathologic correlation. J Am Acad Dermatol. 2010;63 (4):721-2.
33. Toledo-Pastrana T, Hernandez MJ, Camacho Martinez FM. Perifollicular erythema as a trichoscopy sign of progression in frontal fibrosing alopecia. Int J Trichology. 2013; 5(3):151-3.
34. Tosti A, Miteva M, Torres F. Lonely hair: a clue to the diagnosis of frontal fibrosing alopecia. Arch Dermatol. 2011; 147(10):1240.
35. Rakowska A, Slowinska M, Kowalska-Oledzka E, et al. Trichoscopy in cicatricial alopecia. J Drugs Dermatol. 2012; 11(6):753-8.
36. Miteva M, Tosti A. Dermoscopic features of central centrifugal cicatricial alopecia. J Am Acad Dermatol. 2014; 71(3):443-9.

CAPILLAROSCOPY

16

Emilia Noemi Cohen Sabban

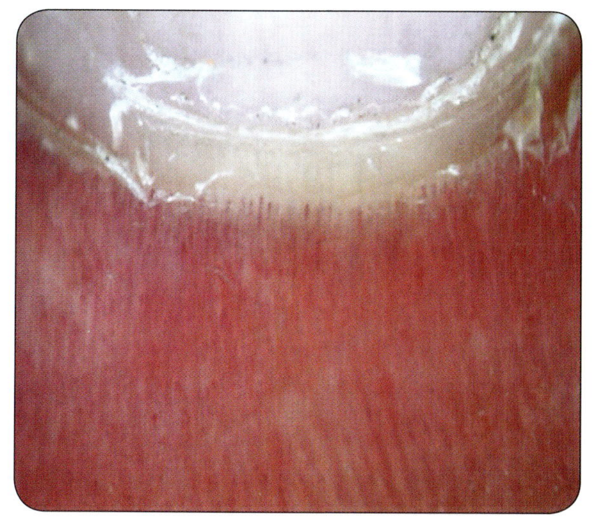

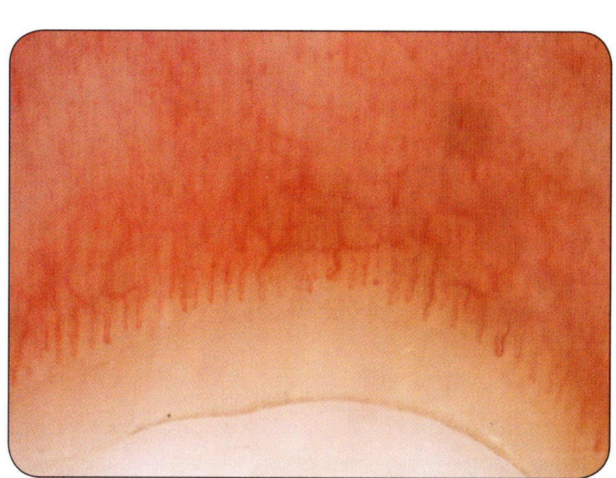

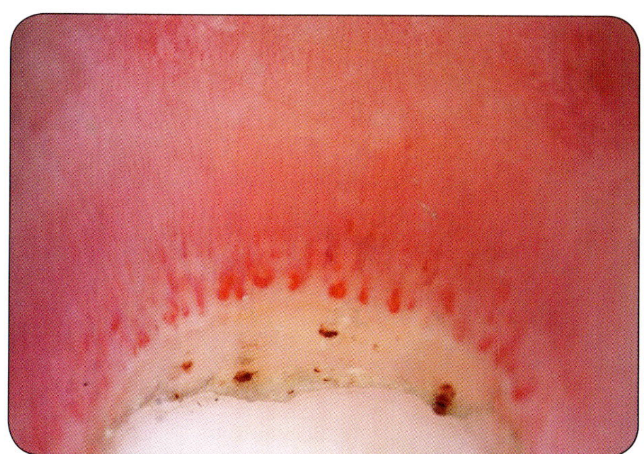

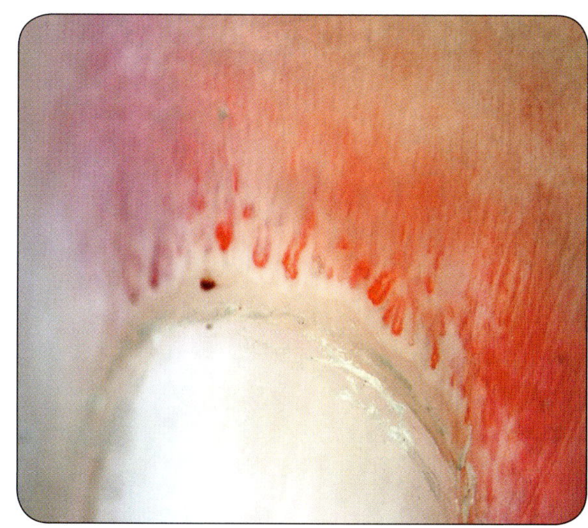

"Capillaroscopy is a noninvasive, safe, in vivo study of the capillaries morphology, which can be assessed by using a magnifying system, enabling the early recognition of morphological and functional abnormalities in microcirculation, the most distal area of the circulatory tree. Cutaneous microcirculation is easy to explore; it is localized at dermal level, and composed of two interconnected plexuses: the subpapillary plexus or superficial plexus, parallel to the epidermis, from which capillary loops branch up; and the deep, dermohypodermal plexus. In vivo study of the capillaries is performed preferably in the nailfold, since in this anatomical region the capillaries lie parallel to the cutaneous surface as opposed to what happens in other skin areas, where they lie perpendicularly, and consequently appear as red dots on a light background."

INTRODUCTION

Capillaroscopy is a noninvasive, safe, in vivo study of the capillaries morphology, which can be assessed by using a magnifying system, enabling the early recognition of morphological and functional abnormalities in microcirculation, the most distal area of the circulatory tree.

Cutaneous microcirculation is easy to explore; it is localized at dermal level, and composed of two interconnected plexuses: the subpapillary plexus (SP) or superficial plexus, parallel to the epidermis, from which capillary loops branch up; and the deep, dermohypodermal plexus.[1]

In vivo study of the capillaries is performed preferably in the nailfold, since in this anatomical region the capillaries lie parallel to the cutaneous surface as opposed to what happens in other skin areas, where they lie perpendicularly, and consequently appear as red dots on a light background.[2]

Nailfold capillaroscopy (NC) consists, therefore, in the direct visualization of the distal line of the periungual capillaries.

The procedure was described more than a century ago, but only in recent decades it has gained popularity and come to play an important role in the diagnosis and monitoring of different illnesses.

Some conditions that cause changes in the shape and density of the capillaries are systemic sclerosis (SSc), dermatomyositis (DM), mixed connective tissue disease (MCTD), Raynaud's phenomenon (RP), overlap syndromes, systemic lupus erythematosus (SLE), as well as conditions involving microcirculation such as diabetes mellitus (DbM) and hypertension (HT).[3]

This procedure has the following advantages:

- Harmless, noninvasive
- Repeatable/reproducible
- Low cost
- High sensitivity
- Good specificity
- Easy interpretation.

There are several instruments used for the observation of capillaries in the periungual fold, such as a stereomicroscope, an optic microscope, an ophthalmoscope, a 40× magnifier, and an adaptor to obtain images. At present, there are also videocapillaroscopes with a software that allows dynamic studies of microcirculation by counting capillary number and assessment of the capillary loops and their branches.

According to some authors, videocapillaroscopy (VC) outperforms conventional capillaroscopy not only in the visualization of moving images but also in sharpness, scope, detail, register, and imaging study.[4]

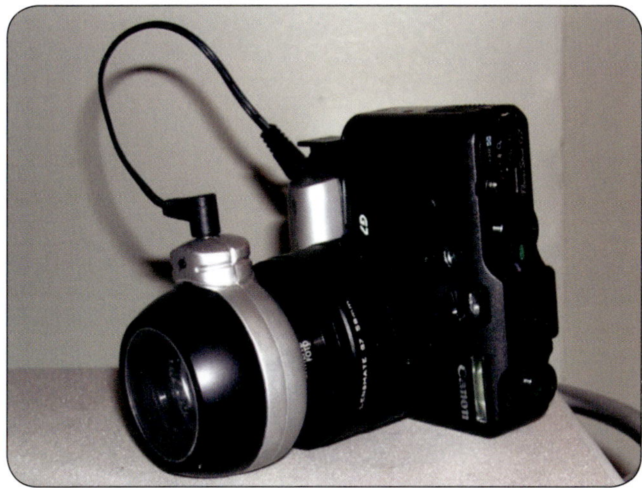

Fig. 16.1: A dermoscope (Dermlite polarized light 10×) attached to a photographic camera.

Dermatologists, having been trained in the use of the dermoscope for the diagnosis of melanocytic and nonmelanocytic lesions, perform capillaroscopy with this instrument attached to a photographic camera to record images, like the ones included in this chapter (Fig. 16.1). A study comparing VC with dermoscope concluded that dermoscopy was efficient enough to identify pathognomonic changes.[5]

It is important to remark that this instrument is inexpensive, easy to use and carry, and that with proper training, it may substitute more sophisticated devices and systems.[6,7]

NORMAL CAPILLAROSCOPY

Even though normality has not yet been defined due to individual variations, it could be said that the normal aspect is characterized by a regular capillary distribution of homogeneous size. This arrangement has been described as the "capillary comb" or "palisade" (Fig. 16.2). Subtle morphological alterations, such as tortuosity, are common and lack pathological value.

In healthy subjects, the capillary density, defined as the number of loops per surface unit, is 9–17 capillary per linear millimeter; at this level, the capillaries have their main axis parallel to the cutaneous surface, as has already been mentioned. Each papilla has 1–3 U-shaped or hairpin capillary loops, in which it is possible to visualize the erythrocyte column. The length of the loops varies between 200 and 400 μm.[6]

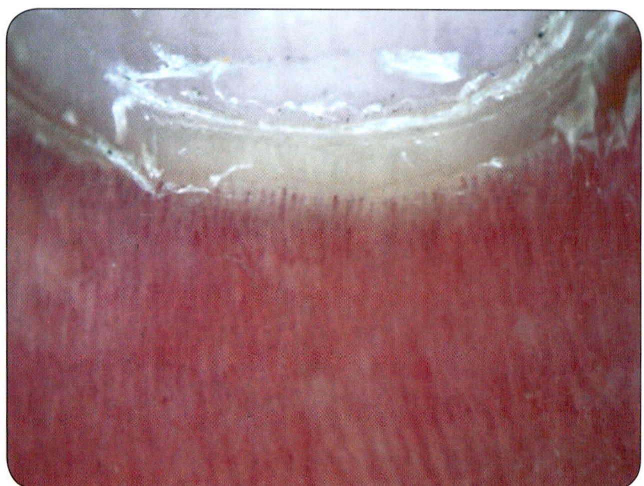

Fig. 16.2: Normal capillaroscopy with the typical "capillary comb" or "palisade" arrangement.

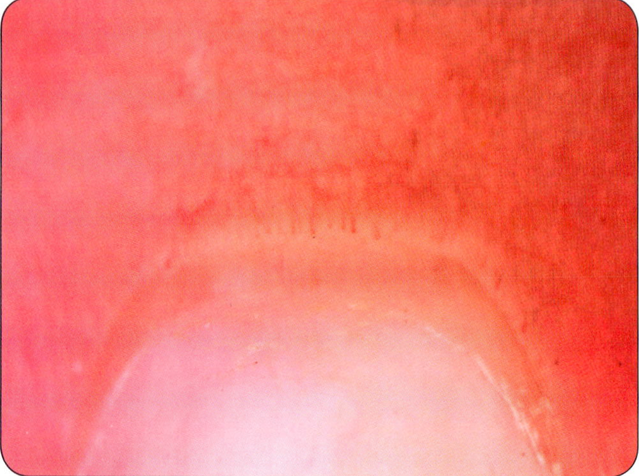

Fig. 16.3: Subpapillary plexus. Vessels with their main axis perpendicular to the capillaries.

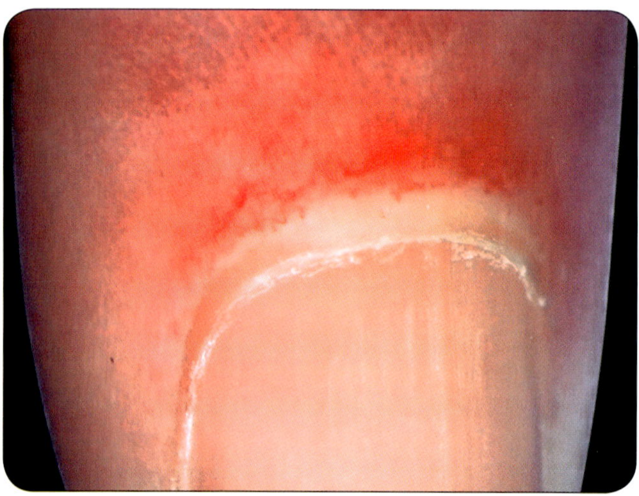

Fig. 16.4: Subpapillary plexus. Vessels with their main axis perpendicular to the capillaries.

Each capillary loop has three parts, an arterial afferent branch (A), around 5–20 μm diameter, and another one venous efferent (V), longer and thicker, which reaches 8-30 μm. Index V:A < 2.1. The transition or middle area corresponds to the union of the two. Both branches run parallel and straight, although some tortuosity is possible.[8]

The SP under the papillary dermis appears like a mesh or a network of larger vessels with their main axis perpendicular to the capillaries. In prepubers and elderly people, whose skin is more translucent, it is much more visible than in young adults, where it is clear in one-third of healthy population (Figs. 16.3 and 16.4).

There are interindividual variations depending on a number of specific factors such as age, race, sex, physical type, occupation, and differences between fingers of the same patient. For example, the capillaries of the second finger are shorter than those of the fourth and fifth fingers.[9]

In patients with dark skin or high phototypes, the cutaneous pigmentation absorbs much more light, decreasing visibility, which renders the technique impracticable.[1]

Manual laborers, due to constant microtraumatism, have a slightly modified capillaroscopic pattern, with tortuous capillaries or traumatic microhemorrhages, which are considered normal findings among them. Constant manicures and cuticle trimming are associated with the appearance of very short capillaries or multiple traumatic hemorrhages without pathological correlation.[10]

We have previously described personal variations, depending on the individual, but there are also external factors that may affect the results of this procedure. Among these, we must mention environmental temperature; the lower the temperature, the lower the number of capillaries, which may be mistaken for loss of capillaries or avascular areas.

The presence of nail polish traces may simulate inexistent hemorrhages, so it is recommended to suspend its application 15–21 days prior to NC.[8]

Lastly, smoking is forbidden to the patient, at least 2 hours prior to the study.[1]

In brief, in healthy subjects there may be isolated abnormalities concerning the distribution, morphology (Chart 16.1) and orientation of the capillaries, which must be taken into account to avoid interpretation mistakes.

Chart 16.1: Most frequent morphological variations in healthy individuals.

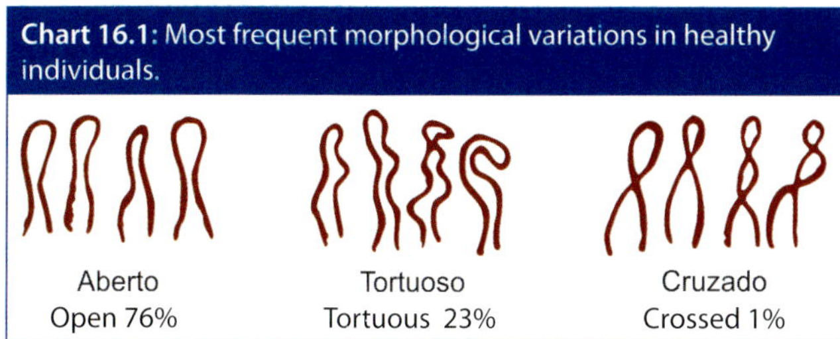

Aberto Open 76%	Tortuoso Tortuous 23%	Cruzado Crossed 1%

Adapted from da Silva LSM, Lima ARAG, Pucinelli MLC, et al. Capilaroscopia panorâmica periungueal e sua aplicação em doenças reumáticas. Rev Assoc Med Bras. 1997;43(1):69-73.

INDICATIONS

At present capillaroscopy is indicated in the following cases:

- To distinguish between primary and secondary RPs
- As adjuvant technique for the diagnosis of diseases such as SSc, SLE, DM, and MCTD
- For the differentiation between active and quiescent diseases
- For follow-up
- For prescription of treatment, dosage adjustment
- Because of its prognosis value (the presence of dilated capillaries in RP is highly indicative of evolution toward SSc).[3,5]

TECHNIQUE

Capillaroscopy is not the same on all fingers; on the contrary, the best results are obtained from the observation of the fourth and fifth fingers, owing to greater skin transparency. The nondominant hand is preferred because its capillaries are longer and the SP is more visible. No pressure must be placed on the skin, so as not to modify the image (Fig. 16.5). The optimal magnification is between 30× and 100×. The patients must feel comfortable and relaxed, their hands warm, to avoid mistakes.[11]

QUALITATIVE AND QUANTITATIVE CAPILLAROSCOPY

Although initially capillaroscopy consisted in a qualitative description, focusing on the morphological abnormalities of the capillaries, it is precisely in SSc and related disorders that its findings started to be quantified, in order to correlate them to the disease activity, its evolution and prognosis based on the involvement of the internal organs, etc.

In this manner, quantitative capillaroscopy was born more recently, focusing on the number and caliber of the capillaries besides their morphology; considering not only the loss of its normal architecture but also the extent of such destructuration; quantifying the number of microhemorrhages and megacapillaries rather than considering just their presence. All this makes it possible to find a capillaroscopic score, which is, in turn, useful for disease follow-up.[12,13]

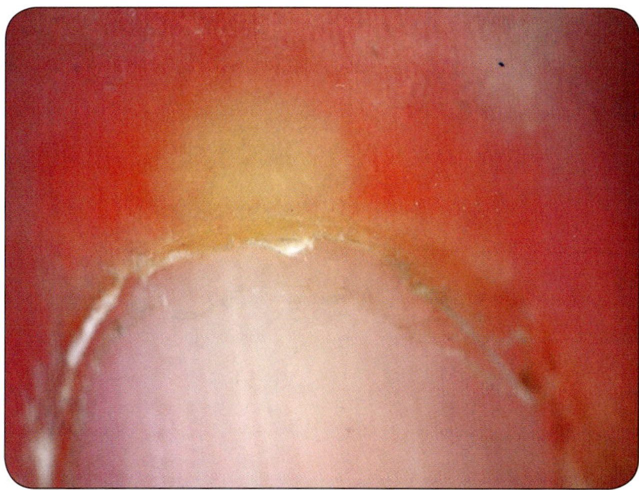

Fig. 16.5: Technique mistake.

MORPHOLOGICAL ALTERATIONS

In capillaroscopy, we can find changes in number, morphology, and architecture of the microcirculation.

The most frequent morphological alterations are tortuosity, homogeneous vasodilation, microhemorrhages and capillary thrombosis, and neoangiogenesis.[14]

Tortuosity

It is frequent in healthy subjects and has little diagnostic value, since the existence of tortuosity does not necessarily imply microcirculation alterations (Figs. 16.6 and 16.7).

Only when tortuosity appears in >20% of the capillaries, it is considered pathological and found in SSc and related disorders (MTCD and DM), SLE, and DbM.

It may be considered a sign of neoangiogenesis, e.g. in psoriasis.

Capillary Dilation

Normal and dilated capillaries may coexist within a papilla. A capillary diameter of >20 µm defines a dilated capillary, which, depending on shape, may be classified as *homogeneous* or *irregular*. Dilated capillaries may be found in multiple conditions such as SSc, DM, MTCD, RP, DbM, acrocyanosis, and hereditary hemorrhagic

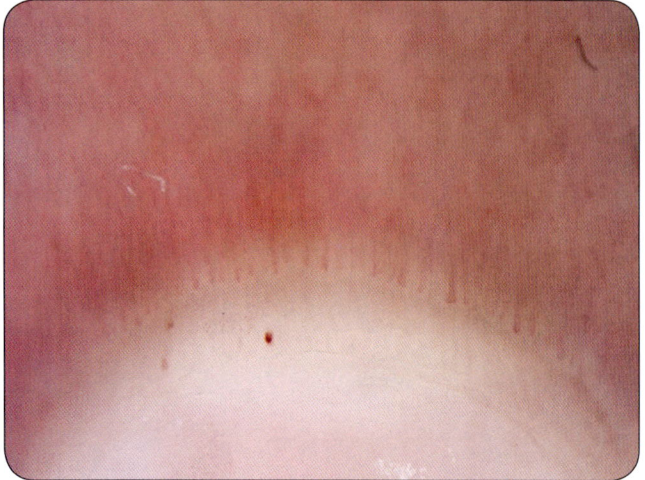

Fig. 16.6: Tortuosity.

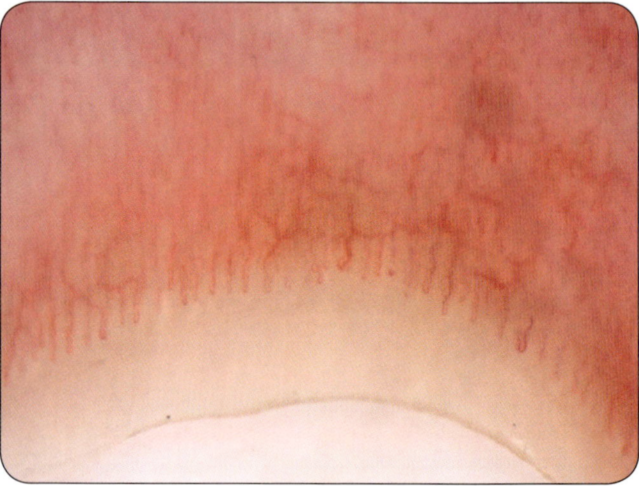

Fig. 16.7: Tortuosity. Subpapillary plexus visualization.

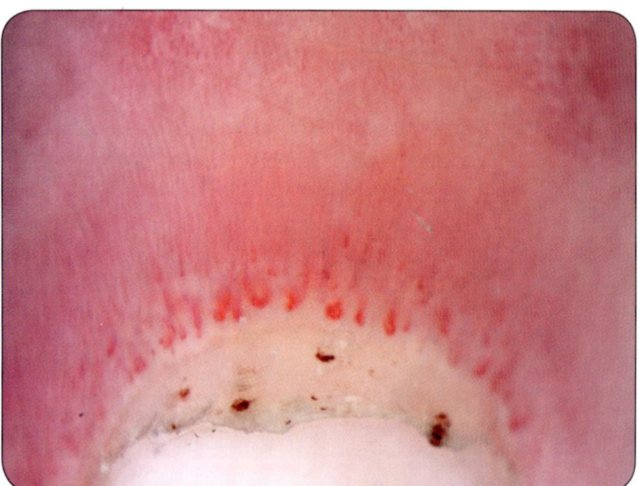

Fig. 16.8: Capillary dilation.

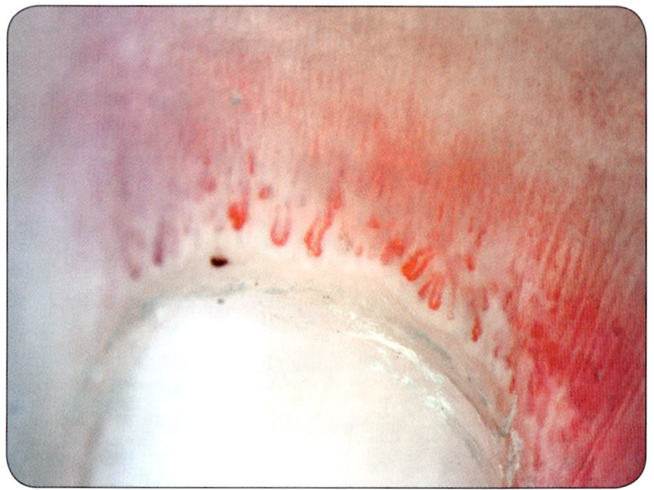

Fig. 16.9: Capillary dilation.

telangiectasia or Rendu Osler's disease, where, apart from variations in size, a wide range of capillary morphologies and orientations may be observed (Figs. 16.8 and 16.9).

A homogeneous enlargement of capillary diameter over 50 µm is known as megacapillary (Fig. 16.10); whereas within the irregular type there is the *microaneurysm*, which is the circumscribed enlargement in a capillary diameter.

Maricq et al. have put forward a classification of vasodilation in grades, where *grade 1* corresponds to no dilation whatsoever; *grade 2* to moderate dilation (4–10 times the regular diameter), and *grade 3* is >10 times the normal size or megacapillary.[15,16]

Megacapillaries are among the early alterations of the "scleroderma (SD) pattern", and in some cases the first manifestation of disease microvascular involvement, then followed by the other alterations composing this pattern.

Furthermore, their presence acquires a *predictive value* since in patients with RP whose capillaroscopy is almost normal, the isolated presence of two or more dilated capillaries in one or two digits or of a megacapillary is highly indicative of an evolution toward scleroderma with 83.1% sensitivity and 100% specificity.[9,17]

Microhemorrhages and Capillary Thrombosis

Microhemorrhages manifest capillary injury, whether post-trauma in normal subjects (manicure and onychophagia) or in patients with disorders within the scleroderma

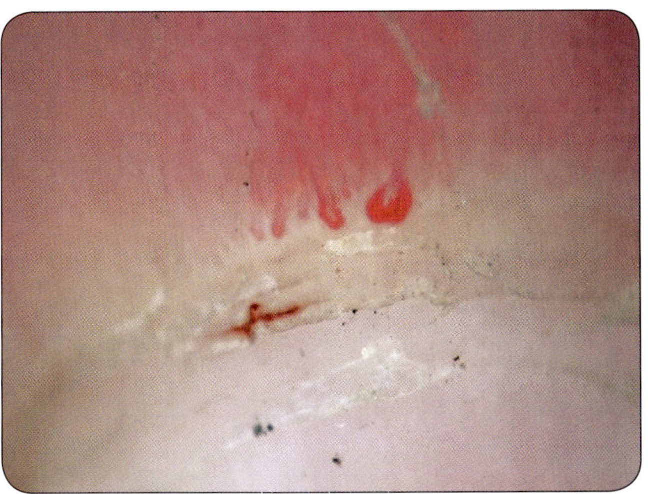

Fig. 16.10: Megacapillary.

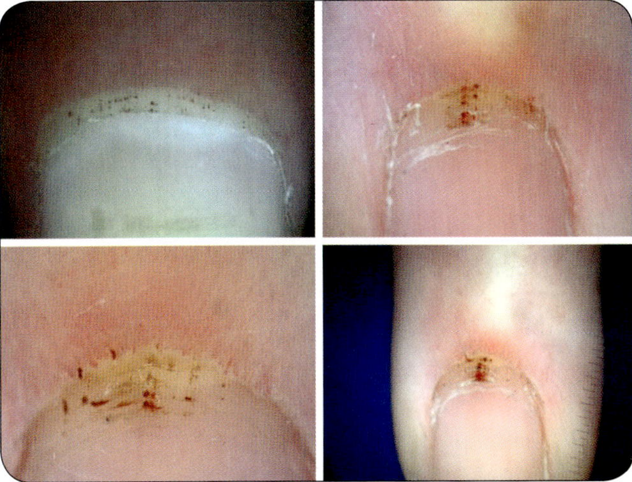

Fig. 16.11: Different examples of microhemorrhages.

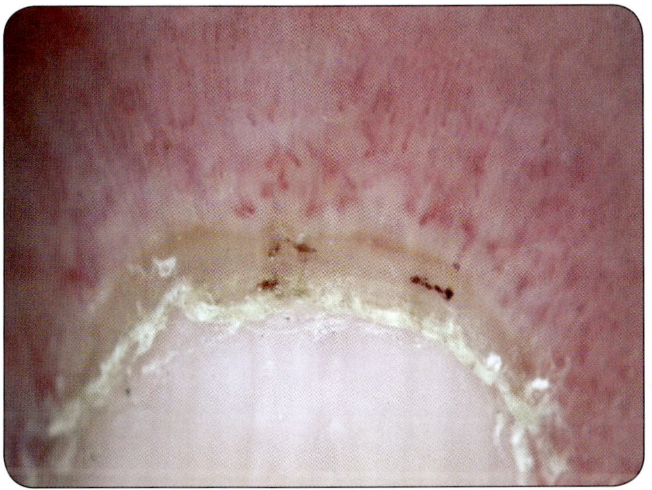

Fig. 16.12: Avascular areas. Neoangiogenesis at the periphery of the avascular areas. Neoformed vessels are thinner, more branched, and with different shapes.

spectrum, due to its close relation with the dilation of the capillary loops.

Capillary erythrocyte extravasation deposits inside the cuticle, distally to the compromised vessel. A "comb-like hemorrhage" has been described in antiphospholipid syndrome.

Both thrombosis and microhemorrhages are dark masses, but it is their shape that tells them apart. Recent hemorrhages have a crescent shape, as opposed to older ones, which are more rounded; besides, in thrombosis the dark stain resembles the shape of the capillary loop, which does not happen in hemorrhages (Fig. 16.11).[4]

Capillary Density

The regular number of capillaries is 9–17 per linear mm (10–30 per mm^2) in adults and 5–9 per mm in children. Fewer than 5 capillaries per mm is considered a decrease in capillary number.

The loss of capillaries correlates with the duration of the disease and this applies not only to SSc but also to DM, DbM, and HT.

If an area larger than 500 μm (0.5 mm) is affected by capillary loss, it is called "avascular area," a component of the SD pattern, which first insinuates in the active pattern, but is highly typical of the late one. Its presence has a prognostic value for progressive and more aggressive disease, involvement of the internal organs, etc., which makes it useful as a warning signal (Fig. 16.12). Avascular areas also represent the most important risk factor for the development of cutaneous ulcers (a frequent vascular complication of SSc), as much as for its healing and for the prescription of aggressive treatments to improve angiogenesis.[18]

Capillary Neoangiogenesis

It is defined by the presence of four or more capillary loops in one single dermal papillae and is one of the alterations present in the SD pattern, indicative of DM and MCTD, but also seen in DbM, psoriasis and cutaneous tumors. It may present in normal subjects, but in isolation.

Neoangiogenesis is usually found in the periphery of avascular areas, since it reflects an attempt at compensating capillary loss and is generally accompanied by some irregularity and increase in capillary size. The newly formed vessels (neoformed vessels) are thinner, more branched

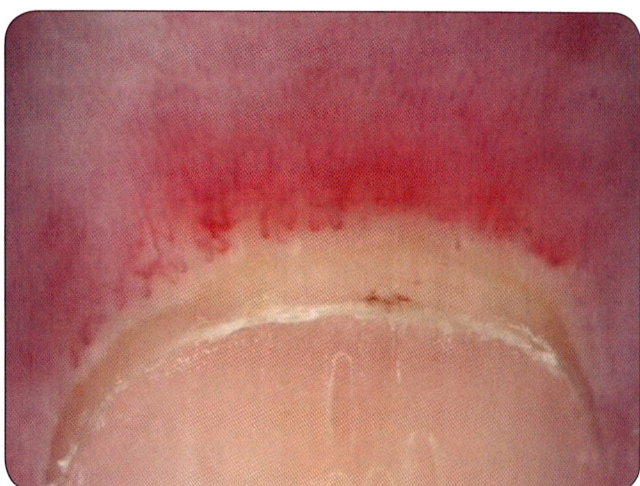

Fig. 16.13: Loss of architecture. Disorganization.

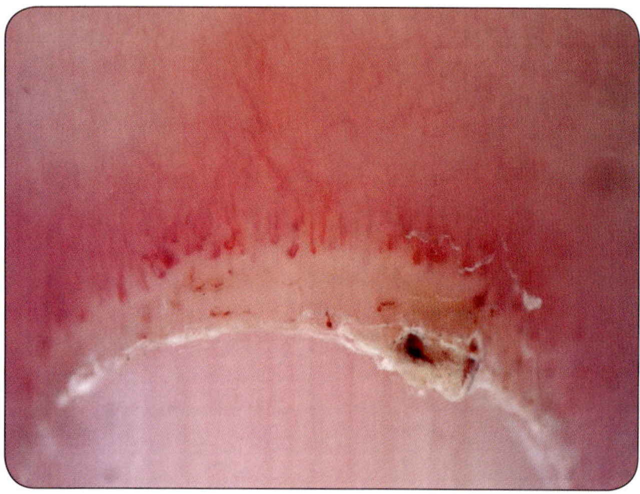

Fig. 16.14: Active scleroderma pattern.

and with different shapes, e.g., arborizing or "bushy capillary" in DM, glomerular, and corkscrew (*see* Fig. 16.12).

Loss of Architecture

It is the characteristic of advanced SSc and includes changes in capillary distribution, shape, diameter, and orientation axis. There is a clear polarity alteration, resulting in the disorganization of the normal order of the capillary bed (Fig. 16.13).[4]

SCLERODERMA PATTERN

The SD capillaroscopic pattern is considered a marker of vascular injury with a high positive predictive value (PPV) for the development of scleroderma, involvement of internal organs, etc. The sensitivity of the SSc classification criteria of the American College of Rheumatology increased from 67% to 99% with the recognition of the SD capillaroscopic pattern. There is a correlation between clinical manifestations, serologic markers, and capillaroscopy.[16]

Table 16.1: The SD pattern.

Pattern	*Predominant changes*	*Less prominent*
Early	Dilated capillaries and megacapillaries	Microhemorrhages
Active	Dilated capillaries, megacapillaries and microhemorrhages	Capillary loss
Late	Capillary loss, avascular areas, angiogenesis, ramification, disorganization	Dilation and megacapillaries

It takes into account the dilated capillaries and megacapillaries, microhemorrhages, avascular areas and angiogenesis, and ramified vessel.[19] Three evolutionary stages have been described according to which of these elements prevails in the capillaroscopic scenario (Table 16.1).[20]

- *Early SD pattern*: Prevalence of dilated and megacapillaries and few microhemorrhages
- *Active pattern*: Dilated and megacapillaries, frequent microhemorrhages and little capillary loss and onset of the loss of normal architecture. It has an evolving picture (Fig. 16.14)
- *Late pattern*: Severe capillary loss—extensive avascular areas, neoangiogenesis with arborizing capillaries and architectural disorganization.

Therefore, it is possible to infer that the longer the duration of the disease, the smaller the number of dilated capillaries and microhemorrhages.

Based on the SD capillaroscopic pattern, it is estimated that about ~15% of patients go from a primary RP (PRP) to a secondary RP (SRP) within 29.4 ± 10 months.[21]

Those patients with PRP who will develop SRP to SSc can be detected at present before the disease manifests clinically.[22] Moreover, in patients without any clinical sign of the disease, with typical SD capillaroscopic changes and positive antibodies, it is possible today to predict that 47% of patients will develop SSc within 5 years; 69% in 10 years, and 70% in 15 years.[23] In patients with an early pattern rapidly progressing to an active pattern, in approximately less than a year, close monitoring is recommended, since evidence suggests a high risk of progression to a late or advanced stage, which in turn correlates with clinical manifestations of SSc.[24]

Table 16.2: Capillaroscopic patterns.
Normal pattern:
• Regular palisade pattern
• Homogeneous distribution
• Normal density, no loss of capillaries.
SD pattern:
• Capillary dilation and megacapillaries
• Microhemorrhages
• Avascular areas.
SLE pattern:
• Tortuosity
• Elongation and curling of capillaries: "Meandering capillaries"
• Capillaries with dilation of afferent branch
• SP prominent.
Traumatic microangiopathy:
• Short capillaries
• Microhemorrhages.

(SD: Scleroderma; SLE: Systemic lupus erythematosus; SP: Subpapillary plexus).

CONSIDERATIONS FOR SPECIFIC PATHOLOGIES

The most validated capillaroscopic pattern is the SD pattern, but there are others, although not equally typical (Table 16.2). The SD pattern is a characteristic of different diseases, but it differs in the percentage of appearance in them:[4,19]

- 80–100% in SSc
- 55–100% in DM
- 25% polymyositis
- 40–80% MTCD.

Systemic Sclerosis

The SD pattern is characteristically found at different stages of the disease (Fig. 16.15). There is a correlation between plasma levels of endothelin-1 (ET-1), clinical manifestations [e.g. digital ulcers (DU)], and capillaroscopic changes (capillary density, ramified, and dilated capillaries) in these patients. The highest plasma levels for ET-1 were detected in the advanced stage or late SD pattern, characterized by loss of capillaries and important tissue fibrosis.[25]

Digital ulcers, present in 50% of scleroderma patients, are the cause of high morbidity, limitation, and impact the quality of life, with pain and discomfort, demanding local and systemic treatment. Recently, the capillaroscopic skin ulcer risk index has been validated as a useful tool to predict the development of new ulcers and/or persistence of unhealed lesions, within 3 months of capillaroscopic evaluation, with statistically significant sensitivity, specificity, and PPV.[26,27]

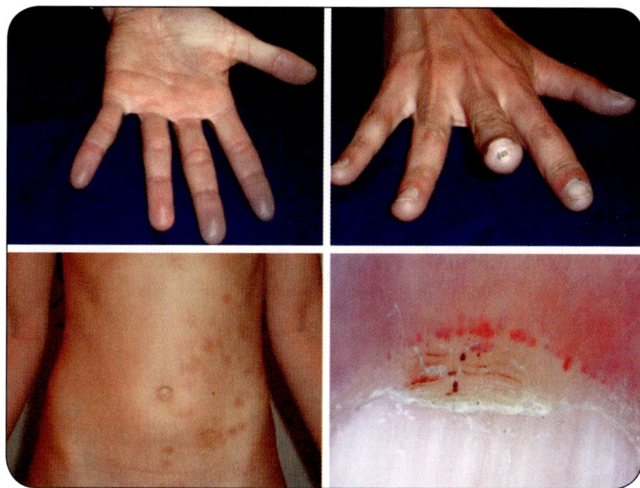

Fig. 16.15: Patient with systemic sclerosis, Raynaud´s phenomenon, digital ulcers, cutaneous involvement, and capillaroscopic scleroderma pattern.

Dermatomyositis

It has an SD pattern indistinguishable from SSc, although according to some authors, the changes in morphology and architecture are not only as significant as in SSc but also faster and more progressive, especially as regards microhemorrhages, avascular areas, and angiogenesis. However, no relevant differences from SSc were found with reference to homogeneous dilation and megacapillaries (Fig. 16.16).[28]

As regards angiogenesis, the presence of "bushy capillaries" or neoformed capillaries with arborizing shape is the characteristic of this disease (Fig. 16.17).[29,30] Finally, it is noteworthy that capillaroscopic changes reflect disease activity, and a correlation has been found between muscle involvement, phosphocreatine kinase serum values, and capillary loss, as opposed to microhemorrhages, which were associated with cutaneous lesions. The capillary dilation, microhemorrhages, and the capillary loss decreased after treatment.[31]

Systemic Lupus Erythematous

In 50% of lupus patients, capillaroscopic findings have SLE pattern, and in 73.3% of cases the antinuclear antibodies

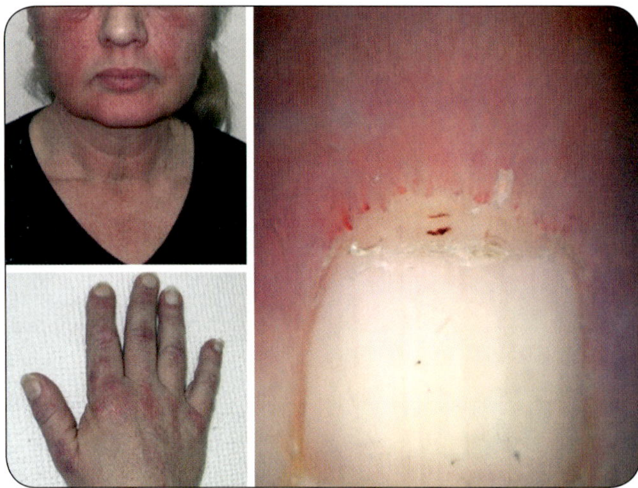

Fig. 16.16: Patient with dermatomyositis. Erythema on the face and anterior neck. Gottron papules on the dorsum of the hand. Scleroderma pattern with dilated capillaries and microhemorrhages.

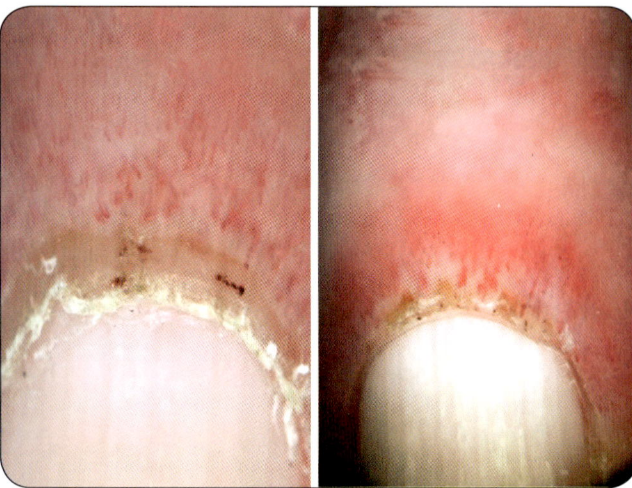

Fig. 16.17: Dermatomyositis. Capillaroscopic scleroderma pattern with avascular areas and neoformed vessels.

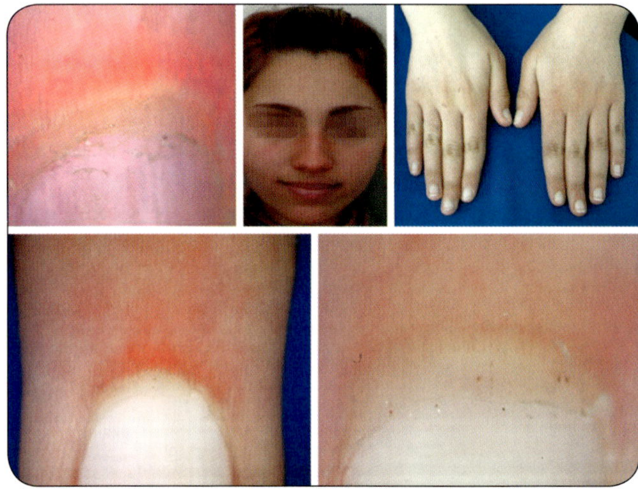

Fig. 16.18: Patient with systemic lupus erythematosus. Loss of the most distal line of capillaries. Malar erythema. Raynaud´s phenomenon. Dilated capillaries, elongated and tortuous, subpapillary plexus visualization.

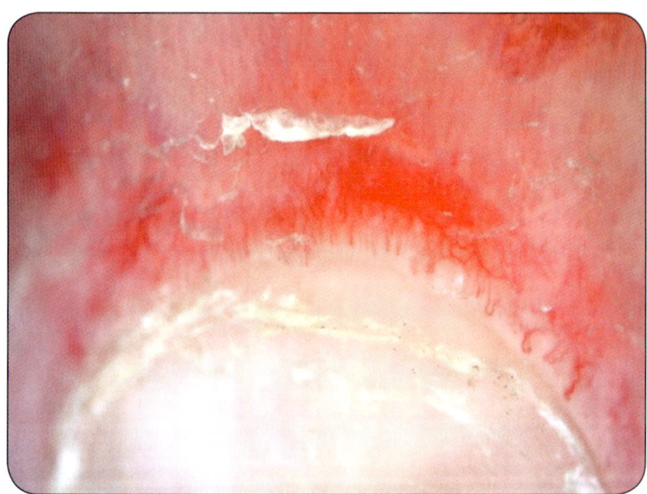

Fig. 16.19: Systemic lupus erythematosus. Loss of the most distal line of capillaries, dilated capillaries, elongated and tortuous, subpapillary plexus visualization, and meandering capillaries.

are positive. In 30% of cases, capillaroscopy is nonspecific; next in frequency comes SD pattern in 13.3% of cases, and lastly, for 6.6% cases the pattern is normal (Fig. 16.18).[19]

The characteristic SLE pattern consists in dilated capillaries, elongated, and tortuous, some of them crossing each other or "meandering"' (a combined effect of waving and curling) and others arborized (Fig. 16.19). Also, in this disease, SP may be prominent, and the afferent branch may be highly dilated. The absence of the most distal line of capillaries has also been described.[4,32]

In a study, it was observed that out of 30 lupus patients, 80% had dilated capillaries, and 6.6% were megacapillaries, while 43% were elongated. Tortuous capillaries were recorded in 70% of cases and SP was prominent in 60% cases. Finally, microhemorrhages were present in 16.6% of studied cases.[19]

An interrelation has been detected in patients with SLE between clinical activity (Systemic Lupus Erythematosus Disease Activity Index), capillaroscopic score, and vascular endothelial activation markers [vascular endothelial

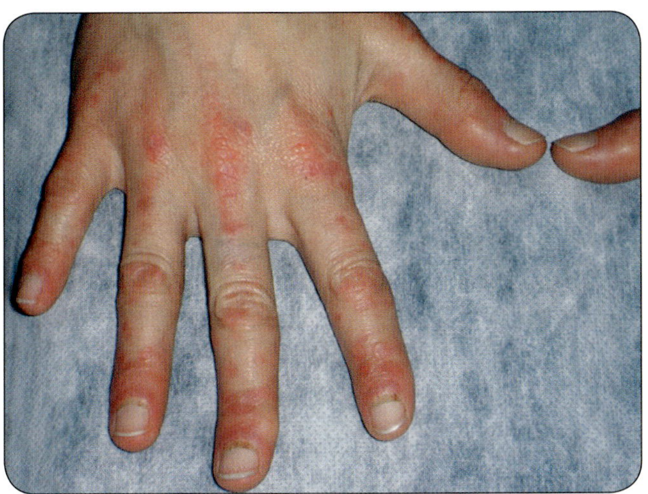

Fig. 16.20: Patient with mixed connective tissue disease.

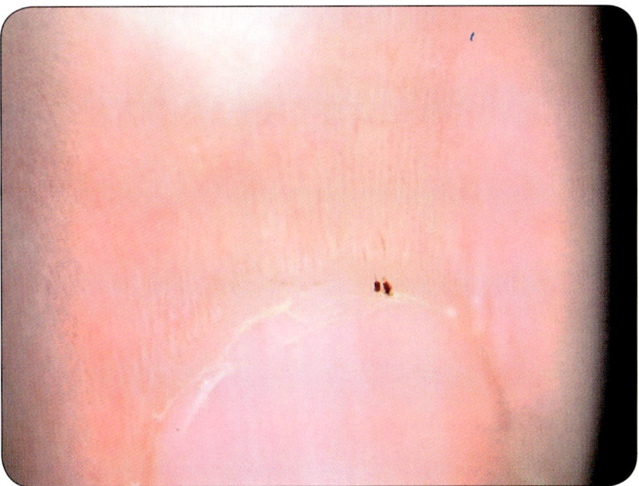

Fig. 16.21: Dilated capillaries on an edematous background and microhemorrhages.

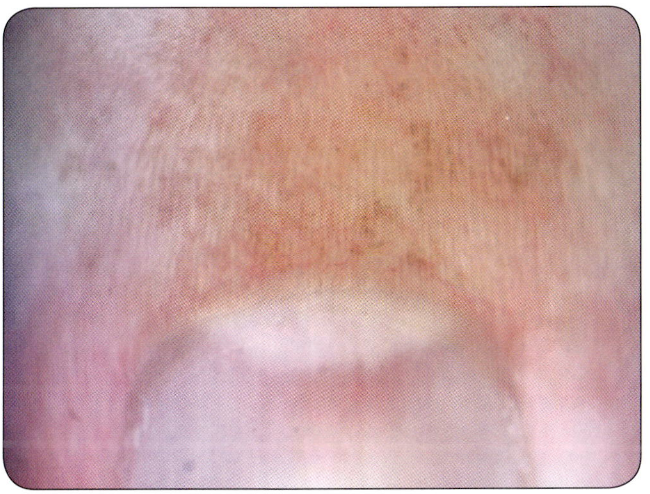

Fig. 16.22: Capillaroscopy in a patient with rheumatoid arthritis: visualization of the subpapillary plexus on a light background.

growth factor (VEGF), ET-1, sTM, and sE-selectina].[33] In a study including 80 patients with SLE, 92.5% cases had capillaroscopic alterations. In 41.25% cases, capillaroscopy was almost normal or presenting slight changes, and in 58.75% cases, the changes observed were mild/severe.[34]

The higher the lupus activity index, the more active the endothelial markers (VEGF) and the higher the capillaroscopic score.[35]

Mixed Connective Tissue Disease

In almost 40% of cases, capillaroscopic changes correspond to SD pattern, while in the rest, the changes are rather nonspecific.[19] The more active the disease, the more the capillaroscopic changes are observed, like arborizing capillaries similar to those of DM (Figs. 16.20 and 16.21).[4,36-38]

Rheumatoid Arthritis (RA)

The most common capillaroscopic image consists in the visualization of the SP on a light background, due to the presence of edema (Fig. 16.22). Capillaries may be tortuous and dilated.

Out of 62 RA patients, 30.6% presented with RP. With regard to the capillaroscopic pattern, SP was prominent in 69% cases, while 58% cases showed elongated capillaries. In 14.5% cases, the capillaroscopic pattern corresponded to scleroderma-like pattern or SD pattern.[39]

Psoriasis

In this case too, SP visualization is a main finding too, but also the capillaries are shorter and their number increased.[40]

Diabetes

Microvascular involvement results in lower density of capillaries with diminished blood flow.[4]

CONCLUSION

Nailfold capillaroscopy is a procedure yields a fast,innocuous, and affordable diagnosis, which reaches extremely high levels of sensitivity and specificity in diseases such as RP and SSc. It also has prognostic value and contributes to a therapeutic response follow-up. Patients with this kind of diseases demand an interdisciplinary team, in which dermatologists, rheumatologists, and clinicians may count on this very helpful technique. It is important to know the capillaroscopic patterns to acquire and transmit a common language among physicians from different specializations for the benefit of our patients.

REFERENCES

1. Clavaguera T, Reyner P. Capilaroscopia en el sujeto sano. Semin Fund Esp Reumatol. 2010;10(Supl 1):11-3.
2. Martínez Sánchez FG. Historia de la capilaroscopía. Semin Fund Esp Reumatol. 2010;11(Supl 1):3-4.
3. Cutolo M, Sulli A, Smith V. How to perform and interpret capillaroscopy. Best Pract Res Clin Rheumatol. 2013;27(2):237-48.
4. Leroux MB. Actualización: *Capilaroscopia* y Videocapilaroscopia su utilidad para el Dermatólogo Práctico. *PIEL-LATINOAMERICANA* 17/04/2009 -AÑO IX- EDICION 337 |Septiembre, 06 - 2013.
5. Dogan S, Akdogan A, Atakan N. Nailfold capillaroscopy in systemic sclerosis: Is there any difference between videocapillaroscopy and dermatoscopy? Skin Res Technol. 2013;19 (4):446-9.
6. Bergman R, Sharony L, Schapira D, et al. The handheld dermatoscope as a nail-fold capillaroscopic instrument. Arch Dermatol. 2003;139:1027-30.
7. Muroi E, Hara T, Yanaba K, et al. A portable dermatoscope for easy, rapid examination of periungual nailfold capillary changes in patients with systemic sclerosis. Rheumatol Int. 2011;31(12):1601-6.
8. da Silva LSM, Lima ARAG, Pucinelli MLC, et al. Capilaroscopia panorâmica periungueal e sua aplicação em doenças reumáticas. Rev Assoc Med Bras. 1997;43(1):69-73.
9. Petry DG, Terreri MT, Len CA, et al. Nailfold capillaroscopy in children and adolescents with rheumatic diseases. Acta Reumatol Port. 2008;33(4):395-400.
10. Carreira PE. ¿Es realmente útil la capilaroscopia? Semin Fund Esp Reumatol. 2010;11(Supl 1):1-2.
11. Sormani de Fonseca ML, Ríos C. Capilaroscopia. Ed. Producere McDowell S.A. Septiembre 2000.
12. Herrick AL, Moore TL, Murray AK, et al. Nailfold capillary abnormalities are associated with anti-centromere antibody and severity of digital ischaemia. Rheumatology (Oxford). 2010;49:1776-82.
13. Herrick AL, Cutolo M. Clinical implications from capillaroscopic analysis in patients with Raynaud's phenomenon and systemic sclerosis. Arthritis Rheum. 2010;62:595-604.
14. Grassi W, Del Medico P. Atlas of Capillaroscopy. Ed. EDRA. Mayo; 2004.
15. Maricq HR. Widefield capillary microscopy. Technique and rating scale for abnormalities seen in scleroderma and related disorders. Arthritis Rheum. 1981;24(9):1159-65.
16. Cutolo M, Pizzorni C, Secchi ME, et al. Capillaroscopy. Best Pract Res Clin Rheumatol. 2008;22(6):1093-108.
17. Secchi ME, Sulli A, Grollero M, et al. Role of videocapillaroscopy in early detection of transition from primary to secondary Raynaud's phenomenon in systemic sclerosis. Reumatismo. 2008;60(2):102-7.
18. Alivernini S, De Santis M, Tolusso B, et al. Skin ulcers in systemic sclerosis: determinants of presence and predictive factors of healing. J Am Acad Dermatol. 2009;60(3):426-35.
19. Lambova SN, Müller-Ladner U. Capillaroscopic pattern in systemic lupus erythematosus and undifferentiated connective tissue disease: what we still have to learn? Rheumatol Int. 2013;33(3):689-95.
20. Cutolo M, Sulli A, Pizzorni C, et al. Nailfold videocapillaroscopy assessment of microvascular damage in systemic sclerosis. J Rheumatol. 2000;27:155-60.
21. Ingegnoli F, Boracchi P, Gualtierotti R, et al. Prognostic model based on nailfold capillaroscopy for identifying Raynaud's phenomenon patients at high risk for the development of a scleroderma spectrum disorder: PRINCE (prognostic index for nailfold capillaroscopic examination). Arthritis Rheum. 2008;58(7):2174-82.
22. Olivé A, García-Melchor E. On Raynaud's phenomenon. Med Clin. 2010;134(10):470.
23. Cutolo M, Smith V. State of the art on nailfold capillaroscopy: a reliable diagnostic tool and putative biomarker in rheumatology? Reumatology. 2013;52(11):1933-40.
24. Sulli A, Pizzorni C, Smith V, et al. Timing of transition between capillaroscopic patterns in systemic sclerosis. Arthritis Rheum. 2012;64(3):821-5.
25. Sulli A, Soldano S, Pizzorni C, et al. Raynaud's phenomenon and plasma endothelin: correlations with capillaroscopic patterns in systemic sclerosis. J Rheumatol. 2009;36 (6):1235-9.
26. Sebastiani M, Manfredi A, Lo Monaco A, et al. Capillaroscopic Skin Ulcers Risk Index (CSURI) calculated with different videocapillaroscopy devices: how its predictive values change. Clin Exp Rheumatol. 2013;31(2 Suppl 76):115-7.
27. Sebastiani M, Manfredi A, Vukatana G, et al. Predictive role of capillaroscopic skin ulcer risk index in systemic sclerosis: a multicentre validation study. Ann Rheum Dis. 2012;71(1): 67-70.
28. De Angelis R, Cutolo M, Gutierrez M, et al. Different microvascular involvement in DM and SS. A preliminary study by a tight videocapillaroscopic assessment. Clin Exp Rheumatol. 2012;30(2 Suppl 71):S67-70.
29. Silver RM, Maricq HR. Childhood dermatomyositis: serial microvascular studies. Pediatrics. 1989;83(2):278-83.
30. Maricq HR, LeRoy EC, D´angelo WA, et al. Diagnostic potential of in vivo capillary microscopy in scleroderma and related disorders. Arthritis Rheum. 1980;23(2):183-9.
31. De Angelis R, Cutolo M, Gutierrez M, et al. Association between nail-fold capillary findings and disease activity in DM. Rheumatology (Oxford). 2011;50(6):1091-8.
32. Kuryliszyn-Moskal A, Ciolkiewicz M, Klimiuk PA, et al. Clinical significance of nailfold capillaroscopy in systemic lupus erythematosus: correlation with endothelial cell activation markers and disease activity. Scand J Rheumatol. 2009;38(1):38-45.
33. Ciolkiewicz M, Kuryliszyn-Moskal A, Klimiuk PA. Analysis of correlations between selected endothelial cell activation markers, disease activity, and nailfold capillaroscopy microvascular changes in systemic lupus erythematosus patients. Clin Rheumatol. 2010;29(2):175-80.

34. Ingegnoli F. Capillaroscopy abnormalities in relation to disease activity in juvenile systemic lupus erythematosus. Microvasc Res. 2013;87:92-4.
35. Moneib HA, Salem SA, Aly DG, et al. Assessment of serum vascular endothelial growth factor and nail fold capillaroscopy changes in systemic lupus erythematosus with and without cutaneous manifestations. J Dermatol. 2012;39(1):52-7.
36. Nagy Z, Czirják L. Nailfold digital capillaroscopy in 477 patients with connective tissue disease and Raynaud´s disease. *J* Eur Acad Dermatol Venereol. 2004;18:62-8.
37. Belini MA. Fenómeno de Raynaud. Rev Arg Reumatol. 2004;15 (1):19-39.
38. Leroux MB, Rinaldi M, Palatnik S, et al. Raynaud primario y secundario a síndromes esclerodermiformes. Comunicación de 97 pacientes estudiados por capilaroscopía periungueal. Arch Argent Dermatol. 2000;50:15-9.
39. Lambova SN, Müller-Ladner U. Capillaroscopic pattern in inflammatory arthritis. Microvasc Res. 2012;83(3):318-22.
40. Bhushan M, Moore T, Herrick AL, et al. Nailfold video capillaroscopy in psoriasis. Br J Dermatol. 2000;142:1171-6.

REFLECTANCE CONFOCAL MICROSCOPY

17

Giovanni Pellacani, Caterina Longo, Elvira Moscarella

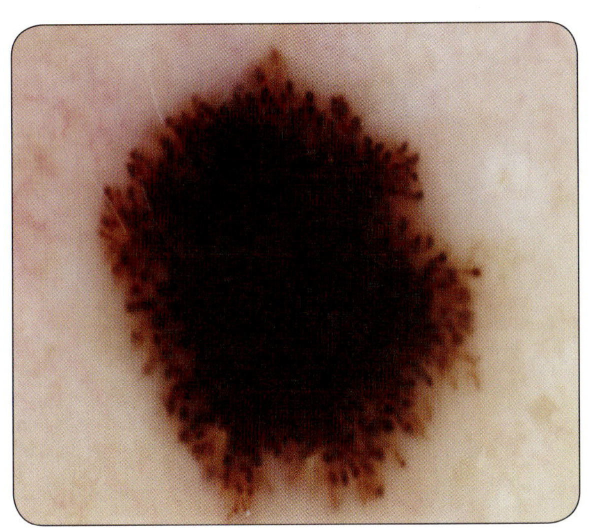

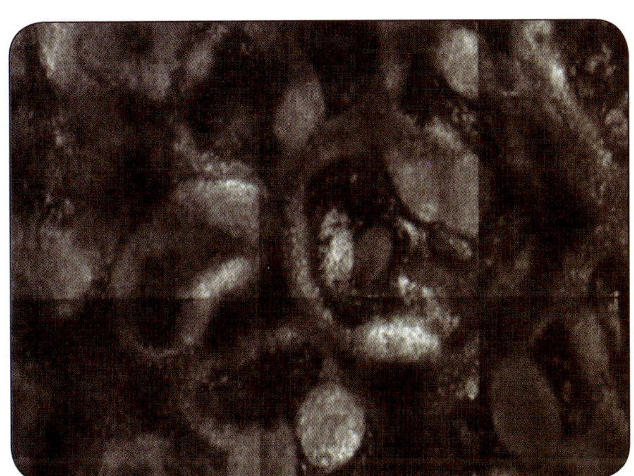

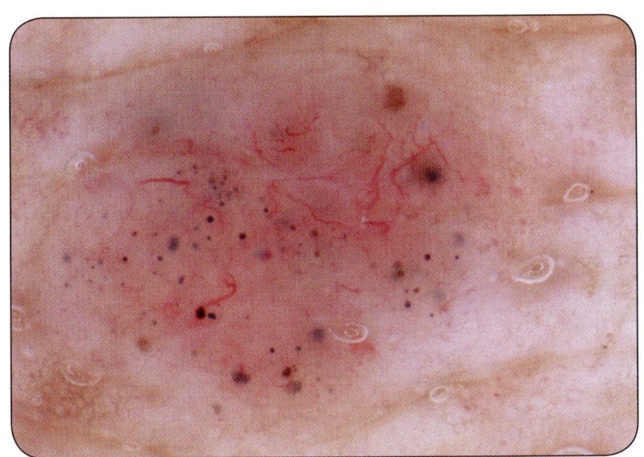

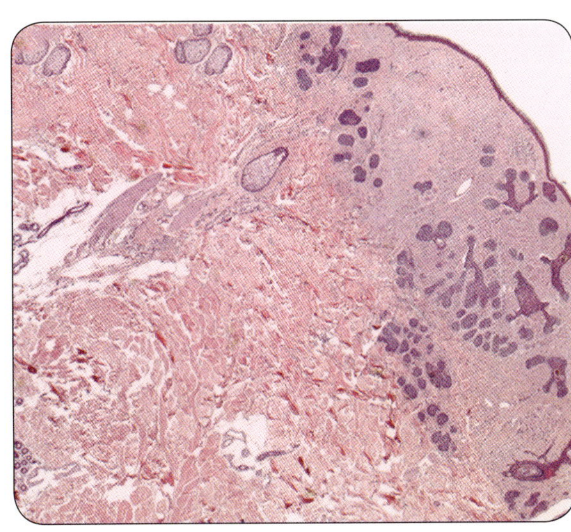

"Reflectance confocal microscopy (RCM) is a noninvasive imaging technique that produces horizontal images of the skin in a cellular level resolution and in real time.
This instrument uses a diode laser with a nearinfrared wavelength of 830 nm that penetrates the skin up to a depth of 200–300 μm, which corresponds to the superficial dermis.
The construction of the images is dependent on the refractive index of the tissue, which changes according to its chemical and molecular structures.
The refractive structures, such as melanin, keratin, collagen fibers, inflammatory cells, and blood cells, appear in white color with different degrees of intensity on the gray-scale, melanin and melanosomes being the most important sources of contrast."

17. 1 THE UTILITY OF CONFOCAL MICROSCOPY IN THE DIAGNOSIS OF SUPERFICIAL SPREADING MELANOMA

Giovanni Pellacani, Nathalie De Carvalho

Melanoma is the most worrisome skin tumor and its early diagnosis reflects on a higher rate of survival, remaining the main key to guarantee a lower risk of mortality. Dermoscopy enhances the diagnosis of melanoma but, in early stages, specific dermoscopic patterns may lack.[1-3]

Reflectance confocal microscopy (RCM) is a noninvasive imaging technique that produces horizontal images of the skin in a cellular level resolution and in real time. This instrument uses a diode laser with a near-infrared wavelength of 830 nm that penetrates the skin up to a depth of 200–300 μm, which corresponds to the superficial dermis. The construction of the images is dependent on the refractive index of the tissue, which changes according to its chemical and molecular structures. In RCM, the refractive structures, such as melanin, keratin, collagen fibers, inflammatory cells, and blood cells, appear in white color with different degrees of intensity on the grayscale, melanin and melanosomes being the most important sources of contrast.[4] An excellent applicability of RCM is in the field of dermoscopically difficult-to-diagnose melanocytic lesions improving the diagnostic accuracy of melanoma and reducing the number of excisions of benign melanocytic lesions.[5] Classically, lesions are analyzed in three different layers: epidermis, dermal-epidermal junction (DEJ), and papillary dermis.

In the study of melanocytic lesions, some considerations must be taken regarding the classification of confocal patterns for each of the three layers evaluated. In the epidermis (stratum spinosum/granulosum), regularity and pigmentation of keratinocytes and the presence of atypical melanocytes (pagetoid cells) will be evaluated. Keratinocytes are seen as polygonal cells with a dark central nucleus and bright cytoplasm (honeycombed pattern) or as polygonal bright cells fulfilled with melanin (cobblestone pattern), the last being present in more pigmented lesions. Normal melanocytes are usually not distinguishable from pigmented keratinocytes at the basal layer, but clustered melanocytes into melanocytic nests are detectable both at the junction and in the upper dermis in melanocytic nevi. Atypical melanocytes, usually detectable in melanoma, are large cells (usually at least twice the size of keratinocyte) with a dark central nucleus and a bright periphery corresponding to high refractive cytoplasm. Shape could be roundish, dendritic, or pleomorphic, usually presenting enlarged thick dendrites or stellate to bizarre shapes with long dendritic arborization (Figs. 17.1A to C).

The RCM aspects in superficial spreading melanoma **and Differential Diagnosis with Benign Melanocytic**

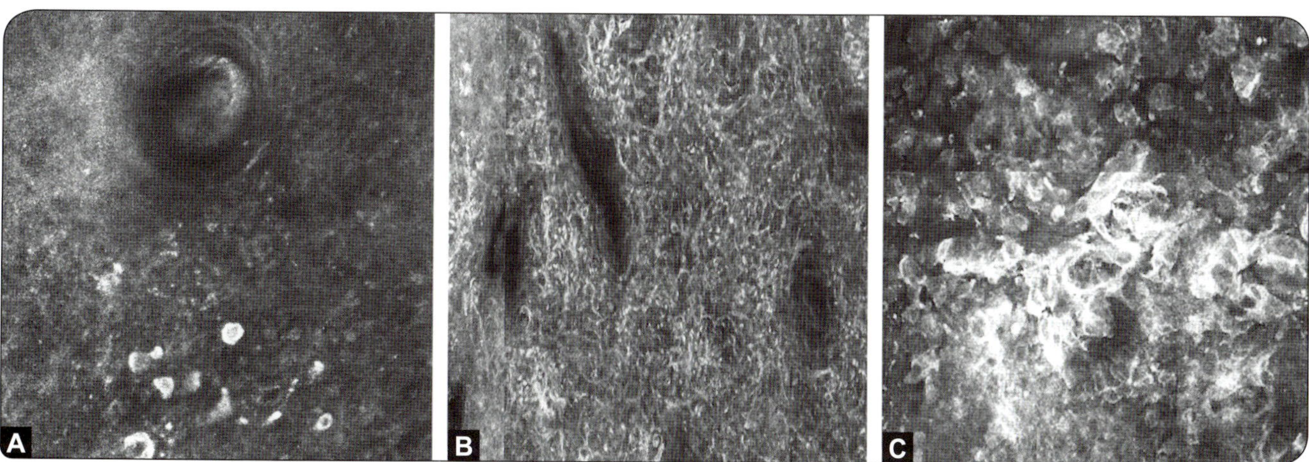

Figs. 17.1A to C: Reflectance confocal microscopy of the granular/spinous layer in melanomas presenting different shapes and sizes of atypical melanocytes infiltrating epidermis in a pagetoid fashion. (A) Presence of roundish pagetoid cells represented by bright large well-defined polygonal structures with a dark central portion corresponding to the nucleus. (B) Presence of a pagetoid infiltration constituted by dendritic cells. Cell body is barely visible, whereas all epidermis looks characterized by bright tangled lines corresponding to the dendritic branches of melanocytes. (C) Pleomorphic pagetoid cells. Some look roundish, others present short-thickened dendrites, stellate, and bizarre shapes.

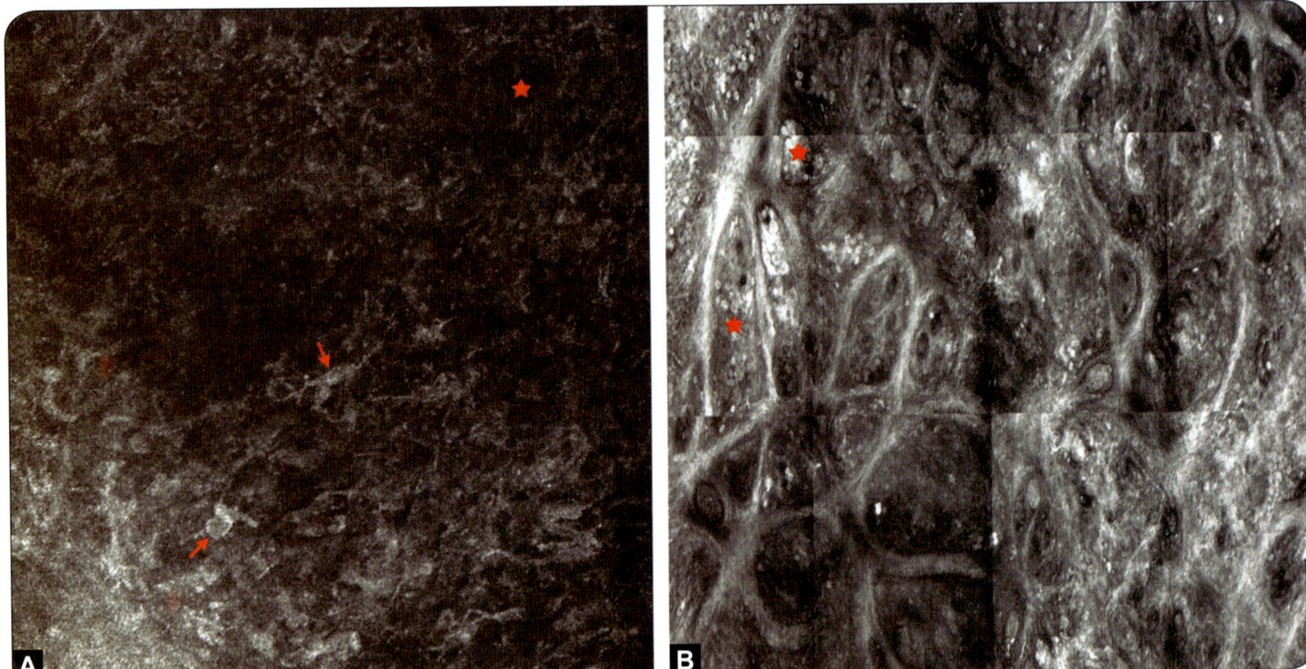

Figs. 17.2A and B: Reflectance confocal microscopy of a superficial spreading melanoma. (A) Epidermal layer altered by the presence of numerous pleomorphic cells (arrows). (B) Irregular architecture at dermal–epidermal junction with papillae infiltrated by large aggregates of atypical cells, and areas of architectural disarrangement (stars).

Lesions. In the last decades, the importance of RCM for the diagnosis and classification of melanomas into subtypes have been developed.[6] Reflectance confocal microscopy is able to detect early melanomas when differential diagnosis with benign melanocytic proliferations is still difficult upon clinical and dermoscopic examinations. Overall, upon RCM the most relevant criteria for melanoma diagnosis are epidermal disarrangement with pagetoid cells (mainly when those cells are roundish and show a widespread distribution), atypical cells in the DEJ, altered junctional architecture (resulting in the so-called nonedged papillae pattern), atypical cells aggregated into irregular/dishomogeneous nests (Figs. 17.2A and B).[5]

According to the melanoma progression model, the architecture of the junction is progressively disarranged by the intraepidermal accumulation of malignant melanocytes in single cells and/or in nests, and subsequent alterations lead to the microinvasion of the superficial dermis, followed by nodular proliferation characterized by vertical growth and deep tumor invasion.[7]

Upon confocal microscopy, different predominant aspects can be observed in melanomas. Overall four different subtypes of melanomas have been described, namely "pagetoid melanoma," "dendritic cell melanoma", "large clustered melanoma," and "mixed type." Each subtype resulted characterized by a predominant cellular population, also correlated with patient's phenotypic aspects and sun behavior. "Pagetoid melanoma" and "dendritic cell melanoma," in fact, corresponded to predominant intraepidermal proliferations of malignant cells and thus they usually corresponded to superficial spreading melanoma (SSM) type upon histopathologic examination, except for lesions located on the face that were frequently classified as lentigo maligna and lentigo maligna melanomas. On the other hand, "large-clustered melanoma" usually corresponded to nodular type, and in the case of histopathologic classification into SSM, nodular component, and vertical growth pattern was always predominant. "Mixed type" represents a combination of the three subtypes, with no predominance of a single pattern.[6]

Thus, RCM characterization of SSM can be summarized into two main categories, joined by the predominant intraepidermal and junctional proliferation.

PAGETOID MELANOMA

Pagetoid melanoma is characterized upon RCM by the presence of numerous roundish and or polygonal cell proliferation as single cells, mainly detectable within the

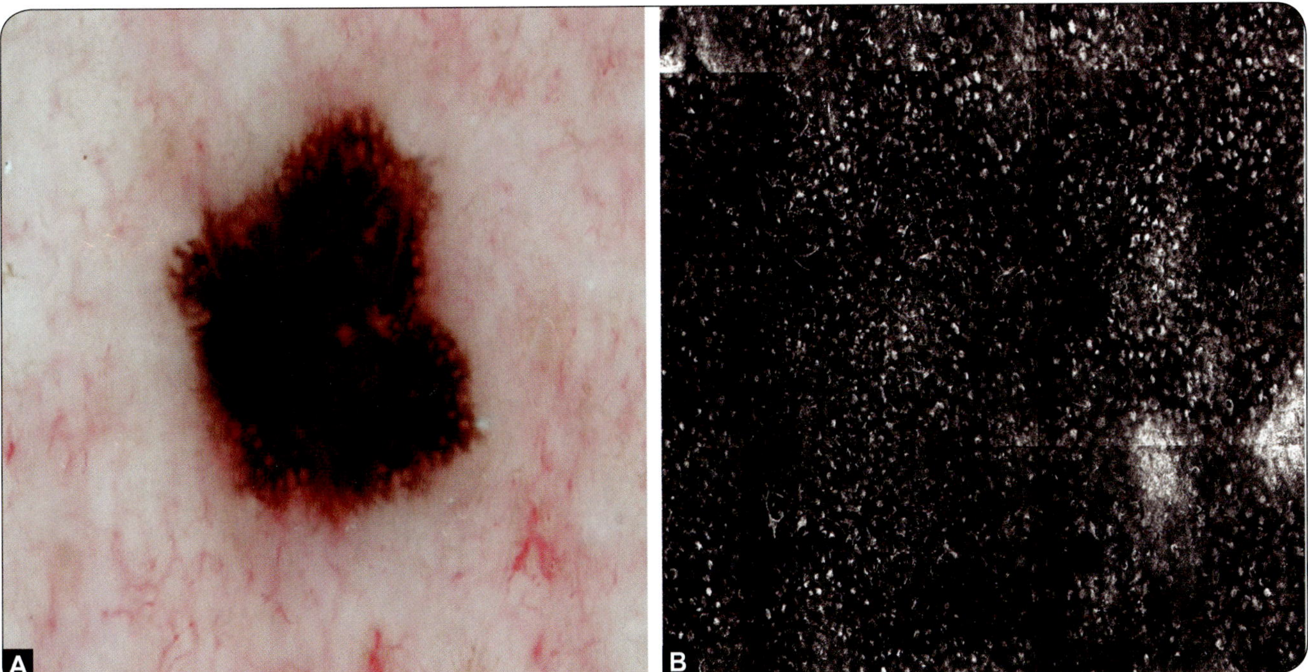

Figs. 17.3A and B: Superficial spreading melanoma, in situ. (A) Upon dermoscopy, atypical network in the periphery and a central dark brown-to-black structureless pattern. (B) Reflectance confocal microscopy at the level of the epidermis showing numerous predominantly roundish pagetoid cells, widespread throughout the entire epidermis.

epidermis in a pagetoid fashion (Figs. 17.3A and B) or proliferating at the DEJ, with a tendency to form irregular clusters (Figs. 17.4A and B), sometimes infiltrating the dermal papillae. This uneven cell proliferation is responsible for the disarrangement of the junctional architecture.

From a clinical point of view, pagetoid melanoma usually appears in adults with many nevi and intermittent solar exposure. In the early stage, during the radial growth phase, atypical melanocytes are still confined to the epidermis. Lesions are usually dark and flat (or slightly elevated), and in dermoscopy, atypical reticular and/or globular pattern, and structureless areas are commonly present.

Due to its clinical-dermoscopic presentation, pagetoid melanoma in its early phase represents a difficult differential diagnosis with atypical/dysplastic nevus. Reflectance confocal microscopy showed the possibility of improving diagnostic accuracy in these lesions.[8] Histopathologic grading of dysplasia resulted correlated with RCM cytoarchitectural disorder. In mild dysplastic nevi, RCM shows few roundish pagetoid cells at the epidermal layer and at the level of the DEJ, which are characteristically located in the center of the lesion. The architecture of the DEJ is slightly irregular with the predominance of elongated nests in the center of the lesion and an overall ringed pattern at the periphery. When atypical cells are pleomorphic and widespread, and disarrangement of the architecture is marked, those lesions can be classified as severely dysplastic nevi upon histopathology, but melanoma cannot be ruled out upon RCM, thus excision is recommended.[4,8]

According to melanoma progression, tumor growth can switch from radial to vertical phases, with deep invasion of the dermis. At this moment, lesions are clinically palpable or present a nodular component, and several dermoscopic patterns characteristic of melanoma are usually visible. Upon RCM, along with numerous roundish to pleomorphic cells into the epidermis, marked alterations of the DEJ and irregular and dishomogeneous clusters of atypical melanocytes, sometimes fulfilling dermal papillae, are visible. On histology, remodeling and flattening of the DEJ, and proliferation of malignant melanocytes at the junction and in the dermis are present.[9]

DENDRITIC CELL TYPE MELANOMA

In this type of melanoma, the following RCM features are present: Epidermal disarray with melanocytic infiltration mainly composed of dendritic atypical cells (Figs. 17.5A and B) and at the DEJ presence of edged and/or nonedged

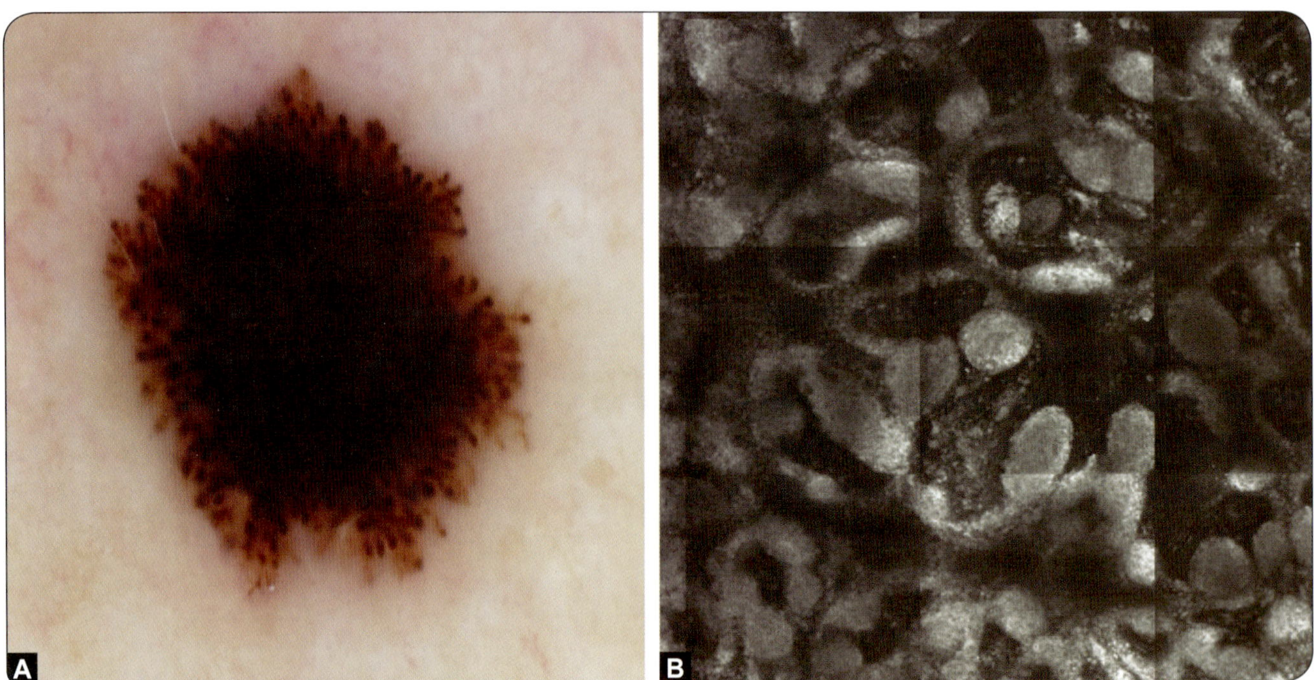

Figs. 17.4A and B: Superficial spreading melanoma, Breslow's thickness 0.3 mm. (A) Upon dermoscopy, the lesion is composed of a dark central structureless area and dark brown-to-black pseudopods in a starburst distribution. (B) Upon reflectance confocal microscopy lesion is composed, at the level of the dermal-epidermal junction, by numerous nests of melanocytes.

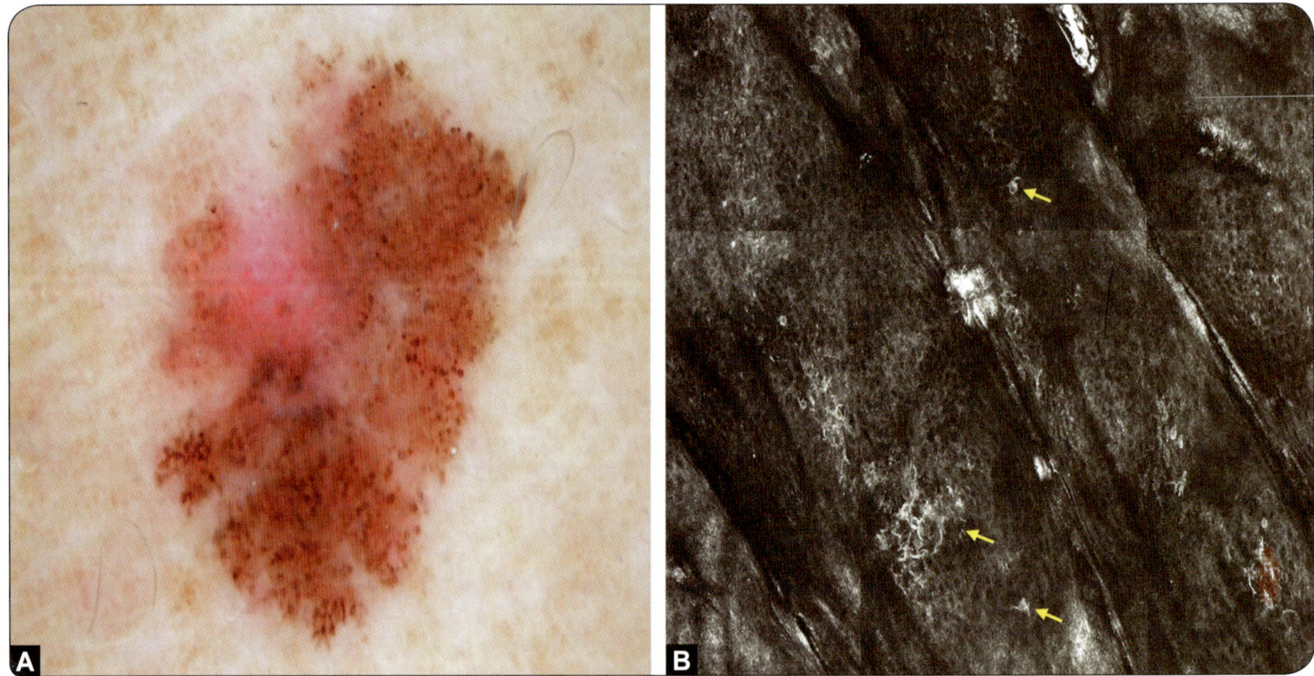

Figs. 17.5A and B: Superficial spreading melanoma, Breslow's thickness 0.5 mm. (A) Upon dermoscopy, the lesion is represented predominantly by a globular pattern with heterogeneous and irregularly distributed globules, and a pinkish area with atypical vessels. (B) Reflectance confocal microscopy at the level of the granular–spinous layer shows irregular honeycombed pattern with a predominance of dendritic pagetoid cells, isolated or clustered in small groups (arrows).

papillae, usually characterized by irregular contours and tangled lines (corresponding to dendrites) in interpapillary spaces. Sometimes some elongated nests are also visible, usually located at the junction.

This subgroup of melanomas frequently occurs in sun-damaged skin, in elderly patients, with few melanocytic nevi. Dendritic cell melanoma diagnosis is sometimes challenging for clinicians because of the overlapping of dermoscopic features with other pigmented macules, such as lentigo simplex, solar lentigo, and/or lichen planus-like keratosis.[10,11]

Reflectance confocal microscopy has been shown to improve the diagnostic accuracy in these lesions especially because of the presence of numerous dendritic cells both within upper epidermal layers and junction, compared with regular honeycombed pattern and ringed/polycyclic pattern in benign lesions.[5]

However, in the diagnostic process, it should also be considered that abundant dendritic cell proliferation is also accounted in some inflamed lesions, due to Langerhans cell proliferation, and in pigmented actinic keratosis, as a consequence of melanocytic hyperplasia with large dendritic melanocytes detectable in the epidermis.

Thus, in the case of large lesions or lesions located in cosmetically sensitive areas, which are exclusively characterized by dendritic cell proliferation, a punch biopsy or shaving, eventually driven on the most suspicious area of the lesion, is recommended.

During tumor progression, appearance of roundish/polygonal cells and aggregates of atypical melanocytes is usually detectable in dendritic cell melanoma, progressively giving rise to the so-called mixed type. Though, usually, these tumors present a slow pattern of growth, it is possible for the development of an invasive clone that results in a nodular component, which is characterized by large aggregates of atypical cells upon RCM. Thus, in case of diagnostic uncertainty in flat lesion, a short- and long-term follow-up is warranted in order to avoid misdiagnosis.

In conclusion, in vivo RCM is very useful in the field of difficult-to-diagnose melanocytic lesions and, at the same time that, benign lesions are saved from unnecessary excisions, early melanomas are also diagnosed. Its systematic application can also represent a cost-effective strategy, enabling accurate diagnosis of melanoma, and saving over the 50% of excision of benign lesions. Adequate training and experience are required for optimal interpretation of confocal images, but this technology should be considered as an adjunct for difficult dermoscopic cases.[12]

REFERENCES

1. Kittler H, Pehamberger H, Wolff K, et al. Diagnostic accuracy of dermoscopy. Lancet Oncol. 2002;3:159-65.
2. Argenziano G, Cerroni L, Zalaudek I, et al. Accuracy in melanoma detection: a 10-year multicenter survey. J Am Acad Dermatol 2012;67:54-9.
3. Ferrari B, Pupelli G, Farnetani F, et al. Dermoscopic difficult lesions: an objective evaluation of reflectance confocal microscopy impact for accurate diagnosis. J Eur Acad Dermatol Venereol. 2015;29:1135-40.
4. Hofmann-Wellenhof R, Pellacani G, Malvehy J, et al. (Eds). In: Reflectance Confocal Microscopy for Skin Diseases. Berlin: Springer-Verlag; 2012.
5. Pellacani G, Guiterra P, Longo C, et al. The impact of in vivo reflectance confocal microscopy for the diagnostic accuracy of melanoma and equivocal melanocytic lesions. J Invest Dermatol. 2007;127:2759-65.
6. Pellacani G, De Pace B, Reggiani C, et al. Distinct melanoma types based on reflectance confocal microscopy. Exp Dermatol. 2014;23:414-8.
7. Clark WH Jr, Elder DE, Van Horn M. The biologic forms of malignant melanoma. Hum Pathol. 1986;17:443-50.
8. Pellacani G, Farnetani F, Gonzalez S, et al. In vivo confocal microscopy for detection and grading of dysplastic nevi: a pilot study. J Am Acad Dermatol. 2012;66:e109-21.
9. Scope A, Zalaudek I, Ferrara G, et al. Remodeling of the dermoepidermal junction in superficial spreading melanoma: insights gained from correlation of dermoscopy, reflectance confocal microscopy, and histopathologic analysis. Arch Dermatol. 2008;144:1644-9.
10. de Carvalho N, Farnetani F, Ciardo S, et al. Reflectance confocal microscopy correlates of dermoscopic patterns of facial lesions help to discriminate lentigo maligna from pigmented nonmelanocytic macules. Br J Dermatol. 2015; 173:128-33.
11. de Carvalho N, Guida S, Cesinaro AM, et al. Pigmented globules in dermoscopy as a clue for lentigo maligna mimicking non-melanocytic skin neoplasm: a lesson from reflectance confocal microscopy. J Eur Arad Dermatol Venereol. 2015 Feb 17 [Epub ahead of print].
12. Pellacani G, Witkowski A, Cesinaro AM, et al. Cost-benefit of reflectance confocal microscopy in the diagnostic performance of melanoma. J Eur Acad Dermatol Venereol. 2016; 30(3):413-9.

17.2 THE UTILITY OF CONFOCAL MICROSCOPY IN THE DIAGNOSIS OF BASAL CELL CARCINOMA

Caterina Longo, Simonetta Piana, Elisa Benatti, Stefania Borsari, Giuseppe Albertini, Aimilios Lallas, Elvira Moscarella

INTRODUCTION

Reflectance confocal microscopy (RCM) is a relatively novel imaging tool that enables the identification of cells and tissues with nearly histologic resolution. Although several noninvasive tools have been explored to test their potential application in the clinical field, RCM has emerged as a unique instrument because it can visualize the skin tissue with a resolution that is comparable with conventional histopathology. It allows a horizontal scanning (en face) of the imaged tissue, with the advantage of exploring a larger field of view compared with vertical sectioning.

Herein, we report the RCM diagnostic features of distinct basal cell carcinoma (BCC) subtypes and their application in clinical setting.

TECHNICAL DETAILS

The commercially available confocal microscope (VivaScope 1500, Mavig, GmbH, Munich, Germany) contains a probe (the head of the microscope), which is attached to the skin by using a disposable plastic window, which is, in turn, taped to a metal ring. A confocal microscope consists of a point source of light, a condenser, objective lenses, and a point detector. The pinhole collects light emanating only from the in focus plane. The mechanism of bright contrast in RCM is backscattering. In gray scale confocal images, structures that appear bright (white) have components with high refractive index compared with their surroundings and are similar in size to the wavelength of light. Backscattering is primarily governed by the refractive index of the structure compared with the surrounding medium. Highly reflective skin components include melanin, collagen, and keratin. The confocal scanning produces high-resolution black-and-white horizontal images (0.5 × 0.5 mm) with a lateral resolution of 1.0 mm and an axial resolution of 3–5 mm. A sequence of full-resolution individual images at a given depth is acquired and stitched together to create a mosaic ranging in size from 2 × 2 mm to 8 × 8 mm. Besides the horizontal mosaic, a vertical VivaStack can be imaged. It consists of single high-resolution images acquired from the top skin surface up to 200 mm, corresponding to the papillary dermis, to obtain an optic biopsy. The VivaStack modality is useful for the assessment of epidermal thickness either under physiologic condition or in the presence of dysfunctional epidermis.

Recently, a handheld RCM has been introduced on the market (VivaScope 3000). This version is a smaller, flexible device, which is useful in areas that are difficult to access (e.g. skin folds and ears). Unlike the 1,500 version, it has an on-instrument control for laser power, imaging depth, and capture, but it does not allow scanning of a large field of view, which is needed, for example, in some tumors to obtain an overview of the architecture. However, it is a promising tool, which can be used for surgical premapping or when multiple site imaging is requested.

BCC CONFOCAL FEATURES

Reflectance confocal microscopy is an excellent tool that provides an accurate noninvasive diagnosis of BCC. The RCM features of BCC have been extensively described and are well-correlated to the histopathological diagnostic criteria of BCC.

González et al.[1] first described the confocal criteria for the diagnosis of BCC. They include the presence of elongated monomorphic nuclei, the polarization of these nuclei along the same axis, a prominent inflammatory infiltrate, increased number of vessels, and the pleomorphism of the overlying epidermis. However, the presence of tumor islands and cords is considered the RCM hallmark of the tumor.

Distinct RCM features are linked mainly to the different histopathologic subtypes although pigmentation may also influence the RCM pattern in terms of refractivity. In fact, pigmented tumors appear highly refractive upon RCM with basaloid islands that are readily identifiable whereas hypopigmented or pink lesions result in darker tumor silhouettes, which are challenging to be recognized. More specifically, in pigmented BCC, the shape of the tumor islands/cords is clearly outlined by a dark contour (clefting)[2] in contrast to the brightness of the peripheral palisading of cells. In hypopigmented BCC, these structures are called "dark silhouettes," because of their dark footprint-like shadow appearance, which is due to the hypopigmented tumor proliferation in a context of bright compact collagen. Additionally, in pigmented BCC, it is possible to observe the presence of dendritic cells

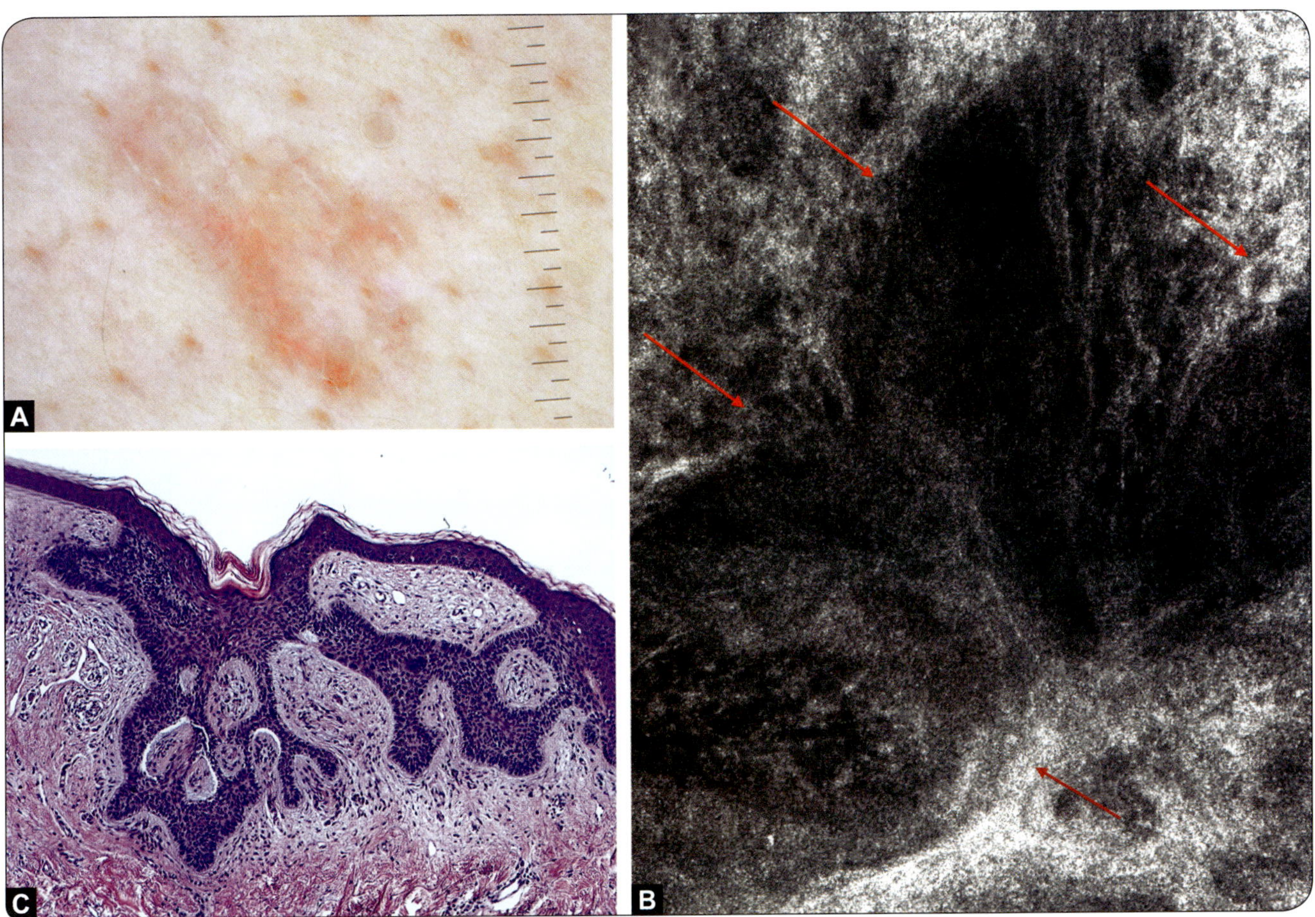

Figs. 17.6A to C: Superficial basal cell carcinoma. (A) Dermoscopy reveals a pink lesion with a few erosions. (B) Reflectance confocal microscopy image shows the presence of dark cords (arrows) connected to the epidermis that correspond to (C) the ones observed on histopathology.

inside the tumor islands that correspond to melanocytes entrapped into the basaloid islands. Along with melanocytes, the pigmentation of BCC upon RCM is linked to the presence of inflammatory infiltrate showing up as bright spots or as ill-defined plump bright cells (corresponding to melanin-laden melanophages).

Our research group recently has identified the RCM criteria to distinguish three main histological subtypes of BCC: Superficial, nodular, and infiltrative.[3] Namely, superficial BCCs revealed the presence of streaming of the epidermis, cords connected to the epidermis with peripheral palisading, and collagen surrounding the cords (Figs. 17.6A to C). On RCM big tumor islands with clefting and peripheral palisading characterize nodular BCCs (Figs. 17.7A to C). Pigmented nodular BCCs are typified by the presence of bright tumor islands and florid inflammatory infiltrate (Figs. 17.8A to C). Infiltrative BCCs were typified by the presence of dark silhouettes with peripheral palisading and collagen surrounding the islands (Figs. 17.9A to C). In all BCC subtypes, it is possible to observe an increased vascularization.

Apart from the three main histopathologic subtypes, the RCM pattern of fibroepithelioma of Pinkus has been described. Upon RCM, it is characterized by a "fenestrated pattern,"[4] consisting of tumor islands or cords with palisading cells at the periphery that outline hyporefractive holes corresponding, histopathologically, to the fibrous stroma (Figs. 17.10A to C).

DIAGNOSTIC ACCURACY OF RCM IN BCC DIAGNOSIS

The presence of elongated monomorphic nuclei, the polarization of these nuclei along the same axis, a prominent inflammatory infiltrate, increased number of vessels, and the pleomorphism of the overlying epidermis

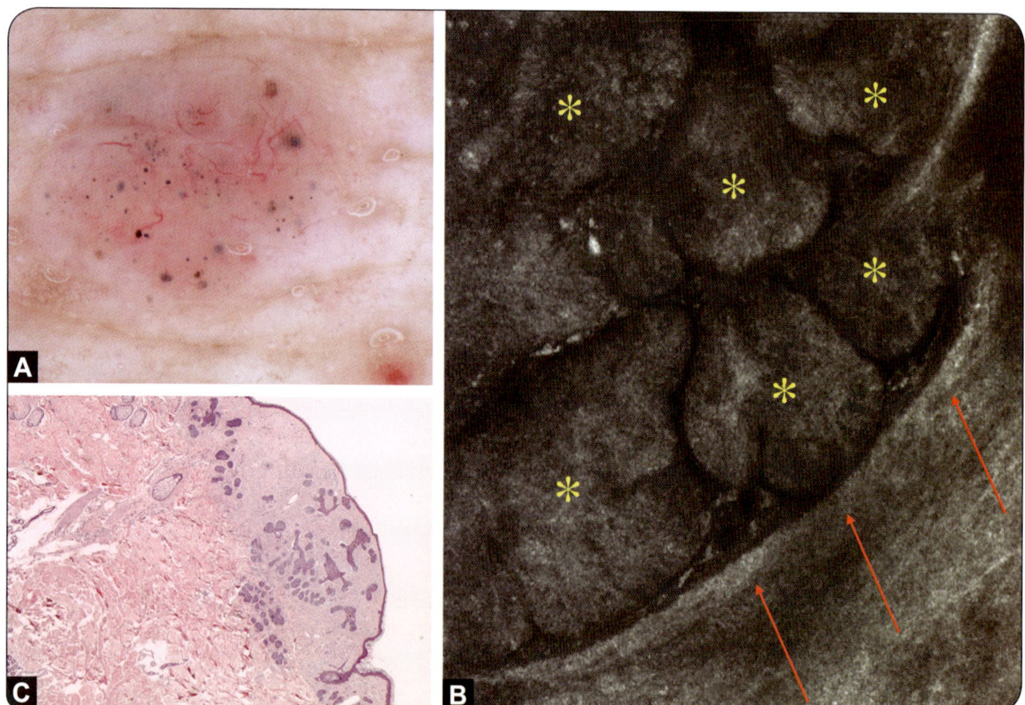

Figs. 17.7A to C: Nodular basal cell carcinoma (BCC). (A) Dermoscopy shows the presence of multiple in-focus blue gray dots, ovoidal globules, and arborizing vessels. (B) Reflectance confocal microscopy image reveals the presence of tightly packed hyporeflective basaloid islands (asterisks) with peripheral clefting (arrows). (C) Histopathology shows the silhouettes of a micronodular BCCs.

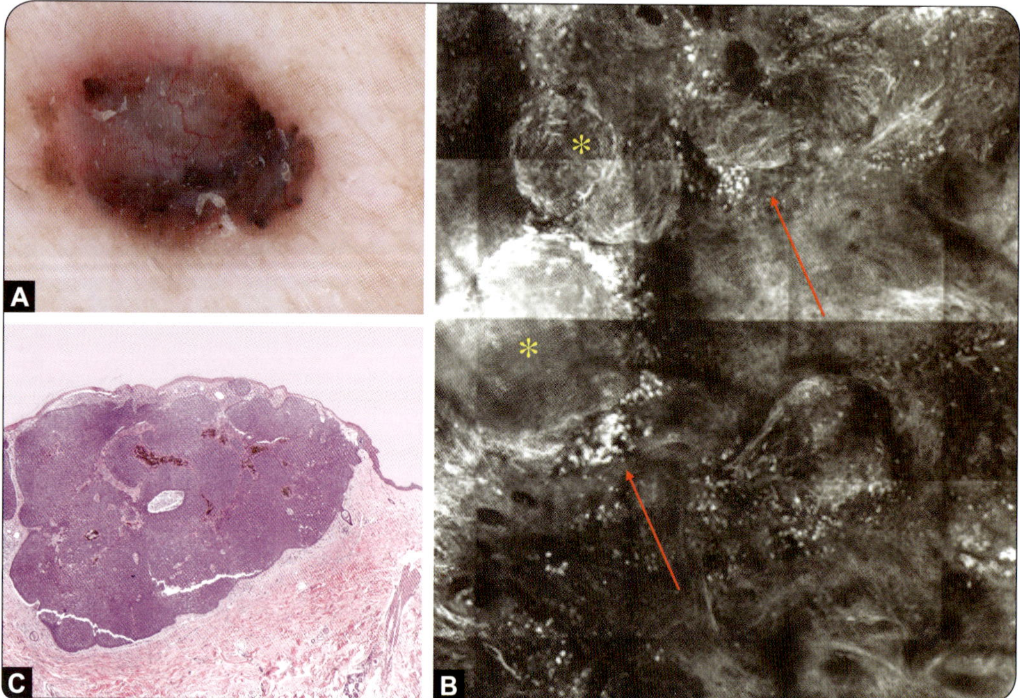

Figs. 17.8A to C: Pigmented nodular basal cell carcinoma (BCC). (A) Dermoscopy shows the presence of arborizing vessels. (B) Reflectance confocal microscopy image reveals the presence of bright and refractive basaloid islands (asterisks) along with clumps of melanophages (arrows). (C) Histopathology shows the silhouettes of pigmented nodular BCCs.

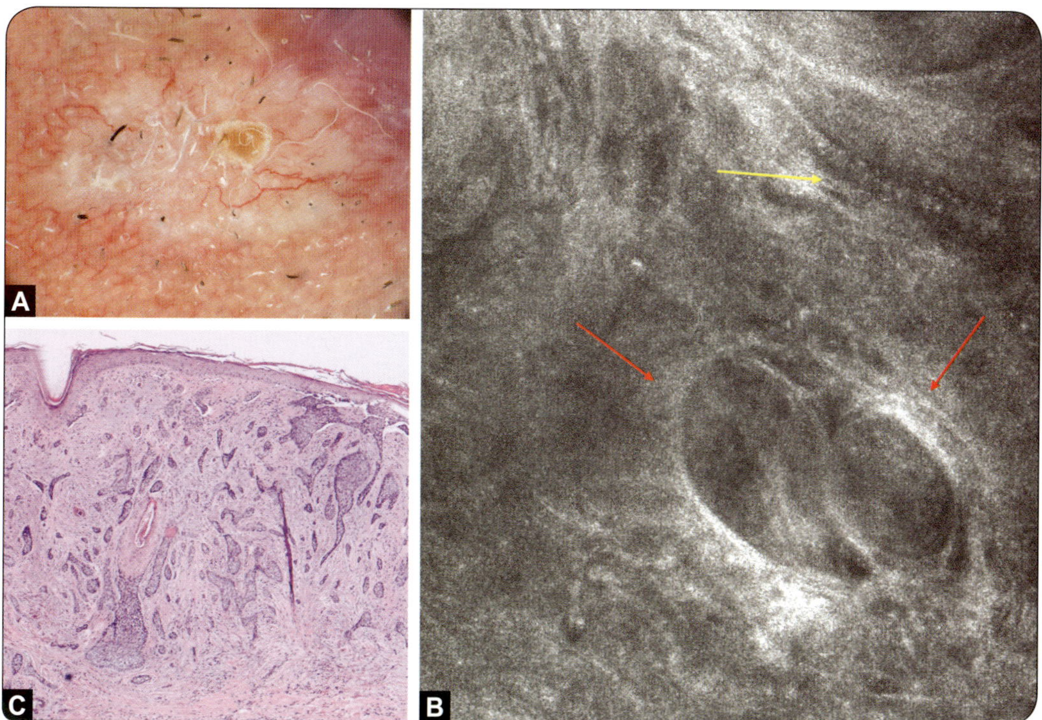

Figs. 17.9A to C: Infiltrative basal cell carcinoma (BCC). (A) Dermoscopy of this case reveals a whitish plaque with linear-arborizing telangiectasia. (B) Reflectance confocal microscopy shows dark silhouettes with peripheral palisading and collagen surrounding the islands (red arrows) along with enlarged vessels (yellow arrow). (C) Histopathology shows the stereotypical pattern of infiltrative BCC.

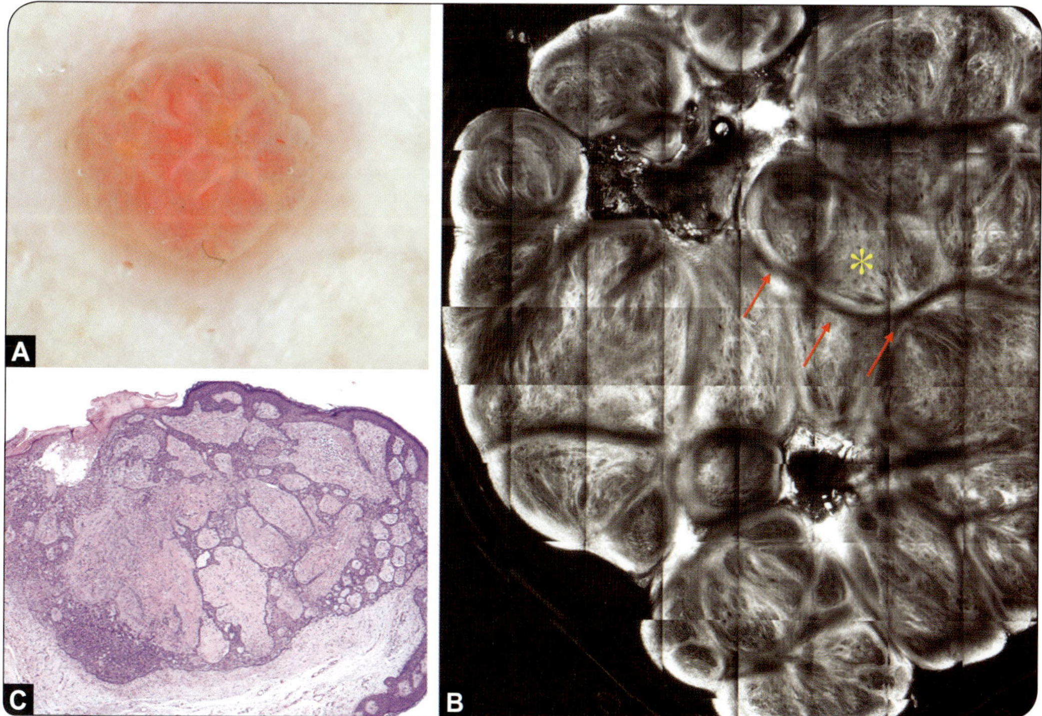

Figs. 17.10A to C: Fibroepithelioma of Pinkus. (A) Short white lines and erosion typify this tumor upon dermoscopy. (B) A typical fenestrated pattern with bright basaloid cords (arrows) and fibrous stroma (asterisk) is seen on reflectance confocal microscopy (RCM) image. (C) Histopathology confirms the RCM diagnosis of a fibroepithelioma of Pinkus.

have been reported as RCMs diagnostic features. It has been demonstrated that the presence of two or more of these criteria is 100% sensitive for BCC, and the presence of four or more of these criteria guarantees a specificity of 95.7% in the diagnosis of BCC.[1] Recently, Guitera et al.[5] described two algorithms to diagnose BCCs and melanomas using in vivo RCM. A total of 710 consecutive cutaneous lesions excised to exclude malignancy were imaged by RCM. Reflectance confocal microscopy features were correlated with pathology diagnosis to develop diagnostic algorithms. The diagnostic accuracy of the BCC algorithm defined on multivariate analysis of the training set (50%) and tested on the remaining cases had 100% sensitivity and 88.5% specificity. Positive features were polarized elongated features, telangiectasia, and convoluted vessels, basaloid nodules, and epidermal shadowing corresponding to horizontal clefting. Negative features were nonvisible papillae, disarrangement of the epidermal layer, and cerebriform nests. Other research papers highlighted the role of RCM in providing a fast diagnosis for pink papules located on the face and for nodular BCCs that could be in differential diagnosis with melanoma.

CONCLUSION

Reflectance confocal microscopy is an accurate tool to diagnose BCCs in clinical settings. Besides diagnostic purposes, RCM found its applications in tumor margin assessment, identification of BCC remnants or recurrence after treatment, and in Mohs micrographic surgery. In our experience, a minimal training is required for novices to recognize BCC structures upon RCM although the diagnosis of pink superficial BCCs may result more challenging compared to pigmented tumors. To conclude, RCM is a fast imaging tool that can provide a reliable diagnosis for those BCCs that are dermoscopically and clinically challenging.

REFERENCES

1. González S, Tannous Z. Real-time, in vivo confocal reflectance microscopy of basal cell carcinoma. J Am Acad Dermatol. 2002;47:869-74.
2. Ulrich M, Roewert-Huber J, González S, et al. Peritumoral clefting in basal cell carcinoma: correlation of in vivo reflectance confocal microscopy and routine histology. J Cutan Pathol. 2011;38:190-5.
3. Longo C, Lallas A, Kyrgidis A, et al. Classifying distinct basal cell carcinoma subtype by means of dermatoscopy and reflectance confocal microscopy. J Am Acad Dermatol. 2014;71:716-24.
4. Longo C, Soyer HP, Pepe P, et al. In vivo confocal microscopic pattern of fibroepithelioma of pinkus. Arch Dermatol. 2012;148:556.
5. Guitera P, Menzies SW, Longo C, et al. In vivo confocal microscopy for diagnosis of melanoma and basal cell carcinoma using a two-step method: analysis of 710 consecutive clinically equivocal cases. J Invest Dermatol. 2012;132: 2386-94.

17.3 THE UTILITY OF CONFOCAL MICROSCOPY IN THE DIAGNOSIS OF SQUAMOUS CELL CARCINOMA

Elvira Moscarella, Simonetta Piana, Marco Manfredini, Stefano Gardini, Giuseppe Albertini, Aimilios Lallas, Caterina Longo

INTRODUCTION

Squamous cell carcinoma (SCC) is the second most common malignant neoplasia of the skin. It derives from the epithelial squamous cells, and affects more commonly fair skinned individuals in areas of chronic sun exposure.[1] Classically, SCC presents as a pink-to-red scaly papule or plaque, at times ulcerated. Pigmented forms can occur, although less frequently. Histopathologically, invasive SCC can be divided into the following three histologic grades, based on the degree of nuclear atypia and keratinization found.[1] Well-differentiated SCC is characterized by more normal-appearing nuclei with abundant cytoplasm and extracellular keratin pearls. Moderately differentiated SCC exhibits features intermediate between well-differentiated and poorly differentiated lesions. Poorly differentiated SCC shows a high degree of nuclear atypia with frequent mitoses and less keratinization. Squamous cell carcinoma in situ, also referred to as Bowen's disease or intraepithelial carcinoma, is the intraepidermal form, which may ultimately progress to an invasive SCC.

Clinical diagnosis of the tumor is usually readily, even if initial forms may be difficult to distinguish from actinic keratoses that are often numerous in the background of severely sun-damaged skin.

DERMOSCOPY

Dermoscopy features of intraepidermal and invasive SCC have been recently described.[2] The dermoscopic hallmark of nonpigmented intraepidermal carcinoma is the presence of dotted and/or glomerular vessels, usually combined with white-to-yellow surface scales and a red-yellowish background color.[2] This pattern is associated with a 98% diagnostic probability of intraepidermal carcinoma. Pigmented Bowen's disease may dermoscopically reveal several pigmented structures, including structureless brown to gray areas, brown dots in linear arrangement, thick, pigmented lines, or a combination of these patterns. Invasive SCC can display several different morphologic types of vessels, including peripheral hairpin, dotted, and/or linear irregular vessels. In addition, signs of keratinization can be present in well-to-moderately differentiated SCC. These include amorphous, structureless white-to-yellow areas, or targetoid-appearing follicular openings consisting of an opaque, yellow center surrounded by a white halo (white circles).[2] Poorly differentiated SCC lacks the signs of keratinization and, instead, shows a polymorphous vascular pattern consisting of small-caliber linear, hairpin, or glomerular vessels over a reddish background.

Reflectance Confocal Microscopy of Squamous Cell Carcinoma

Confocal features of SCC have been described only in a few reports up to now.[3-5] The hallmark of SCC in reflectance confocal microscopy (RCM) examination is the presence of atypical keratinocytes, forming a disarranged epidermal pattern. However, because of the presence of marked hyperkeratosis and/or ulceration, RCM is not always suitable for imaging SCC. Both hyperkeratosis and ulceration represent a limit for the deep penetration of laser light, so that in many cases RCM is not a feasible imaging tool. In explorable lesions, however, RCM may represent an adjunct tool in the differential diagnosis with other skin tumors and with inflammatory diseases.

Squamous Cell Carcinoma In Situ (Bowen's Disease) (Figs. 17.11 to 17.16)

Starting from the upper layers of the epidermis, superficial disruption at the level of the stratum corneum with single detached keratinocytes can be seen, corresponding to scale crust. Detached keratinocytes appear as bright polygonal cells with high reflectance. Polygonal nucleated cells at the stratum corneum represent parakeratosis. At the level of the spinous and granular layers, the epidermal honeycomb is formed by keratinocytes of variable size and shape, forming an atypical to disarranged honeycombed pattern. Round nucleated cells can be seen at the level of the spinous layer, corresponding to dyskeratotic keratinocytes.[3-5] At the dermal layer, round blood vessels traversing through the dermal papillae perpendicular to the skin surface can be seen.

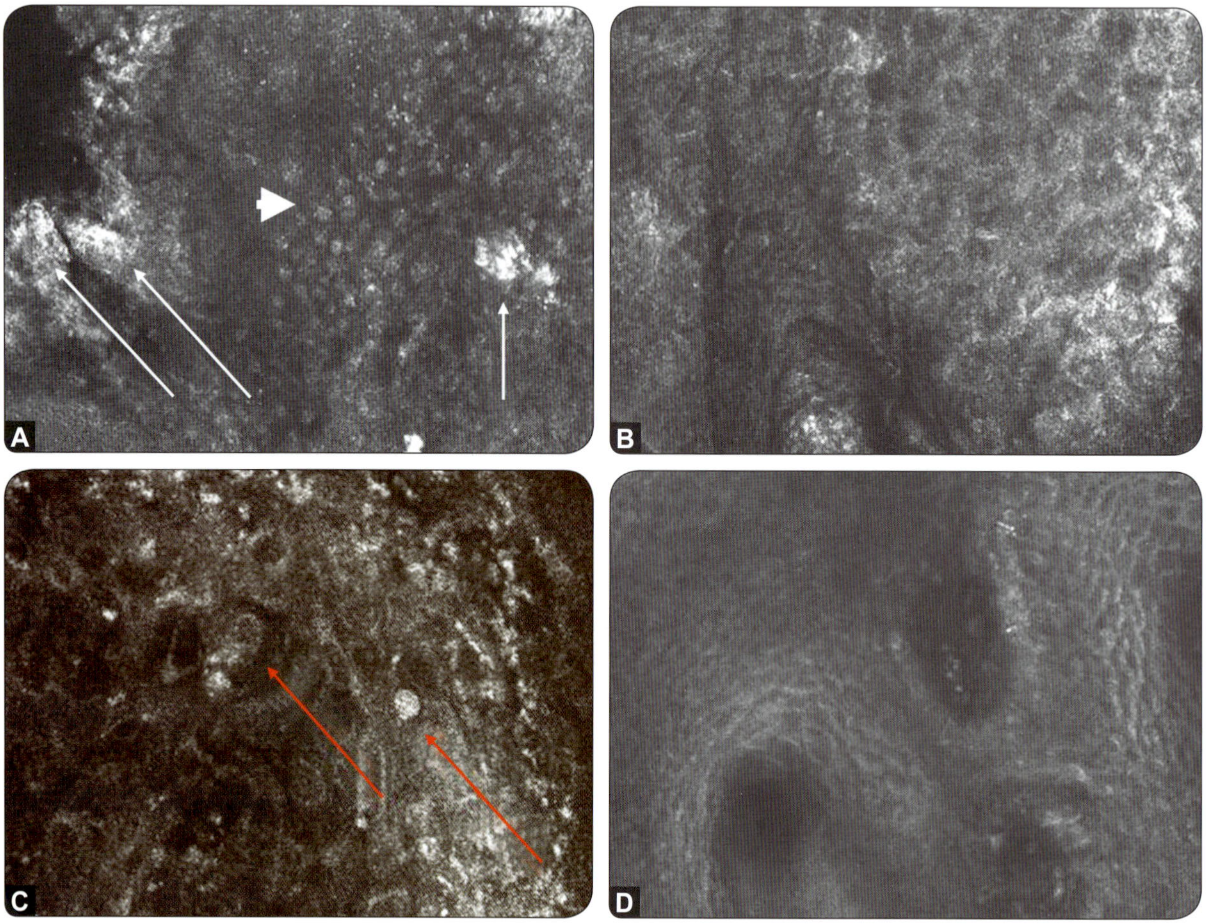

Figs. 17.11A to D: Confocal features of squamous cell carcinoma. Reflectance confocal microscopy single images 0.5 × 0.5 mm. (A) At the level of the corneal layer, scale crust appears as brightly reflective amorphous islands (arrows), polygonal nucleated cells represent parakeratosis (arrowhead). (B) Atypical honeycombed pattern at the level of the spinous granular layer, composed of keratinocytes of different size and shape. (C) Example of a disarranged epidermal pattern, with the presence of multiple round nucleated cells, corresponding to dyskeratotic cells (arrows). (D) Small edged papillae at the dermal layer, with round blood vessels traversing through the dermal papillae perpendicular to the skin surface.

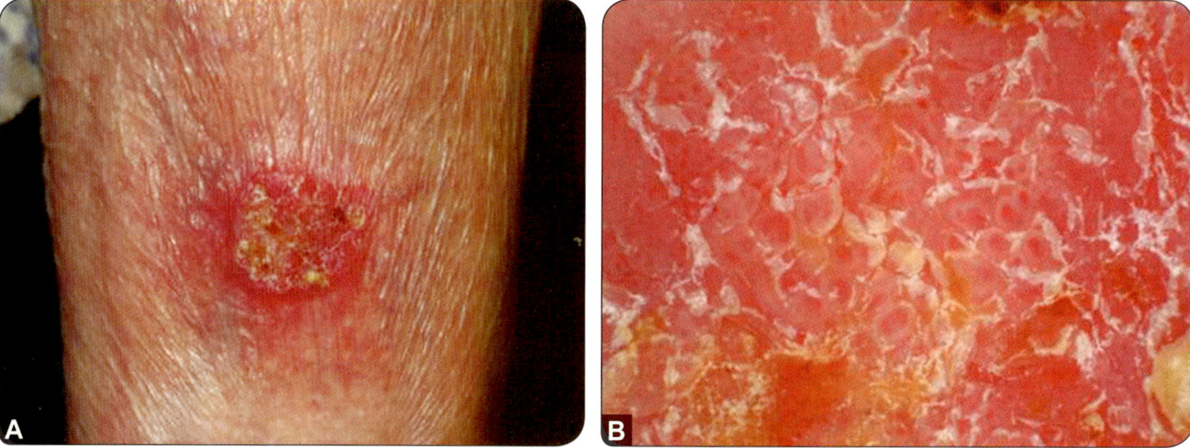

Figs. 17.12A and B: In situ squamous cell carcinoma arising on the leg of an 80-year-old man. (A) Clinically, the lesion appeared as an erythematous plaque with scaly surface. (B) In dermoscopy, multiple white-to-yellow scales, erythematous background and multiple dotted vessels surrounded by a whitish halo.

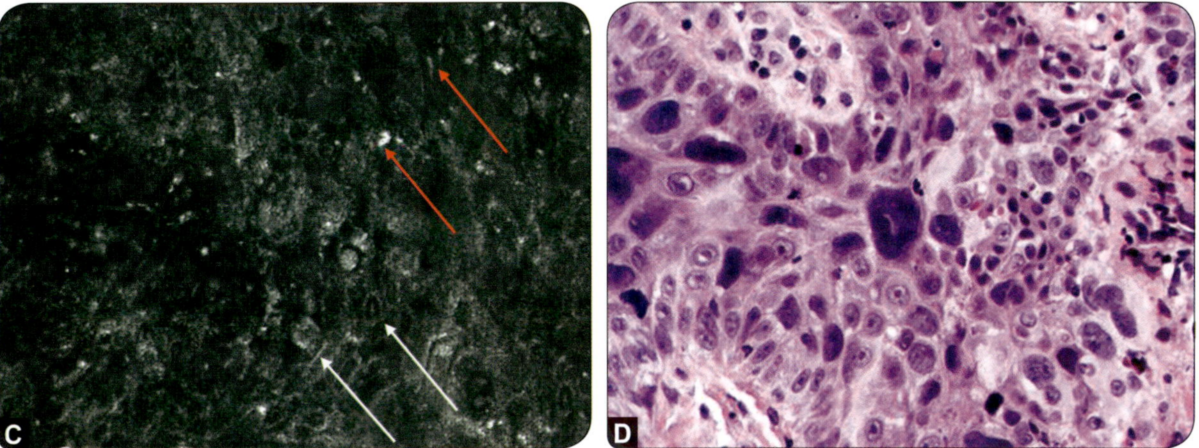

Figs. 17.12C and D: (C) Reflectance confocal microscopy image (0.5 × 0.5 mm) at the level of the spinous layer, highlighting the presence of a disarranged epidermal pattern, with the presence of multiple round nucleated cells, with a targetoid appearance (white arrows) corresponding to dyskeratotic cells, and small bright cells corresponding to inflammatory cells (red arrows). (D) Histopathologically, the same dyskeratotic cells show large atypical nuclei with dense chromatin or irregularly round cells with evident nucleoli. Occasional inflammatory cells are evident.

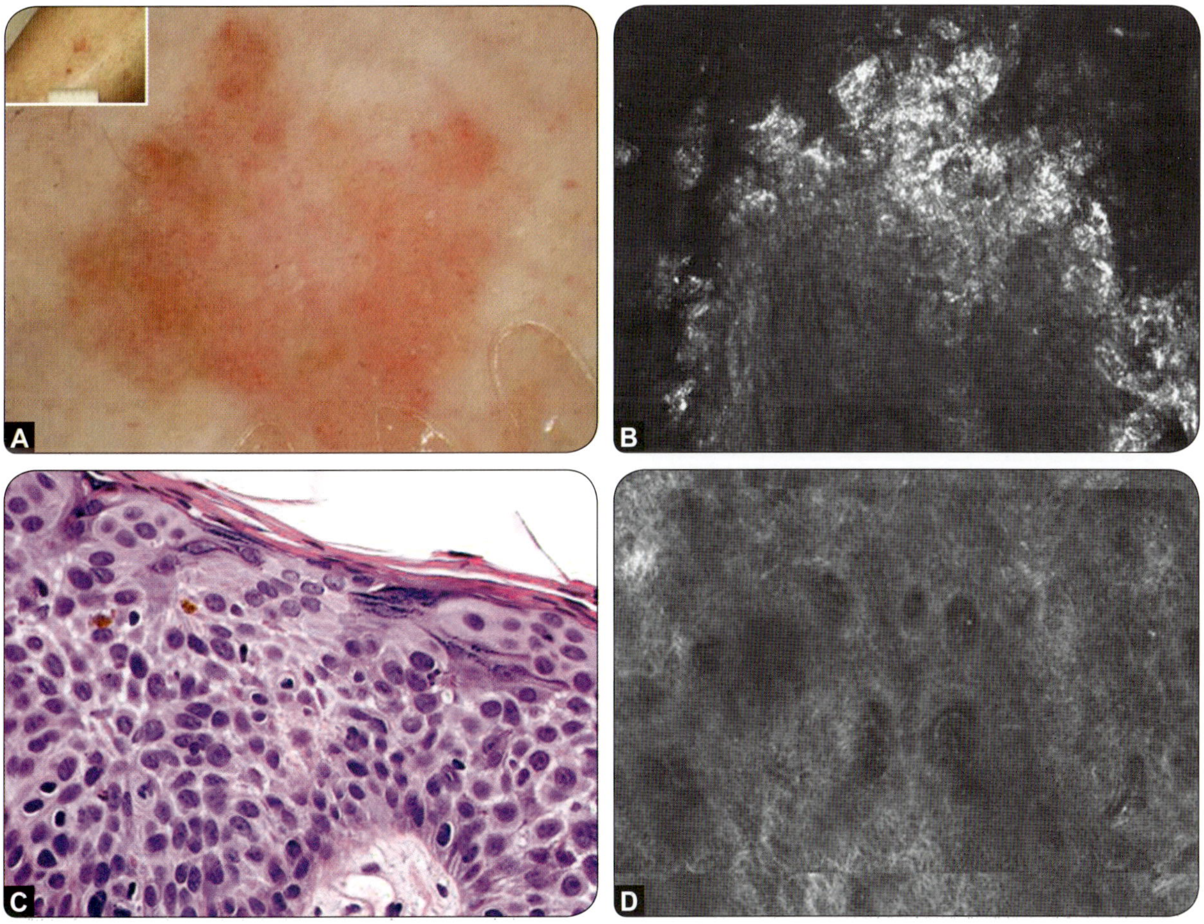

Figs. 17.13A to D: In situ squamous cell carcinoma arising on the upper arm of a 72-year-old woman. (A) In dermoscopy, a structureless white center and multiple dotted vessels at the periphery of the lesion. Clinical picture is in the inset. (B) Reflectance confocal microscopy single image (0.5 × 0.5 mm) taken at the level of the corneal layer, showing the presence of brightly reflective amorphous islands corresponding to hyperkeratosis. (C) On histopathological examination, underneath a hyperparakeratotic layer, neoplastic cells are irregularly round and sometimes arranged in ill-defined nests. (D) Reflectance confocal microscopy image at the level of the dermal-epidermal layer with round blood vessels traversing through the dermal papillae perpendicular to the skin surface.

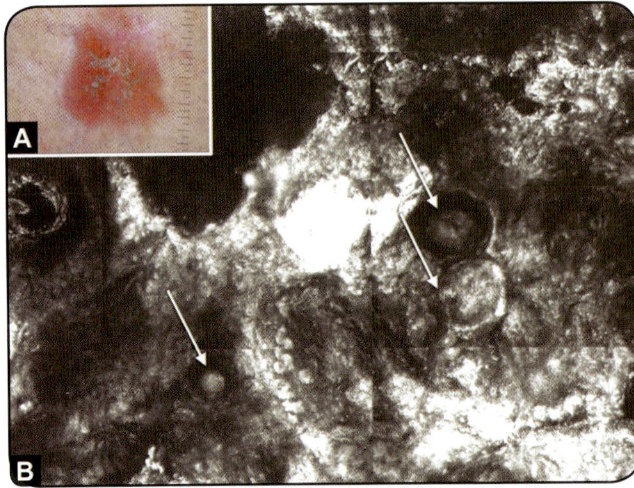

Figs. 17.14A and B: Pigmented squamous cell carcinoma in situ. (A) Dermoscopy showing a scaly surface, clustered dotted vessels, and brown dot in a line at the periphery of the lesion. (B) Reflectance confocal microscopy mosaic image at the level of the superficial epidermis (2.5 × 1 mm) highlighting the presence of hyperkeratosis, with brightly reflective amorphous islands, round, bright aggregates of keratotic material corresponding to keratin pearls (arrows).

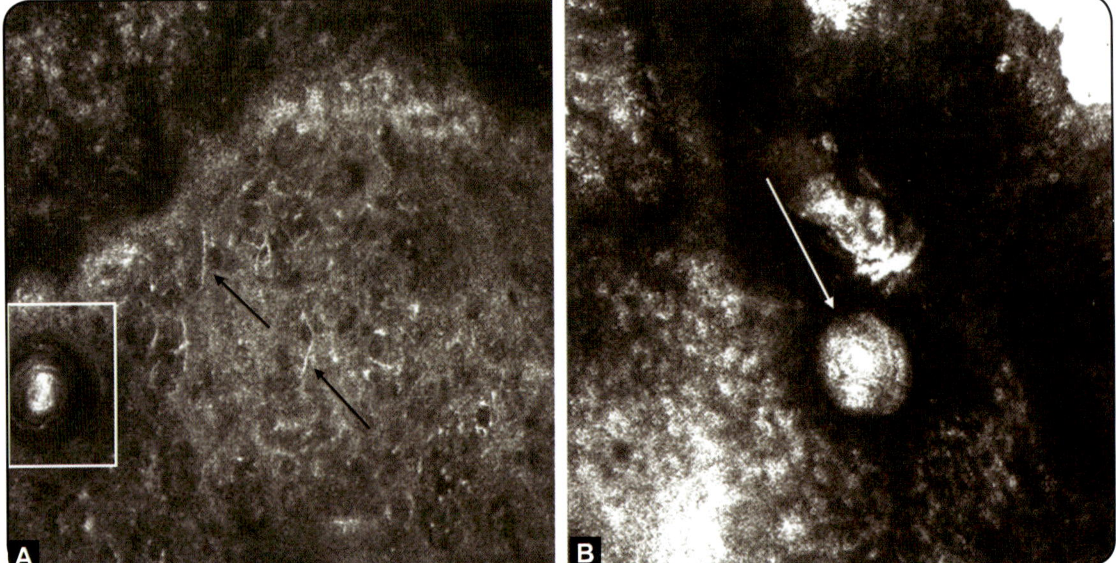

Figs. 17.15A and B: Pigmented squamous cell carcinoma in situ. (A) Reflectance confocal microscopy image (0.5 × 0.5 mm) of an atypical honeycombed pattern, with multiple highly reflective dendritic cells (arrows). A milia-like cyst is also detected, appearing as a brightly reflective onion-shaped structure (white square). (B) Bright aggregates of keratotic material corresponding to keratin pearls (arrow).

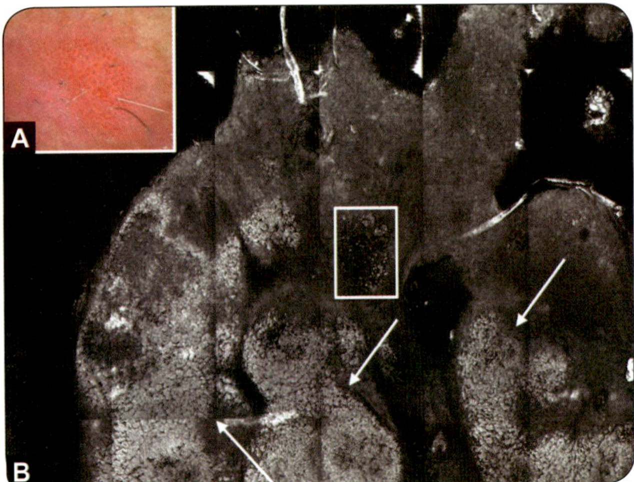

Figs. 17.16A and B: Invasive, poorly differentiated squamous cell carcinoma. (A) In dermoscopy, a prevalence of red color is seen, with multiple glomerular vessels. (B) Reflectance confocal microscopy mosaic image (3 × 2.5 mm) at the spinous layer. An extensive area composed of bright, compact, hyper-reflective particles (white arrows) is visible on the lesion surface, corresponding to ulceration, and not allowing the visualization of the deeper layers of the epidermis. A focal area of spongiosis is detected (white square).

In pigmented Bowen's disease, large round and dendritic cells can be present in the granular layer, representing pigmented keratinocytes or melanocytes. In severely sun-damaged skin, Bowen's disease may arise in an area of solar lentigo, so that edged papillae can be the seen at the level of the dermal-epidermal junction.[3-5]

Invasive SCC

Invasive SCC can display all the features that are visible in the in situ form. In addition, in hyperkeratotic lesions, keratin pearls can be detected, appearing as round, bright aggregates of keratotic material. At the dermal level, nest-like structures with surrounding fibrosis can be visualized by RCM. However, the presence of hyperkeratosis represents a limit in the deep visualization of the tumor, thus establishing that the level of invasion of the tumor is difficult in the majority of cases. In addition, ulceration, sometimes present on the lesion surface, represents an additional limit for confocal examination.[3-5]

REFERENCES

1. Yanofsky VR, Mercer SE, Phelps RG. Histopathological variants of cutaneous squamous cell carcinoma: a review. J Skin Cancer. 2011;2011:210813.
2. Lallas A, Argenziano G, Zendri E, et al. Update on non-melanoma skin cancer and the value of dermoscopy in its diagnosis and treatment monitoring. Expert Rev Anticancer Ther. 2013;13(5):541-58.
3. Rishpon A, Kim N, Scope A, et al. Reflectance confocal microscopy criteria for squamous cell carcinomas and actinic keratoses. Arch Dermatol. 2009;145(7):766-72.
4. Ulrich M, Kanitakis J, González S, et al. Evaluation of Bowen disease by in vivo reflectance confocal microscopy. Br J Dermatol. 2012;166(2):451-3.
5. Peppelman M, Nguyen KP, Hoogedoorn L, et al. Reflectance confocal microscopy: non-invasive distinction between actinic keratosis and squamous cell carcinoma. J Eur Acad Dermatol Venereol. 2015;29(7):1302-9.

DERMATOSCOPY—CHAOS AND CLUES

18

Philipp Tschandl, Cliff Rosendahl

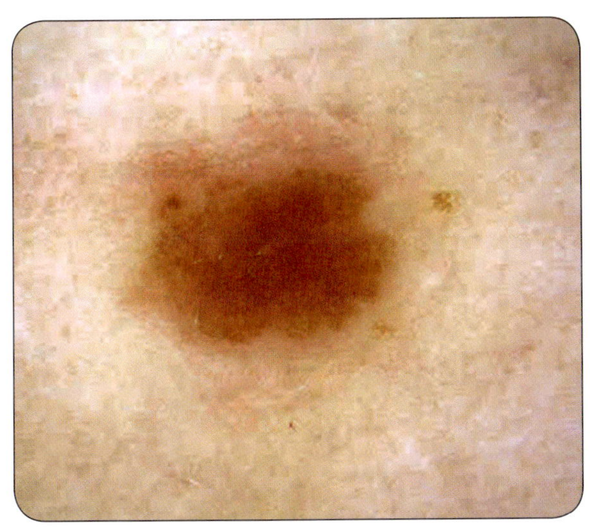

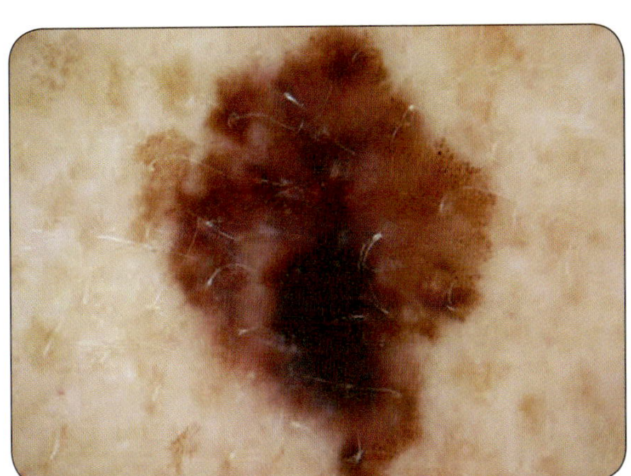

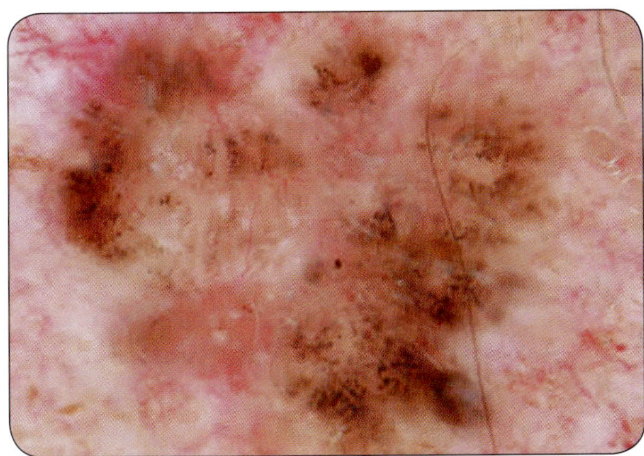

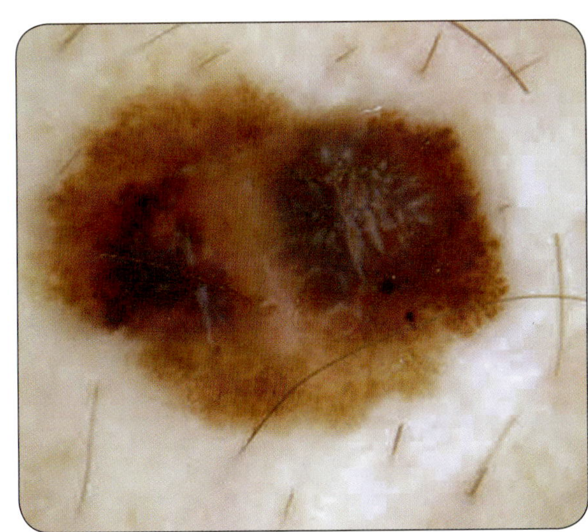

"Since pattern analysis takes up a lot of time to master pattern analysis to its full extent, and to be able to give beginners a method for quickly examining patients, a short method in algorithmic layout has been formed.
This was initially called "short pattern analysis" but became generally known as the method "chaos and clues" (C&C).
Three main advantages in comparison to the other algorithms were hoped for: applicability to melanocytic as well as nonmelanocytic lesions, quick application, and more easy progression to the "full" pattern analysis method."

BACKGROUND

The application of dermatoscopy to differentiate melanoma from nevi has been a focus of this technique since the late 1980s. Since it seemed complicated for beginners to identify every possible morphologic feature and integrate them to a diagnosis, other approaches have been made. Algorithms containing a limited amount of features to be evaluated have been constructed and tested. The most popular and commonly used ones have been reported in a consensus paper of the International Dermoscopy Society in 2003: the ABCD rule, Menzies method, 7-point checklist, and the 3-point checklist.[1] Almost all of them calculate a score by evaluating different morphologic features and using a certain cut off classify a lesion as a melanoma or nevus. This is already one downside as this takes up time and cannot be performed to many lesions on a patient. Since many patients at high risk for melanoma are characterized by having many pigmented skin lesions, these algorithms quickly become less useful in daily practice. Another major downside of the algorithms is their assumption that only melanocytic lesions are being tested with them. To fulfil this assumption, a "two-step" procedure has been promoted in which the first step involves screening for many morphologic features to determine melanocytic status and the second step determines whether the lesion is a melanoma. This first step not only takes up additional time but is also prone to error in regard to diagnostic accuracy, which has been discussed in the literature.[2]

In sum, the mentioned algorithms take up a lot of time, and are only applicable for melanocytic lesions and are prone to be erroneous due to their necessity for a two-step procedure. For this reasons, the need for a different approach emerged. Since the revival of dermoscopic research in the late 1980s, pattern analysis was regarded as the very basis of this technique, and has been refined by modification to more objective terms by Harald Kittler.[3] Since it takes up a lot of time to master pattern analysis to its full extent, and to be able to give beginners a method for quickly examining patients, a short method in algorithmic layout has been formed. This was initially called "short pattern analysis" but became generally known as the method "chaos and clues" (C&C) Three main advantages in comparison to the other algorithms were hoped for: applicability to melanocytic as well as nonmelanocytic lesions, quick application, and more easy progression to the "full" pattern analysis method.

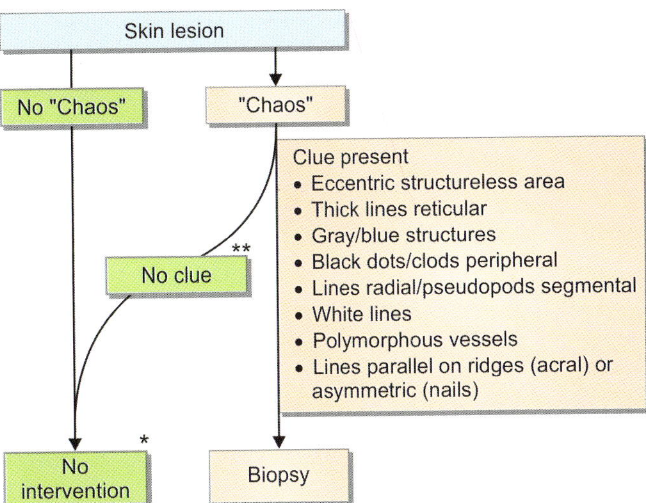

Fig. 18.1: Algorithm "chaos and clues."

"Chaos and clues" algorithm has been initially tested against the other commonly known algorithms in regard to interobserver agreement and diagnostic accuracy of melanocytic lesions and showed comparable results (unpublished data by the authors). After that, its application for all lesions regardless of melanocytic nature has also been tested in a consecutive series of patients in a geographic area of high ultraviolet exposure.[4] A sensitivity of 98.6% for basal cell carcinoma, 86.5% for squamous cell carcinoma, and 79.3% for melanoma was found, with an overall sensitivity to find any kind of malignancy of 90.6% paired with a specificity of 62.7%. The highest rate of false-positive cases was due to lichen planus like keratoses, by nature often being chaotic and difficult to differentiate from malignant lesions morphologically.

CHAOS AND CLUES—THE METHOD

The algorithm uses the basic terminology of modified pattern analysis; for details on basic elements and their arrangement, refer to the respective chapter of this book (*see* Chapter 12).

The chaos and clues algorithm consists of two questions (Algorithm, Fig. 18.1), the first being "Is chaos present in the lesion"?

Chaos

The first step in the algorithm is to scan a lesion for asymmetry in color or structure, in short: "chaos." This step is

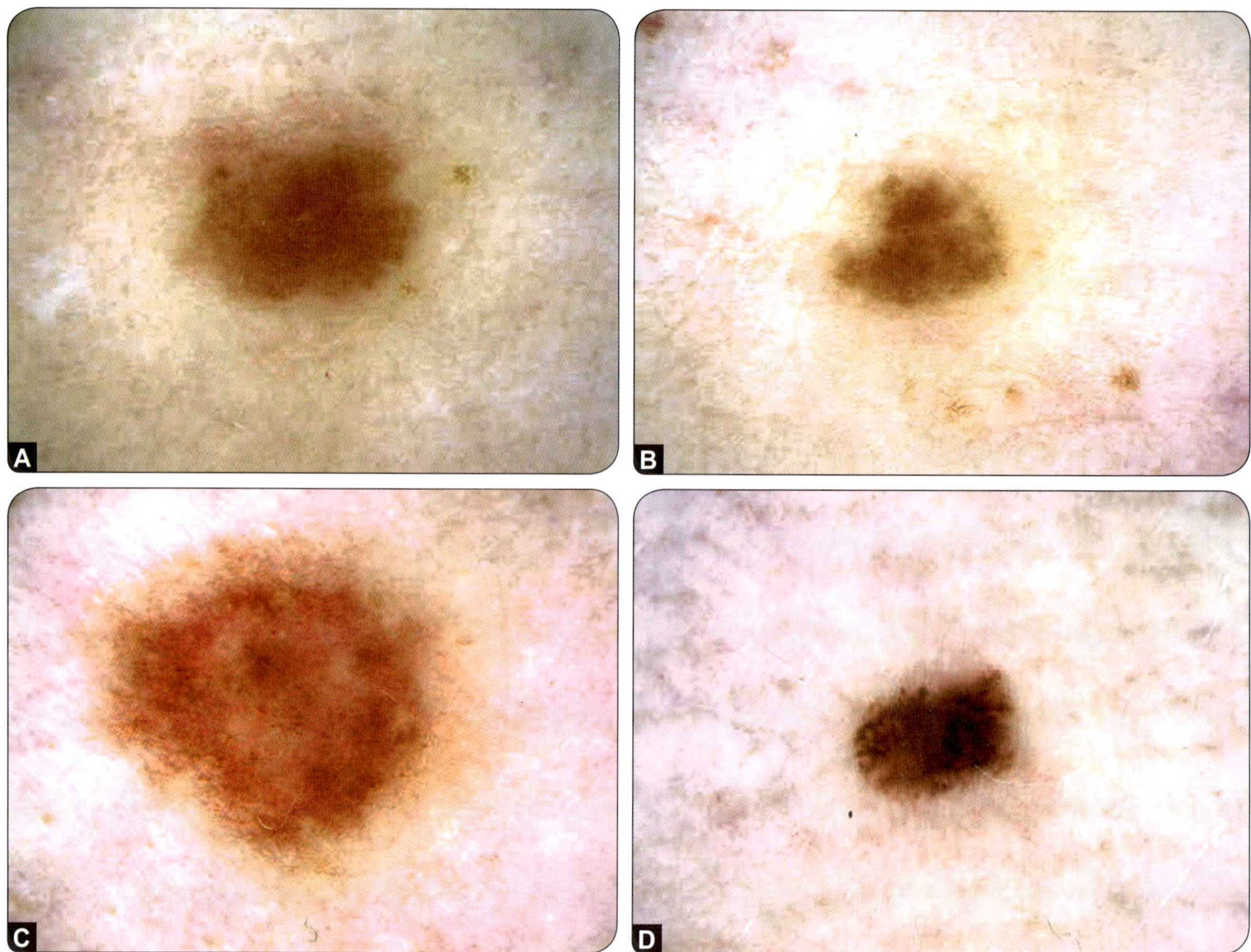

Figs. 18.2A to D: Four lesions on the same patient. Lesions A to C are symmetrical; lesion D is asymmetrical (Chaos) and shows pseudopods as a clue. Lesion D was diagnosed as an in situ melanoma.

designed to be intuitive and quick to enable the physician to evaluate many lesions and quickly skip those which are unequivocally benign. Though seeming very straightforward, the exact evaluation of "chaos" needs some explanation and training of the eye. The reason for this is that one should not expect perfect architectural symmetry, as this is extremely rare in biologic systems. A helpful approach to train the eye on what is "chaotic" and what is not is to compare many lesions of the same patient, which usually show similar patterns. This—also known as the "comparative approach"—is often able to distinguish the "chaotic" lesion on a patient from the regular ones (Figs. 18.2A to D). Another important point is not to confuse structure with form: a lesion with an asymmetric outline can still be "not chaotic" if the inner dermoscopic structures are evenly and symmetrically distributed. Last, one should be cautious in some special situations: nodular, especially fast growing or changing lesions, should always be biopsied if no unequivocal benign diagnosis can be made. Flat pigmented lesions on the face with gray color are always suspicious for being malignant, even if symmetric. Acral lesions with a symmetric pattern of parallel lines on the ridges are always suspicious for being an acral melanoma.

If no "chaos" is present, the lesion can be omitted and the examiner can move on to the next lesion.

If "chaos" is present, the examining physician evaluated the lesion further by moving on to the second step/question of the algorithm: "Is there a clue to malignancy present in the lesion?"

DERMATOSCOPY— CHAOS AND CLUES

18

Philipp Tschandl, Cliff Rosendahl

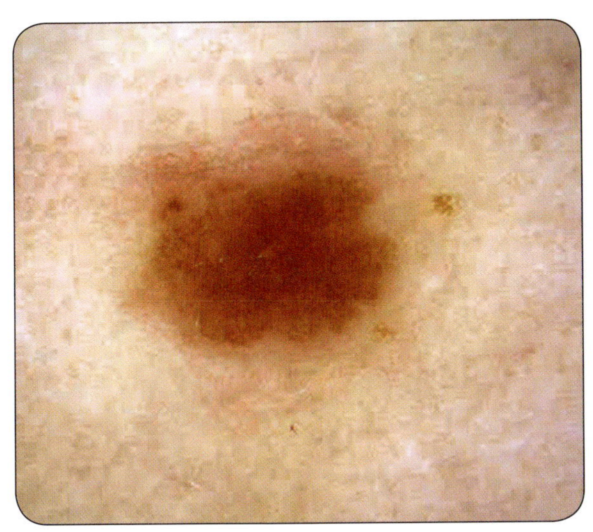

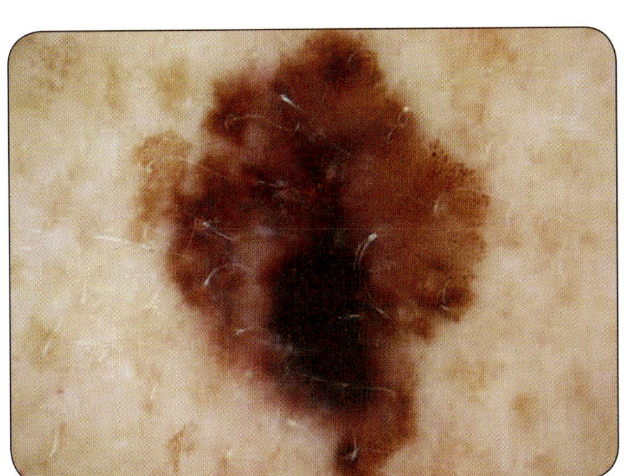

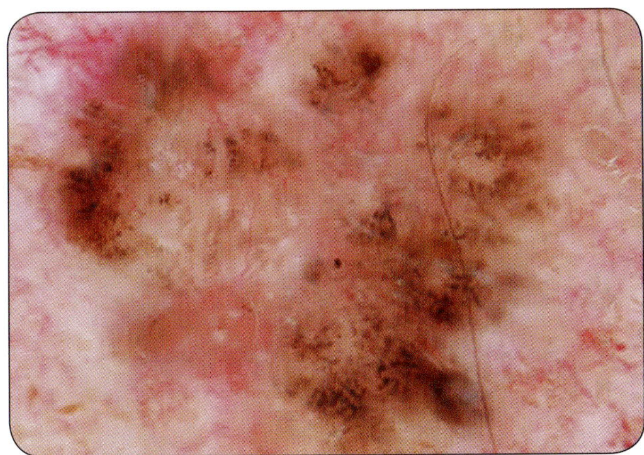

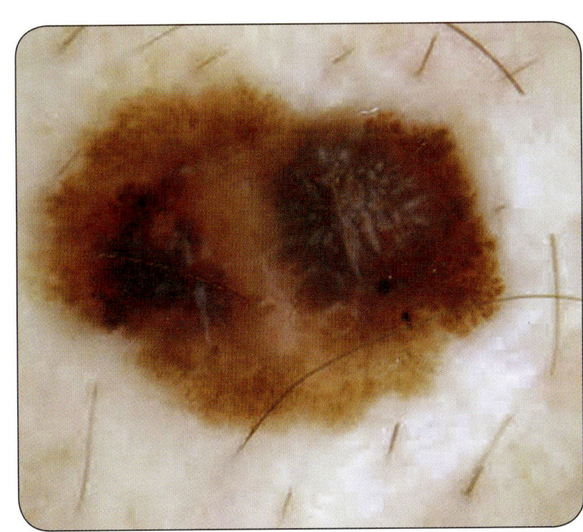

"Since pattern analysis takes up a lot of time to master pattern analysis to its full extent, and to be able to give beginners a method for quickly examining patients, a short method in algorithmic layout has been formed.
This was initially called "short pattern analysis" but became generally known as the method "chaos and clues" (C&C).
Three main advantages in comparison to the other algorithms were hoped for: applicability to melanocytic as well as nonmelanocytic lesions, quick application, and more easy progression to the "full" pattern analysis method."

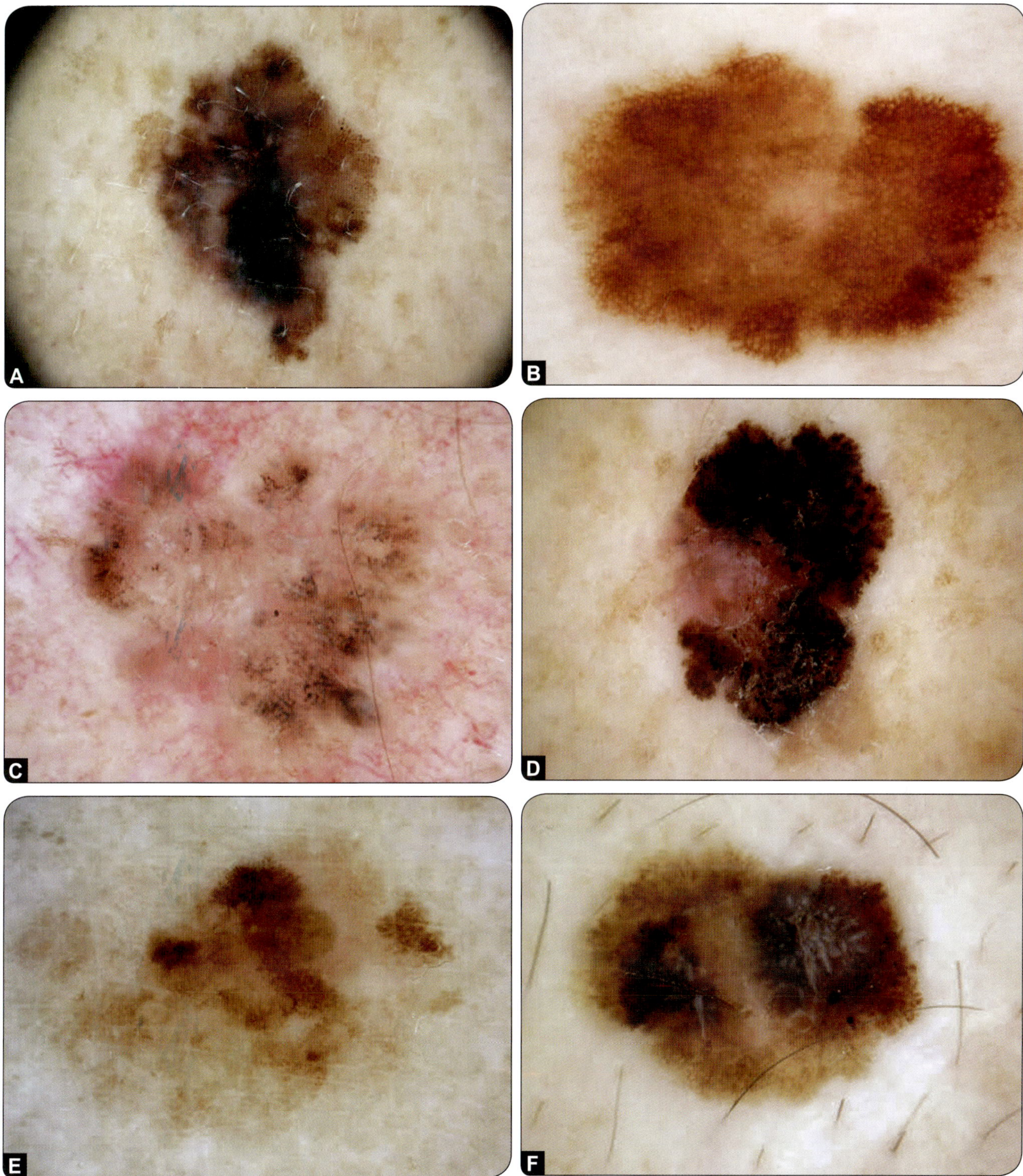

Figs. 18.3A to F: Different dermoscopic clues suggesting malignancy. Lesions A to H depict melanomas except lesion C, which is a basal cell carcinoma: (A) Eccentric structureless area. (B) Focal thick lines reticular. (C) Gray dots. (D) Black clods peripheral. (E) Lines radial/pseudopods segmental. (F) White lines.

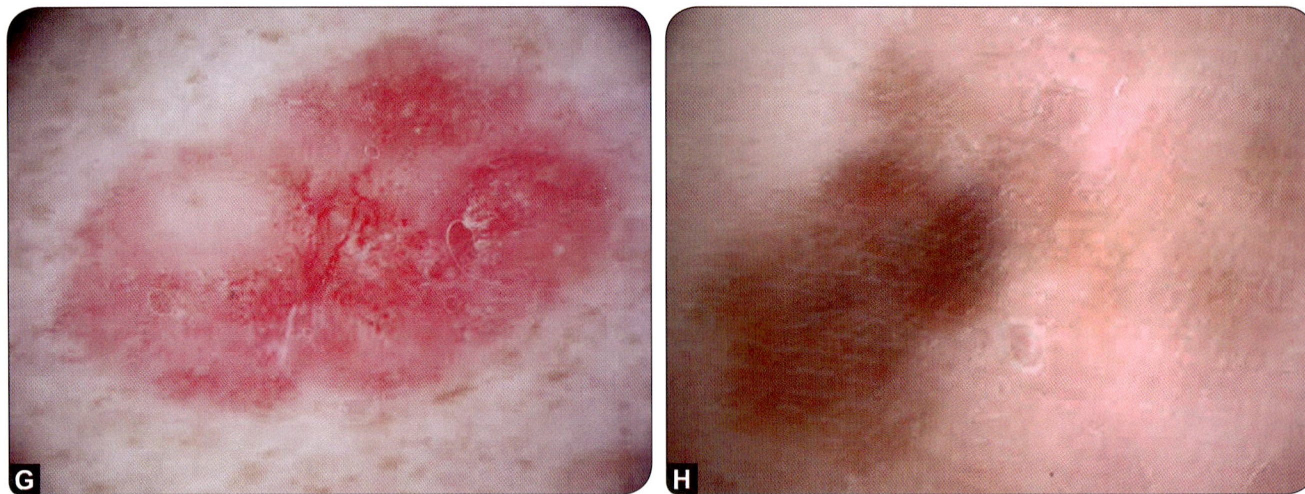

Figs. 18.3G and H: (G) Polymorphous vessels. (H) Lines parallel on the ridges.

Clues

The second step of the algorithm screens the lesion for the presence of at least one of the further described "clues to malignancy" (Figs. 18.3A to H). If one of those clues is present, this suggests the presence of a malignant lesion and mandates (excision) biopsy of the lesion:

- *Eccentric structureless area (Fig. 18.3A)*: Area at the edge of a lesion without any discernible structure that can hold any color except skin color
- *Thick lines reticular (Fig. 18.3B)*: Reticular or branched lines where lines are thicker than the nonpigmented holes in between
- *Gray or blue structures (Fig. 18.3C)*: Any known structure (dots, clods, or circles) with blue or gray color
- *Black dots or clods, peripheral (Fig. 18.3D)*: Dots or clods at the border of the lesion, distributed asymmetrically
- *Lines radial or pseudopods, segmental (Fig. 18.3E)*: Lines or pseudopods (line with a clod at one end) directing outside the lesion or to a common base; those lines/pseudopods do not encompass the whole perimeter but are arranged segmentally.
- *White lines (Fig. 18.3F)*: White lines, often perpendicular to each other. The color "white" is defined as being brighter than the surrounding skin.
- *Polymorphous vessels (Fig. 18.3G)*: Vessels can appear in different ways dermoscopically, as dots, clods, lines, looped, curved, serpentine, helical, or coiled. If in a single lesion, at least two of these appearances are combined, this is called "polymorphous.".
- *Lines parallel, on ridges (acral), or asymmetric (nails) (Fig. 18.3H)*: On acral skin parallel lines can appear in the furrows, on the ridges, or perpendicular to those. If they are present on the ridges (parallel ridge pattern) this is a clue to malignancy. Though this clue is exclusive to acral skin, all other clues can also appear on this anatomic site. If longitudinal/parallel pigmentation on a nail has an asymmetric distribution of color or structure, this is a clue to malignancy.

REFINEMENTS

Though not being included in the initial description of the presented algorithm, it has been proposed to add one layer in the beginning to further quicken the screening of patients in daily practice. Before assessing the lesion for "Clues," morphologically unequivocal seborrheic keratoses should be omitted because of their abundance and ability to being easily diagnosed. This additional step is potentially increasing performance and speed of the examination dramatically with growing experience of the physician.

REFERENCES

1. Argenziano G, Soyer HP, Chimenti S, et al. Dermoscopy of pigmented skin lesions: results of a consensus meeting via the Internet. J Am Acad Dermatol. 2003;48(5): 679-93.
2. Tschandl P, Rosendahl C, Kittler H. Accuracy of the first step of the dermoscopic 2-step algorithm for pigmented skin lesions. Dermatol Pract Concept. 2012;2(3):203a08.
3. Kittler H. Dermatoscopy: Introduction of a new algorithmic method based on pattern analysis for diagnosis of pigmented skin lesions. Dermatopathol Pract Conc. 2007;13(1).
4. Rosendahl C, Tschandl P, Cameron A, et al. Diagnostic accuracy of dermatoscopy for melanocytic and nonmelanocytic pigmented lesions. J Am Acad Dermatol. 2011;64(6): 1068-73.

INDEX

Page numbers followed by *f* refer to figure and *t* refer to table

U

V

W

Z